VISUAL PERCEPTION

THE NEUROPHYSIOLOGICAL FOUNDATIONS

VISUAL PERCEPTION
THE NEUROPHYSIOLOGICAL FOUNDATIONS

EDITED BY

Lothar Spillmann
Neurologische Klinik
Universität Freiburg
Freiburg i. Br., Federal Republic of Germany

John S. Werner
Department of Psychology
University of Colorado
Boulder, Colorado

ACADEMIC PRESS, INC.
Harcourt Brace Jovanovich, Publishers
San Diego New York Boston London Sydney Tokyo Toronto

COVER: Illustration demonstrates illusory motion in depth when moved to and fro. The original design is by the Japanese op-artist, Hajime Ouchi. (Ouchi, 1977. Reprinted with permission.)

This book is printed on acid-free paper. ∞

Academic Press, Inc.
San Diego, California 92101

United Kingdom Edition published by
Academic Press Limited
24–28 Oval Road, London NW1 7DX

Library of Congress Cataloging-in-Publication Data

Visual perception : the neurophysiological foundations / Lothar Spillman and John S. Werner, editors.
p. cm.
Bibliography: p.
Includes index.
ISBN 0-12-657675-0 (alk. paper) ISBN 0-12-657676-9 (paper)
1. Visual perception. 2. Neurophysiology. I. Spillman, Lothar. II. Werner, John Simon.
[DNLM: 1. Nervous System--physiology. 2. Visual Perception--physiology. WW 105 V83416]
QP475.V58 1989
612.8'4--dc20
DNLM/DLC
for Library of Congress 89-6858
CIP

Printed in the United States of America
90 91 92 93 9 8 7 6 5 4 3 2

Dedicated to Richard Jung (1911–1986),
Donald M. MacKay (1922–1987),
and
Hans-Lukas Teuber (1916–1977)

CONTENTS

CONTRIBUTORS

Numbers in parentheses indicate the pages on which the authors' contributions begin.

Israel Abramov (163), Department of Psychology, Brooklyn College, Brooklyn, New York 11210

Anthony J. Adams (381), School of Optometry, University of California, Berkeley, California 94720

Munehira Akita (163), Psychology Laboratories, Kyoto Institute of Technology, Kyoto 606, Japan

Richard A. Andersen (23), Department of Brain and Cognitive Sciences, Whitaker College, Massachusetts Institute of Technology, Cambridge, Massachusetts 02139

Stuart Anstis (205), Department of Psychology, York University, Downsville, Ontario M35 1P3, Canada

Janette Atkinson (349), The Psychological Laboratory, University of Cambridge, Cambridge, CB2 3EB, England

Martin S. Banks (349), School of Optometry, University of California, Berkeley, California 94720

Günter Baumgartner (129), Neurologische Klinik, Universitätsspital, 8091 Zürich, Switzerland

Randolph Blake (23), Department of Psychology, Vanderbilt University, Nashville, Tennessee 37240

Ivan Bodis-Wollner (381), Department of Neurology, Mount Sinai School of Medicine, City University of New York, New York, New York 10029

Oliver J. Braddick (205), The Psychological Laboratory, University of Cambridge, Cambridge CB2 3EB, England

Thomas Brandt (205), Neurologische Klinik, Klinikum Grosshadern, Ludwig-Maximilians-Universität, D-8000 München 70, West Germany

Terrence Caelli (417), Department of Psychology, Queens University, Kingston, Ontario K7L 3N6, Canada

Patrick Cavanagh (273), Département de Psychologie, Université de Montréal, Montréal, Quebec H3C 357, Canada

Alan Cowey (163), Institute of Experimental Psychology, Oxford University, Oxford, OX1 3PT, England

M. L. J. Crawford (23), Sensory Sciences Center, University of Texas, Graduate School of Biomedical Sciences, Houston, Texas 77030

Otto D. Creutzfeldt (449), Neurobiologische Abteilung, Max-Planck-Institut für Biophysikalische Chemie, D-3400 Göttingen-Nikolausberg, West Germany

Russell DeValois (231), Department of Psychology, University of California, Berkeley, California 94720

Jay M. Enoch (381), School of Optometry, University of California, Berkeley, California 94720

Christina Enroth-Cugell (53), Biochemical Engineering Center, Technological Institute, Northwestern University, Evanston, Illinois 60201

Adriana Fiorentini (129), Laboratorio di Neurofisiologia del C.N.R., I-56100 Pisa, Italy

Burkhart Fischer (273), Neurologische Klinik, Universität Freiburg, D-7800 Freiburg i. Br., West Germany

John P. Frisby (317), Department of Psychology, University of Sheffield, Sheffield, S10 2TN, England

Stephen Grossberg (417), Department of Mathematics, Institute for Adaptive Systems, Boston University, Boston, Massachusetts 02215

Richard M. Held (349), Department of Psychology, Massachusetts Institute of Technology, Cambridge, Massachusetts 02139

K.-Peter Hoffmann (349), Lehrstuhl für Allgemeine Zoologie und Neurobiologie, Ruhr-Universität, D-4630 Bochum, West Germany

Donald C. Hood (53), Department of Psychology, Columbia University, New York, New York 10027

Gerald H. Jacobs (23), Department of Psychology, University of California, Santa Barbara, California 93106

Marc Jeannerod (381), I.N.S.E.R.M., Laboratoire de Neuropsychologie Expérimentale, Unité 94, F69200 Bron, France

Peter Lennie (103), Department of Psychology, Center for Visual Studies, University of Rochester, Rochester, New York 14627

Dennis Levi (231), College of Optometry, University of Houston, Houston, Texas 77004

Margaret Livingstone (163), Department of Neurobiology, Harvard Medical School, Boston, Massachusetts 02115

Donald I. A. MacLeod (53), Department of Psychology, University of California at San Diego, La Jolla, California 92093

Lamberto Maffei (231), Laboratorio di Neurofisilologia del C.N.R., I-56100 Pisa, Italy

Svein Magnussen (129), Psykologisk Institutt, Universitetet i Oslo, Blindern 0317, Oslo 3, Norway

Donald E. Mitchell (381), Department of Psychology, Dalhousie University, Halifax, Nova Scotia, B3H 4J1, Canada

Michael Morgan (417), Department of Psychology, University College, London WC1E 6BY, England

J. Anthony Movshon (205), Department of Psychology, New York University, New York, New York 10003

Christa Neumeyer (23), Institut für Zoologie, Johannes Gutenberg-Universität, D-6500 Mainz 1, West Germany

Guy Orban (205), Laboratorium voor Neuroen Psychofysiologie, Katholieke Universiteit, B-3000 Leuven, Belgium

Gian F. Poggio (317), School of Medicine, The Johns Hopkins University, Baltimore, Maryland 21210

V. S. Ramachandran (273), Department of Psychology, University of California at San Diego, La Jolla, California 92093

David Regan (317), Department of Psychology, York University, Downsville, Ontario M35 1P3, Canada

Ingo Rentschler (417), Institut für Medizinische Psychologie, D-8000 München 2, West Germany

Jyrki Rovamo (231), Department of Psychology, University of Helsinki, SF-0017 Helsinki 17, Finland

Peter H. Schiller (129), Department of Brain and Cognitive Sciences, Whitaker College, Massachusetts Institute of Technology, Cambridge, Massachusetts 02139

Julie L. Schnapf (53), Department of Ophthalmology, University of California Medical School, San Francisco, California 94143

Clifton M. Schor (317), School of Optometry, University of California, Berkeley, California 94720

Robert Sekuler (205), Department of Psychology, Brandeis University, Waltham, Massachusetts 02254

Robert Shapley (417), Department of Psychology, New York University, New York, New York 10003

Carla J. Shatz (349), Department of Neurobiology, Stanford University School of Medicine, Stanford, California 94305

Lothar Spillmann (1), Neurologische Klinik, Universität Freiburg, D-7800 Freiburg i. Br., West Germany

Davida Y. Teller (11), Department of Psychology, University of Washington, Seattle, Washington 98195

James P. Thomas (129), Department of Psychology, University of California, Los Angeles, California 90024

Anne Treisman (273), Department of Psychology, University of California, Berkeley, California 94720

Colwyn Trevarthen (103), Department of Psychology, University of Edinburgh, Edinburgh EH8 9TA, Scotland

Christopher W. Tyler (317), Department of Visual Science, Smith-Kettlewell Institute of Visual Science, San Francisco, California 94115

Arne Valberg (163), Fysisk Institutt, Biofysikkgruppen, Universitetet i Oslo, Blindern 0317, Oslo 3, Norway

David Van Essen (103), Biology Division, California Institute of Technology, Pasadena, California 91125

Richard C. Van Sluyters (349), School of Optometry, University of California, Berkeley, California 94720

Rüdiger von der Heydt (273), Neurologische Klinik, Universitätsspital, 8091 Zürich, Switzerland

Jan Walraven (53), Institute for Perception-TNO, 3769 DE Soesterberg, The Netherlands

Heinz Wässle (103), Max-Planck-Institut für Hirnforschung, D-6000 Frankfurt 71, West Germany

John S. Werner (1), Department of Psychology, University of Colorado, Boulder, Colorado 80309

Gerald Westheimer (5), Department of Physiology-Anatomy, University of California, Berkeley, California 94720

Hugh R. Wilson (231), Department of Pharmacology and Physiology, The University of Chicago, Chicago, Illinois 60637

Eberhart Zrenner (163), Universitäts-Augenklinik, Abteilung für Physiologie und Pathophysiologie des Sehens, 8000 München 2, West Germany

PREFACE

Visual Perception: The Neurophysiological Foundations presents many of the main facts and theories that guide contemporary research on visual perception. The chapters cover virtually all aspects of visual science, from philosophical postulates to computational algorithms, and from photoreceptor processes to neuronal networks. The aim was to present these specific areas under a global theme: the correlations between perceptual phenomena and the underlying neurophysiological processes and mechanisms.

The contributors to this volume were initially brought together at a conference in Badenweiler, near Freiburg, Federal Republic of Germany (June 29–July 3, 1987). The conference was organized to take stock of the achievements made in the past 25 years in the field of visual science, and to discuss ways of presenting these discoveries in an advanced textbook. Some seventy internationally known vision researchers from thirteen countries participated. They were divided into fifteen working groups, each of which was responsible for one major topic in vision research. While the Badenweiler Conference served to focus the interests of the participants and provided much stimulating discussion, the chapters that were subsequently written went beyond the findings presented there. Each working group had a chairperson who integrated the contributions of the group into a cohesive chapter that could be understood by graduate students and nonspecialists in vision research. Each chapter was subsequently reviewed by a number of experts for its scope and clarity.

Rarely has as much enthusiasm and effort been devoted to describing the psychology and physiology of vision from all possible approaches: psychophysics, neurophysiology, neuroanatomy, neuropharmacology, and clinical visual science. Although there had been a scientific journal dedicated to this goal already in the last century, the *Zeitschrift für Psychologie und Physiologie der Sinnesorgane,* the tradition was temporarily lost. It is clear from this volume, however, that this quest is once again a major concern in the field and the approach can resume with new procedures, sounder concepts, and a broader knowledge-base from supporting disciplines. We thus hope that the readers of this book will be stimulated to use a more multidisciplinary approach in their own research in the future.

ACKNOWLEDGMENTS

We are indebted to our many colleagues who gave generously of their time and expertise in providing outside reviews of the chapters in this volume. These were: Thomas D. Albright, Richard Aslin, Horace B. Barlow, Mark A. Berkley, Robert M. Boynton, Doris Braun, Bruno G. Breitmeyer, David Burr, John Clavadetscher, Robert Desimone, Walter H. Ehrenstein, Rhea Eskew, Robert Fox, Kenneth Fuld, Mark A. Georgeson, Alan Gilchrist, Mark W. Greenlee, Peter Hammond, John P. Harris, Lewis O. Harvey, Jr., Ronald S. Harwerth, Mary M. Hayhoe, Robert F. Hess, Chris Johnson, Stanley Klein, Kenneth Knoblauch, Janusz J. Kulikowski, David N. Mastronarde, John D. Mollon, Jeremiah I. Nelson, Hans-Christoph Nothdurft, Richard K. Olson, Tatiana Pasternak, Ido Perlman, Scott Raney, Christoph Redies, Brian Rogers, Brooke Schefrin, Lindsay T. Sharpe, Ruxandra Sireteanu, William Skaggs, Charles E. Sternheim, Lesley Ungerleider, Jackie van Hof-van Duin, Vicki J. Volbrecht, Michael Wertheimer, and Jeremy Wolfe.

Many people assisted in the making of the book: in Freiburg, Debbie Johnson, Joachim Obergfell, and Clemens Fach; in Boulder, Vicki Steele, Beth Smith, and David Peterzell. We thank them all. Thanks go also to Franz Rombach and Petra Krüger in Freiburg for mailing services, and to Peter Kaiser at York University for making the electronic mail network accessible to the vision community, thereby greatly facilitating our task as editors. We also wish to thank Joe Ingram, our editor at Academic Press, for his active encouragement, patience, and understanding.

Gerald Westheimer, Christina Enroth-Cugell and Otto Creutzfeldt are gratefully acknowledged for advising us on organizational matters; Jeremiah I. Nelson's informed, witty, and constructive criticism was of great help to us in shaping the scientific contents of the book; and Lyle E. Bourne, Jr. and Andreas Zschoch deserve special mention for lowering administrative hurdles. The great success of the Badenweiler conference was significantly aided by its location in the Grandhotel Römerbad. The exceptional atmosphere that prevailed provided an important catalyst for the planning and completion of this book. On behalf of all participants, we wish to express our gratitude for the kind hospitality of Director Klaus Lauer and his staff.

We would like to thank our sponsors whose support made this book possible. These are: the United States Air Force Office of Scientific Research (grant 87-0146); the Deutsche Forschungsgemeinschaft in Bonn; the Max-Planck Institut für Hirnforschung in Frankfurt/Main; the Alexander von Humboldt Stiftung in Bonn; the Fritz Thyssen Stiftung in Köln; the Ministerium für Wissenschaft und Kunst in Stuttgart; Daimler Benz A. G. in Stuttgart; Sonderforschungsbereich 325 in Freiburg, Main; the National Institute on Aging (AG04058) and National Institute of Child Health and Human Development (HD19143).

Finally, we would like to thank our families, especially Jutta and Kris, for tolerating the many long hours away from home.

Lothar Spillmann
John S. Werner

1

INTRODUCTION

Lothar Spillmann and John S. Werner

This book provides an overview of visual science, emphasizing current attempts to correlate neurophysiological mechanisms and human perception. The main questions addressed by the individual chapters are reminiscent of those posed by Lettvin, Maturana, McCulloch, and Pitts (1959) in their famous paper: "What the Frog's Eye Tells the Frog's Brain." The chapters ask: What are the relevant perceptual phenomena to be understood? What is it that we perceive, and what are the visual stimuli that give rise to this experience? What are the quantitative characteristics of the stimulus–response relations as defined by careful psychophysical experiments? What can single-cell studies in cat and monkey tell us about human visual perception? Which neural mechanisms might explain the behavioral data, and how can these be related to the known physiological properties of single-unit receptive fields or an ensemble of cellular responses?

These questions, deceptively simple and seemingly straightforward, have inspired a great deal of research that is not easily summarized for the nonspecialist. Although excellent introductory texts of neurophysiology and of perception are available, there are large gaps between the textbooks for the undergraduate student and the technical reports in scientific journals. This book was written to bridge these gaps for the graduate student and vision researcher who seek a summary of the scientific developments outside their own specialized area of expertise. The reader should not expect a complete account of modern visual science; rather, the purpose of this book is to elucidate, as did Jung (1973), some of the most important correlations between human perception and the underlying neuroanatomical and neurophysiological mechanisms. The chapters combine data from perception, psychophysics, neurophysiology, neuroanatomy, neuropharmacology, comparative and developmental psychology, and artificial intelligence. In short, this book is an attempt to summarize what is known about the brain mechanisms that mediate our visual experience.

I. THE HISTORICAL CONTEXT OF MODERN VISUAL SCIENCE

Visual scientists interested in the relations between neural coding and perception can point with pride to landmark successes over more than a century. Among them are the achievements of Purkinje (1823) and Schultze (1866) in clarifying the duplicity of visual sensitivity made possible by rods and cones; of Mach (1865) in furthering our understanding of border and contrast perception; of Maxwell (1856), Helmholtz (1867), and Hering (1878) for advancing our understanding of color receptors and opponent-color processes; of Exner (1888) for elucidating the principles underlying our perception of motion and motion aftereffects; and of von Kries (1905) in proposing mechanisms of light and dark adaptation. These celebrated discoveries were based on careful observations of the nature of visual experience directed at uncovering essential properties in presumed neural networks. One general assumption was that constraints on the nature of what we experience must reflect some of the constraints on the neural code. Of course, attempts to correlate brain and behavior have not always been successful, as Westheimer points out in Chapter 2 of this volume, so one does well to be mindful of the linking propositions, described by Teller in Chapter 3, that are implicit in any argument extending from one domain to another.

The data of visual science have not accumulated in a linear manner over the last century. Validation of most nineteenth century proposals had to await the advent of modern physiological techniques. The intervening years did, of course, witness the emergence of Gestalt psychology, an influential movement that provided conceptual advances as well as a rich description of the complex organization of visual perception. The Gestalt notions, however, were even more difficult to relate to neurophysiology than those of Purkinje, Mach, Hering, and Exner. Classic observations made in the 1800s are now commonly used in investigations at the level of the individual neuron (Chapters 7, 8, and 9), but we are only beginning to understand the cellular basis of light adaptation (Chapter 5) and to identify the pathways that might mediate Gestalt observations (Chapter 11).

Shortly after the second World War, Richard Jung, a clinical neurologist and neurophysiologist in Freiburg, West Germany, Hans-Lukas Teuber, a neuropsychologist at New York University and later The Massachusetts Institute of Technology, and Donald M. MacKay, a communications engineer from Keele, England, independently advocated the further development of psychophysical experiments that would yield data that could be correlated with results from visual neurophysiology. Their efforts culminated with the joint editing of the *Handbook of Sensory Physiology,* which is widely regarded as the authoritative treatise of research in this area up to the mid-1970s. From today's perspective, it appears that their work provided an important influence in the transition from the methodologies and theories of the nineteenth century to those of the present (Chapter 16).

II. CURRENT TRENDS

It is instructive to compare the proceedings of the first, much acclaimed, Freiburg Conference on the Neurophysiology and Psychophysics of the Visual System held in 1960 (Jung & Kornhuber, 1961) with the state of the field represented by the chapters in this volume. Much of the emphasis on certain topics has shifted since the 1960s. Whereas some issues seem to have dropped out of sight, others have emerged and provided new frames of reference.

Single-unit recording in cats and monkeys, relatively new in 1960, continues to be a fundamental method for understanding the information transmitted at various levels in the visual system. But while the emphasis was once almost exclusively on the information processed by single cells, in 1989 there is greater emphasis on the specialized parallel pathways and cortical modules that collectively carry visual information (Chapter 6). Moreover, modern neurophysiological research can be performed with alert, behaving animals to explore complex aspects of visual search and attention (Chapters 4 and 11); or it may be combined with pharmacological agents that temporarily inactivate ON-channels (Chapter 7). These quick advances in visual science once prompted Richard Jung to remark that while it was possible for him to summarize the literature on visual perception and neurophysiology in a single chapter for the *Handbook of Sensory Physiology* in 1973, writing such a chapter only 10 years later would have been an overwhelming task.

The field of vision research is rapidly changing in other ways as well. For example, the study of the Troxler effect, Ganzfelds, and stabilized retinal images was a very active field in the mid-1950s and early 1960s but has ceased to be a central issue in the late 1980s. Similarly, the McCollough effect, a prime example of early evidence for "double-duty" neurons and the subject of several hundreds of papers, has not attracted much recent interest. Masking and metacontrast, topics of substantial interest until the mid-1980s, seem no longer in vogue. Of course, many intriguing questions in these areas remain to be solved, and it is conceivable that interest in these topics will reemerge when neurophysiology advances to a point where the perceptual phenomena can be better addressed.

In the meantime, new topics have taken the place of the old ones. Among them are microspectrophotometry, signal transduction at the receptor level, current recording from the three kinds of cones, psychophysical evaluation of receptor densities in the human fovea, separation of chromatic and achromatic processing, spatial sampling by cortical modules, short- versus long-range interactions, receptive versus perceptive field organization, magnocellular versus parvocellular streams of information processing, cortical magnification and hyperacuity, point-to-point correlation in stereopsis, neurophysiological studies of perceptual constancies, illusory contours, developmental changes in vision and perception from infancy through senescence, single-cell analysis of attention, and application of psychophysics to assessment of diseases of the retina and visual pathways.

In a project such as this, some overlapping coverage is inevitable. The treatment of spatial frequency analysis, for example, is an issue we believed to be sufficiently important to be tackled from different angles (Chapters 4, 7, 10, and 15). Similarly, parallel processing is covered to some extent in three different chapters (6, 8, and 11). In other cases, scientific opinion was intermixed with data in the hope that it would provoke discussion and clarify interpretations of difficult issues that are not yet fully resolved.

It is gratifying to note that in some instances old findings and insights have been revived, such as the Gestalt laws proposed as early as 1912 by Max Wertheimer. The aperture problem (Chapter 9, Fig. 19), depth-from-shading (Chapter 11, Fig. 5), and many examples of complex perceptual phenomena can be found in Wolfgang Metzger's (1953) "Gesetze des Sehens," but without the benefit of today's understanding of the neurophysiological mechanisms that might mediate these phenomena. Although the names of even the most influential Gestalt psychologists (M. Wertheimer, W. Köhler, K. Koffka, K. Duncker, A. Michotte, W. Metzger) are only rarely cited nowadays, the basic questions they posed remain: Which factors constrain our perception of the visual world? Why do we see the way we do and not differently? Modern methods and new ways of interpretation enable today's vision scientist to go beyond the level of mere description. The recent attempts to explain the Kanizsa and Ehrenstein illusions are good examples. Two phenomena first studied by Musatti and Metelli are perceived transparency and kinetic depth effects in rotating (reversible) figures. Undoubtedly, forthcoming understanding of the motion pathways (magnocellular, Area MT, parietal stream) will spark a similar revival in the work of Hans Wallach and Gunnar Johannson.

Other forerunners of modern developments in visual science may be seen in the early pioneers of behavioral plasticity: Donald O. Hebb's discussion of nativism versus empiricism, Ivo Kohler's experiments with reversing goggles, Austin Riesen's sensory deprivation experiments, Eleanor Gibson's and Robert Fanta's studies of infant vision, Robert Weale's analysis of the aging visual system, and Richard Held and Alan Hein's experiments on perceptual development (Chapter 13). With a greater understanding of visual development, it is possible to identify the origins of some anomalies of visual perception and, conversely, to use deficits of perception to infer functional characteristics of the brain. As early as 1971, Bela Julesz coined the term "psychoanatomy" for the study of the visual brain by analysis of perception. Since then a number of noninvasive methods have been found and are being used in basic psychophysics as well as in clinical visual science (Chapter 14).

Many complex perceptual phenomena are simulated today in artificial neuronal networks using computers. J. J. Gibson's work on ecological optics (i.e., textures, gradients, flow fields) in the 1960s can be seen as a forerunner to much of today's research on computational vision. Gibson attempted to define higher-order stimulus dimensions that are related to perception of our natural environment (Chapters 12 and 15). Significant in much of this work is the *global* nature of the stimulus input. This in turn requires processing by *populations* of neurons, if not indeed of entire cortical areas, having large receptive fields and a nontopographic organization so characteristic of the extrastriate areas studied in neurophysiological research today. Receptive fields in some of these cortical modules are often dependent on both sensory and nonsensory variables such as attention and motivation and, therefore, go beyond the classical model of receptive fields.

The present volume attempts to show how knowledge obtained from *both* psychophysical and neurophysiological studies may be applied to a better understanding of vision. While "neurophysiology in search of psychophysics" is becoming widely accepted as a viable strategy in the study of human perception, the opposite approach, "psychophysics in search of neurophysiology," has already gained acceptance.

A major challenge for the future study of visual processing will be to transcend the neuronal analysis of relatively simple stimuli to the perceptual synthesis of biologically significant patterns. Where in the brain are color, motion, and form put together again, if they are? What is the neural basis of perceived invariance and object identity (e.g., in faces)? How is visual information joined by information from other sensory modalities? Is there a sensorium enabling us to "see" via touch, and vice versa? What is the role of memory in identifying the meaning of a stimulus from the "what" and "where" systems? How is this information interlaced with information from eye movements, attention, and motor action?

We thus hope that the process of mutual enlightenment between psychophysics and neurophysiology is promoted by this book and will continue to inspire the vision community, not just for the merit of the empirical science, but also for advancing our understanding of the world. The vast majority of our experiences are derived from the sense of vision. It is therefore necessary to study visual perception if we want to understand the properties of the world around us. The following two chapters point out the possibilities and limits of this approach as seen from an historical as well as epistemological perspective. The succeeding twelve chapters provide empirical tests of these propositions, and the last chapter is a personal tribute to three inspiring scientists who prompted us to accept the challenge of editing this book.

2

RELATING NEURAL MECHANISMS TO VISUAL PERCEPTION

Historical and Philosophical Considerations

Gerald Westheimer

Whatever our persuasion of science, we are agreed on the goal: a concise and universal description of natural phenomena. When it comes to human vision, it is clearly not possible to reach this goal by itemizing individual experiences. Abstractions are needed.

The approach to this abstracting procedure favored in modern times is to embed visual phenomena within a physical structure. Good examples are the concepts of visual direction and lines of sight as handles of spatial vision, leading to such sophisticated structures as the Vieth-Mueller circle and the horopter. In the brightness domain, we have the candle, the inverse-square law; in color, the trichromatic principle, Grassmann's laws, and spectral curves of fundamentals. Research with these tools can be conducted with simple apparatus and with the experimenter obtaining data on himself. The amount of knowledge acquired by these means is truly staggering—so much so that the results of current research obtained by these techniques can often be found in the literature decades, sometimes even more than a century, ago.

Just the same, the analytical goal of many scientists is not satisfied with a good abstraction of a visual phenomenon in such terms. Somehow, it is not enough to lay down the scotopic luminosity curve, or the fall-off of visual acuity with retinal eccentricity, or a threshold-versus-intensity curve. The wish to penetrate more deeply into these matters developed about the middle of the nineteenth century, with the burgeoning knowledge of anatomy and physiology. The microscope revealed rod and cone receptors and their distribution in the retina (Schultze, 1866). One visualized visual purple, a pigment contained in the rods. A greater sense of unity of knowledge arose from matching the scotopic luminosity curve with the absorption curve of visual purple (König, 1894). Current visual scientists and several generations before us have been immersed in this spirit, including psychologists. It is no coincidence that Wundt, the father of experimental psychology, worked for years in the laboratory of Helmholtz, the greatest sensory physiologist of the nineteenth century.

The underpinning given to the observed visual phenomena by these early anatomicophysiological findings is, however, not really firm. For example, it was accepted for a long time that the psychophysically determined dark-adaptation curve was simply related to the regeneration curve of visual purple; or that the grain of the eye's spatial sense was limited by the spacing of the retinal receptors. But research in the last decades has shown that this is not the case. So the attempts to uncover foundations go on.

In this quest for a foothold, sooner or later one gets to the nervous system. Now, while the gross layout of the nerves and the brain had been described centuries ago, knowledge of the finer points of neurohistology is comparatively recent. It is not often remembered that it was Helmholtz, in his doctoral thesis in 1841, who discovered that nerve fibers arise from nerve cells. Only a hundred years ago, the raging controversy was whether the nervous system was composed of discrete cells. The term "synapse" was coined by Sherrington, who died as recently as 1952.

The search for neural substrates of behavior has been a most lively endeavor. The beginning was immensely promising. We need to remind ourselves of the excitement caused by E. D. Adrian's observations on impulse coding of sensory events. The title of his book (Adrian, 1928) alone conveys the message, *The Basis of Sensation.* One of the formative experiences of my generation of visual scientists was exposure to Hartline's figure (see Fig. 1) demonstrating the Bunsen–Roscoe–Bloch law in the activity of single optic nerve fibers in limulus (Hartline, 1934).

For the sake of fairness and historical accuracy, I should, however, not conceal other formative experiences, which in retrospect were not nearly so lasting in their impact. Examples included the sequence, at one time included in all lecture courses and textbooks on the eye, of the breakdown products of rhodopsin (rhodopsin, lumirhodopsin I, lumirhodopsin II, metarhodopsin), which had little meaning to those who did not know much chemistry, and, one suspects, even to those who did. That the quest for an anatomicophysiological substrate of psychophysical findings can lead into a cul-de-sac should neither surprise nor dishearten us; it must, however, make us cautious.

At the outset one needs to confront the whole issue of reductionism. This concept became a serious issue in the 1840s after the laws of conservation of energy were formulated and the question raised whether they were applicable to the living organism. If so, physiological laws could be reduced to chemical ones, and vitalism could be abandoned. A logical consequence of reducing physiological laws to chemical ones is that the former, if all went well, could in principle be deduced from the latter.

The theme of this book is really a special version

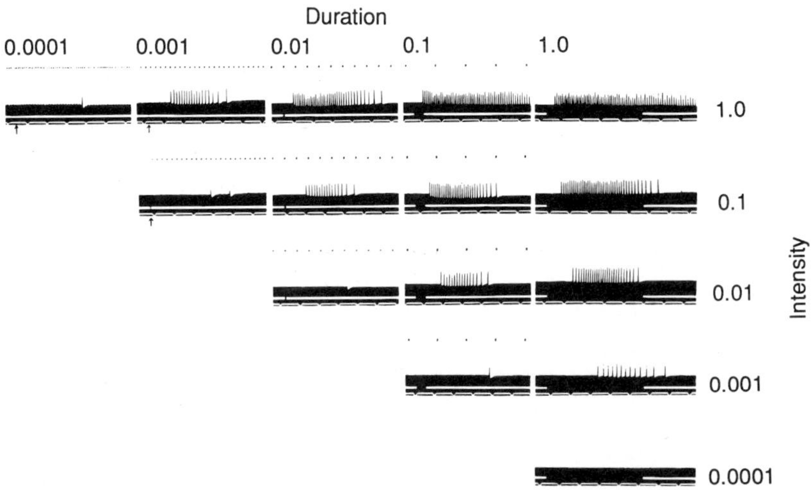

Fig. 1 Impulses from a visual cell of limulus, the horseshoe crab, in response to light flashes of various intensities and durations. The responses obey almost perfectly the Bunsen–Roscoe–Bloch law, a psychophysically based rule, according to which there is a reciprocal relationship between light intensity and flash duration for the perception of a constant brightness. From Hartline (1934). (© 1934 Alan R. Liss, Inc., with permission.)

of reductionism, namely, the reduction of the phenomena of visual perception to those of neurophysiology. Two extremes of the spectrum of views in this matter can be easily identified. The first has support from the most important philosophers, Hume and Kant, to whom we owe the insight that the existence of a world outside of us is merely a supposition, based on indirect evidence obtained through our senses. There is no arguing about this stance; metaphysics is with us, whether we like it or not.

Taking just a purely phenomenological viewpoint without benefit of a coherent thought structure is, however, not an option available to us, certainly not in our Western civilization. No one lets the world pass by their eyes without constructing some theories of what is going on, and that applies to animals as well as the human. Preaching about the falsity of the scientific enterprise is a specious undertaking, inconsistent already at the outset because the supposition of the existence of a scientific enterprise is in itself an act not at all different from what goes on within the enterprise.

The other extreme attitude to reductionism can also be unproductive. One is reminded of the historical development in approaching and defining what are perhaps the single most basic pillars of science, the axioms of geometry. It started off with the significant realization that axioms are presuppositions, that is, they come prior to any geometrical proof, and cannot themselves be proved. Thus the statement, "There is one and only one straight line between two points," is a geometrical axiom, whose self-evidence we have to take for granted. But when this train of thought is elaborated too much further, we have to take pause. For example, a succession of mathematical philosophers proceeded to analyze the sentence making up the above axiom into its constituents: what do we mean by "point," how do we define "between," and so on. The most consequential of these thinkers was Husserl. It is a revelation to read his work, but to me it is the end of a road, a beautiful transfiguration, a ride into the sunset.

The healthy, day-to-day activity of a visual scientist—and visual science is very much alive, robust, and growing—lies somewhere between the passive contemplation of phenomena as they pass before our eyes and the obsessive seeking of fundaments in physiology, anatomy, biochemistry, and beyond.

Reductionism as a program has always been more of a dream than a reality. It has been explained to me that the properties of only the very simplest molecules can be deduced from the physics of the atom; with complex molecules, chemists have to start all over again with new laws and rules that cannot immediately be traced to the laws of physics. Genetics did not start with the chemistry of DNA; in fact the phenomena of genetics are vital ingredients in the discoveries of molecular biology. Progress in developmental neurobiology depends as much on knowledge of what the fully grown nervous system looks like and how it operates, as on the mechanisms of cell growth and division and the processes of how growing axons recognize their target cells. Thus, wherever we look in cognate sciences, there are anchor points in less fundamental disciplines as well as more fundamental ones, and not, if one takes a standard view of reductionism, only in the more fundamental ones.

All of this is of relevance to the topic of this volume. It may be that some of the earlier neurophysiologists working in the visual system were more interested in the immediate access it gave to nerve fibers, synapses, easily defined sensory stimuli, the capability to differentiate nature from nurture, or the possibility of discovering universals of cortical organization. But the quarter century that has elapsed between the predecessor book (Jung & Kornhuber, 1961) and this one has changed all that. Once the first discoveries had been made (one can mention the antagonistic organization of retinal receptive fields into center and surround, or the distinction between on- and off-neurons, or the presence of oriented receptive fields in the first cortical projection), single-cell researchers in the mammalian visual system developed categorizations which do little for psychophysicists. For example, there is still no clear differentiation between two kinds of visual responses that can be ascribed to the X-system and Y-system of ganglion cells, respectively.

On the other hand, there is a multitude of visual responses that ought by now to have had their neural substrates mapped out and still have not. I am not referring to complex perceptions that obviously require input from many parts of the brain and from memory, but rather to basic visual responses whose processing is likely to be subserved by the cortical areas that have been under intense scrutiny for decades now: whether one isolated target is laterally displaced as compared with another, or seen nearer or farther, or seen moving in one direction or another, or with one velocity or another. The responses of the cortical receptive fields claimed to be relevant to these abilities often differ by two orders of magnitude from what the intact primate can do.

This raises the question of whether the difficulty is merely an unjustified impatience with the slow pace of the admittedly difficult and time-consuming work of uncovering the circuitry of the visual brain, or whether the expectation of having neurophysiologists unravel the substrates of simple visual behavior is unrealistic.

Finding strong and immediate correlations between the structure and function of the visual nervous system and the visual performance of the whole organism is an expectation that has been fulfilled in only a very few instances. Even in the apparently simple case of the decrease of visual acuity with retinal eccentricity, it becomes difficult to disentangle such factors as cone density versus ganglion cell density, cortical magnification, resolution versus localization acuity, and so on. We have nowhere reached the stage yet where we can predict performance from anatomy and physiology; those who think they can might try their hand at the expected performance in the visual field of one eye that is homologous to the blind spot of the other.

What is wrong is not the overall expectation of arriving at such correlations between neurophysiology and behavior but the use of the word "prediction." We are not dealing with a unidirectional process, in either direction. The tasks confronting the scientist when mapping the visual ability of the whole organism are just that; he might generate strong hints as to what the underlying substrate might be, but, given the diversity of biological hardware and the multitude of ways by which evolution is known to solve a problem, he is not in the position of predicting the actual organic implementation. However, if he listens carefully to what the anatomists or physiologists have really found (as distinct from what is sometimes claimed in the titles of their papers), important clues may emerge that can help decide which approach to follow in the design of experiments. Only very rarely can the phenomenological approach attain such spectacular successes as deciding on the trichromacy of color vision, and on an inherent opponent processing stage, a hundred years before the anatomists and physiologists could reach the same conclusion. Most of the time, progress is only tentative, incremental, needing lots of mid-course corrections. While it is important on the part of the behavioral researcher in vision to be open to cues from genuinely fundamental and singular findings in anatomy and physiology, one is hard pressed to decide what should be regarded as fundamental and singular. In our discipline, practicing reductionism must be done with caution: simply because somewhere there was an attempt to place single unit responses into a few *ad hoc* classes, we should not immediately proceed to categorize visual responses accordingly.

In neurophysiology, the sheer size and complexity of the mammalian visual nervous system surely overwhelm the investigator. It was a heady time when the first scouting reports came in. Those days are past, however, even in the extrastriate cortical areas. In the hard work of detailed analysis there is no hope without outside guidance, and reductionism points in the wrong direction. Help exists only in the opposite path: categorization of performance and behavior as guide to the internal construction of the visual system. But this again must be approached with caution and not dogmatically. Take the case of the internal organization subserving spatial vision. Is it appropriate to use the physicists' structure of a three-dimensional manifold with a euclidean metric? And if so, are three orthogonal axes, *x, y, z;* the best? Or would not a coordinate system be better that is centered on the fovea and uses radii and meridians? If we erect an inappropriate structure, it will be a difficult task to order the data in it, and the results will most likely be confusing. On the whole, the mathematician has been of surprisingly little help in the analysis of the visual system. So we turn to phenomenology to provide suggestions for the categories into which the practicing anatomist and physiologist can order his findings. Is disparity an independent dimension? Are there firm cardinal directions in color space? Can the results of experiments in perception and the constancies help to provide the framework for single-unit studies? And, conversely, are the latter robust enough to be regarded as outlining the substrates for the visually predicated behavior of the whole organism? This is what this volume is all about.

3

THE DOMAIN OF VISUAL SCIENCE

Davida Y. Teller

I. VISUAL SCIENCE AS A SCIENTIFIC DOMAIN

In *The Structure of Scientific Theories*, the philosopher Frederick Suppe (1977) describes the concept of a scientific domain, as introduced by Dudley Shapere (1974), as follows:

> Scientific domains are characterized as a number of *items of information* . . . which come to be associated together as a *body of information* having the following characteristics: the association is based on some well-grounded, significant, relationship between the items of information which are suggestive of deeper unities among the items; there is something problematic about the body so related; the problems are important; and, usually, science is "ready" to deal with them. . . . The very association of items in the domain . . . rationally poses or raises problems. . . . Often it tends to "favor" certain types of solutions to these problems. [Suppe, 1977, p. 687]

Visual scientists come from many parent disciplines, including perception, psychophysics, optics, anatomy, physiology, and the computational sciences. Yet we share a common scientific commitment. We want to know, to quote Koffka (1935, p. 76): "Why do things look as they do?" That is, we want to explain how we see on the basis of the properties of the neural machinery that makes seeing possible. The problem is of course very difficult, in part because of the complexity of both the visual capacities and the visual substrate, and also in part because of the logical and philosophical difficulties involved in explanatory efforts that attempt to unite such different levels of scientific discourse.

Despite the difficulties, the first Freiburg symposium (Jung & Kornhuber, 1961) and the Badenweiler conference (on which this book is based) provide existence proofs that, for some of us at least, visual science constitutes a unified, workable scientific domain. Yet it is a domain whose shared premises and reasoning patterns have not often been articulated in detail. The purpose of this chapter is to attempt to examine some of these shared premises, beginning with the very general domain criteria provided by Shapere and proceeding through analogies, general and specific linking propositions, and finally a few examples of current patterns of reasoning which involve these and other elements.

II. DOMAIN CRITERIA

To return to Shapere's criteria: The psychophysics and physiology of vision are united by a *well-grounded, significant relationship*. It is an old and fundamental premise of visual science that visual experience is, one way or another, a manifestation of the workings of the eye and brain. The first of G. E. Müller's Axioms of Psychophysical Correspondence, articulated in 1896 (see below), states that "The ground of every state of consciousness is a material process . . . to whose occurrence the presence of the conscious state is joined." And, in discussions of the mind-body problem, philosophers go so far as to debate the question of in what sense the mind and the brain are "identical." It is hard to imagine a greater affirmation of a "deep unity" between these disciplines.

More specifically, the concept of information flow is common to and unites the two fields. If we learn from a psychophysical experiment that two physically different visual stimuli are indiscriminable, we know that the information that they differ is lost somewhere along the physiological information-processing chain. On the other hand, if the two stimuli are psychophysically discriminable, we know that the information that the stimuli differ must be represented (carried) at every step of at least one continuous information-processing chain. We also know that sensory information is recoded within that chain, and it makes sense to presume that there are critical loci (Teller & Pugh, 1983) and critical recodings that leave their marks on our perceptual capacities and subjective perceptual experiences. Without question, sensory encoding and recoding processes limit and shape perception.

Furthermore, the *association of items in the domain rationally poses or raises problems*. These problems automatically take the form, what is it about the neural substrate of vision that makes us see as we do? When information is lost, we ask, how and where and why is it lost? When information is retained, we ask, along what chain of substrate elements does this information make its way, how is it carried at each stage, and at what levels does it undergo major recodings? And, when and how do critical information transformations leave their marks on perception?

The *form of acceptable explanations within the domain* is also clear. If the question is, what is it about the neural substrate of vision that makes us see as we do, the only acceptable kind of answer is, we see *X* because elements of the substrate *Y* have the property *Z* or are in the state *S*.

We now come to the question, what is the *thing that is problematic*? There are at least two answers here. The first is probably common to all scientific domains: our understanding of how to go about finding the answers to the questions is incomplete. With some important exceptions, the finding of fully satisfying explanations of psychophysically defined phenomena on the basis of substrate properties has proved to be remarkably difficult. This is doubtless largely because the two subdomains are complex, and (like the question, why are there two unequal tides every day?), conceptually simple questions do not always have simple answers. But it may also be because our conceptual patterns are unclear or unreliable. If we cannot state the criteria for what counts as an acceptable explanation, we may not be able to tell a sloppy attempt at explanation from a successful one.

The second problematic aspect is a special one for sensory and perceptual domains: how shall we deal with the mind–body relationship? It has historically been argued that perceptual states and brain states come from different realms of discourse; sensations and neurons are made of different stuff. If this is true, the concept of *explanation* of perceptual by physiological events may prove elusive in all but the simplest cases. We may be stuck with a domain that has at best a seam, and at worst a permanent chasm, down the middle.

This leaves us with the final criterion: *usually, the science is "ready" to deal with the questions*. Of this one is less certain, but then apparently so are Suppe and Shapere, judging by the qualifier "usually." On the one hand, we are surely more ready to deal with these questions now than we have ever been before, because more and more detailed knowledge of the properties of the substrate—especially of the quantitative anatomical characteristics and the detailed response properties of individual neurons at many levels of the visual projection system—is becoming available. In addition, there has been much coevolution (Churchland, 1986) between studies of function and studies of substrate, and many interesting analogies have been made between phenomena at different levels. And yet the incomplete articulation of our reasoning patterns and our criteria of success remains.

One approach is to examine the work of current visual scientists and to try to glean the common logical structures from the common practice. As Suppe (1977) suggests,

> The key to developing an adequate philosophical understanding of science as an epistemic enterprise is the detailed examination of actual scientific practice, from which one generalizes and evaluates the reasoning patterns encountered. . . . As science progresses, it has to develop new, more sophisticated patterns of reasoning if it is to continue expanding knowledge of its phenomena [pp. 683, 696]

The present chapter constitutes an attempt to engage the reader's mind in the "detailed examination of actual scientific practice," that is, in the articulation of premises and the exploration of reasoning patterns by means of which hints are exchanged and explanations established between psychophysical and physiological realms. It is also an invitation to the reader to engage in historical and philosophical research on the evolution of reasoning patterns in visual science and on the nature of explanatory efforts that attempt to unite the mental with the material realm.

III. ANALOGIES

A time-honored pattern of reasoning between psychophysical phenomena and the visual substrate has been the making of pictorial or graphical analogies. The general technique involved, which can only be stated with tongue partially in cheek, is to try to make sketches, or other descriptions of the psychophysical and physiological phenomena, that *look alike*. The reasoning pattern is, roughly, that if psychophysical and physiological data can be manipulated in such a way that they can be plotted on somewhat similar axes, such that the two graphs have more or less similar shapes, then that physiological phenomenon can be taken to be a major causal factor in producing that psychophysical phenomenon. The use of such analogies as a form of argument has been common in the past few decades of visual science, and the imprecise statement of what analogies are is intended to capture the rough and ready use of analogies which sometimes occurs in attempts to link the two different realms.

Some specific examples may serve to communicate the general flavor of reasoning by pictorial analogy. The explanation of the shape of the scotopic spectral sensitivity curve by the shape of the absorption spectrum of rhodopsin (in combination with absorption in the optic media) is an example of a well-established analogy, bolstered as it can be by many other elements of fact and logic. At the other extreme, the common textbook explanations of Mach bands and other contrast phenomena by unsupported pictorial analogy to the spatial pattern of activity across a row of ommatidia, or even prototypical ganglion cells, often provide examples of weak and unsupported uses of analogy which do not stand up well to rigorous analysis (cf. Teller, 1984).

Explicit analyses of specific analogies have been made occasionally in the vision literature. For example, the explanation of the existence of opponent colors by analogy to chromatically opponent cells, while encouraging in principle, overlooks many failures of fit between the detailed properties of color perception and the detailed properties of currently known peripheral cells; other difficulties with "textbook" examples of opponent color theory have been discussed by Hood and Finkelstein (1983). The early, explicit use of analogy in relating the states of central neurons to perceptual phenomena is well exemplified by the work of DeValois and colleagues (e.g., DeValois, 1965) and is well worth careful study; and the explanation of the Westheimer phenomenon by appeal to the center–surround antagonism of individual ganglion cells has been examined in detail by Teller (1980).

There is, of course, no quarrel with the use of analogies in scientific thinking; many useful and potentially rigorous explanations doubtless enter the discipline by this route (cf. Suppe, 1977, p. 687). Ideally, the initial analogy will be followed up by exploring its ancillary assumptions and implications, and subjecting the whole logical structure to the usual kinds of tests—face validity, range of applicability, mutual consistency, acceptability of *ceteris paribus* conditions, and so on (cf. Teller, 1980, 1984)—that lead to the acceptance or rejection of other scientific propositions.

On the other hand, we have passed the point at which the similarity of curve shapes per se can be accepted as an explanation of psychophysical by physiological phenomena. The job by now is to explore the depth and quality of each specific analogy between psychophysical and physiological data sets, the strength of the pattern of reasoning within which the analogy is embedded, and the general and specific linking propositions involved in its use. It is to the discussion of linking propositions that we now turn.

IV. LINKING PROPOSITIONS

The disciplines of perception and psychophysics deal with the description of mental events, while physiological studies of the visual projection system seem much more readily tied to the major continuum of the physical and biological sciences. The fact that physiological and perceptual data arise from such seemingly disparate origins and deal with such different levels of phenomena has often led to the presumption that some special kinds of bridge laws, or bridging statements, will be needed to bring them into a single realm of discourse.

Over the past century there has been a series of attempts to explicate the logical and philosophical nature of such special bridging statements. Such statements have been variously called psychophysical axioms (Müller, 1896, cited in Boring, 1942), psychophysical linking hypotheses (Brindley, 1960), and linking propositions (Teller, 1984; Teller & Pugh, 1983). Recent definitions propose that a *linking proposition is a claim that a particular mapping occurs, or that a particular mapping principle applies, between perceptual states and states of the visual substrate* (cf. Teller & Pugh, 1983; Teller, 1984, p. 1235).

A linking proposition can be *general*, as are Müller's Axioms and Brindley's (1960) treatment of Identity propositions (see below). Alternatively, it can be *special*, or specific to a particular perceptual phenomenon or to a particular set of optical, photochemical, anatomical, or physiological elements. The location of the neural elements can be unspecified, and a claim made only that, since a particular perceptual state occurs, visual information must or might somewhere be encoded in a particular form. Alternatively, the linking proposition can involve the dependence of specified visual phenomena on the properties of specified neural elements or on the occurrence of a critical transformation at a particular stage of the visual information-processing chain. It is argued below that general and special linking propositions play very different roles in scientific logic.

A. General Linking Propositions

General linking propositions are best exemplified in their classic form, the Axioms of Psychophysical Correspondence articulated by G. E. Müller in 1896. Boring (1942) quotes the first three Axioms as follows:

> 1. The ground of every state of consciousness is a material process, a psychophysical process so-called, to whose occurrence the presence of the conscious state is joined.
>
> 2. To an equality, similarity or difference in the constitution of sensations . . . there corresponds an equality, similarity, or difference in the constitution of the psychophysical process, and conversely. Moreover, to a greater or lesser similarity of sensations,

> there also corresponds respectively a greater or lesser similarity of the psychophysical process, and conversely.
>
> 3. If the changes through which a sensation passes have the same direction, or if the differences which exist between series of sensations are of like direction, then the changes through which the psychophysical process passes, or the differences of the given psychophysical process, have like direction. Moreover, if a sensation is variable in *n* directions, then the psychophysical process lying at the basis of it must also be variable in *n* directions, and conversely. [p. 89]

In more recent times, Brindley (1960) argued against the scientific rigor of logical arguments that involved judgments of any characteristic of sensations other than their identity or nonidentity. Judgments of identity or nonidentity—detection and discrimination experiments—were accorded "Class A" status, and deemed to be relevant to the study of visual physiology. All other subjective reports, including judgments of the similarity, mutual exclusiveness, or uniqueness of sensations, were accorded "Class B" status. For some schools of visual science, Brindley's influential treatment provided an excuse for limiting drastically the range of psychophysical phenomena included in the scientific domain. For example, by this view the uniqueness and mutual exclusiveness of certain hues neither require nor allow physiological explanation. Boynton and Onley (1962) protested this narrow treatment, but it was strongly influential in the subsequent decades.

The present author (Teller, 1984) has proposed a systematization of the original, broader range of general linking propositions. She articulates four general families of linking propositions, namely, Identity, Similarity, Mutual Exclusiveness, and Simplicity, and for each family identifies an Initial proposition and its Contrapositive, Converse, and Converse Contrapositive forms. These concepts, and many examples, are fully developed in the original article, and space constraints prevent their repetition here. Other families, such as Directionality and Dimensionality, could also be added to cover the full range of Müller's Axioms.

Although Brindley (1960) referred to linking statements as *hypotheses*, this nomenclature may be misleading, because it suggests that all linking propositions are falsifiable or confirmable by means of experimentation. In fact, history and present usage both suggest that general linking propositions usually play the part of axioms (Müller, 1896, cited in Boring, 1942) or premises, if not analytic truths or tautologies (cf. Brindley, 1960). In any case, they are probably not subject to empirical confirmation or disconfirmation, at least not in any simple way or by any single experiment or set of experiments.

In sum, general linking propositions would most typically seem to play the role of premises in visual science. Refusal to accept a particular family of linking propositions would seem simply to exclude the corresponding subset of phenomena from tractability within the scientific domain. For many (but not all) modern visual scientists, the current trend is to accept the broader range of linking propositions, and define the domain inclusively, although not always without a certain degree of cognitive discomfort. The pejorative sting of the "Class B" label dies hard.

B. Special Linking Propositions

In addition to discussing general linking hypotheses, Brindley (1960) drew attention to a second category which he called *special linking hypotheses*. He identified several very specific ones that seemed to him well established; for example, that the perceptual "retinal tree" is caused by the shadow cast by the retinal blood vessels on the receptors. He also argued that, unlike general linking propositions, special linking propositions were at least in principle subject to empirical test; and that the truth of special linking propositions could be established by "correlating very many features of a sensory phenomenon with corresponding features of an objectively determined one" (p. 149).

Special linking propositions take forms like the following:

> We see *X* because elements *Y* at level *L* of the visual projection system have the property *Z* or are in the state *S*.

or,

We see X if and only if . . . .

or, reversing the direction,

Whenever we see X, elements Y of the substrate will have the property Z. . . .

The concept of a special linking proposition brings us back to our initial discussion of argument by analogy. In fact, the term *linking analogy* would seem an appropriate unification of the two discussions, and it underlines the point that special linking propositions can play a variety of roles in scientific argument. While they remain incompletely articulated, they are no more than analogies. In better formulated cases, special linking propositions seem to play the role of hypotheses or predictions. In fact, Brindley even suggested that some could be so well established that they could be called linking *conclusions*.

For example, statements that the phenomena of light and dark adaptation are caused by changes of input–output relationships in particular classes of retinal neurons; that disparity-tuned cells of Area 18 form the neural basis of stereopsis; that particular classes of cells in Area 17 correspond to the channels of psychophysical multiple-channels theory; that alias patterns are caused by the geometrical characteristics of the photoreceptor mosaic; or that chromatically opponent bipolar cells provide the opponent channels required by psychophysically based opponent process theory are all examples of specific linking propositions. Many others appear in the pages of this book.

It is left to the reader to take these propositions one at a time, and ask, what role is each one playing in the particular reasoning pattern in which it is embedded? To what extent is each one in principle subject to empirical test? What would be the most definitive way to try to "correlate very many features" of the psychophysical with the physiological phenomenon? Are there other criteria than the ones Brindley proposed? And, what is the current status of each argument?

V. PATTERNS OF REASONING

We now proceed to offer a few comments on a series of reasoning patterns that have traditionally enjoyed some success, and/or are currently coming into use, in attempts to relate vision to the visual substrate. The different reasoning patterns variously involve analogies, general and special linking propositions, and other patterns of logic and intuition. The list is obviously not exhaustive, and the intent is to be provocative. The goal of the exercise is to challenge working scientists to become more explicitly aware of such patterns of reasoning, so that we can sort them out, make them mutually consistent, keep the best ones, and improve the mix over time.

A. Reasoning from Psychophysics to Physiology: Trivariance and the Categorization of Cells

In relation to modern neuroscience, psychophysics is an ancient discipline, and, for at least a half century after Müller's time, reasoning patterns were unidirectional: from psychophysics to physiology. For example, both the trichromacy of color mixture and the three-dimensional nature of subjective hue/brightness space have been known for over a century. These psychophysical descriptions, in combination with dimensionality propositions, have greatly influenced the design of physiological experiments and the description of the resulting data.

The trichromacy of color-mixture data strongly suggests that color/brightness information is limited by passing through a three-channel stage, and it is generally believed, although not logically necessary (Brindley, 1960), that the bottleneck is imposed by the existence of three and only three cone types. Thus, when it became possible to estimate the action spectra of single photoreceptors, the earliest published cone action spectra were categorized into three classes, with the expectation that no other classes would be found (e.g., Brown & Wald, 1964), although this scheme could not possibly have been derived from the data themselves. Similarly, the tridimensionality of subjective color space, with its canonical chromatic axes defined by the pairings of unique hues, led at a slightly later historical stage to the somewhat forced categorization of single cells into three types: luminance, red/green, and yellow/blue (e.g., DeValois, 1965).

It is true that if there are only three cone types there can be only three independent channels at later levels. However, there can in principle be any number of (not fully independent) channels at each level, made from any number of different combinations and weightings of photoreceptor types, and any number of recodings of the information. Nowadays it is argued that there need not be an explicit "luminance" channel at peripheral levels, and at least some modern physiological data argue that there is not. Furthermore, the fit between the unique and mutually exclusive hues and the specific chromatically coded cells found at peripheral levels is not good; and there may be no current consensus as to whether cells that correspond to the unique hue coding need exist at a more central level.

Even though the tridimensionality of color/brightness vision is psychophysically clear, we do not know a priori how good or bad an approximation of the truth it will be to categorize cells at any given level into three types. The use of formal classification criteria rather than initial theoretical presumption would seem important in establishing the objectivity of cell categorizations, even in the presence of established psychophysical theory.

B. Reasoning from Physiology to Psychophysics: "Custom-Designed Stimuli" for Psychophysical Experiments

Single unit recording allows direct observation and description of the functional characteristics of individual neurons. Once such descriptions become available, it is possible to custom design the stimuli for psychophysical experiments, with the intent that the signals generated by the stimulus would be processed by, and challenge or reveal additional properties of, particular cells within the visual system.

The Westheimer phenomenon (Westheimer, 1965) provides an early example. The center–surround antagonism of individual neurons in mammalian retina had been discovered, but was not readily revealed by experiments on spatial summation at detection threshold. But when stimuli were tailored exactly right—a tiny test spot, presented against background disks of varying diameter—the threshold for the test spot was seen to first rise, and then fall again, as the diameter of the background field increased. An analogy was born.

The epitome of this pattern of reasoning is the concept of silent substitution (Estévez & Spekreijse, 1982). Since photoreceptors are univariant, they have *null sets* or *equivalence classes*: sets of stimuli which all lead to the same activation of the individual photoreceptor, and are thus indiscriminable for that photoreceptor. If the action spectra of all photoreceptor types are known, spatial or temporal stimulus patterns can be designed which are invisible to some cone types while providing suprathreshold contrast for others. Thus, one should be able to provide stimulus patterns that traverse, say, only the long-wavelength-sensitive (LWS) cones, and thus study the range of psychophysical performance that is available via solely LWS-cone-initiated signals.

The same reasoning can be extended, although with an increasing baggage of assumptions, to later levels of the visual system. Later neurons, like photoreceptors, are univariant and have equivalence classes. If, for example, there were three and only three linear, independent, color/luminance channels at a given physiological level, and their spectral characteristics were known, then one could in principle design stimuli to fall in the equivalence classes of any two of them, activate only a single cell type at that level, and study the vision of a subject seeing through only the remaining class of cells. The current interest in vision at isoluminance provides an example of work that may fit into this paradigm, and the possible sequential recodings provide a wealth of additional possibilities.

Unfortunately, the load of excess characteristics required to make such isolation work is large, including the requirement of homogeneity within cell classes. Further, the larger the number of classes, the smaller the range of stimuli that will null all but one of them;

and artifacts that activate unintended channels will have to be tracked down. In short, there is no way to tell at this moment the degree to which postreceptoral silent substitution paradigms will work out in practice.

C. Quasi-Physiological Models and Machine Vision

Another common activity in visual science is to develop mathematical models intended to explain psychophysical data. One of the logic patterns involved in many such modeling efforts has been that the models must be at least *quasi-physiological*, that is, constrained to incorporate modules or elements whose properties are consistent with our current concepts of the properties of substrate elements (Donald Hood, personal communication). In general, purely mathematical models have been of lesser interest. A corollary of this rule is that psychophysically derived models are to some degree amenable to support, or vulnerable to disconfirmation, by means of new physiological evidence.

For example, the similarities of bandwidth between Wilson and Gelb's (1984) psychophysically derived multiple-channels model and the cortical cells studied by DeValois, Albrecht, and Thorell (1982) lead to the suggestion that these cells form the substrate for the psychophysically derived channels. Demonstration of discrete classes of cells tuned to different spatial frequencies would seem to be the next step in establishing Brindley's identity of detail between the two levels, and demonstration of a continuous series of cell types would seem to disconfirm it.

There has been much coevolution between visual psychophysics and visual physiology, particularly in the convergence of the choice of stimuli and the choice of paradigms. In particular, visual psychophysicists have tended to study phenomena for which intuitively appealing analogies could be made between early sensory processing and psychophysical phenomena, and to ignore more global perceptual topics for which believable physiological analogies are less readily invented. Similarly, at least some physiologists have studied single units with specific functional questions firmly in mind.

One of the more newly arriving aspects of visual science, machine vision, forms an interesting contrast in modeling approaches. Marr (1982), for example, advocates the study of global aspects of perception, regardless of whether physiological analogies are readily available; and the development of computational algorithms, which need not be physiologically constrained, as models of visual processing. Despite the inclusion of machine vision in modern conferences on relating psychophysics to physiology, it may well be that, at least in the short run, machine vision approaches will take us away from, rather than toward, a coevolving, unified domain.

D. Analogies between Anatomy and Psychophysics

Another relatively recent trend in visual science is the resurgence of reasoning patterns that involve direct analogies between anatomical (as opposed to physiological) and psychophysical domains. Three examples are listed briefly, along with a few comments about the partially developed reasoning patterns that seem to be involved.

The first example concerns theories of the constraints that the numbers and spatial sampling characteristics of cells in the various visual processing layers place on spatial vision. The initial stage of this processing concerns the photoreceptor *mosaic*, with the term mosaic itself chosen to invoke the image of covering the retina with contiguous, nonoverlapping sampling areas. The constraints that passage through such a discrete sampling mosaic place on spatial information are coming to be relatively well understood. However, one sometimes hears mention of later processing levels referred to casually as resampling by, say, the ganglion cell mosaic. Since ganglion cell bodies can be displaced considerably from their receptive fields, and since receptive fields overlap, the mosaic analogy may serve our intuitions poorly. One also hears the presumption, which cannot be quite right, that a decrease in the number of cells from one level to the next necessarily constitutes a loss of spatial information.

The second example concerns the concept of *magnification factors*: changes in the numbers of cells per degree of visual angle at different anatomical processing levels, especially as these changes vary with retinal eccentricity. The question is, can these changes be used to model or explain variations of visual function with retinal eccentricity? An underlying reasoning pattern in this field is that the same number of square or cubic centimeters of neural tissue, or the same number of cells, will always be required to perform a given neural analysis or underlie a particular psychophysical performance. One trend in psychophysical experimentation that may lead to difficulty in this field is the variation of stimulus parameters with eccentricity, based on a prior estimate of magnification factors, rather than the collection of enough data to reconfirm (or disconfirm) these factors within each individual experiment.

The third example of analogies between psychophysics and anatomy concerns *parallel processing:* the concept that relatively independent, anatomically separated physiological modules or processing streams carry out different aspects of visual processing and that, conversely, the independence of different visual functions can be used as an indicator of anatomical isolation. A major linking proposition in this area seems to be that visual functions which are processed in the same stream can interact and, conversely, visual functions which interact must be processed in the same stream. The information that stays together, plays together, and vice versa.

A troublesome area for parallel processing models remains the question, to what degree must the information carried and processed in the various streams be reintegrated within the neural substrate? In other words, what form must visual information take in order to provide the subjectively integrated perceptual world and/or to allow integrated responses to external stimuli? There appears to be no consensus on even a working premise in this area.

E. Developmental Data: An "Orthogonal Dimension?"

As a final case, the author may perhaps be forgiven for introducing a pattern of reasoning that has influenced much of her own work. In studying even the best established analogies between vision and substrate, one is often struck by the fact that even a good analogy is a beginning, and not an end. As Brindley argued, we gather evidence in support of a specific linking proposition by comparing very many details of the psychophysical with the physiological phenomenon. It seems possible that developmental data could be useful in this context, as a new dimension with which to challenge specific linking propositions. That is, suppose one believes that a certain set of cells or synapses is a necessary condition for the occurrence of a certain psychophysical phenomenon. Similarity of onset times would provide support for such a belief, while the ontological antedating of the physiological by the psychophysical phenomenon would provide a powerful reason to reject or modify the original theory.

In fact, developmental work proceeds slowly, and generation of data clean enough and powerful enough to challenge theory has proved difficult. There has been a recent increase in the number of theoretical treatments of the data on infant vision, but most of them have to do with applying sampling theory to model changes in acuity, more as an extension of sampling theory than as a challenge to it. Whether developmental data will ever have the power to provide major challenges to theories of the dependence of visual function on visual substrate remains an open question for the future.

VI. BRIDGES

Finally, we return to the question of linking propositions, in order to reexamine the initial assumption on which the whole putative need for linking propositions is based: Are psychophysical and physiological terms truly from different realms of discourse, necessarily and for all time? Does the mind–brain dichotomy necessarily insert a unique chasm down the middle of visual science, such that special bridging statements will always be needed? Or might the simple fact that psychophysicists and physiologists talk to each other result eventually in a single linguistic fabric—a single realm of discourse—with the ghost of the mind–body dichotomy restrained to a harmless whispering within its warp and woof?

One reason for optimism comes from the reexamination of special linking propositions. Linking hypotheses or predictions of the form "We see *X* if and only if elements of the substrate *Y* . . ." or "Since substrate elements *Y* have the property *Z*, we should see *X*" do not seem at face value to be particularly different from hypotheses seen in many other contexts. Brindley's (1960) argument that they are subject to empirical support or disconfirmation strengthens the apparent similarity to other disciplines. The larger the body of explicit and empirically well-established special linking propositions, perhaps the less will be the need to see the domain as importantly divided into two distinct sources. The stronger the bridge, the less the need for bridge laws.

A second reason comes from a comparison of the possible bridge laws, or concept reductions, in visual science to classical examples from other disciplines. Classical examples of successful concept reductions are the identification of table salt with sodium chloride and of the temperature of a gas with the mean kinetic energy of its molecules. In discussions of the mind–body problem, philosophers of a reductive materialist persuasion often argue that specific mental events will be similarly identifiable with specific brain states. Yet, for many of us, the gap between mental and material states seems bigger than the gap between natural language and chemical or physical language, and the potential reduction of perceptual states to brain states somehow produces a sense of personal loss. One feels, rightly or wrongly, that something fundamental has been overlooked in the reduction; and for this reason, one resists the reduction in principle. But what, exactly, has been overlooked?

Actually, one might argue that the similarity among the three examples is greater than it seems. On further inspection, none of these three reductions is fully satisfying, because in each case, some of the connotative meaning of the natural language term has been lost. For most of us, salt is not connotatively equivalent to sodium chloride; the properties left out are the prescientific innocence of one's knowledge of salt, and the direct sensory experience of whiteness and salty taste. Similarly, the ontological origin and the sensory experience of temperature are left out of the reduction to mean kinetic energy. But these losses of connotative meaning can seem strikingly similar to the loss one feels in identifying perceptual states with brain states. What is left out in a reduction of perceptual states to neural activity would be (at least) the direct and scientifically innocent access one has to one's own perceptual states.

Perhaps it is always true that the reduction of scientific concepts entails an initial, and sometimes permanent, loss of context and connotative meaning. Such a realization can make the proposed perception–brain identity more palatable than it is otherwise and reduce one's psychological resistance to it. In any case this realization has set the present writer's mind considerably to rest on acceptance of reductive materialism as a philosophical persuasion.

A final reason for optimism comes from the fact that we are beginning to get some much needed help from modern philosophers of science. For example, Churchland (1986) provides important and relevant discussions of such concepts as coevolution and intertheoretic reduction, and Hardin (1988a) has begun the task of "unweaving the rainbow"—introducing scientific perspectives into philosophical discussions of the nature of color. With luck we shall soon learn much more, in much more sophisticated terms, about the possible uniqueness or ordinariness of visual science as a unified scientific domain. Perhaps the need for the concept of linking propositions will pass behind us entirely, and/or perhaps our attempted explanation of mental by material events will have implications for other disciplines, or even for advances in philosophical treatments of the mind–body relationship (cf. Hardin, 1988b).

In summary, the chapters of this book provide a

rich resource for further detailed analyses of the reasoning patterns of the domain called visual science in the decade of the 1980s and the ways in which these reasoning patterns have shaped the choice of experiments and research paradigms. In some chapters, the logic of the approach to relating vision to the visual substrate may be primitive, while in others it is advanced. In some, the reasoning patterns are clearly and elegantly presented; in others, sound but quite implicit; and in yet others, obscure. Some chapters will stand up well over time, while others may not. In one way or another, all will doubtless form fuel for the musings of future historians of science, concerning the quaintly limited ways in which working scientists understood the logic of the scientific problems in which they were so very deeply involved.

ACKNOWLEDGMENTS

Preparation of this chapter was supported by National Institute of Health Research Grants EY 02920 and EY 07078. I thank many colleagues, especially Delwin Lindsey, Donald Hood, and Peter Lennie, for valuable discussions.

4

INTERSPECIES COMPARISONS IN THE UNDERSTANDING OF HUMAN VISUAL PERCEPTION

M. L. J. Crawford, Richard A. Andersen, Randolph Blake, Gerald H. Jacobs, and Christa Neumeyer

I. INTRODUCTION

A. Why Study Other Species?

The history of the advance of knowledge in the biological sciences is replete with examples of how the study of other species has been indispensable to scientific progress. No area of biology would have developed to any significant degree without the contributions made by observations and research carried out on animals. Since the time of Galen, the study of the anatomical and physiological systems in animals has established the foundation for inferences drawn concerning possible physiological substrates for human perception, and has provided, as well, the basis for speculation about mechanisms underlying behavioral and perceptual processes in the species itself.

This information transfer has not always been unidirectional, that is, from animal physiology to human perception. It has also worked the other way around. The study of human perception through visual psychophysics has often guided the study of anatomy and physiology in animals. For example, consider stereopsis, the appreciation of depth from binocular viewing (see Chapter 12, this volume). The perceptual aspects of stereopsis have been recognized since Aristotle and have received sporadic attention throughout history. In the last century, Wheatstone (1838) demonstrated that horizontal disparity of the binocular images was sufficient to produce the perception of depth, and Herman Wilbrand speculated rather accurately about the anatomical substrate of stereopsis at least 60 years before it was actually demonstrated. Wilbrand concluded that the two homononymous hemiretinas were represented in the same overlapping area of the cortex, and that retinal point-pairs, from the left and right eye, interacted to provide the basis for stereopsis (Polyak, 1957). Through continuing psychophysical study (e.g., Ogle, 1950; Julesz, 1960) the requirements of the neural substrates for stereopsis became increasingly evident. The actual demonstration came from the experiments of Barlow, Blakemore, and Pettigrew (1967) and Pettigrew, Nikara, and Bishop (1968) in their electrophysiological studies of cat cortex. Since then, the work of Bishop (see Bishop & Pettigrew, 1986), Poggio (see Chapter 12, this volume), and Crawford (Crawford et al., 1983, Crawford, Smith, Harwerth & von Noorden, 1984) leaves little doubt that cortical binocular cells provide the physiological basis for stereopsis.

From this example it can be seen that the study of other species serves at least four valuable purposes: (1) to determine the anatomical and physiological *substrate* of perceptual processes; (2) to gain better *experimental control* over the subject of study, for example, being able to manipulate the kind and degree of visual experience during visual development; (3) to work out the *rules* for how anatomical, physiological, developmental, and behavioral variables determine the function of a sensory or perceptual system; and (4) to test the *generality* of these rules across species. The closer the species, phylogenetically, the more likely the solutions to the problem have common elements between the species.

B. What Makes a Good Animal Model for Human Visual Perception?

Ideally one would want an animal research model for visual perception to have the same anatomical, physiological, and behavioral attributes as that of humans. Of course, practical animal models may approximate only one or more characteristics of the human visual system. Bearing in mind that, in the absence of language, it is virtually impossible to equate perceptual phenomena between human and animal observers, sensory parameters can be explored in both humans and other animals, often using the same measurement apparatus and procedures. Some of the more obvious desirable and practical characteristics of an animal model are as follows:

1. The species should exhibit the visual behavior of interest in its natural environment.
2. The species should possess anatomical characteristics which permit extrapolation to comparable structures in humans.
3. The species should demonstrate discriminative behaviors suggestive of comparable processes in humans (e.g., color-matching, hue discrimination, stereopsis, visual development).
4. The species should be an "appropriate" experimental subject according to the following criteria:
   a. Predictability: The animal should give a consistent behavioral response, that is, a low variance of response.
   b. Availability: The animal should be available in sufficient numbers, and at an affordable cost, so as to permit replication of experimental research.
   c. Convenience: The animal should be of a size and disposition conducive to handling.
   d. Ethical considerations: The animal should merit use as a research model. Sacrifice of rare or endangered species should not be acceptable.

The following sections are intended to illustrate these considerations in selecting the particular species of animal subject, and in the interpretations and generalizations of results to processes in other species and to perceptual processes in humans. The reader is urged to refer to the logical constraints described in Chapter 3 of this volume in order to better interpret the conclusions drawn about the relations between brain function in experimental animals and human visual perception.

II. COMPARATIVE ASPECTS OF CAT SPATIAL VISION

Let us begin with a description of the comparative vision of the cat, visual science's most popular nonhuman research species. The cat has contributed enormously to our understanding of the neuroanatomy and neurophysiology of mammalian vision. Indeed, many of the hallmark properties of mammalian visual neurophysiology were discovered and elaborated in the cat. These include the center–surround organization of retinal ganglion cell receptive fields (Kuffler, 1953), the existence of multiple parallel visual pathways (i.e., *X*, *Y*, and *W* pathways) from retina to brain (Enroth-Cugell & Robson, 1966), and the orientation selectivity and binocularity of cortical cells (Hubel & Wiesel, 1962).

This wealth of neurophysiological and neuroanatomical data about the cat's visual system raises two questions: (1) To what extent can the visual capacities of the cat be explained in terms of the sampling constraints and receptive field properties of retinal, geniculate, and cortical neurons? (2) To what extent are cat and human visual performance comparable? The first question, of course, addresses one of the most fundamental issues of sensory neuroscience, the neural basis of perception. The second question relates directly to the first one; to the extent that human and cat vision are comparable, one may reasonably assume that neurophysiological findings in the cat shed light on the neural machinery of human vision. In this section we review evidence that bears on these two questions, with particular emphasis on spatial vision (i.e., the detection and discrimination of objects and displays defined by luminance contours). It is useful to start with a few general comments concerning strategies for comparing psychophysical data with physiological data.

A. Physiology and Psychophysics

In evaluating the relation between cat physiology and cat psychophysics, we shall want to compare measures of neural responsiveness (e.g., firing rate) with measures of behavioral performance (e.g., contrast detection threshold). What conditions must be satisfied for this comparison to be meaningful? To begin, the same stimulus should be employed in both types of measurements. For instance, to learn about contrast coding, we might employ a sinusoidal grating to generate action potentials (the physiological measure) as well as to measure contrast thresholds (the psychophysical measure); it would make little sense to compare neural data collected with spots of light to behavioral data obtained using a grating.

Simply employing the same physical stimulus, however, does not ensure equivalence between the two types of experiments. In physiological experiments, the animal's eyes may be dilated and/or immobilized, whereas in a behavioral experiment natural pupils and freely moving eyes are the rule. Hence, retinal illuminance (determined by pupil size) and temporal frequency (influenced by eye movements) may differ significantly in the two types of experiments; this means that a given physical stimulus may not be truly equivalent in the two experiments. This lack of stimulus equivalence can be minimized by recording from an alert, behaving animal, but this requires training the animal to maintain fixation so that the visual stimulus can be accurately placed in the receptive field of the neuron whose activity is being recorded. An alternative solution is to coordinate the design of stimuli in psychophysical and physiological experiments so that equivalent optical quality, retinal illuminance, etc. are ensured. Still, certain factors will be very difficult to equate.

Next comes the problem of data comparison. How does one compare the responsiveness of a neuron or class of neurons with an animal's performance on a threshold task? Even with the same stimulus providing a common denominator, how can one relate a neuronal response to a given stimulus to a behavioral response elicited by that same stimulus? One strategy might involve measuring the minimum stimulus value that elicits a reliable response, perhaps employing some type of signal detection task to define a physiological threshold (e.g., Bradley, Skottun, Ohzawa, Sclar & Freeman, 1987). However, to the extent that different cells exhibit different thresholds, one must posit some decision rule specifying how signals from these different cells contribute to a psychophysical judgment. Are such judgments based on activity within the most sensitive neuron, on some weighted average of neural activity, or what? And, what is the particular performance level required (e.g., 75% correct) to define threshold? In view of these considerations, it is unrealistic to expect strict equivalence between a physiological threshold and a psychophysical threshold.

A second, more realistic, strategy for relating psychophysics to physiology entails deriving a family of psychophysical thresholds and expressing these thresholds in the form of a psychophysical function. The term "psychophysical function" refers to a plot showing the variation in threshold (e.g., the dimmest light increment that elicits a response) with some stimulus dimension (e.g., wavelength). The resulting spectral sensitivity function (in this example) defines the bandwidth of the system for that stimulus dimension, and, it is hoped, the function will exhibit some characteristic shape, or signature (e.g., nonmonotonicity). Now one can compare this psychophysical function to the same sort of function defined physiologically. The two functions can be compared in terms of their shapes and bandwidths. This comparison provides a more compelling test of the equivalence hypothesis, because it involves comparing changes in threshold over some common stimulus dimension. Interestingly, for some stimulus dimensions, the bandwidth determined behaviorally greatly exceeds the bandwidths of individual neural elements. To give an example, the cat can resolve spatial frequencies spanning roughly a 5-octave range (Blake, Cool & Crawford, 1974), yet individual neurons typically respond over a much narrower range of frequencies (Movshon, Thompson & Tolhurst, 1978a). The upper and lower limits of this range vary from cell to cell, however, and the total range encompassed by a large sample of cells matches the 5-octave bandwidth measured behaviorally.

A third strategy for relating psychophysics to underlying neural processes involves generating quantitative predictions of visual performance derived from anatomy. For instance, sampling theory specifies the highest resolvable frequency that can be unambiguously registered by an array of neural elements. This so-called Nyquist limit (see Chapter 10, this volume) can be computed from density estimates for, say, retinal ganglion cells, and this limit, in turn, can be compared against behavioral performance. Similarly, one can compute Nyquist limits for two different species to predict the extent to which the two species should perform differently on a visual task.

A fourth, potentially powerful strategy is to correlate deficits in behavioral performance with disorders in the visual nervous system. These disorders could occur naturally (e.g., reduced cortical binocularity in Siamese cats) or could be experimentally induced (e.g., reduced binocularity from alternating monocular deprivation early in life). This strategy has been employed with great success (e.g., Lehmkuhle, Kratz & Sherman, 1982), in part because so much has been learned about the effects of early visual deprivation (e.g., Movshon & Van Sluyters, 1981). In effect, physiologists have devised recipes (i.e., early rearing techniques) for altering the visual nervous system in interesting and suggestive ways. Psychophysicists were quick to capitalize on these recipes to study the behavioral concomitants of these neural deprivation effects. Moreover, it has been possible to find and study humans with comparable histories of early visual deprivation, thereby forging a link between clinical ophthalmology and visual neurophysiology (e.g., Holopigian, Blake & Greenwald, 1986).

These, then, are some strategies for extrapolating from physiology to psychophysics and for generalizing from an animal species to humans. Versions of these strategies have been employed in the study of cat spatial vision, and results from those studies are the major focus of this section of the chapter. In evaluating behavioral data on cat spatial vision, it is useful to keep in mind those factors, optical and neural, that could influence the quality of cat spatial vision and its comparability to human spatial vision. Accordingly, a summary of those factors is given in the next subsection.

B. Optical and Neural Determinants of Cat Spatial Vision

The design of any visual system involves a compromise between light sensitivity and spatial resolution—those adaptations that favor one almost always detract from the other. In the case of the cat, this compromise between sensitivity and resolution leans in favor of sensitivity, at least by human standards, a compromise that makes sense given this animal's nocturnal leanings. It is useful to keep this thought in mind as we consider the optical and neural factors that govern cat spatial vision.

1. Optics of the Cat Eye

Looking first at the optical system in the cat, the eyeball itself is relatively large, with a broad light-gathering cornea, a pupil with an enormous dynamic range, and a globular lens placed relatively far back in the eye. Assuming average values for the dioptric components of the eye (Vakkur & Bishop, 1963), one degree of visual angle subtends 0.218 mm on the retina, a value approximately 30% smaller than that estimated for the human. The retinal illuminance associated with this smaller image, however, will be brighter, by as much as 5 times under dim light conditions when the pupil is fully dilated. The total range of accommodation in the cat has been estimated to be 4 D (diopters) (Vakkur, Bishop & Kozak, 1963), and its near point falls around 25 cm (Bloom & Berkley, 1977). Interestingly, accommodation in the cat appears to be accomplished by actual movement of the principal planes of the lens (Hughes, 1973), not by an increase in lens power.

Turning next to the optical performance of the cat's eye, Robson and Enroth-Cugell (1978) have derived a modulation transfer function (MTF) for the cat's optics (i.e., a plot of the ratio of image contrast to target contrast at different spatial frequencies). When the test target was imaged through a 4 mm artificial pupil, the cutoff spatial frequency (i.e., the highest spatial frequency passed by the optics) equaled approximately 20 cycles/degree. Under natural viewing conditions, the cat would have to view a surface whose average luminance was approximately 500 cd/m^2 for its pupil to be equivalent in area to that produced by an artificial pupil 4 mm in diameter (Hammond & Mouat, 1985). While this light level is easily realizable under daylight viewing conditions, it is unusual to work at light levels as high as 500 cd/m^2 in the laboratory. This means that during most behavioral work the cat's pupil will be larger than 4 mm, and, therefore, the quality of the image on the cat's retina will be somewhat poorer because of the enlarged pupil. To illustrate, when viewing a surface luminance of 40 cd/m^2 (a value within the range typically used in behavioral work), pupil size in the cat increases to approximately 55 mm^2, which would be equivalent to viewing through a circular artificial pupil a little over 8 mm in diameter. Optical quality in the cat has not been measured with an artificial pupil so large, therefore, we can only speculate about the quality of the retinal image produced under these conditions. Robson and Enroth-Cugell (1978) did measure the line-spread function through the cat's natural pupil (size unspecified), and the cutoff frequency of the derived MTF fell around 15 cycles/degree. Thus, knowing nothing else about the cat's visual system, we can expect the optics of the cat's eye to impose a limit on the cat's acuity somewhere between 15 and 20 cycles/degree.

2. The Cat Retina

The cat, like the human, possesses a duplex retina in which rods far outnumber cones (Steinberg, Reid and Lacy, 1973). Even within the region of maximum cone density, the area centralis, rods are 10 times more numerous than cones, in marked contrast to the rod-free human fovea. The density of cones within the area centralis is about 27,000 cones/mm^2; rod density in the area centralis equals about 275,000 rods/mm^2. Recalling that 1 degree visual angle corresponds to 0.218 mm, we can express cone and rod density in angular units: a 1 degree^2 region centered on the area centralis contains approximately 1225 cones and 13,000 rods. On average, neighboring cones are separated by 1.7 arc min, while rod separation is about 0.54 arc min. The visual significance of these figures is considered when we discuss acuity. Incidentally, the degree of regularity in the spatial distribution of the mixed photoreceptor mosaic has been described by Steinberg et al. (1973) and Wässle and Riemann (1978). Both groups have noted a significant departure from strict regularity in the cone array, and Wässle and Riemann have contrasted this with the rather precise mosaic of cones in the monkey fovea.

Because the entire cat retina, including the area

centralis, contains a mixed photoreceptor population, it is important to know something about the luminance conditions at which a single photoreceptor system exclusively contributes to visual performance in the cat. Only by working above the upper luminance level for mesopic vision can visual performance be unambiguously related to sampling properties of the cat's cone mosaic, or only by working below the lower luminance level for mesopic vision will performance be exclusively rod based. Ganglion cell data and pupil area data can be used to estimate the upper and lower bounds on the mesopic range for an awake cat viewing its environment through natural pupils. Enroth-Cugell, Hertz, and Lennie (1977) used a two-color isolation procedure to measure light levels at which ganglion cells received cone input only and rod input only. Over a sample of 11 cells, the upper limit of the mesopic range varied from 2.5 to 3.5 log cd/m^2, and the lower limit varied between -0.8 and 0.2 log cd/m^2. These values were based on a pupil 1 mm^2 in diameter, so they can be interpreted as cat trolands (i.e., estimates of retinal illuminance, the product of luminance and pupil area). Taking average values from Enroth-Cugell et al. for the two extremes of the mesopic range, the curves of Hammond and Mouat (1985) were used to determine the light level that would produce these values of retinal illuminance with natural pupils. According to this analysis, cat ganglion cells should receive pure rod input when the prevailing level of luminance falls anywhere below 0.1 cd/m^2 and pure cone input whenever this level exceeds 50 cd/m^2. The mesopic range in the cat, therefore, spans slightly less than a 3 log-unit range of luminance.

Like the photoreceptors, ganglion cells reach peak density in the area centralis. All ganglion cells receive inputs from both rods and cones, although the β type ganglion cells, which are thought to correspond to the physiologically defined X cells, appear to receive a larger proportion of cone input than do the α cells, thought to be Y cells (e.g., Steinberg et al., 1973). Grouping ON and OFF cells together, β cell density in the area centralis has been estimated to be approximately 6,000/mm^2 (Hughes, 1981). This value is almost 5 times lower than the cone density in the area centralis, implying convergence of many cones onto single ganglion cells. In the primate fovea, there is evidence for 1:1 convergence of single cones onto individual ganglion cells.

3. Cortical sampling

Finally, the packing density of neurons in cat visual cortex (i.e., number of cells/cubic millimeter) is 2.5 times less than in monkey visual cortex (Beaulieu & Colonnier, 1983), and the total number of neurons in Area 17 of cat is estimated to be 6 times less than in Area 17 of the monkey. In view of these numerical disparities, it is natural to expect that the cat's cortex provides less fine-grained reconstruction of the retinal image than does the monkey or human cortex (Barlow, 1979).

C. Visual Resolution in Cats and Humans

1. Visual Acuity

Over the years, a number of laboratories have determined the cat's visual acuity; the consensus of these experiments places that figure in the neighborhood of 6–8 cycles/degree (Smith, 1936; Blake et al., 1974; Jacobson, Franklin & McDonald, 1976; Bloom & Berkley, 1977; Mitchell, Giffin & Timmey, 1977; Vandenbussche & Orban, 1983). Most of these measurements were performed, incidentally, at light levels in the upper mesopic and lower photopic range for the cat. Unlike in man, the cat's threshold acuity does not seem to vary with grating orientation (Vandenbussche & Orban, 1983), which is somewhat surprising given the preponderance of visual cortical cells tuned to the principal meridians (e.g., Rose & Blakemore, 1974). The cat's visual acuity does vary, however, with retinal eccentricity, and, as illustrated in Fig. 1, the falloff in the cat's acuity with eccentricity mirrors rather closely the falloff in human acuity. The human acuity measurements (Berkley et al., 1975) were made using a 60% contrast vertical grating that flickered at 1 Hz; the cat data (Blake & Bellhorn, 1978) were collected using a 45% contrast vertical grating flickering at 1.5 Hz.

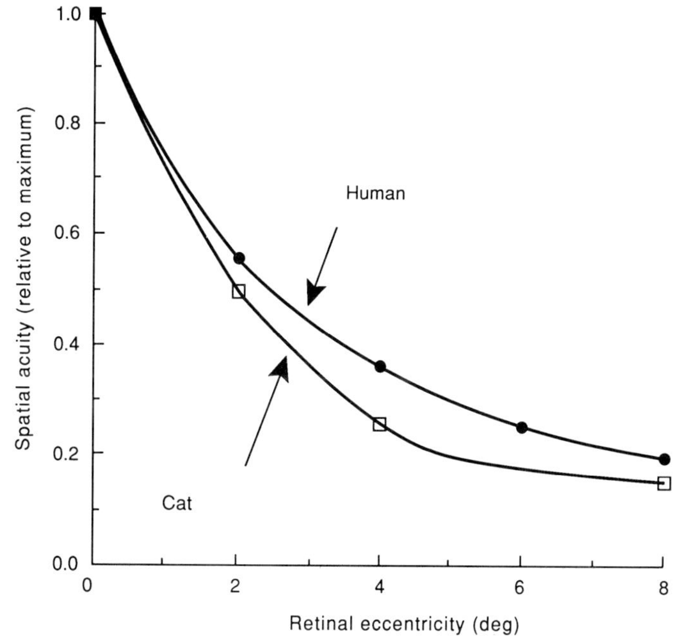

Fig. 1 The falloff in visual acuity with retinal eccentricity for the cat (Blake & Bellhorn, 1978) and human (Berkley et al., 1975). Acuity is defined as the highest resolvable spatial frequency of a grating.

What factors limit spatial resolution in the cat? It is doubtful that the cat's optics are responsible for the animal's acuity, for the high frequency cutoff of the modulation transfer function (Robson & Enroth-Cugell, 1978) is near 20 cycles/degree. Moreover, the Nyquist limit of the cone mosaic of the cat's area centralis comes to about 18 cycles/degree, and the falloff in cone density with eccentricity is more gradual than the falloff in the cat's acuity (see Fig. 2). These two observations strongly suggest that acuity is not being limited by the sampling density of the cones. The falloff in β cell density with eccentricity does, however, dovetail nicely with the progressive loss in the cat's visual acuity with retinal eccentricity, (Fig. 2). This correspondence suggests that convergence of cone signals onto ganglion cells may be a major limit to visual acuity in the cat. At present it is impossible to say whether ON and OFF systems of the β cell population act in concert, or independently, to set limits on acuity (Hughes, 1981).

How does this conclusion compare to the situation in humans? In the human eye, optics, cone sampling density, and β ganglion cell sampling density all yield

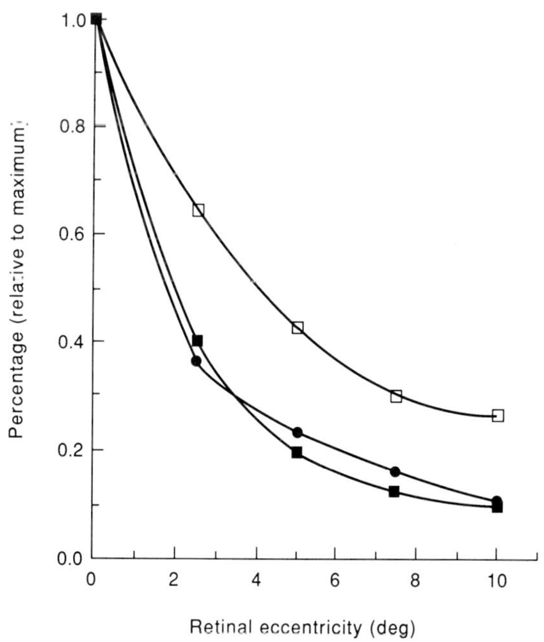

Fig. 2 Grating acuity in the cat at different retinal eccentricities compared with cone and ganglion cell density at the same locations.

approximately the same estimate of foveal acuity, 60 cycles/degree, which closely matches the value actually obtained under optimal conditions (see Chapter 10, this volume). The falloff in acuity with eccentricity, however, correlates well with the change in density of β ganglion cells and does not match the change in density of cones, suggesting that the same factor, pooling of signals by ganglion cells, limits visual resolution in cats and in humans.

How well does the cat's behaviorally measured acuity match the best resolution exhibited by single cells? In the retina, ganglion cells of the brisk-sustained type (thought to be the β type cells) with receptive fields in the area centralis can resolve gratings as high as 9 cycles/degree (Cleland, Harding & Tulunay-Keesey, 1979). Moving away from the area centralis, cutoff frequencies for this class of ganglion cells are systematically lower and, in fact, follow very closely the falloff in β cell density shown in Fig. 2. Comparable acuity values (i.e., approximately 7 cycles/degree) have been reported for X cells in the lateral geniculate nucleus (Lehmkuhle et al., 1980) and for simple cells in Area 17 (Eggers & Blakemore, 1978; Movshon, Thompson & Tolhurst, 1978b). In other visual areas, including Area 18 (Movshon et al., 1978a), the lateral suprasylvian cortex (DiStefano, Morrone & Burr, 1985; Zumbroich & Blakemore, 1987), and the superior colliculus (Bisti & Sireteanu, 1976), cells are unable to resolve spatial frequencies higher than 2.5 cycles/degree. These observations implicate Area 17 as the cortical region crucially involved in the resolution of fine spatial detail. In this regard, it is notable that lesions of Area 17 in the cat produce about a 30% reduction in grating acuity (Berkley & Sprague, 1979) and even greater losses in the ability to detect vernier offsets (Sprague, Berkley & Hughes, 1979).

2. Spatial Contrast Sensitivity

Several laboratories (Bisti & Maffei, 1974; Blake et al., 1974) have measured the cat's contrast sensitivity function (CSF), that is, the curve depicting variations in the reciprocal of contrast threshold with spatial frequency. Representative results are shown in Fig. 3, which shows CSFs measured for the cat and for a hu-

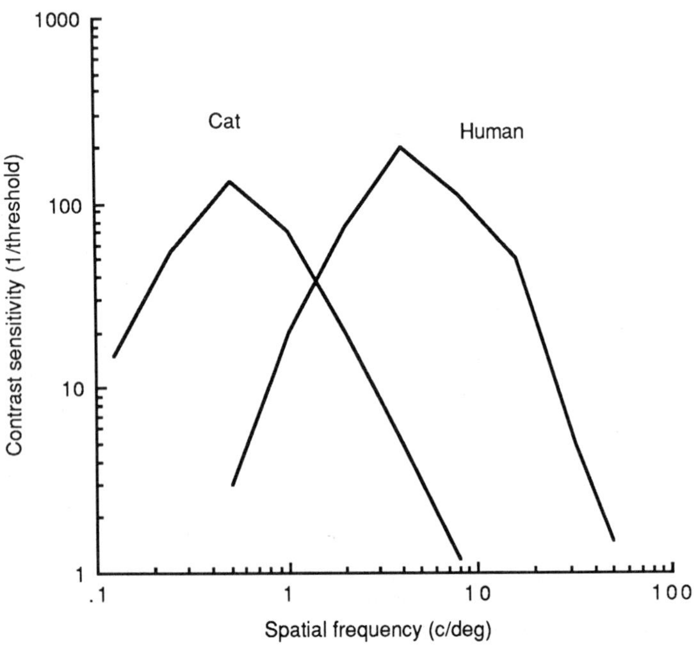

Fig. 3 Contrast sensitivity functions for the cat and human.

man under comparable stimulus conditions (i.e., stationary gratings presented at a low photopic background level). While both functions span roughly a 5-octave range of spatial frequencies, the peak of the CSF for the cat is situated about 3 octaves lower than the peak of the human CSF. Humans, in other words, see high spatial frequencies invisible to the cat, whereas the cat sees low spatial frequencies invisible to humans.

The shape of the cat's CSF varies with the rate of the temporal modulation of the bars of the grating (Blake & Camisa, 1977; Pasternak et al., 1985) as well as with background luminance level (Pasternak & Merigan, 1981). Specifically, drifting or flickering a grating impairs contrast sensitivity at higher spatial frequencies while at the same time improving sensitivity at low spatial frequencies. Lowering the background luminance level depresses sensitivity at all spatial frequencies. These same stimulus variables, luminance and temporal modulation, have an equivalent effect on the shape of the human CSF (e.g., see Robson, 1966; DeValois, Morgan, Polson, Mead & Hull, 1974).

D. The Neural Basis of Contrast Sensitivity in the Cat

Turning to the question of underlying neural mechanisms, some investigators (Blake & Camisa, 1977; Blake & DiGianfilippo, 1980; Lehmkuhle, Sherman & Kratz, 1984) have proposed that X cells are primarily responsible for the cat's contrast sensitivity at high spatial frequencies while Y cells mediate grating detection at low spatial frequencies. Several lines of evidence led to this proposal. First, it was originally thought that Y cells respond to low spatial frequencies that fail to activate X cells, while X cells respond to high spatial frequencies unresolvable by Y cells (e.g., Derrington & Fuchs, 1979; Lehmkuhle et al., 1980). More recently, however, it has been shown that Y cells do exhibit a measurable response to high spatial frequencies (So & Shapley, 1979), so one cannot be certain that resolution of high spatial frequencies is exclusively the province of X cells. Second, several laboratories have measured losses in contrast sensitivity in cats deprived of patterned binocular input during kittenhood and found those losses to be most pronounced at low spatial frequencies (Blake & DiGianfilippo, 1980; Lehmkuhle et al., 1984). This matched well with reports that binocular deprivation early in life reduces the incidence of Y cells in the lateral geniculate nucleus while leaving the number of X cells relatively unaltered (e.g., Kratz, Sherman & Kalil, 1979). Because of electrode sampling bias, however, one must interpret this finding with caution (see Shapley & So, 1980). All things considered, the hypothesis that X and Y cells differentially contribute to the cat's CSF remains largely speculative.

What is clear, however, is that the detection of grating patterns by the cat is mediated by neurons narrowly tuned for spatial frequency and orientation. This conclusion comes from masking experiments in which cats were required to detect sinusoidal gratings that appeared superimposed upon one-dimensional noise (Blake & Martens, 1981; Blake & Holopigian, 1985). The spatial frequency content and the orientation of the noise were varied relative to the frequency and orientation of the test grating, to determine the extent to which the noise impaired detection of the grating. The resulting masked thresholds were plotted in the form of "tuning curves," and some typical results are shown in Fig. 4.

Looking first at the pair of curves in the top panel, notice that noise impaired grating detection only when the spatial frequencies in that noise were within about 2 octaves of the test spatial frequency; noise further removed from the test frequency had no influence on detection, although that noise remained highly visible. The behavioral tuning curves derived from masking were also consistently broader and somewhat asymmetric for the lower test spatial frequency. These tuning width estimates and the somewhat broader, asymmetric tuning at lower frequencies are characteristic of spatial tuning curves for neurons in Area 17 of the cat's cortex. In contrast, cortical cells in Area 18 (Movshon et al., 1978b) and in the lateral suprasylvian cortex (Zumbroich & Blakemore, 1987) exhibit significantly broader spatial frequency tuning than that estimated from the masking experiments and measured in Area 17.

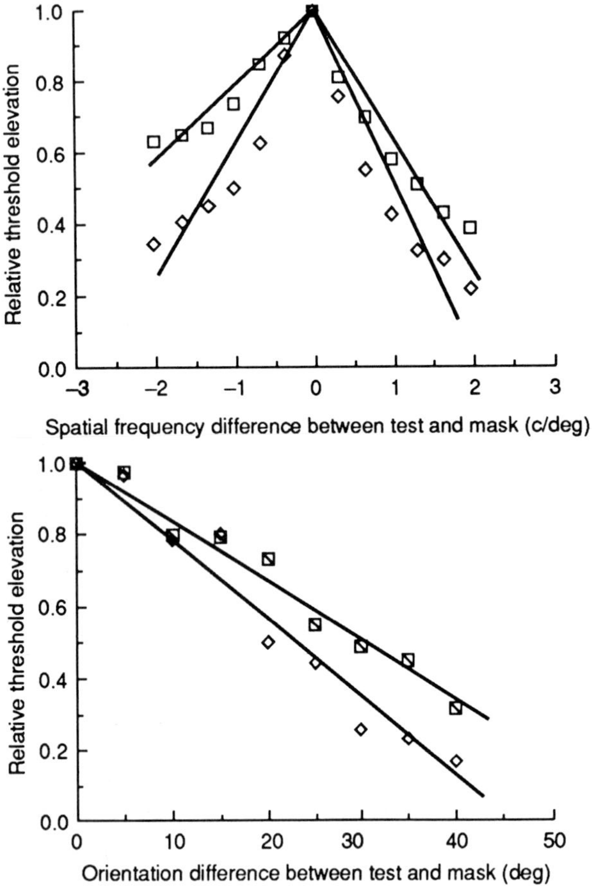

Fig. 4 (Top) □, 0.35 c/deg; ♦, 1.45 c/deg. Elevation in contrast threshold for detection of a grating pattern that appeared within a band of one-dimensional noise whose spatial frequency content was varied relative to the spatial frequency of the test grating. The units along the abscissa are octaves, where an octave is a factor of two difference in spatial frequency. (Bottom) ⧅, 0.35 c/deg; ◇, 1.0 c/deg. Elevation in contrast threshold for detection of a vertical grating appearing within a 1-octave band of noise whose orientation was varied relative to vertical. The values along the abscissa are angular degrees (e.g., a value of 45° corresponds to noise whose contours are oriented diagonally).

Turning next to orientation selectivity, the pair of curves in the bottom panel shows that noise impaired detection of the test grating only when the orientations of the test and noise were within 25–30° of one another. Furthermore, orientation selectivity was consistently narrower at higher spatial frequencies. These values, too, correspond quite well with estimates of orientation tuning for cortical cells (e.g., Rose & Blakemore, 1974). Because there is overlap in the degree of orientation tuning of cells in Areas 17 and 18, however, we cannot draw conclusions about the population of cortical cells (e.g., Area 17 versus Area 18) responsible for the orientation selectivity revealed by masking.

Comparable masking experiments have been performed on humans, and resulting estimates of spatial frequency tuning (Stromeyer & Julesz, 1972) and orientation selectivity (Campbell & Kulikowski, 1966; Phillips & Wilson, 1984; Black & Holopigian, 1985) very closely match the estimates derived for the cat. Some of those results from humans are discussed in Chapter 10. Suffice it to say, this equivalence between human and cat spatial vision point to the involvement of comparable neural mechanisms in grating resolution by humans and by cats.

E. Spatial Discrimination

The two previous subsections focused on tasks involving the *detection* of spatial patterns by the cat. Now let's consider how well the cat can *discriminate between* clearly visible, high-contrast patterns on the basis of orientation or spatial frequency. More to the point, can we predict the cat's discrimination from the spatial selectivity of single cortical neurons?

1. Orientation

Starting first with discrimination between targets which differ only in orientation, the smallest published behavioral threshold for the cat is 2° (Vandenbussche & Orban, 1983). Moreover, the cat (like man) shows an oblique effect for this discrimination, in that differences in grating orientations centered around vertical and horizontal are more finely discriminated than those centered around diagonal (Vandenbussche & Orban, 1983). In absolute terms, however, humans outperform cats: under optimum conditions, humans can discriminate orientation differences as small as a fraction of a degree.

This species difference in orientation discrimination could be explained in several ways. First, cortical neurons in human visual cortex could be more narrowly tuned for orientation than neurons in cat cortex. Recall, however, that masking data (Blake & Holopigian, 1985) point to equivalent tuning in cat and human. Second, cat cortical neurons could be inherently more variable in their responsiveness, thereby requiring a larger change in orientation to yield a reliable response change. At present there is no way to evaluate this possibility. Finally, it could be that the cat's visual cortex, because it contains fewer neurons than the human visual cortex, samples the orientation domain more coarsely (Sakitt & Barlow, 1982). Because the standard error of the sum of N independent measures of a noisy process decreases as the square root of N, a visual cortex with more cells should resolve smaller angular differences. To make quantitative predictions about the expected size of this difference in discrimination thresholds between human and cat requires information (e.g., the dimensions of a hypercolumn in human vision) not currently available.

It is informative to compare the cat's behaviorally measured discrimination threshold with estimates of orientation tuning of cat cortical neurons. Estimates of orientation tuning vary, but even the most narrowly tuned neurons respond over a 40° range of orientations. Clearly, then, discrimination is not limited by the breadth of tuning. Bradley et al. (1987) have shown, though, that a reliable difference in the firing level of narrowly tuned cortical cells can be produced by an orientation difference as small as 1.84°, a value remarkably close to the best behavioral threshold. Bradley et al. point out that the ability of a single cell to signal these kinds of small orientation differences depends on the steepness of the cell's orientation tuning curve and the response variability of the cell.

2. Spatial Frequency Discrimination

To complete this survey of cat spatial vision, let us consider the animal's ability to discriminate patterns on the basis of differences in spatial frequency. For spatial frequencies near the peak of their contrast sensitivity function, cats can discriminate frequencies differing by as little as 20% (Blake, Holopigian & Wilson, 1986). Performance is worse at lower spatial frequencies, but this may have to do with the limited number of cycles actually contained in the test display. Once again, human performance on a comparable task is considerably better: at their best, humans can discriminate frequency differences of the order of 5% (e.g., Campbell, Nachmias & Jukes, 1970).

How well does the cat's behaviorally determined threshold compare to difference thresholds measured physiologically? Within their sample of 18 cat cortical cells, Bradley et al. (1987) found that the average spatial frequency difference reliably signaled was 21%, a value that matches the best performance observed behaviorally. It is noteworthy, though, that their sample of cells included a few that were sensitive to frequency differences as small as 5%, a value surpassing the cat's best performance but equaling the best performance exhibited by human observers. Again, the difference between cat and human discrimination performance may be related to the difference in the number of cells in their visual cortex, that is, the size of the basis set, to use a term borrowed from sampling theory (Sakitt & Barlow, 1982).

F. Conclusion

Cat and human spatial vision are comparable in several important ways. Both species can resolve spatial frequencies spanning about a 5-octave range, with the visible range for the cat situated at a point lower along the spatial frequency axis. When detecting grating patterns, both cats and humans appear to utilize neural channels narrowly tuned for spatial frequency and orientation. Where cat and human spatial vision are dissimilar (e.g., visual acuity), we can point to neuroanatomical differences between the two species (e.g., ganglion cell density) that may account for these dissimilarities in performance.

III. INSIGHTS INTO HUMAN COLOR VISION FROM STUDIES OF OTHER MAMMALS

Color vision is a much studied characteristic of our species. The keenness of the human color capacity and its role in visual perception have been documented in countless psychophysical experiments, and the literature burgeons with details as to how stimulus variation relates to perceived color. Yet, despite all of this effort, there is still only a very limited understanding of the biological mechanisms underlying human color vision. To achieve this understanding one must rely on examination of nonhuman visual systems. This section examines the advantages of studying other mammals as an aid to understanding human color vision and provides one example of how such an approach has proven fruitful. (See Chapter 8, this volume.)

A. General Comments on Color Vision in Mammals

Color vision has been demonstrated in most mammalian species for which compelling investigations have been carried out (for a review see Jacobs, 1981), and there is only a single mammalian species, the rat, for which the evidence indicates a complete lack of color vision capacity (Neitz & Jacobs, 1986b). However, color vision among mammals also varies considerably from humans both in acuteness (i.e., the fineness of color discrimination) and its dimensionality. With respect to the latter, only the primates have shown trichromatic color vision (i.e., color vision based on three cone receptor photopigments in the retina) like that of humans. Rather, most mammals have dichromatic vision (i.e., color vision based on two cone receptor pigments in the retina). This variation from the human color capacity can be turned to a research advantage in comparative color vision studies. Consider the following question: What implications for color vision arise from the spectral positioning and spectral separation of various cone types? An answer to this question would be of interest, both as an aid to understanding the details of chromatic opponent organizations and perhaps for giving insight into why particular cone types and combinations have evolved.

Dichromacy appears to be the normal color vision for many mammals. Among dichromatic mammals, however, the actual cone pigment complement varies considerably. For instance, although ground squirrels, tree squirrels, and tree shrews all have short wavelength cones with roughly the same spectral peaks (435–445 nm), these three species show great variation in the spectral location of their second longer wavelength cone—from 518 to 556 nm (Jacobs, Neitz & Crognale, 1985; Jacobs & Neitz, 1986; Blakeslee, Jacobs & Neitz, 1988). A comparison of the response properties of the spectrally opponent units in the visual systems of these three species could be used to illuminate the advantages and disadvantages for color vision associated with variation in the pairings of different cone pigment sets.

Mechanisms of color vision vary considerably among species, and some nonmammalian vertebrates are known to have good color vision. One might suppose that these species would provide better models for understanding human color vision than the mammals who, as we have noted, mostly do not have very keen color vision. However, problems arise from some very obvious differences in mechanisms used to produce color vision in mammals and nonmammals. Three such differences may be noted: (a) A large number of nonmammalian species, for instance many birds and reptiles, employ an elaborate system of color oil droplets which, in conjunction with multiple classes of cone pigments, provide an initial filtering of spectral input quite unlike that found in humans or any other mammals. (b) The great expansion of the neocortex of mammals means that the central visual projections differ fundamentally between mammals and nonmammals, and, thus, the central nervous system mechanisms for elaborating color information are also quite different. (c) It appears that the means for organizing spectrally opponent pathways may be fundamentally different in mammalian and nonmammalian visual systems. In the latter, at least in certain fishes, birds, and reptiles, the connections between specific cone types and horizontal cells appear rigidly deterministic, whereas in mammalian retinas no evidence for such a specificity of connection is apparent (Boycott, Hopkins & Sperling, 1987). The opponent separation required to produce color vision must, thus, arise quite differently in mammalian and nonmammalian visual systems. All of these features suggest that although many species have color vision capacity, the machinery for its accomplishment varies considerably. That variation appears smaller within mammals than between mammals and other vertebrates.

B. Polymorphism of Color Vision in a Nonhuman Primate

We turn now to an example of the thesis proposed above; that is, a description of a case where the study of color vision in a nonhuman species has significant implications for understanding human color vision. It has long been recognized that color sensitivity varies considerably among humans, namely, there are different forms of color sensitivity, which are best known as the familiar color vision defects and anomalies. The study of atypical color vision cases has been central in many attempts to understand the mechanism for human color vision. Since the mid-1970s it has been discovered that other primate species also have color sensitivities which systematically differ from normal human color sensitivity. This is significant, because in these species the mechanism underlying the different forms of color vision can be directly examined. One such species is the squirrel monkey (*Saimiri sciureus*).

The polymorphism of squirrel monkey color vision was discovered with behavioral tests of the same sort used to reveal polymorphisms of human color vision (Jacobs, 1983a,b, 1984). Figure 5 summarizes results from several behavioral tests on individual squirrel monkeys and illustrates the magnitude of these differences. In formal classification, some monkeys would

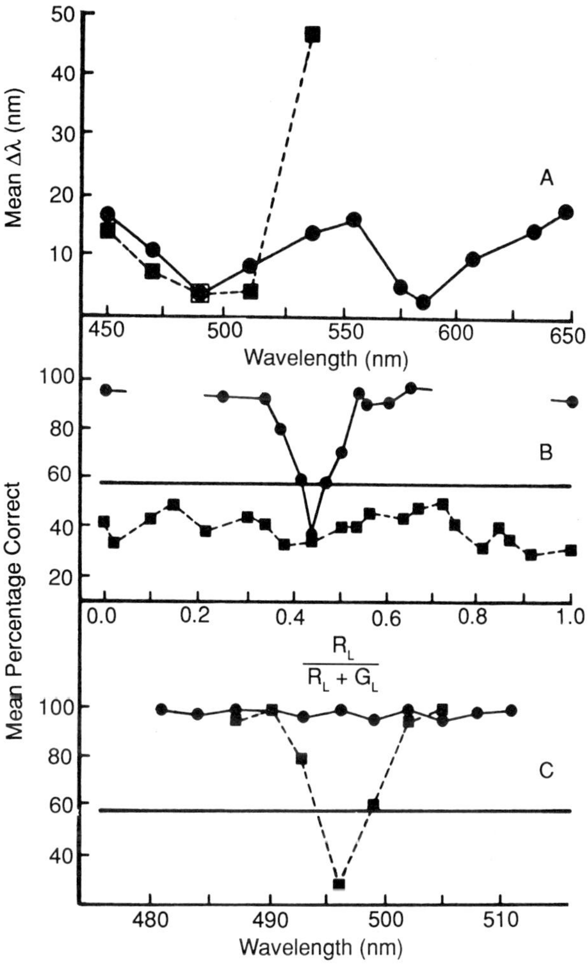

Fig. 5 Examples of results obtained from a dichromatic squirrel monkey (squares) and a trichromatic squirrel monkey (circles) on three tests of color vision. (A) Wavelength discrimination functions. (B) Rayleigh matches. In this test animals were required to discriminate various mixtures of red and green lights from a standard yellow light. The data points are the performance levels obtained from highly trained animals in a three-alternative discrimination task. The horizontal line indicates the 95% confidence level for successful discrimination. Note that the dichromatic animal is unable to make any of the color discriminations. (C) Tests for the presence of a neutral point. In this test animals were required to discriminate monochromatic lights from an equiluminant achromatic light. Other details are the same as for B. (From Jacobs & Neitz, 1985.)

be considered to have trichromatic color vision, and others have dichromatic color vision. Furthermore, just as in the case of the human color vision polymorphism, several subtypes can be discerned in each of these categories. The total range of color vision variation in a large sample of squirrel monkeys encompassed six types; three of these were trichromatic variants and three dichromatic (Jacobs, 1984). Not only does the squirrel monkey share the human characteristic of color vision polymorphism, but also some of the variants appear qualitatively similar. For instance, some squirrel monkeys behaved similarly to human protanopes in sensitivity to the long wavelengths, wavelength discrimination abilities, and color matching.

What accounts for the strikingly different forms of squirrel monkey color vision? To examine this question, measurements of cone photopigments were made in squirrel monkeys whose color vision had been established by behavioral tests (Mollon, Bowmaker & Jacobs, 1984; Bowmaker, Jacobs, Spiegelhalter & Mollon, 1985; Bowmaker, Jacobs & Mollon, 1987). Photopigments were measured with microspectrophotometry (MSP), a procedure that involved the passage of a narrow measuring beam through the outer segments of individual photoreceptors. MSP measurements were made on photoreceptors from a total of 16 squirrel monkeys. From this group of animals absorbance spectra were obtained for more than 600 individual cones.

Five different classes of photoreceptors were found in this sample of squirrel monkeys. One class, having an average peak sensitivity (λ_{max}) at about 498 nm, represents rods, while the other four classes represent cones. One sparsely represented type of cone in these retinas had an average λ_{max} of about 433 nm. The average λ_{max} values for the other three were 536, 549, and 564 nm. Unlike the rods and short wavelength cones, there were striking variations in the presence of these three cone types among the individual animals. That variation corresponded exactly with the measured variation in color vision.

Figure 6 shows spectral sensitivity functions based on the absorbance of the four cone pigments of squirrel monkeys. Animals with dichromatic color vision

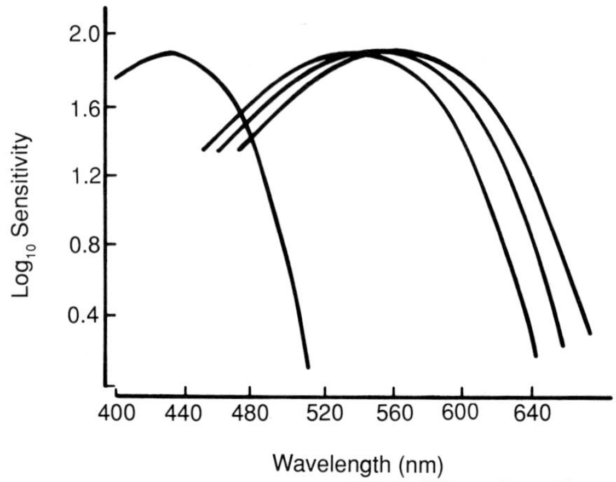

Fig. 6 Smoothed and normalized absorbance curves for the four classes of cone pigment found in the squirrel monkey. These pigments are present in various combinations in individual animals (see text).

have either the 536, 549, or 564 nm cone pigments, each in conjunction with the 433 nm cone pigment. Those monkeys with trichromatic vision may have any pair of the three longer wavelength cone pigments in conjunction with the 433 nm cone pigment, that is, 536 and 549 nm, or 549 and 564 nm, or 536 and 564 nm cone pigments.

The results illustrated in Figs. 5 and 6 indicate that the different forms of color vision in a nonhuman primate, the squirrel monkey, depend entirely on parallel differences in the complement of cone pigments. There are several implications of this discovery for understanding the mechanisms that underlie human color vision.

C. Squirrel Monkey Color Vision: Implications for Human Color Vision

For some issues, the study of squirrel monkey color vision and its mechanisms can make long-held ideas about the mechanisms for human color vision either more or less plausible, but in other cases, new explanations may be suggested. Examples of both follow.

1. Color Vision Variations Due to Photopigment Variations

It has long been believed that the major forms of congenital color vision defects in humans arise from variations in the cone pigments. For example, dichromacy reflects the absence of one of the three normal cone classes (e.g., Boynton, 1979; Pokorny, Smith, Verriest & Pinckers, 1979). That view has been supported by many indirect measurements which were strongly believed to reflect the function of the cone pigments, namely, color matching, measurements of visual sensitivity, reflection densitometry, etc. (Alpern & Pugh, 1977; Alpern & Wake, 1977). However, only in a few cases has it been possible to measure directly cone pigments in individuals whose color vision differed in known ways (Weale, 1959; Baker & Rushton, 1965). The discovery that the cone pigment complements of squirrel monkeys discretely differ, in parallel with their measured differences in color vision, shows clearly that the explanation for variations of human color vision accurately accounts for color vision variations in another primate. As such, that result supports the belief that the major forms of human color vision variation can be traced to individual differences in the cone pigment complement.

2. Explanations for Anomalous Trichromacy

The anomalous trichromacies represent both the most frequent of the congenital color vision variations in humans and the most difficult to explain. Over the years a considerable number of hypotheses have been advanced to account for these anomalies (Pokorny et al., 1979).

Psychophysically, there are three trichromatic phenotypes among squirrel monkeys (Jacobs, 1984). They have been defined in terms of the relative proportions of a red + green mixture required to "match" a standard yellow light. One of the three groups required roughly the same proportions of red and green as a normal human trichromat, but the other two groups behaved somewhat similarly to the two major forms of human anomalous trichromatism, that is, one required relatively more red light in the mixture while the other required relatively more green light. Although the correspondence is by no means perfect (see Bowmaker et al., 1985), a reasonable analogy can be drawn between these latter two squirrel monkey phenotypes and anomalous human color vision.

This analogy sheds light on some of the explanations advanced for human anomalous trichromacy. For instance, it has been suggested that human anomalous trichromacy might result from abnormal variations in optical density of the cone pigment (Ruddock & Naghshineh, 1974) or in the mixing together in a single receptor of two types of photopigment (Baker, 1966). To the contrary, the squirrel monkey trichromatic variations seem to result exclusively from discrete shifts in the spectra of the cone pigments (Fig. 6); there is no evidence either for variation in pigment density or for mixing of pigments within a single receptor. Therefore, these explanations for anomalous trichromacy are rendered much less plausible.

3. Photoreceptor Mosaics in Heterozygous Females

Human color vision defects and anomalies are unequally represented in the two sexes. A similiar distribution of the different forms of color vision can be found in the squirrel monkey. Whereas female squirrel monkeys have been found to have either trichromatic or dichromatic color vision, all male monkeys are dichromats (Jacobs, 1984). This finding has led to the hypothesis that the inheritance of middle to long wavelength cone pigments in squirrel monkeys is produced by the action of three alleles (form of a gene on a chromosome) at a single locus on the X chromosome (Mollon et al., 1984; Jacobs & Neitz, 1985). Each allele accounts for one of the three middle to long wavelength cone pigments. Such an arrangement would account for the universality of dichromacy among males. The hypothesis further supposes that random X-chromosome inactivation occurs in female monkeys, thus allowing the heterozygous animal to have two populations of middle to long wavelength cones. This provides the basis for trichromatic color vision. There is now substantial evidence indicating that this mechanism correctly accounts for the different forms of color vision in the squirrel monkey (Jacobs & Neitz, 1987).

It has long been supposed that in the human, unlike the squirrel monkey, there are two (or more) cone pigment genes on the X chromosome with the middle to long wavelength cone pigments specified at these loci (see Nathans, 1987). Classical theory further suggests that low frequency alleles at these loci specify aberrant photopigments; these will be directly expressed in males, leading to the common forms of color anomaly and color defect. The mother or female child of such a male defective will be heterozygous at a pigment locus, and such individuals will presumably produce an aberrant photopigment in addition to two normal photopigments. In heterozygous females, random X–chromosome inactivation would be expected to lead to a retinal cone mosaic in which some cones express maternally derived chromosomes while others express paternally derived chromosomes. There have been a number of attempts to demonstrate cone mosaicism in heterozygous females (Pokorny et al., 1979), but consistent evidence for the presence of such is lacking.

The results from the squirrel monkey suggest that it may be difficult to demonstrate photoreceptor mosaicism in heterozygous females because the mosaics formed by paternally and maternally derived photoreceptors have a relatively fine grain. There are two arguments in support of this possibility. First, simply to produce trichromacy in the female squirrel monkey, the two middle-to-long-wavelength pigments would each have to be present in regions no larger than the dimensions of individual retinal receptive fields. Second, and perhaps more directly, MSP examination of arrays of 1–2 dozen neighboring photoreceptors from the foveal tissue of a trichromatic squirrel monkey revealed no evidence that the two cone types were systematically arranged into a mosaic pattern (Mollon et al., 1984). Rather, the two cone types seemed to be randomly intermixed. In sum, work with the squirrel monkey suggests that photoreceptor arrays formed by random X-chromosome inactivation are fairly fine grained. This may well be why the presence of such mosaics has been hard to demonstrate in the human heterozygous female.

IV. COLOR VISION IN GOLDFISH: A MODEL FOR HUMAN COLOR VISION?

Color vision is assumed to be adapted to the specific environmental conditions under which an animal lives. The number and spectral sensitivities of the receptor types and the neural organization of the visual system can differ widely across species. Therefore, it seems rather unlikely to find close similarities between color vision systems in humans and animals from different habitats. However, if two color vision systems that have evolved independently reveal similar properties, then general functional principles for the design of any highly effective color vision system may be invoked. For example, color vision in the honeybee is trichromatic, and it resembles human color vision in wavelength discrimination as well as in color contrast and color constancy (von Helversen, 1972; Neumeyer, 1980, 1981). It has a spectral sensitivity function, however, that is different from humans, with a shift into the ultraviolet (UV), and is located between 300 and 650 nm. Whether color vision of the honeybee has the properties of an opponent color vision system, as found in humans (see Chapter 8, this volume), or whether it is more simply organized is still an open question. In vertebrates, highly effective color vision systems based on more than two cone types, and possibly as many as four, are found in fishes, reptiles, and birds (Jacobs, 1981).

A. Why the Goldfish as an Experimental Animal?

Goldfish, carp, and other cyprinid fishes have long been important subjects in studies of photoreceptor cells, retinal physiology, and structure. Early microspectrophotometric measurements of single cone outer segments in the goldfish revealed absorption spectra of three types of photopigments (Marks, 1965), and the first intracellular recordings of vertebrate photoreceptors showed three spectral types of cones in the carp (Tomita, 1965). The results of neurophysiological and neuroanatomical investigations indicated that the cyprinid retina is a highly complicated structure in which important steps of color specific information processing take place (Wheeler, 1982). Investigations of single cones in the goldfish have shown three spectral types with maximal sensitivities at 450, 535, and 620 nm. This, together with the fact that retinal neurons have response properties of "color opponency" as in the primate visual system, suggested that goldfish might have a trichromatic color vision system similar to that of humans.

The perceptual properties of color vision can only be investigated in behavioral experiments. The behavioral testing technique, in which a presentation of color is rewarded with food, was introduced by Karl von Frisch (1913, 1914) to study color vision in the minnow, a cyprinid fish, and in the honeybee. In lower vertebrates, however, this method has been only rarely applied and investigations of color vision in these species have been largely neglected.

B. The Measurement of Wavelength Discrimination

To characterize a color vision system, an understanding of differential wavelength discrimination ($\Delta\lambda$) is of central importance. The $\Delta\lambda$ function can provide insight into the number of photoreceptor types involved and the peripheral steps of information processing. Early measurements of wavelength discrimination were obtained by Wolff (1925) in the minnow (*Phoxinus laevis*) and later in the goldfish by Yarczower and Bitterman (1965). Both experiments failed to equate the color stimuli in brightness for the fish, so discriminations may have been based on either brightness *or* hue. Therefore, wavelength discrimination in the goldfish was reexamined using the following method (Neumeyer, 1986). Freely swimming goldfish could choose between two test fields illuminated by monochromatic light. Choice of the correct color was rewarded with a small amount of a food paste delivered through thin plastic tubes at the test field (see Fig. 7). Test fields were illuminated using slide projectors and fiber optics. The intensity of the monochromatic light was adjusted to equal stimu-

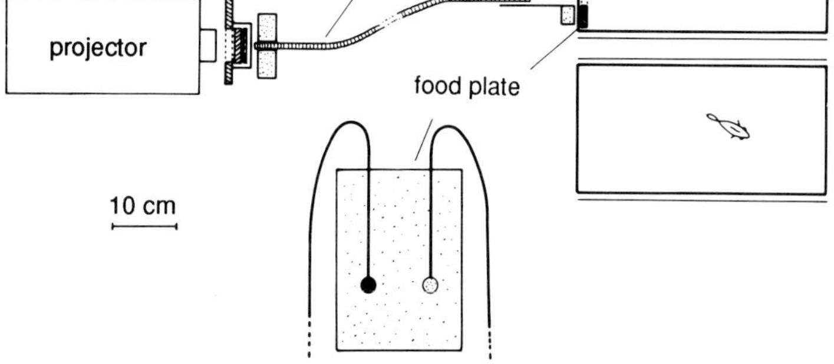

Fig. 7 Experimental setup for wavelength discrimination experiments. The three identical tanks with single goldfish are seen from the top. The optical apparatus could be moved from one tank to the other. The filter wheel contained interference and neutral density filters. The food plate was inserted into the water and contained the two test fields which were illuminated from the outside of the tank. A food paste was given for reward through thin tubes which ended at the test field openings. When measuring spectral sensitivity, the fish was trained to swim to the nonilluminated (dark) test field while the comparison test field was illuminated with monochromatic light of different wavelengths and intensity. In the measurement of wavelength discrimination, the two test fields were illuminated with monochromatic light of different wavelengths, with intensities adjusted to equal "fish-subjective" brightness according to their spectral sensitivity function.

lus efficiency, according to the spectral sensitivity function measured previously under the same experimental conditions (Neumeyer, 1984). The fish were trained using 20 wavelength pairs between 404 and 719 nm. The frequency with which the training wavelength was approached relative to the comparison wavelength was determined. The difference threshold for the two wavelengths ($\Delta\lambda$) was defined as a choice frequency of 70%.

Figure 8 shows the $\Delta\lambda$ function of the goldfish. Small values of $\Delta\lambda$, indicating a keen wavelength discrimination, were found at 400, 500, and 610 nm. This result is surprising, as in other trichromatic color vision systems there are only two ranges of best wavelength discrimination.

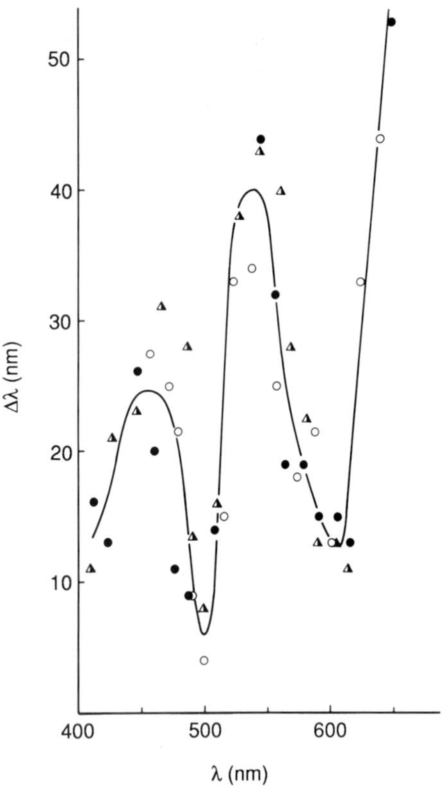

Fig. 8 $\Delta\lambda$ functions for three goldfish. The continuous line represents average values. From Neumeyer (1985).

To understand the processes underlying wavelength discrimination, model computations of the $\Delta\lambda$ function were performed based on the following considerations (for details see Neumeyer, 1986). In the response of a single cone, information about wavelength is lost (i.e., excitation is proportional only to the number of quanta absorbed). To obtain information about "color," the central nervous system has to compare the excitation values of at least two classes of cones having different spectral sensitivities. The effect of each wavelength on the different cone types represents the "input side" of the color vision system, and this effect can be described by a point in color space. The coordinates of this point (color locus) stand for the relative excitation values of the three cone types. The color loci of two wavelengths which can "just be discriminated" by the animal have a distance **R** in color space. According to Helmholtz (1892), this distance is equal for each just discriminable wavelength pair. When **R** is calculated for one such experimentally determined pair, it is possible to ask for each other wavelength, which adjacent wavelength has the same distance **R**. The difference between these two wavelengths is $\Delta\lambda$. To calculate **R**, the metrics of the color space must be defined. In human color vision, Helmholtz (1892) proposed that **R** can be calculated as the line element in the Riemannian space, as the most general case (see Wyszecki & Stiles, 1982). In the goldfish, a special case of distance measure was used; **R** was calculated as the euclidean distance.

It was first determined whether the measured $\Delta\lambda$ function of the goldfish is similar to a $\Delta\lambda$ function calculated on the basis of the animal's cone sensitivity functions, as shown in Fig. 9. Figure 10A shows, however, that the measured and theoretical functions do not match, especially not in the short wavelength range. To obtain small values of $\Delta\lambda$ in this range, an additional sensitivity increase between 400 and 450 nm had to be assumed. Several attempts to model the minimum at 610 nm failed and led to the hypothesis that the cone sensitivity functions do not uniquely determine the $\Delta\lambda$ function (see below).

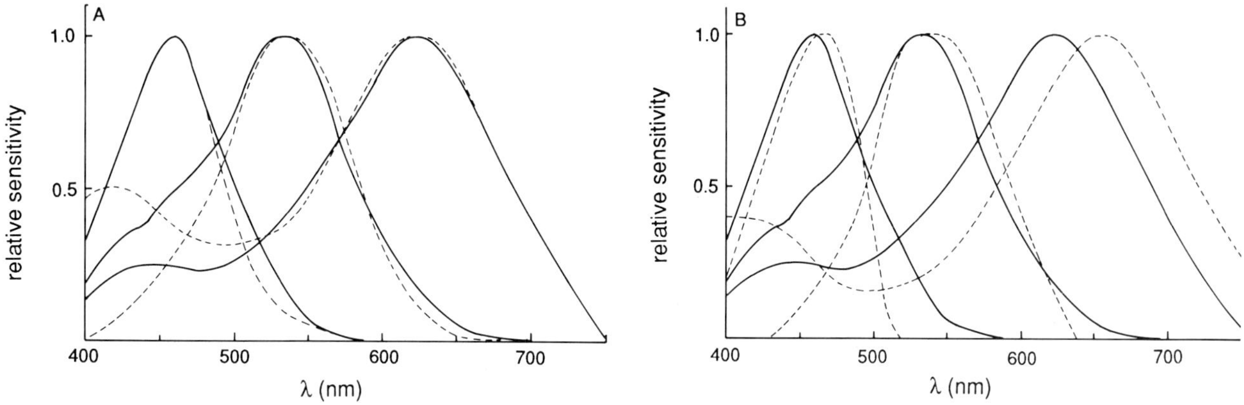

Fig. 9 Spectral sensitivity functions that were used in the model computations of the Δλ function. Continuous lines: Cone spectral sensitivity functions as obtained in direct measurements of photopigment absorption spectra. (The calculated Δλ function based on these functions is shown in Fig. 10A.) Dashed lines: Modified sensitivity functions. (A) Functions which approximated the measured Δλ function in the short and the mid-wavelength spectral range (Fig. 10B). (B) Functions which gave the best approximation in the entire spectral range (Fig. 10C). From Neumeyer (1986).

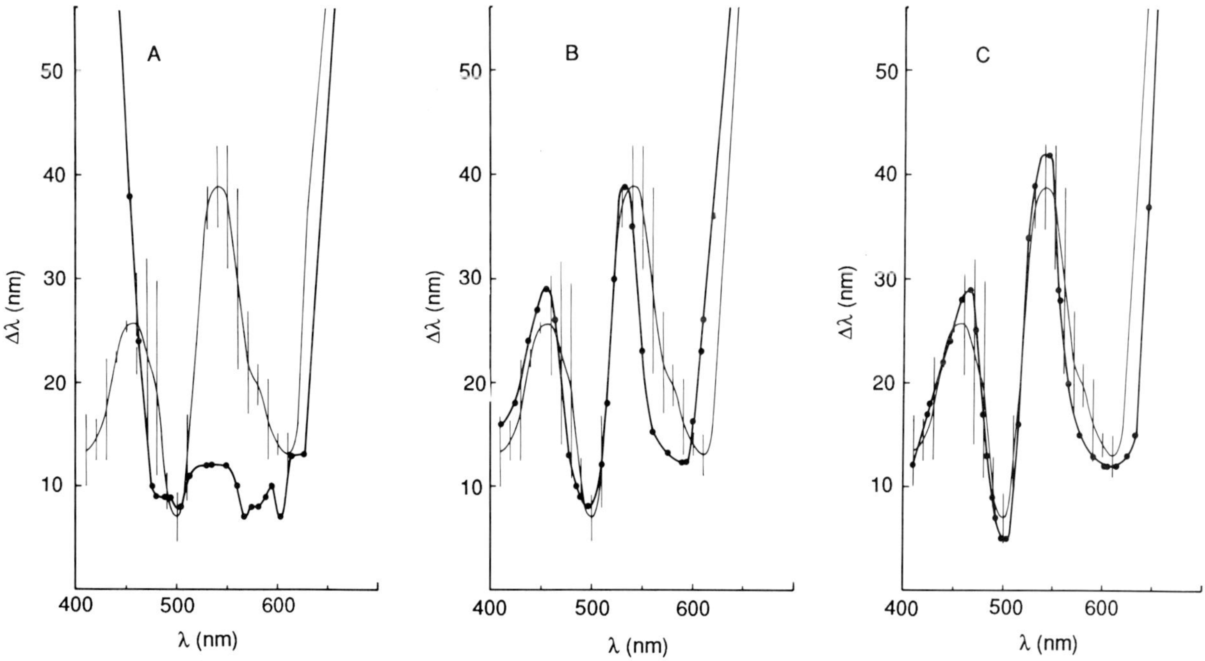

Fig. 10 Calculated Δλ functions (dots) in comparison to the measured Δλ function from Fig. 8. (A) Calculated on the basis of the cone sensitivity functions (continuous lines in Fig. 9). (B) Calculated on the basis of the modified sensitivity functions in Fig. 9A. (C) Calculated on the basis of the modified functions in Fig. 9B. From Neumeyer (1986).

C. Evidence That the Goldfish Has an Ultraviolet-Sensitive Receptor as a Fourth Cone Type

Two explanations may be given for the high discrimination ability in the range of 400 nm: (1) an increase in sensitivity between 400 and 450 nm due to a secondary peak (the β band) of the long wavelength cones; (2) a separate cone sensitivity function which has its maximum in the UV range. To decide between these two possibilities, color mixture experiments were performed (Neumeyer, 1985). The rationale for the procedure was the following: In the first case, short wavelength light of 404 nm should excite the short wavelength cones as well as the long wavelength cones (via their side-maximum). Therefore, a fish trained on a wavelength of 404 nm should not be able to discriminate this wavelength from an additive mixture of 434 nm (blue light) and 683 nm (far red light). In the second case, a wavelength of 404 nm should not be discriminable from a certain mixture of blue and UV light. As shown in Fig. 11, the goldfish could not discriminate a mixture of about 50% blue and 50% UV light from the training wavelength of 404 nm, but it could easily discriminate a mixture of blue and red light. This result suggests that the goldfish uses not only three types of cones in its color vision but a UV-sensitive cone type as well. Additional color mixture experiments have shown (Neumeyer, 1988) that the information from the four cone

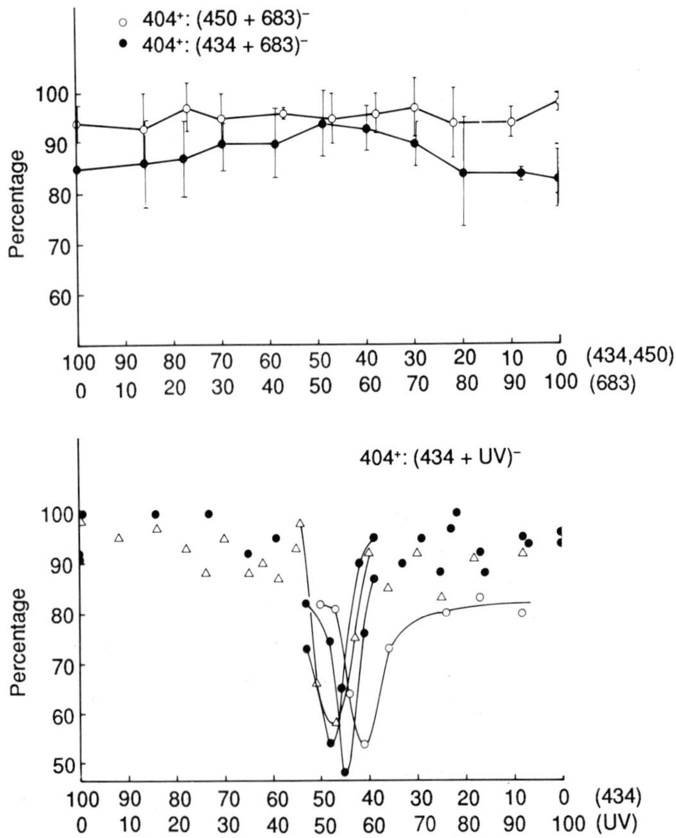

Fig. 11 Results of the color mixture experiment. (Top) The fish were trained on a wavelength of 404 nm and tested against an additive mixture of blue light (450 nm) and far red light (683 nm). (Bottom) Trained as above, but tested against a mixture of blue light (434 nm) and ultraviolet (367 nm) light. Different symbols denote results from different animals.

types is processed separately, that is, the goldfish has tetrachromatic color vision. Thus, for the goldfish, all colors of equal brightness can be represented in a tetrahedron, analogous to the color triangle of human trichromatic color vision.

D. Does the Goldfish Possess an "Opponent" Color Vision System?

As shown in Fig. 10B, the $\Delta\lambda$ function could not entirely be modeled on the basis of three cone sensitivity functions. Best discrimination was always obtained at shorter wavelengths (590 instead of 610 nm). Only when the maximum of long wavelength cone sensitivity was shifted to 660 nm could a good approximation be obtained (Fig. 10C).

Figure 12 shows behavioral measures of goldfish spectral sensitivity measured from 400 to 719 nm compared to the spectral sensitivities of the individual cone classes. The spectral sensitivity function has three pronounced peaks, at 470, 540, and 660 nm. The narrow form of the maxima and their displacement in comparison to the cone spectral sensitivity maxima can be explained by mutual inhibitory interactions between the different cone mechanisms. This was concluded from the results of measurements under chromatic adaptation (Neumeyer, 1984). The interactions are assumed to take place in the retina, and the action spectra of C-type horizontal cells can be interpreted accordingly. It should be noted that the goldfish spectral sensitivity function is similar to the increment threshold function measured on a white background for humans and monkeys and has been modeled with inhibitory neuronal interactions (Sperling and Harwerth, 1971). Since wavelength discriminations in goldfish can be similarly described, information processing in the color vision of cyprinid fish might be similar to that in primate visual systems.

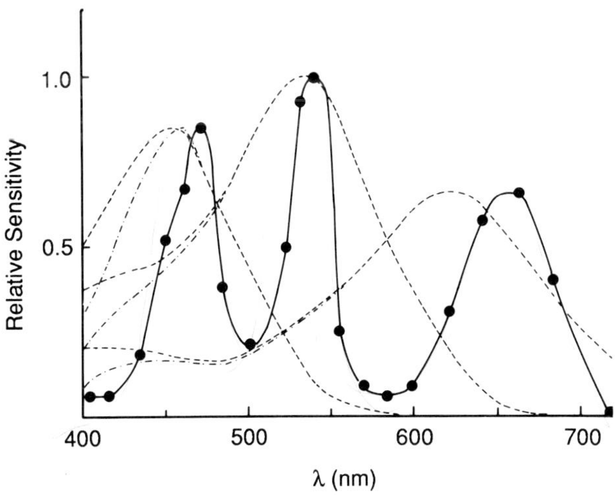

Fig. 12 Relative spectral sensitivity function of the goldfish (dots) in comparison with the sensitivity functions of cones (dashed lines, after Harosi, 1976). From Neumeyer (1984).

V. SPECTRAL SENSITIVITY OF HUMANS, RHESUS MONKEYS, AND NEURONS

Surface electrodes and noninvasive physiological measurements are limited in resolution and sensitivity, often resulting in a poor correlation with visual perception in the human observer. To place a probe inside the brain and sample the behavior of specific neurons in response to a specific visual input clearly increases the correlation between stimulus input and the informational content in the neuronal response of the brain. Of course, this cannot be done in human subjects, but on morphological, physiological, and behavioral grounds, the macaque monkey has proved to be an excellent research substitute.

On the basis of morphological similarities within the visual system, humans and the higher primates are thought to possess similar physiological mechanisms. The classic work of Polyak (1957) showed that the retinal elements of humans and macaque monkeys are very similar, and that there is a close morphological similarity in the way visual space is represented throughout the central nervous system. Finally, psychophysical comparisons between macaque monkeys and human observers have shown striking similarities in the vision of the two species (Blough & Schrier, 1963; Sidley & Sperling, 1967; DeValois & Jacobs,

1968; DeValois, Morgan, Polson, Mead & Hull, 1974; Crawford, 1976, 1977; Harwerth & Smith, 1985; Oehler, 1985; Spillmann, Ransom-Hogg & Oehler, 1987). In short, the macaque monkey (in particular, the rhesus monkey, *Macaca mulatta*) appears to meet all criteria as a psychophysical, anatomical, and physiological research surrogate for the human visual system.

Even though the psychophysical evidence on the comparability between the visual capacities of the macaque and human has been compelling, data have been presented for only a small number of experimental conditions. Color or spectral sensitivity data for the macaque monkey has been shown to be similar to that of humans under photopic levels of light adaptation (Grether, 1939; Sidley & Sperling, 1967; DeValois & Jacobs, 1968; Sperling, Sidley, Dockens & Jolliffe, 1968; DeValois et al., 1974; Harwerth & Smith, 1985), while Blough and Schrier (1963) demonstrated similar scotopic sensitivities in the two species. However, these data were obtained without control over where the test flash fell upon the retina. Moreover, with the exception of the work by Sperling, the test stimuli have been projected on reflective or rear-projection surfaces, thus making it difficult to compare monkey sensitivity with that of man on an absolute quantum scale. The use of a Maxwellian-view optical system (Sidley, Sperling, Bedarf & Hiss, 1965) obviates this problem. Finally, with development of additional behavioral procedures to control fixation (Crawford, 1976, 1977) spectral sensitivities can be obtained for a variety of retinal loci and under a variety of luminance and chromatic adaptation conditions.

Fixation control, increment-threshold measurement, and microelectrode recording from single neurons have been combined to study the visual signals from the lateral geniculate nucleus (LGN) to the cortex when the monkey is responding to the visual stimulus. These combined techniques have permitted the *perceptive field* (Jung & Spillmann, 1970) of the alert behaving monkey to be brought into spatial registry with the *receptive field* of the LGN neuron. The neuronal receptive field was conventionally defined as the area of the retina (and visual space) that, when stimulated, produced a change in the response rate of the neuron. The perceptive field, on the other hand, referred to the area of the retina (and visual space) that, when stimulated by a visual stimulus, produced a change in the behavioral response of the monkey. Therefore, both the monkey and the neuron alike could be instructed: "Tell us if you can see the test flash." By systematically reducing (in 0.2 log-unit steps) the number of quanta contained in the test flash, the threshold sensitivities of the monkey and the neuron were determined for 22 wavelengths across the visible spectrum, each at the same retinal locus and under the same viewing conditions, and in the absence of any confounding effects of anesthesia.

Threshold for the monkey was operationally defined as the log of the reciprocal of the number of quanta contained in a test flash detected half the time. Similarly, threshold for the neuron was defined as the number of quanta in the test flash that evoked a "just observable change" in response rate of the neuron compared to the ongoing spontaneous discharge rate. This could be either an increase or decrease in response rate, as color-opponent neurons were often encountered, responding with excitation to stimulation with one wavelength of the test flash and with response inhibition to a different wavelength.

A. Threshold Spectral Sensitivity of Human and Monkey Observers

Spectral sensitivity of monkey and human observers were measured behaviorally for central and peripheral retinal locations under both photopic and scotopic conditions (Figs. 13 and 14). The data for the two species were quite similar for both photopic and scotopic adaptation levels; that is, humans and macaque monkeys seem to have color vision systems that are virtually the same.

What is the physiological basis for these sensitivity functions? How do neurons process and convey visual information throughout the visual system? And, what information does a single neuron convey about the colors of objects of the visual world? It is possible to

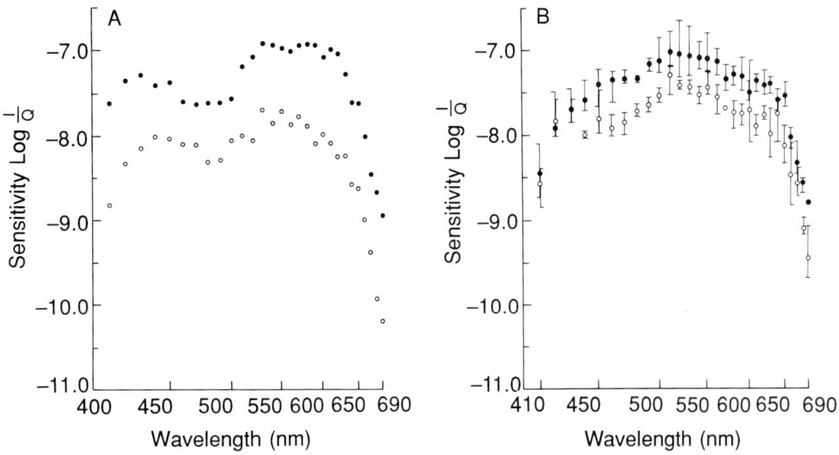

Fig. 13 (A) Photopic increment-threshold spectral sensitivity curves for a human observer taken at center fovea (filled) and at 14° away in the temporal retina (open). Note that there is a drop of about 1.0 log unit in sensitivity, with only minor differences in the shapes of the curves. (B) Photopic increment-threshold spectral sensitivity curves for a rhesus monkey taken under identical conditions as for (A). Note that the peak threshold sensitivity of the monkey is virtually identical to that of the human observer, and that the shape and drop in sensitivity with peripheral viewing are quite comparable to the human.

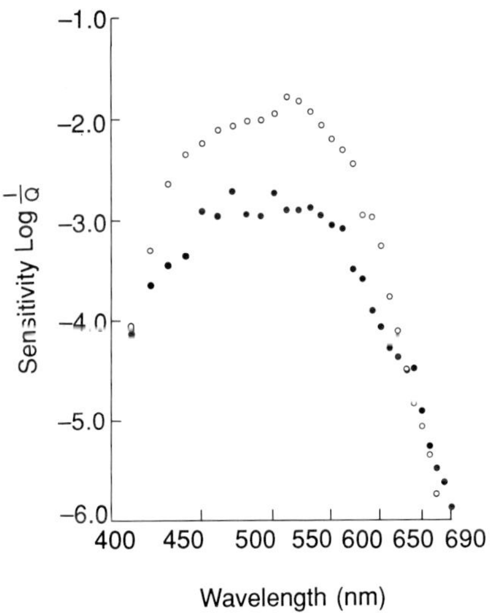

Fig. 14 Scotopic increment-threshold spectral sensitivity curves for a rhesus monkey for two retinal locations. Note that the rod-dominated sensitivity curve is about 1 log unit less sensitive in the fovea (filled) compared to that at 6° away in the temporal retina (open). This is comparable to changes seen in human observers (Crawford, 1977).

examine the visual brain directly using the combination of electrophysiological and behavioral techniques for insight as to how these mechanisms operate at the single-cell level to generate these behavioral functions.

B. Threshold Spectral Sensitivity of Monkey and Neurons

Rhesus monkeys were implanted with a stainless steel cylinder which accepted a head-mounted stereotaxic holder (Evarts, 1966). Varnished tungsten microelectrodes were then driven to the LGN of the alert behaving monkey by a micrometer-activated hydraulic system. Single neurons were isolated, and thresholds for monochromatic test flashes were measured for 22 wavelengths over the visible spectrum. Neurons were occasionally held for several hours, though responses (and thresholds) for single neurons were usually recorded for only a few minutes each. The tactic was to locate the receptive field for an LGN neuron and then, by shifting the fixation point, bring the perceptive field of the monkey into spatial registry so that both monkey and LGN neuron were "attending" to the same stimulus. The test stimulus was then reduced in intensity until the threshold was reached for the neuron and for the monkey (see Sperling et al., 1978).

The center of the receptive field of the LGN neuron was located by moving the fixation target in small steps and using a large 6° diameter test light, usually of 620 nm and high intensity. The experimenter rapidly covered the 18° field for a number of positions of the fixation target. The test light was then reduced to

2° for a finer determination of the receptive field location. Smaller stimuli could then be employed to map the center–surround characteristics of the receptive field. Thresholds were obtained with the 2° test field for comparison with behaviorally obtained thresholds using the same stimulus.

Threshold spectral sensitivities of 50 LGN neurons were compared on the same scale with the behavioral sensitivity of the monkey. Most neurons showed a threshold sensitivity selective for a limited range of wavelengths and exhibited color opponency, being excited at one portion of the spectrum and inhibited at another. The opponency seen most often was to some combination of red and green wavelengths.

Figure 15 shows a comparison of the excitatory component of several color-opponent units with the behaviorally measured threshold spectral sensitivity curve. It is clear that most of the peak sensitivities of the single units are less than the monkey's psychophysical sensitivity (all units had their receptive fields within 6° of the fovea), while the upper profile of their collective neuronal thresholds approximates the shape of the spectral sensitivity curve. Moreover, an LGN neuron having its input from the most sensitive color-opponent neurons at threshold would have both the same breadth of response and absolute sensitivity as the monkey. These neurons would be rarely sampled since there are few at threshold (Barlow, 1972b).

Neurons of this type have been recorded from the pulvinar (Crawford & Espinoza, 1978) and LGN. An example of a parvocellular LGN unit appears in Fig. 16 (Sperling et al., 1978). This neuron had a broad spectral sensitivity which matched the behavioral threshold of the monkey. Thus, this neuron would be able to signal reliably whether a test flash had occurred.

These results show that at a very early stage in the primate visual system, single neurons display a threshold spectral sensitivity comparable to the behavioral response of the monkey. That is, in the response of a single neuron there is sufficient information to serve as the neural substrate for the monkey's

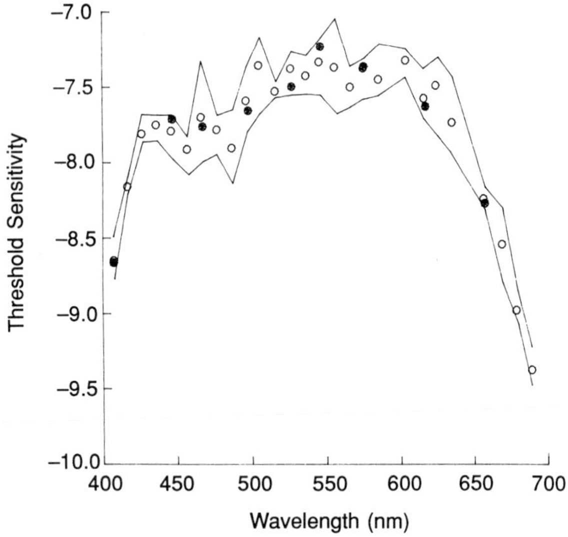

Fig. 16 Photopic increment-threshold spectral sensitivity curves for a rhesus monkey (○, ± 1SD) and a parvocellular LGN broad-band neuron taken under identical conditions from the same retinal locus (●). Note that the threshold for the monkey and the neuron are the same throughout the spectrum (Redrawn from Sperling et al., 1978).

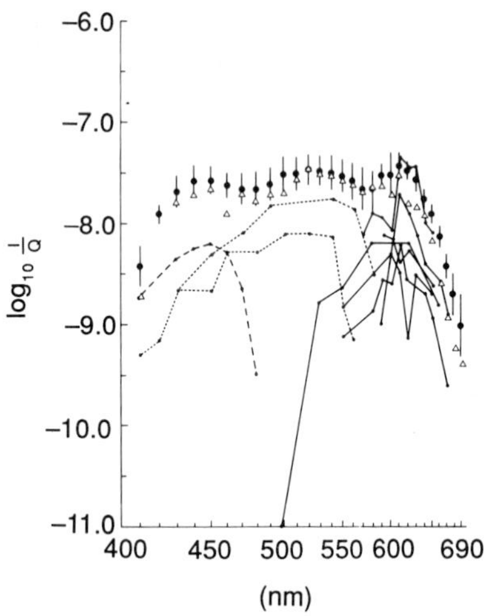

Fig. 15 Photopic increment-threshold spectral sensitivity curves for a 2° test flash at the center fovea (filled) and at 6° away (triangles). These curves are compared to the excitatory component of nine opponent-color neurons recorded from the parvocellular layers of the LGN. Note that the peak neuronal sensitivities are generally less than that of the psychophysical measures. The collective upper profile of these units approximates the shape, but not the sensitivity, of the behavioral curves.

detection of a test light. This suggests that the gain of the visual system for photopic threshold detection must be determined at or before the fourth order neuron of the primate visual system.

VI. COMPARISON OF HUMAN AND MONKEY VISUAL MOTION PERCEPTION

Physiological and anatomical experiments have implicated a presumed motion processing pathway in the extrastriate cortex of macaque monkeys (Van Essen, 1985; Andersen, 1987; Maunsell & Newsome, 1987; Chapter 9, this volume). Understanding this pathway is an important first step in elucidating neural mechanisms for motion processing. One approach for studying this pathway is to train monkeys and humans in psychophysical tasks that test motion thresholds. These experiments have indicated that, for all aspects of motion perception so far tested, monkeys and humans have the same psychophysical thresholds (Golomb, Andersen, Nakayama, MacLeod & Wong, 1985; Siegel & Andersen, 1988). This suggests that the neural mechanisms underlying these percepts in the two species are the same, and it points to the macaque monkey as an ideal animal model for studying motion perception in humans.

A. Structure-from-Motion Perception in Monkeys and Humans

Siegel and Andersen (1987) developed a novel stimulus display for studying the perception of structure from motion. This display is designed to provide movement cues without position cues. These displays for studying motion perception are somewhat analogous to random dot stereograms used to study stereopsis in the absence of feature cues.

Figure 17 shows one of the displays used to study structure from motion. The display consists of randomly distributed moving dots that form the percept of a hollow, revolving cylinder. Each dot is present for a minimum period of time before being replotted at another random location on the surface of the cylinder. The minimum point life (exposure duration) serves several purposes, the most important being

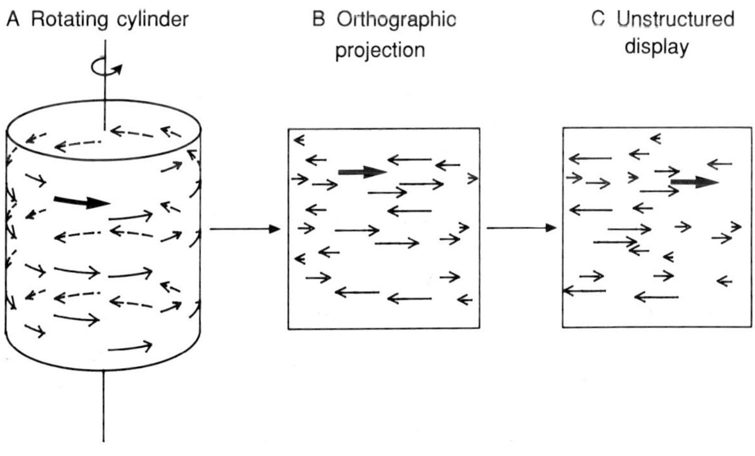

Fig. 17 Method for generating three-dimensional structure from motion displays. Each vector represents the direction and speed of moving dots. (A) The percept that is generated by the moving dot display is one of a hollow, rotating cylinder. (B) The parallel (orthographic) projection of the cylinder onto the display screen. This two-dimensional velocity field gives rise to the three-dimensional percept in A. (C) The unstructured display that is computed by displacing each point by a random amount up to the limit of the entire width of the display. The fate of an individual trajectory is shown by the bold arrow. The point density on the surface of the display is kept constant by displaying each moving dot for a finite amount of time. New dots appear at random locations on the display and follow new trajectories. From Siegel and Andersen (1988). Reprinted by permission from *Nature*, **331**, pp. 259–261. Copyright © 1987 Macmillan Journals Limited.

the removal of position cues when the display goes through a transition from no structure to structure.

The subjects perform a reaction time task in which they must detect the transition from an unstructured noise pattern to the revolving cylinder. The noise pattern has all the same vectors as the structured stimulus, the only difference being that the vectors are randomly shuffled, thus destroying the structure. If the transition is made to a display that is only partially structured, often the cylinder can still be perceived, but with more difficulty. For example, a cylinder with a fraction of structure of 0.5 has each of its points perturbed by a random amount up to a limit of 0.5 of the diameter of the display. By varying the fraction of structure in the test stimulus, psychometric functions can be generated.

Figure 18 shows psychometric functions for one monkey and one human performing the three-dimensional cylinder task. The curves in each panel are similar, indicating that the two species have similar abilities to detect structure from motion in the three-dimensional display. Monkeys and humans also had similar thresholds for the two-dimensional structures of rigid rotation and nonrigid expansion. Control experiments indicated that the subjects were using the global structure of the display to do the task and not local cues such as a change in the local distribution of speeds or directions of movement.

It is difficult to know if humans or monkeys are truly using three-dimensional percepts to perform the cylinder tasks or if they are using the two-dimensional structure of the velocity field. This problem is particularly acute in monkeys, who cannot verbally report their perceptions. However, reaction times provided indirect evidence that the monkeys as well as humans were, in fact, using three-dimensional neural representations.

Reaction times for the three-dimensional cylinder task were long for both monkeys and humans, averaging around 1000 msec. On the other hand, reaction times for the two-dimensional tasks of rotation and expansion were considerably shorter, averaging around 600 msec. A difference of 400 msec in terms of neural computation time is quite significant. If one examines the two-dimensional cues available in the

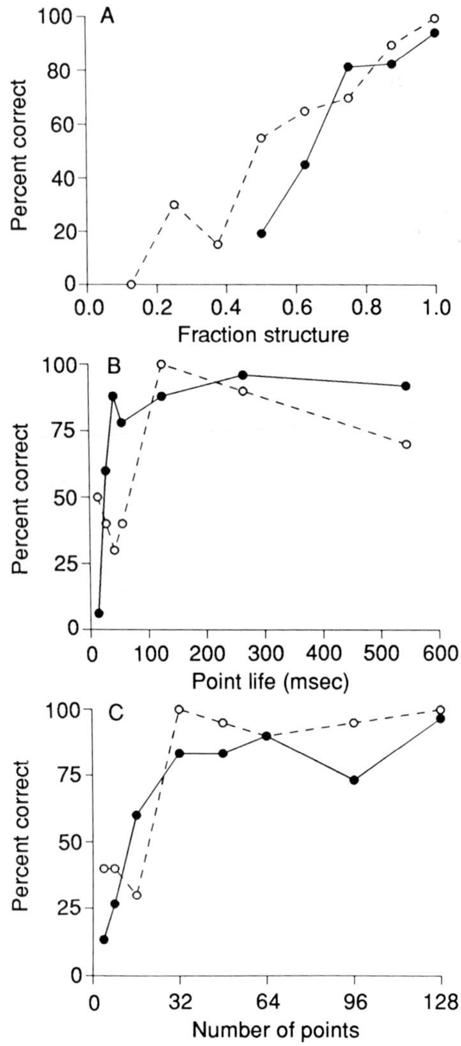

Fig. 18 (A) Plot of performance of one monkey and one human as a function of the fraction of structure in the three-dimensional cylinder display. In this experiment 128 points were visible at any one time, and each point was on for 532 msec. The cylinder revolved at 35 degrees/sec, and the screen refresh rate was 35 Hz. (B) Task performance as a function of point life. For 128 point displays, point lives of under 100 msec reduced performance in detecting the transition from noise to a three-dimensional cylinder of 0.875 fraction structure. Refresh rate was 70 Hz, and the angular velocity was 35 degrees/sec. (C) Task performance as a function of the number of dots. The same parameters as in B were used, but the point life was held constant (532 msec) and the number of points varied. Performance deteriorated below 32 points. From Siegel and Andersen (1988). Reprinted by permission from *Nature*, **331**, 259–261. Copyright © 1987 Macmillan Journals Limited.

three-dimensional cylinder and two-dimensional rotation tasks, those cues are found to be very similar; the cylinder has fast speeds in the center of the display and slow speeds in the surround, whereas the rotation has slow speeds in the center and fast speeds in the surround. Thus one would assume that if the subjects were using only two-dimensional cues available in the velocity field, then the reaction times should be more similar. The increased reaction time could not be accounted for by the fact that the cylinder was hollow and required the segregation of two surfaces, whereas the two-dimensional rotation had only one surface. In tasks where two two-dimensional rotations in opposite directions were used, the reaction time increased at most by 50 msec. In conclusion, these experiments suggest that monkeys (and humans) use three-dimensional neural representations to perform these tasks.

B. Characteristics of Spatio-Temporal Integration

Having developed the three-dimensional structure-from-motion task, it was possible to ask how motion information is integrated in space and time to form the three-dimensional percepts. This issue had already been approached from a theoretical perspective by Ullman (1979), who showed that "given three distinct orthographic views of four non-coplanar points in a rigid configuration, the structure and motion compatible with the three views are uniquely determined." Obviously, 4 points and 3 frames are only a theoretical limit, and the brain is likely to require more points and time since there is much noise in neural signals. Also, the brain is likely to use an algorithm for retrieving structure from motion that does not perform at the theoretical optimum. To examine temporal integration, the exposure duration of the individual points was changed, and the spatial integration was studied by changing the number of points.

Figure 18B shows that in both monkeys and humans performance in the three-dimensional cylinder task is reduced when the lifetime falls below 100 msec for 128 points. Figure 18C indicates that both species do poorly when there are less than 32 points with point lives of 500 msec. Moreover, a trade-off between point life and point number was found with shorter point lives requiring more points and vice versa.

C. Structure-from-Motion Computation Involves Formation of Three-Dimensional Surface Representations

There are three elements in the above experiments suggesting that three-dimensional percepts of surfaces result from integration of information from the velocity field. The first bit of evidence derives from masking experiments and shows that information is used from the entire surface for performing the task. The second kind of evidence concerns the reaction time data and indicates that the computation time varies with the type of surface being computed. Yet, the most compelling evidence for surface representations comes from the third piece of evidence, the time integration experiments. Recall from the reaction time data that it requires 1000 msec to perform the three-dimensional surface task. However, the individual points are visible for only 100 msec before being plotted at a new, random location. Thus, any algorithm that requires the exact position of individual points throughout the computation period would fail under these conditions. Rather, the brain appears to compute surfaces so that the appearance of a dot anywhere on the surface can be used for the computation.

D. Effects of Middle Temporal Area Lesions on Motion Perception

The effects of restricted Area MT lesions on motion and structure-from-motion thresholds have been examined in rhesus monkeys (Siegel & Andersen, 1986). Motion thresholds were tested using a shear motion detection task. This was a reaction time task in which the animal had to release a lever with the onset of a shear motion stimulus in a previously static random dot display (Golomb et al., 1985). The structure-from-motion task was the three-dimensional cylinder task described previously. Psychometric functions were generated by varying the amplitude of the shear motion.

Prior to the lesions, motion thresholds were determined at different retinal locations. In this procedure the animal fixated a small point at the start of each trial, and the test stimuli were then presented at different locations in the visual field. Next, the retinotopic representation in Area MT was mapped using microelectrodes. Area MT contains a representation of the contralateral visual field that results from the systematic anatomical mapping of the retinas via the lateral geniculate nucleus and earlier visual cortical Areas V1 and V2. A small lesion was made at a selected location in this retinotopic map using the neurotoxin ibotenic acid. Motion thresholds were then retested to measure the effects of these lesions on motion perception.

The use of ibotenic acid is an important control. This compound destroys cell bodies but not fibers of passage. This selectivity is important because the optic radiation (the projection from the lateral geniculate nucleus to primary visual cortex) passes directly below Area MT. A surgical ablation of Area MT would likely also damage these fibers, producing a nonspecific lesion. The nonspecificity of the lesion would complicate the interpretation of lesion induced deficits.

Figure 19 shows the results of an MT lesion made in the lower visual field contralateral to the side of the lesion. Shear motion thresholds show a dramatic increase confined largely to the area of the visual field that corresponds to the retinotopic locus of the lesions. An important observation is that this deficit recovered in 3 to 4 days. Control experiments showed that contrast thresholds were not affected by these lesions. Thus, the increased motion thresholds were not due to the animal's being blind at the locus of the lesion. Rather, the deficit was selective for motion perception.

Another experiment tested the effect of Area MT lesions on three-dimensional structure-from-motion perception. The animal was not able to perceive the cylinder even at 100% structure. Again the deficit was restricted to the area of the visual field that corresponded to the retinotopic locus of the lesion. Interestingly the deficit remained long after the shear thresholds had recovered and was still prominent at 23 days post lesion.

E. Summary of Motion Experiments

The psychophysical experiments indicate that monkeys and humans have similar abilities to detect structure from motion. Several lines of evidence further suggest that in our three-dimensional tasks the brain is forming representations of surfaces by integrating information from the velocity field over space and time.

Lesion experiments indicate that Area MT is important for perceiving motion and structure from motion. However, there is rapid recovery in motion deficits following the lesions, suggesting that the brain undergoes a functional reorganization. There are two possible mechanisms for this recovery: (1) reorganization within Area MT and (2) reorganization of parallel pathways around Area MT. Experiments that totally ablate Area MT can distinguish between these two possibilities. Another question is the role of training and visual experience on recovery. Would visual deprivation prevent recovery? These and many other interesting experiments examining plasticity in adult brain are made possible because the connectivity, and increasingly the function, of the visual extrastriate cortex is becoming better understood.

VII. CONCLUSIONS

These contributions demonstrate the enormous value in the use of research animals to model physiological processes thought to underlie sensory and perceptual processes in humans. These are only examples of animal research on topics which are covered in more detail in subsequent chapters.

Relative to the linking propositions, and their atten-

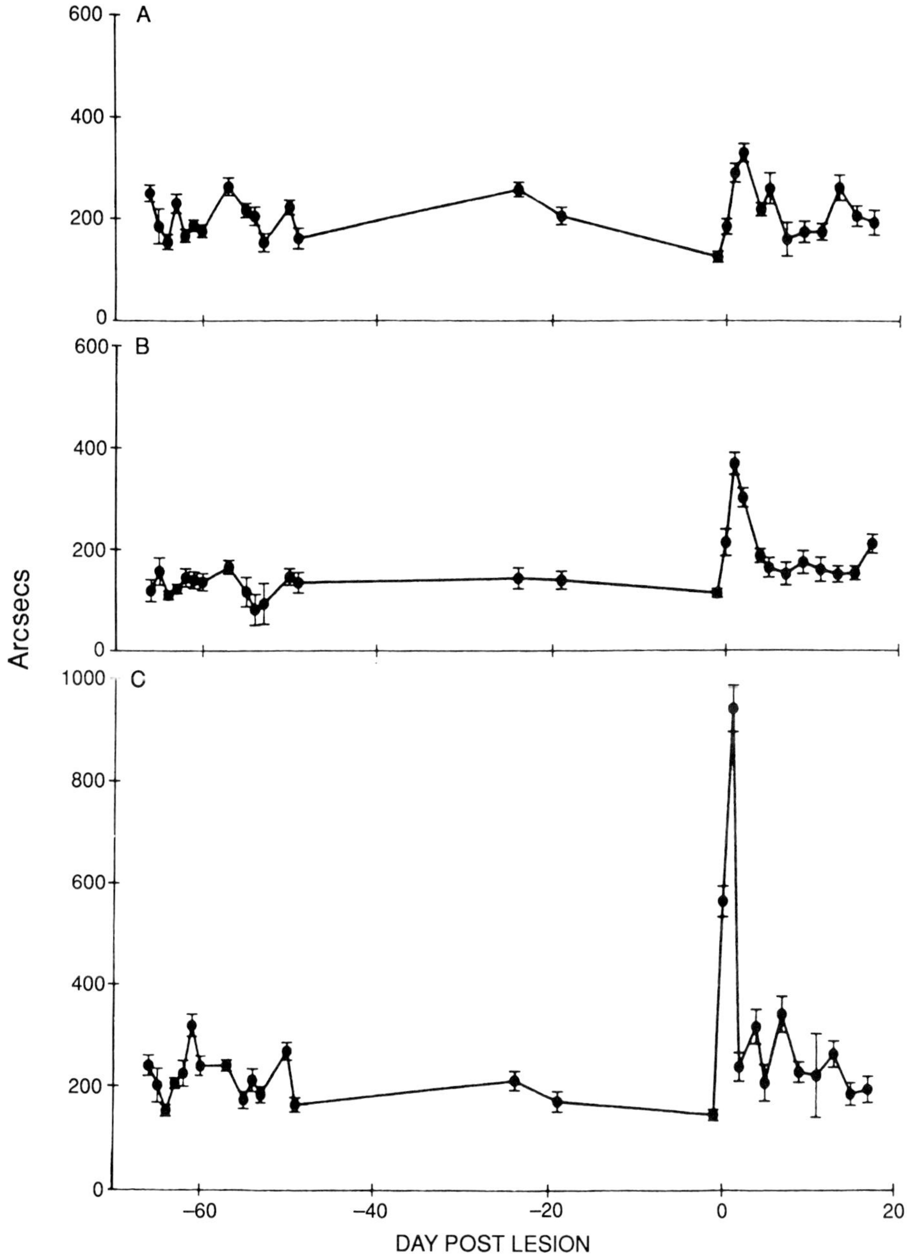

Fig. 19 The effect of ibotenic acid lesions in visual Area MT on shear motion thresholds of the monkey for three visual field locations. Fifty percent hit rates are plotted from psychometric curves in which spatial and temporal frequency is held constant and amplitude is varied. The lesion was placed in the lower visual field representation of Area MT in the contralateral (right) hemisphere. Little effect is seen for central and upper field locations (top and middle), and the greatest effect is focused at the lower field location (bottom) with thresholds increasing after 1 day to over 900 arc sec. Also note that the thresholds recover rapidly in a few days.

dant precautions described in Chapter 3, there are at least two sets of linking propositions employed in the examples cited here. First, there are the propositions which relate the sensory process in humans to some sensory process in the animal model, a sort of sensory–sensory proposition which expresses how monkey spectral sensitivity compares to human threshold color vision and/or how contrast sensitivity functions are comparable between cats and humans. The second sort of linking proposition utilizes the assumption of commonality, namely, the two sensory/perceptual processes appear similar enough to assume similar underlying physiological processes. This assumption relates the sensory function in humans to some neural substrate in the animal model. It is the latter linking proposition which most commonly expresses the correlative relationship between brain function and sensory/behavioral processes. These are explicit propositions on the role of inhibitory interactions between retinal neurons and wavelength discrimination in goldfish; on the role of cone pigments in anomalous primate color vision; on the role of LGN cells in determining the threshold spectral sensitivity curve; on the role of MT neurons in primate sensitivity to motion; and on the role of narrowly tuned cat cortical neurons determining sensitivity to spatial frequency and orientation. These propositions stand as working hypotheses to be supported, rejected, or supplanted by other such propositions as physiological and psychophysical evidence accumulates.

5

THE CONTROL OF VISUAL SENSITIVITY
Receptoral and Postreceptoral Processes

Jan Walraven, Christina Enroth-Cugell, Donald C. Hood,
Donald I. A. MacLeod, and Julie L. Schnapf

I. INTRODUCTION

The world we see is a reconstructed world, a clever deduction based on information transmitted by light. That information is carried as changes in the quantity and quality of the light after it has left its source and interacted with matter. Thus, light provides the medium in which objects make their energy imprints, like footprints in the sand, as Wright (1967) put it so beautifully.

To extract the information contained in the retinal image, the eye must be able to respond over the full range over which the light can be modulated within that image. These modulations are produced by both the light source and the reflectance properties of objects. The latter produce intensity variations that have to be simultaneously sampled and thus require a certain dynamic range of the visual system. Fortunately, the (cyclic) variations due to the natural light source are very slow and, therefore, do not impose heavy demands on the dynamic response of the system. These changes do, however, require large adjustments of steady-state sensitivity—nearly 10 decades from starlight to sunlight at noon.

In addition to variations in the level of illumination, we also have to consider the variations in the spectral composition of the light. During the course of the day the spectral variations involved are quite substantial, as one may realize when looking at the vivid colors of the sky at sunset. There is also the problem that, on clear days, the world is actually illuminated by two entirely different light sources, the sun and the sky, providing white and blue illumination, respectively. Furthermore, in more or less screened dwellings, either natural (like the tropical rain forest) or artificial (inside buildings), the color of the filtered and reflected light may strongly depart from that of the original light source. The wide range of more or less colored artificial light sources we use in our environment constitutes the most recent challenge the visual system has to meet.

The upshot of all this is that our visual system has to deal with information modulated in a medium, light, that itself is subject to considerable changes, both with respect to its amplitude and wavelength. This poses formidable problems, not only with regard to sensitivity control, but also with respect to disentangling the variables of light and matter, so thoroughly confounded in the retinal image profile. The latter problem, the discounting of the illuminant as Helmholtz (1867) called it, has an obvious link with sensitivity control; whenever the eye adjusts its sensitivity to compensate for a change in illumination, it is actually trying to eliminate the light source as a variable.

Sensitivity control implies that the response to a stimulus can be modified by the visual system. This can be implemented in various ways, depending on what the system is interested in. This brings us back to Wright's metaphor of footprints in the sand. The way in which these are produced, that is by absorption of light by objects, is not equivalent to subtracting fixed amounts of energy, but rather to a fractional or proportional reduction. Thus, an object is characterized by a relative rather than absolute energy profile, that is, by the fraction of incident light that it reflects toward the eye. This fraction, which is constant, is called reflectance. This is the physical invariant that the visual system should capture in order to register a stable world in which objects appear the same, regardless of the absolute amount of incident light they reflect. This implies that sensitivity control should be such that it does not interfere with the processing of relative luminance variations, or contrast (see also Chapter 15, this volume).

The eye's sensitivity control has to operate at both high and low illumination levels and, therefore, employs two different strategies. At high light intensities the goal, so to speak, is to reduce the light and decrease sensitivity. At low light levels, the system cannot be so wasteful and may even sacrifice spatial and temporal resolution in order to make the most of each photon it can catch. The result is an exquisite sensitivity regulation, closely following, albeit at some distance, the limit imposed by the intrinsic noise (photon fluctuations) of the physical stimulus.

The mechanisms that enable the eye to operate optimally under all stimulus conditions can be studied with different tools and methods. These have in common that a visual response is measured as a function of some stimulus variable. What the main stimulus variables are, and how they can be quantified, are briefly discussed in the following section.

II. THE LIGHT STIMULUS

A. Measuring the Stimulus

There are many units and concepts related to the measurement of light (Wyszecki & Stiles, 1982). Here, however, only the most relevant ones are introduced (see also Chapter 7, this volume).

The "strength" of the light stimulus, subjectively experienced as brightness, is measured in the unit of luminance, the candela per meter squared (cd/m^2). This is a photometric unit, that is, a radiometric unit (here, radiance) corrected for the spectral efficiency of a standardized eye. The spectral efficiency is defined by the so-called luminosity function, either $V(\lambda)$ or $V'(\lambda)$, for cone (photopic) and rod (scotopic) vision, respectively. These are bell-shaped functions, that define the relative luminous efficiency of light as a function of wavelength (λ). The functions have their maximum at 555 nm, for cones, and at 507 nm, for rods. (It should be added that brightness is affected not only by luminance, but also by other variables, as discussed in Chapter 7.)

In vision research it is important to make allowance for the fact that the luminance of the light incident on the retina varies with pupil size. This had led to the definition of a unit of retinal illuminance measured in troland (td), or troland value (T). The troland value is defined as

$$T = Lp \tag{1}$$

with L (luminance) expressed in cd/m^2 and p (pupil area) in mm^2. There is a photopic and a scotopic troland, based, respectively, on $V(\lambda)$ and $V'(\lambda)$. The conversion from trolands to photons or quanta (at the cornea of the eye) is given by

$$N = T[(\lambda/V(\lambda)]2.25 \times 10^3 \quad (2)$$

for photopic trolands, and

$$N = T'[(\lambda/V'(\lambda)]9.02 \times 10^2 \quad (3)$$

for scotopic trolands.

Here, N is specified in photons per second per square degree (deg^2) and λ in nm (10^{-9} m). For conversion from deg^2 to cm^2 on the (human) retina, T has to be multiplied by a factor 8.5×10^{-4}. Due to differences in the anatomy of the eye, human trolands and animal trolands are not equivalent. In particular, differences in the focal length are important because they determine the size of the retinal image, and hence, the light concentration per unit retinal area. To put it more precisely: the retinal illumination given by Eq. (1) varies inversely as posterior nodal distance squared. Thus, for a monkey, the retinal illumination corresponding to a troland is about 1.4 times greater than in man; the cat troland is even 1.8 times more effective.

The determination of the actual retinal illumination, in terms of absorbed photons, requires assumptions about transmission losses in the ocular media and extrareceptoral space, and also about the probability of (effective) photon absorption. For scotopic vision, the fraction of photons at the cornea that ultimately excites the rods is estimated to be of the order of 0.17 to 0.48, with 0.25 as the best estimate (Hallett, 1987). However, due to neural noise and, possibly, transmission thresholds (a criterion level that has to be surpassed before signals are transmitted to the brain), the eye behaves as if it uses only 5% of the incident photons (e.g., Barlow, 1977) or even less, of the order of 1 to 2% (Sakitt, 1972; van Meeteren, 1978). Recent estimates from electrical recordings in single rods indicate that 1 scotopic troland corresponds to about 4 effective photon absorptions per second (Baylor, Nunn & Schnapf, 1984), as is also consistent with psycho-physical estimates (Denton & Pirenne, 1954).

In addition to photometric units there are also colorimetric units. These relate to the spectral composition of the light. Color can be represented by a vector in a three-dimensional (color) space in which the three axes plot quantities, so-called tristimulus values (X, Y, and Z), that define (although rather indirectly) how the light is registered in the three cone photopigments (Vos, 1978; Wyszecki & Stiles, 1982).

For the specification of color the relative amounts of X, Y, and Z rather than their absolute values are of interest. These relative values, x, y, and z, defined as $x = X/(X + Y + Z)$ etc., are called chromaticity coordinates. Since $x + y + z = 1$, it is sufficient to specify the chromaticity of a light stimulus with only two of the three chromaticity coordinates. The convention is to use x and y, the coordinates of the standardized CIE chromaticity diagram. This is just one of the many ways to represent color information and, actually not the most relevant one from the physiological point of view. A more appropriate representation, reflecting basic physiological mechanisms of color discrimination, is given by MacLeod and Boynton (1979).

B. Stimulus Range

The eye has to deal with variations in both the luminance and the color of the light source. The luminance range and various other visual variables are shown in Fig. 1. Also shown are the stimulus–response characteristics of single rods and cones, hereby assuming that the photoreceptor response reaches its half-maximum value at about 4 log photopic trolands, for cones, and at about 1.4 log scotopic trolands, for rods (see also Fig. 20). Note that the small dynamic range covered by the cones and rods necessitates adaptation mechanisms for moving that range, either to low levels for rods or high levels for cones.

The variations in the spectral composition of the light illuminating our world may seem less impressive than the variations in luminance, but they are large enough to produce appreciable shifts in the color of objects. Figure 2 provides a representative example of some of the extremes that may be encountered under

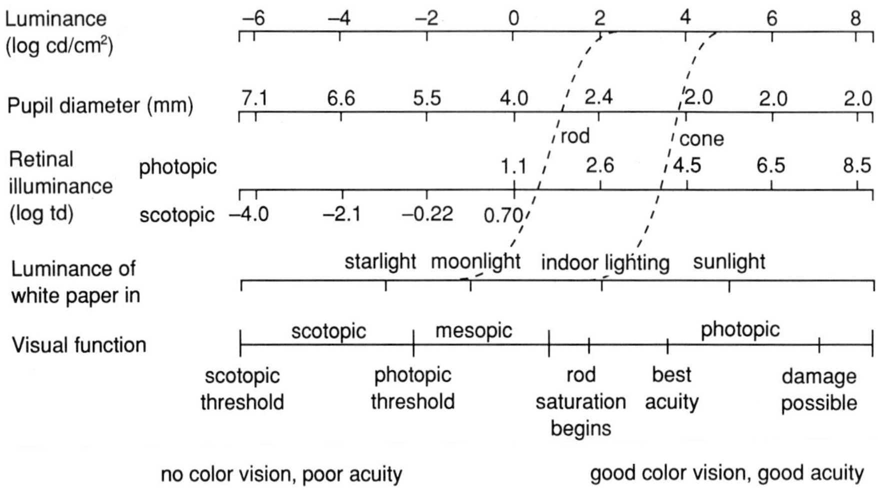

Fig. 1 Operating range of the visual system. The dashed curves represent rod and cone stimulus–response functions derived from recordings of membrane current in single primate photoreceptors (Baylor et al., 1984, 1987). The troland units can be converted to photons absorbed per receptor per second by multiplying by factors 4 and 10 for scotopic and photopic trolands, respectively. After Hood and Finkelstein (1986); © Wiley.

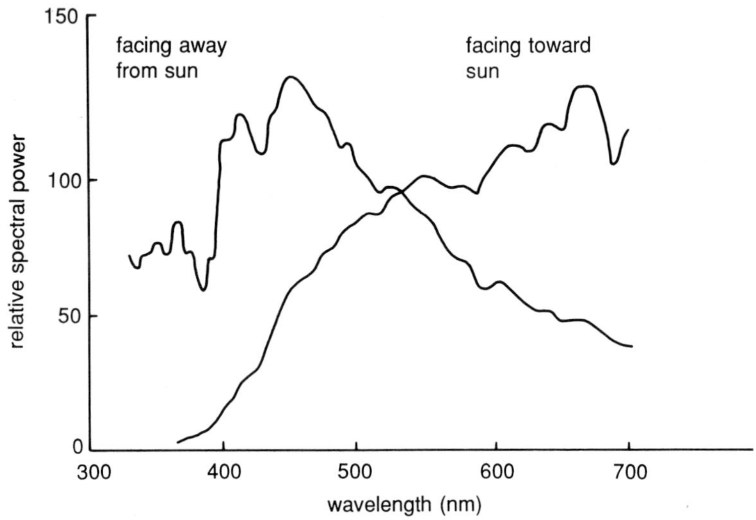

Fig. 2 Relative spectral power distributions of a bluish and reddish sample of daylight, reflected by a surface facing away from the sun (at 30° solar altitude) or directed at it (at 8° solar altitude). After Condit and Grum (1964).

natural lighting conditions. Without chromatic adaptation, that is, separate sensitivity controls in the cone pathways, the reddish and bluish lights shown in Fig. 2 would profoundly affect our perception of object colors. For example, the reddish light would make green grass look brown, whereas the bluish light would turn a yellow banana into a green one.

C. Contrast

As discussed in the introduction, sensitivity control is more than adjusting the visual response to variations in the intensity and color of the light source. The mechanisms involved should also allow the visual system to respond to reflectance rather than to absolute luminance (the product of reflectance and incident illumination). This means that an increase in illumination, which leaves contrast unchanged, should be processed in such a way that the visual response, or at least certain aspects of that response, remain unchanged as well. It can be shown that physiological data are indeed consistent with such a response mechanism (Section IV, C).

As can be seen in Fig. 3, there are different ways to vary contrast in a psychophysical stimulus. This has resulted in different nomenclatures and definitions. The contrast indicated by C_W is the type usually associated with Weber's law ($\Delta L/L$ = constant), whereas C_M relates to the Michelson contrast definition. Other definitions may sometimes be needed, particularly when dealing with light decrements (Whittle, 1986). The simplest contrast profile (C in Fig. 3) suggests a definition in terms of

$$C = L_{\text{high}}/L_{\text{low}} \tag{4}$$

The same definition might be applied to Weber contrast, which, when using the Weber nomenclature, would translate into

$$C = (\Delta L + L)/L \tag{5}$$

However, this is rarely done. Rather, contrast in this configuration is expressed as

$$C_W = \Delta L/L \tag{6}$$

Notice that this definition specifies the spatial transient (the luminance difference, ΔL) as the relevant variable, rather than $\Delta L + L$. Later we present an argument for doing so (Section III, B, 2). The Michelson contrast (C_M), which is usually used in conjunction with sine-wave gratings, is also defined as a transient, namely, peak-to-peak an
tive to an average backg
the expression

$$C_M = (L_{\max} - L$$
$$= (L_{\max} - L$$

Actually it does not ma
definition is used, as long a
definitions given in Eqs. (4, ... will all yield invariance of contrast when the corresponding luminance profiles are multiplied by a certain factor, as would result from a change in illumination level. By the same token, invariance of the visual response to contrast can be achieved if sensitivity control is such that its action is equivalent to a multiplicative reduction of the light input. Changing the pupil size would be the most direct way to implement that principle. However, the dynamic range of the pupil, a little more than 1 log unit, is no match for the environmental changes in light level (See Fig. 1). So, additional adaptation mechanisms, preferably mimicking the action of the pupil, are required. Without such mechanisms, high light levels would drive the visual response to its maximum (response saturation), and thus severely limit the range over which contrast can be recorded.

The range of contrasts produced by reflecting objects is relatively small, spanning a factor of about 20. However, for specular (mirrorlike) reflections or direct viewing of the light source the range is limited only by the intensity range of the source in question. Such a stimulus is usually recognized by the visual system for what it is, that is, light instead of matter. The corresponding perceptual attribute is called brightness and may be interpreted as the psychological correlate of luminance. In the case of reflected light,

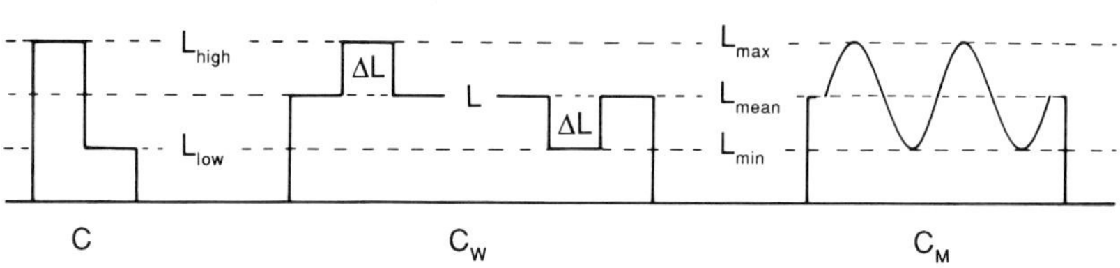

Fig. 3 Luminance profiles illustrating the contrast definitions given in the text. C, High/low luminance ratio, Eq. (4); C_W, Weber contrast, Eq. (6); C_M, Michelson contrast, Eq. (7).

.. expressed as a percentage (relative .. surface), the appropriate term is light- ..ightness or grayness thus relates to reflectance ..ich puts it in the context of perception of matter (gray paint, for example) rather than light. Most of the psychophysical research on visual adaptation is based on experiments that involve contrast perception at the threshold of vision, where one does not have to consider the implications of the light or matter distinction. In experiments employing suprathreshold stimuli, as in studies on lightness or brightness constancy, the proper response measures for dealing with the duality of light/matter perception is far from simple (cf. Gilchrist, Delman & Jacobsen, 1983; Flock & Nusinowitz, 1984).

In this section the three major variables of the light stimulus were introduced: luminance, color, and contrast. All three have to be dealt with by the visual system's sensitivity control. In the following, some of the major principles and basic facts relating to these three different aspects of sensitivity regulation are discussed, starting with what can be gleaned from psychophysical findings.

III. PSYCHOPHYSICAL FINDINGS

Before discussing sensitivity control in the context of psychophysics, the definition of "sensitivity" should be made clear. So far we have used this concept only to refer to the visual system's ability to discriminate small changes in stimulus strength. When it comes to more specific definitions (based on measurements), "sensitivity" may have different connotations. As pointed out by Shapley and Enroth-Cugell (1984), in psychophysics sensitivity usually refers to the reciprocal of the minimum stimulus strength required for the stimulus to be reliably detected (1/threshold). It may thus be related both to the noise in the system and to other mechanisms that determine the gain or responsivity of the system.

However, when sensitivity is measured in physiological experiments, the contribution of noise is usually eliminated by averaging over many identical stimulus–response cycles. Physiological sensitivity, then, is solely a measure of gain. It would be much less confusing, therefore, to use the word gain for physiologically measured sensitivity, defining it as the ratio of a noise-free criterion response (ΔR) to the stimulus magnitude (ΔS), in the small signal range where the response is still proportional to the stimulus. The latter proviso (linear response range) is necessary to distinguish "true" gain changes from the effect of response saturation. That is, the effect that may occur when a too strong stimulus and/or lack of sufficient gain control forces a neuron to operate along the lower sloped portion of its stimulus–response characteristic, close to its response ceiling (see the response functions in Fig. 1). This is in itself an adaptation mechanism, but the gain reduction that may be obtained has to be paid for by a progressive shrinkage of available response amplitude (response compression). This is hardly a desirable means for sensitivity control. Arguably, the main goal of sensitivity control is actually to avoid this "saturation catastrophe," as Shapley and Enroth-Cugell (1984) called it.

A. Luminance Adaptation

1. Threshold-versus-Intensity Function

In most experiments on visual adaptation, a conditioning or adaptation stimulus is used for altering the state of adaptation, and a test stimulus is used for probing the resulting changes in sensitivity. A typical example of such an experiment is one in which the minimal stimulus strength is measured for detecting a 1° test field presented as a flash, say, 200 msec, superimposed on a large homogenous 10° adaptation field. One thus obtains a threshold-versus-intensity (t.v.i.) function, probably the most frequently used characteristic for studying adaptation processes (see Blackwell, 1972).

The typical result for photopic (cone) vision, as obtained under the aforementioned conditions, is shown

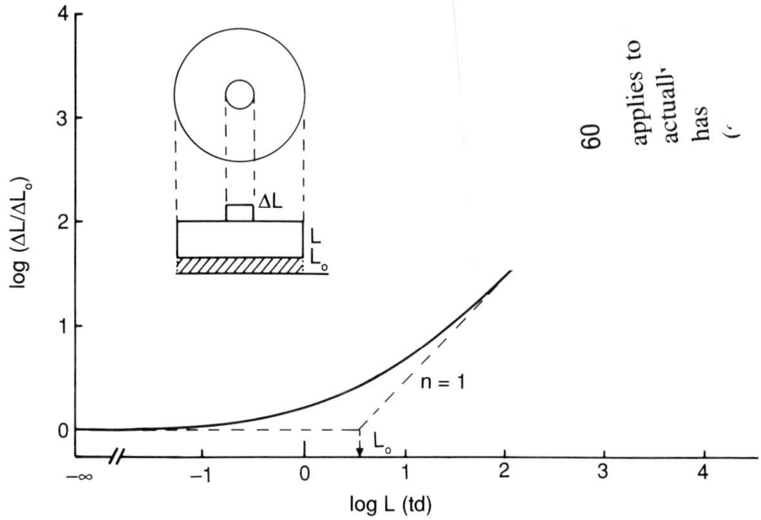

Fig. 4 Generalized threshold-versus-intensity (t.v.i.) function or Weber–Fechner function based on the tabulated data of Wyszecki and Stiles (1982). See text for further details.

in Fig. 4. This curve, also called the Weber–Fechner relation, is based on averaged data from the work of Stiles (1978), as tabulated by Wyszecki and Stiles (1982).

The curve shown in Fig. 4 traces the change in incremental threshold luminance (ΔL) relative to the threshold in the dark, or absolute threshold (ΔL_0), as a function of the luminance of the background (L). The function can be described, to a fair approximation, by

$$\Delta L/\Delta L_0 = k(L + L_0)^n \tag{8}$$

The constant k represents the Weber fraction (of the order of a few percent), L_0 stands for "dark" light or Fechner's (1860) Eigengrau, and n is an exponent that may vary between 0.5 and 1. Note that for $n = 1$ and $L >> L_0$, one obtains Weber's law ($\Delta L/L = c$), as represented by the 45° asymptote in Fig. 4. At low luminance levels, where L falls below L_0 and ΔL approaches the (absolute) threshold in the dark (ΔL_0), the normalized threshold ($\Delta L/L_0$) approaches 1, as indicated by the horizontal asymptote in Fig. 4. The intersection of the asymptotes defines the value of L that corresponds to L_0 (arrow).

The gradual increase in detection threshold (or decrease in sensitivity) with increasing luminance level might reflect the effect of an increase in noise and/or a reduction in gain. The possible effect of noise is discussed in the next section. Now we first address the possible involvement of gain mechanisms. It is of interest in this respect that the Weber–Fechner relation has actually been found to be compatible with such gain changes in photoreceptors (e.g., Boynton & Whitten, 1970; Hood & Hock, 1974; Fain, 1976; Normann & Anderton, 1983; Valeton, 1983). In view of the limited operating range of the photoreceptors, there seems to be an obvious need for adaptation at that level. However, in contrast to what is found in cold-blooded animals, the gain changes proper (i.e., those not due to response compression) that can be deduced from recordings from primate cones seem to be quite limited. The main mechanism involved appears to be inactivation of the photopigment (bleaching). This does not become effective until relatively high light levels are reached (in excess of 10^4 td), which would imply that most of the gain control has to take place "downstream" from the photoreceptors. This is also evident from the fact that the gain changes inferred from psychophysical data usually start at lower light levels than would be expected on the basis of recordings from primate photoreceptors.

The Weber–Fechner relation (t.v.i. function) also

cotopic (rod) vision. However, this may be due to interaction with the cone system. It een shown that Weber's law is not achieved ope of $n < 0.8$) in the visual system of the complete achromat who has no cone vision (Sharpe, Fach, Nordby & Stockman, 1989); nor is it achieved by the isolated rod system of the normal trichromat (Sharpe *et al.*, 1989; Sharpe, 1989). It appears from these studies, which are consistent with others (e.g. Makous & Boothe, 1974; Makous & Peeples, 1979), that Weber's law is only attained for rods when using backgrounds strongly stimulating the cones as well as the rods.

At a retinal illuminance in excess of about 100 scotopic td, sensitivity rapidly starts to decrease (indicated by an increase in the Weber fraction), and the slope of the t.v.i. function becomes progressively steeper. This effect, first documented in the classical studies of Stiles (1939) and Aguilar and Stiles (1954), is shown in Fig. 5. This so-called rod saturation is an interesting phenomenon because it possibly reflects the absence of adequate gain control in mammalian

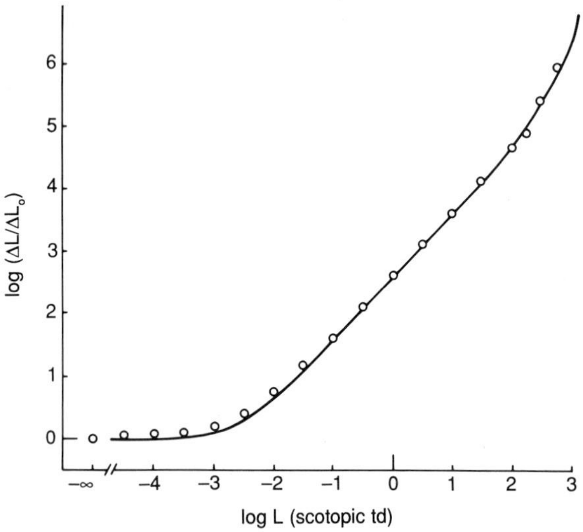

Fig. 5 Scotopic threshold-versus-intensity (t.v.i.) function showing the effect of rod saturation. The data, averages of four observers, are from Aguilar and Stiles (1954). The curve fitted to the data is a theoretical function (Walraven & Valeton, 1984).

rods. The observed threshold increase is what one would expect if the background light drives the rods to their maximum response, a limit that cannot be exceeded, whatever the intensity of the test flash. Actually this might be advantageous because it effectively prohibits the rod system from interfering with the signal processing of the (high resolution) photopic system.

The absence of gain control in individual rods seems at odds with the impressive 5 log unit range over which the rod t.v.i. function follows Weber's law before saturation sets in. The possibility that single rods can cover such a range may be safely excluded, and one has to think therefore, in terms of rod pools rather than individual rods (Rushton, 1965). The tremendous amplification that can thus be achieved has to be kept under control by adaptation mechanisms operating within the neural network subserving the rod pool (Virsu, 1978). How the network adaptation is implemented is still largely unknown, but its effect, as reflected in the shape of the t.v.i. function, can be reasonably well described by a variety of models. The theoretical function fitted to the data in Fig. 5 may be considered as a case in point.

The fact that rods, in contrast to cones, can be saturated by steady backgrounds is a consequence of their high sensitivity and lack of gain control. The only mechanism that might protect the rods from response saturation is bleaching of the photopigment. However, due to their high sensitivity, the rods already reach their maximum response at light levels that produce negligible bleaching. Cones, on the other hand, reach only half their maximum response at a retinal illuminance (about 4 log td) that already bleaches about 50% of the photopigment. Above that light level, bleaching increases in proportion with intensity and, thus, by actually bringing the effective photon catch to a standstill, enables the cones to operate indefinitely.

The shape of t.v.i. functions is affected by the temporal and spatial parameters of test and adaptation stimuli, but also by the type of discrimination task involved. When the discrimination of a luminance difference is measured with two separate fields, presented (simultaneously) side by side, one obtains Weber's law for the whole range over which the stimuli are visible (Cornsweet & Pinkser, 1965; Whittle & Swanston, 1974). Note, however, that in this condition the visual system does not have to detect a single transient, relative to a steady background signal, but that it has to establish the difference between two separate transients. Thus, the discrimination of the two stimuli involves the comparison of the outputs of spatially separated channels. It is of interest, though, that here too a fractional rather than an absolute difference is required for discriminating the stimuli. This would be consistent with a mechanism that compares signals on a logarithmic rather than a linear scale. Alternatively, one might assume that noise is at the root of this particular manifestation of Weber's law. However, one would expect then, that the discrimination of the signals would become more difficult when the flashes are presented on a background, just as in the case of a single flash on a background. This is not observed. The mutual discriminability of the flashes remains unaffected (as long as the individual flashes are above threshold) when background intensity is increased (Thijssen & Vendrik, 1971; Whittle & Swanston, 1974).

2. Noise Considerations

At low light levels the visual system is confronted with the problem of extracting signals from a noisy stimulus (Poisson distributed photons), noisy receptors (thermal breakdown of photopigments), and noisy transmission lines (spontaneous random release of neurotransmitters). Many studies have addressed this problem (Barlow & Pelli, 1987), especially with respect to photon noise (e.g., Bouman, 1961; Barlow, 1964b). The photon density (i) of a light stimulus shows fluctuations that increase in proportion with the square root of i. So, the input to the photoreceptors is given by $i \pm i^{0.5}$. This means that the threshold for seeing a change in signal strength (Δi) will be proportional to $i^{0.5}$, provided, of course, that photon noise is the only factor that limits visual sensitivity. Psychophysical evidence for a square-root relationship in t.v.i. functions, generally known as the de Vries–Rose law (DeVries, 1943; Rose, 1948), has been obtained with small, short flashes, detected by the rod system only (Barlow, 1957; Van den Brink & Bouman, 1957).

Despite a variety of psychophysical data that are consistent with the de Vries–Rose law (see also Walraven and Bouman, 1966), it is not very likely that photon noise is the sole determinant of visual sensitivity (Barlow, 1977). Nevertheless, it would be a sound strategy of the visual system to adjust sensitivity in proportion with the square root of the light input. This kind of signal compression is optimal in the sense that it would reduce the photon noise term to a constant, irrespective of stimulus strength (Bouman, 1961; Barlow & Levick, 1969). On the other hand, scaling in proportion to n, rather than $n^{0.5}$, thus implementing Weber's law, provides a mechanism for extracting contrast, and hence reflectance, as discussed below. One might speculate that reflectance is at the root of (invariant) color vision, either chromatic or achromatic. Weber's law would be useful, therefore, in conditions that allow good color vision, that is, relatively high luminance (photopic vision) and relatively large fields. When that is not the case, noise may become an important consideration (the noise term becomes relatively large at low light levels), thus leading to prevalence of the de Vries–Rose law. It is of interest in this respect that varying the statistical characteristics of the light source has been found to affect visual threshold (Teich et al., 1982).

With increasing light level the photon noise becomes relatively unimportant and, therefore, less relevant for explaining contrast discrimination thresholds (except for very small stimuli, where photon flux has to be considered). On the other hand, one might postulate that physiological noise is always an important factor, both at low and high light levels. This is a rather difficult area, because one also has to consider that noise may be reduced by gain control. Nevertheless, there are various arguments that would at least caution against introducing noise as a major explanatory principle for the effect of backgrounds on visual sensitivity. First, the effect of gain control, as measured by noise-free physiological data, is by itself already sufficient to predict the general characteristic of the t.v.i. function. Second, the results from the side-by-side discrimination experiment discussed above, showing no effect of adding a background, argue against a noise explanation. (Whereas a gain control, affecting the two fields in the same way, would predict this result.) Finally, "t.v.i." functions obtained with suprathreshold criteria, like the equibrightness curves measured by Whittle and Challands (1969), are similar in shape to the function measured at threshold. This suggests that the same (gain) mechanism that determines the shape of the t.v.i. function at suprathreshold, where a noise explanation is irrelevant, is also involved at threshold.

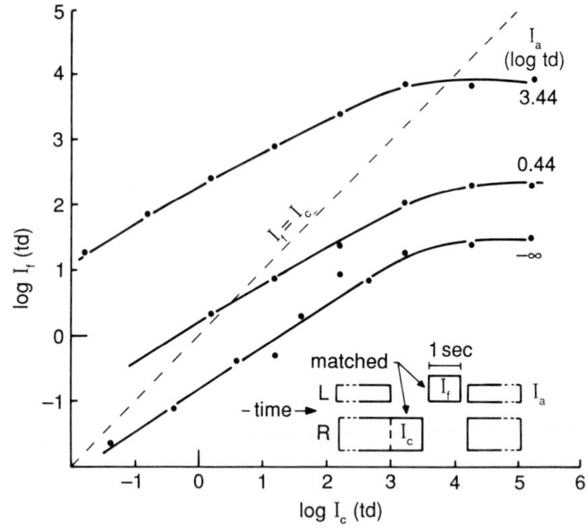

Fig. 6 Retinal illuminance of a *flashed* stimulus (I_f), presented to the left eye, that matches the brightness of an identical *continuous* stimulus (i_c), presented to the right eye. Different curves relate to different levels of preadaptation (I_a) of the eye viewing the flashed stimulus. The inset shows the temporal arrangement of the stimuli seen by the left (L) and right (R) eye, respectively. Data redrawn from Craik (1940).

3. Range Selection

Sensitivity control is not solely determined by what happens in single photoreceptors. Other functional units, in particular receptive fields or even more extensive networks have to be considered as well. Examples of global interactions are: the periphery effect (McIlwain, 1966; Krüger & Fischer, 1973; Breitmeyer *et al.*, 1980), long-range chromatic induction (Valberg *et al.*, 1985; Pöppel, 1986) and orientation-selective inhibition beyond the conventional (cortical) receptive field regions (Nelson & Frost, 1978).

Still, although visual adaptation must involve post-receptoral interaction, it seems clear from Fig. 1 that there should at least be some degree of sensitivity control at the level of the photoreceptors—even if the mechanisms in question may be partly controlled from outside the receptor. The sensitivity control should be such that the dynamic operating range of the receptor can be shifted along the intensity axis (see Fig. 1). The presence of such a range-selecting principle was probably first made explicit by Craik (1940), who backed it up with an important experiment. Using haploscopic stimulation (i.e., different stimuli for the two eyes) he compared the brightness of a light seen either as a flash (left eye) or as the tail end of a steady light (right eye). The rationale behind his experiment is that adaptation is not instantaneous, so the flashed and steady stimulus may be assumed to produce responses that measure, by their difference in magnitude, the effect of adaptation. Some of Craik's data, which have been confirmed by Geisler (1978), are reproduced in Fig. 6.

The curves shown in Fig. 6 reveal various interesting points, but for the present purpose we only want to point out that the curves are similar in shape and shifted vertically with increasing adaptation level. Such behavior implies that adaptation affects the response to the flashed light in the same way as a neutral density filter in front of the eye would do. It is for that reason that this type of adaptation has been dubbed "dark-glasses" adaptation (MacLeod, 1978). The same general principle can be inferred from a study by Onley and Boynton (1962) in which flashed stimuli, presented to eyes adapted to different adaptation fields, were matched in brightness.

The "dark-glasses" adaptation principle revealed

in Craik's experiment enables the visual system to extend its operating range without loss of dynamic responsiveness. This means that it can always employ its full response potential for registering the luminance variations in the retinal image. An important characteristic of this principle of gain control is that its action can be described by an attenuation of the input to the neuron in question. Thus, the maximum attainable response (dynamic range) of the neuron is not affected; it only takes more signal at the input to generate it. Alternatively, a gain reduction can also be implemented by attenuation of the signal at the output of a neuron. This means that the response range becomes compressed, since the response "ceiling" can be lowered but not the response "floor" (the response cannot become less than zero). Such a mechanism does not increase the operating range of the neuron in question, but if its output provides the input to another neuron, the latter will now have its input scaled, just as with "dark-glasses" gain control.

Craik's results show that the 3 log unit range over which the flashed stimulus had to vary in order to match increasing intensities of the steady comparison stimulus is not reduced by presenting the flash on a 3.4 log td background. This lack of compression indicates that the adaptation produced by a (steady) background is consistent with dark-glasses adaptation. The dark-glasses attenuation increases with increasing luminance of the background. If this would occur in proportion with background luminance, an increment (ΔL), added to the background luminance (L), would have its efficacy reduced in proportion with L. So, in order for ΔL to remain just visible with increasing L, as is the case for a t.v.i. experiment (Fig. 4), ΔL would have to grow in proportion with L. Thus, Weber's law ($\Delta L/L = c$) would be in evidence.

Although it is an attractive idea to implement Weber's law by means of the same "dark glasses" that protect the system from response compression, it is not necessary to do so. It can be shown that a dark-glasses control, followed by a gain mechanism that aims at a constant output, also produces Weber's law even if the dark-glasses attenuation is not proportional with light level (Walraven & Valeton, 1984). As discussed below, such a two-stage system may be related to the different tasks of range selection and contrast processing.

4. Contrast Processing

As argued above, contrast is the key to maintaining invariance of visual perception in conditions of varying illumination. Sensitivity control should be implemented in such a way, therefore, that the response to a particular light ratio (contrast) remains constant when, due to an increase in illumination, the luminances of the lights defining that ratio are increased in the same proportion. One way to keep the response constant is to undo the increase in illumination, that is, reduce the (effective) retinal illumination. Pupil constriction, pigment depletion, and reduction of spatial and/or temporal light integration provide different means to achieve that goal. In addition, there is physiological evidence showing that photoreceptors and other visual neurons are able to shift their operating range in order to accommodate changes in illumination (see Fig. 23, for example). Again, this is a mechanism mimicking the effect of light reduction. Thus, the general principle of the visual system's adaptation machinery is consistent with the dark-glasses principle reflected in Craik's data. Since this implies multiplicative signal reduction it is referred to as multiplicative adaptation, to distinguish it from subtractive processes discussed later.

Multiplicative adaptation provides the means for preserving contrast, but that by itself is not sufficient for *responding* to contrast. Somehow the visual system must be able to behave like a logarithmic analyzer, that is, produce responses that correlate with ratios rather than with differences. For example, a luminance step of 100 units should yield the same responses as a 10 unit step, if they both relate to the same luminance ratio, say, 1000 to 900 and 100 to 90. If, on the other hand, the 10 unit step would represent the difference between 15 and 5 units, then that same step, now representing a larger contrast ratio, should yield a larger response than the 100 unit step.

Such a ratio or contrast processer will behave in

accordance with Weber's law since it will produce the same response to an increment (ΔL) on a background (L), as long as the luminance ratio ($\Delta L/L$) remains constant. A simple way to explain Weber's law, therefore, is to assume a (near) logarithmic transformation, somewhere in the pathway from stimulus to response (Cornsweet, 1970). The idea of this kind of response compression goes back to Fechner (1860) but has also been proposed in more recent times (e.g., Cornsweet & Pinsker, 1965; Kelly, 1969). However, the problem with the idea is that physiological evidence for a logarithmic stimulus–response function is lacking.

There is actually no need to invoke a logarithmic transducer function, since Weber's law can also be implemented by other means. All that is needed is a (fast) gain control that aims at a constant output, by changing the gain in proportion to signal strength. Such a mechanism, also called automatic gain control (Rushton, 1965) or proportional gain adjustment (Ullman & Schechtman, 1982), has to act very fast in order to be able to follow the continuously changing light profile on the retina. Koenderink, Van de Grind, and Bouman (1971), who discussed such a "Weber-machine" in detail, estimated the adaptation time constant to be of the order of 10–30 msec. It is questionable whether this type of signal processing should still be considered a gain control in the same sense as the dark-glasses mechanism discussed before. It might just as well be interpreted as a contrast processor. Walraven and Valeton (1984) made that distinction in a model incorporating two attenuation stages, one for range selection, by means of dark-glasses adaptation, and one for contrast processing.

To summarize the main message of this section, the visual system not only has to respond over a wide range of light levels, but it should also be able to extract contrast. These are different tasks, that may involve different mechanisms.

5. Brightness versus Lightness Constancy

If visual perception were dictated by Weber's law, we would see a world varying in contrast, but we would not be aware of changes in illumination. By abstracting relative luminance changes (contrast), information about absolute light level is lost. This prediction is at odds with the fact that we are perfectly capable of discriminating between dim and bright illumination, both with respect to overall light level and local distribution (shades and shadows). At the same time, we experience constancy of color and lightness of the surface of objects, as determined by their (spectral) reflectance. So, what actually is constant, reflectance, is perceived as invariant, whereas that which is not invariant, the illumination and its distribution, is indeed recognized as such.

Gilchrist et al. (1983) discuss in this context possible differences in the physical properties of edges produced by changes in reflectance, as opposed to changes in illumination (shadows), as cues for the corresponding perceptions of lightness and brightness. The same authors also confirm the constancy of lightness and, in the same experiment, the absence of constancy for brightness (Jacobsen & Gilchrist, 1988). Similar results were obtained by Heggelund (1974) and Arend and Goldstein (1987). These studies indicate the importance of discriminating between lightness and brightness. It is of particular interest moreover, that the perceptual constancy predicted by Weber's law is found only for lightness, our perceptual correlate for reflectance. That link between Weber's law, which predicts invariance, and reflectance, which is indeed invariant, suggests that the Weber mechanism is specifically involved in the perception of matter rather than the perception of light.

If we pursue this line of thought, then it follows that illumination, rather than reflectance, is the variable in our visual world that has to be controlled. That control should not aim at invariance because that would imply loss of information. On the other hand, it should provide sufficient signal reduction (without interfering with contrast processing) to protect the system against response compression. Dark glasses that do not completely compensate for the illumination level could provide the means for complying with both demands. It is of interest in this respect that the vertical shifts of the curves in Fig. 6 indicate that dark-glasses adaptation does not attenuate in proportion with adaptation level. To appreciate this, note that a 3 log unit increase in background luminance (from 0.44 to 3.44 log td) is accompanied by a vertical shift of less than 2 log units. The relationship between gain factor and background luminance can be inferred from the lateral distance between the dark-adapted curve and the 45° diagonal. This distance measures the logarithm of the factor by which the (adapted) continuous stimulus (I_c), has been dimmed (by gain control) relative to the flashed (unadapted) stimulus (I_f).

Notice in Fig. 6 that it is not until the dark-adapted curve starts to run horizontally (at about 4 log td), that the separation increases in proportion with the luminance of I_c. So, as has also been documented by Geisler (1981), it is only at relatively high luminances of I_c that Weber's law comes to the fore. Considering the light levels involved, this Weber behavior can almost entirely be attributed to the depletion of photopigment, the depletion becoming proportional with light intensity at retinal illumination in excess of about 4 log td. In other words, the attenuation due to dark-glasses adaptation does not yield invariance until bleaching takes over and thereby produces Weber's law. It is of interest that this occurs in the range of 3.5–5 log td, which is the range of retinal illuminations typically produced by a light colored object in daylight under out-of-doors conditions (Le Grand, 1957).

In this section, which deals with a complex and still only partly understood area of visual perception, we introduced the idea that Weber's law does not necessarily reflect the action of "dark-glasses" adaptation. We would rather place it in the context of the visual system's response to contrast. This view may be incorrect, and it certainly is not fashionable, but it seems worthwhile to consider this possibility in relation to the problem of separating the two main variables of our visual world, reflectance and illumination.

B. Color Control

1. Spectral Sampling Problems

The problem the visual system faces in chromatic sensitivity control is actually not that much different from the one encountered in the luminance domain. The main difference is that, instead of one channel, there are now three channels to be controlled, each looking at the world through a different color filter.

It would have been nice if the objects in this world were illuminated with light confined to three, non-overlapping wavebands and if the three types of cones were exactly tuned (also without overlap) to each of those bands. In that case spectral variations in the illuminant could be completely described with three independent variables, detected in three independent systems. It would be possible then, to fully compensate for changes in this three-primary illuminant and thus have perfect color constancy.

Unfortunately, the visual system has to deal with illuminants that have complex spectral power density (SPD) distributions. The same applies to the spectral reflectance curves of object colors, even if these can be reasonably well described with additive combinations of only 2–4 basis spectral distributions (Cohen, 1964; Maloney, 1986). To further complicate matters, the visual system, giving up on the idea of monitoring every wavelength in the spectrum, is equipped with cones that have broadly overlapping rather than separated spectral absorption functions.This simplifies the spectral analysis and also boosts sensitivity.

Part of the price to be paid for this incomplete sampling is that we cannot have perfect color constancy. This can be intuitively appreciated by realizing that the light captured in the photoreceptor is spectrally modulated by various filters, introduced by the light source, the objects, and the photopigments. Spectral changes due to the light source can be compensated for only by opposite changes at the photopigment level. Such changes can be implemented only by altering the effective densities of the three cone pigments by selective bleaching or equivalent neural adaptation. However, one can imagine that such compensatory changes will not always be successful in negating the spectral changes introduced by the illuminant. For example, if the latter is a monochromatic light, there is no way by which the visual system can recover the difference in spectral reflectance of objects seen under broadband illumination. Those interested in the mathematical treatment of this and related problems are referred to Buchsbaum and Gottschalk (1984), Brill and West (1986), and Worthey and Brill (1986).

2. Two-Process Mechanism

There is a vast amount of literature on chromatic sensitivity control or chromatic adaptation. Useful entries, in particular to the older literature, can be found in the reviews by Graham and Brown (1965) and Jameson and Hurvich (1972). In this field there are still many riddles to be solved, but in general the so-called von Kries coefficient law (Von Kries, 1905) may still be considered the main principle involved in sensitivity control. This law postulates multiplicative gain control applied to separate cone systems. It has been shown that the coefficient law may be seemingly invalidated, due to its confounding the effect of another mechanism, operating in a subtractive rather than multiplicative fashion (Hurvich and Jameson, 1972). This so-called second process, often referred to as chromatic induction, may actually not be isolated that easily (Walraven, 1973). However, if the test stimulus is presented as a (suprathreshold) increment on a background, then the observed hue shift can be described by two processes, a multiplicative one and a subtractive one. The latter actually enables the visual system to "discount" the additive contribution of the background (Walraven, 1976, 1977) or at least nearly so (Shevell, 1978). When the incremental stimulus is flashed, the discounting is complete (Werner and Walraven, 1982; Davies, Faivre & Werner, 1983), and one can measure then the isolated effect of multiplicative adaptation. In fact, the separation of stimulus transient (ΔI) and background (I) has always been implicitly recognized in definitions of contrast (see Fig. 2).

The discounting effect, which was already observed by Whittle and Challands (1969) in studies of brightness adaptation, is possibly achieved in the visual system through antagonistic center–surround units in the retina (see receptive fields, Section IV, C, 3) which make spatially uniform inputs ineffective and selectively emphasizes spatial transients. Also, time-differentiating mechanisms (e.g., Arend, 1973, 1976) are probably involved. The discounting effect can be readily observed when viewing a small green increment on a bright red background. When adaptation is complete, the incremental light will always appear greenish, even near threshold, although it should appear yellowish or reddish due to color mixing with the background.

3. Two-Color Thresholds

Sensitivity control, as manifested in the t.v.i. characteristic for luminance discrimination, is also found under conditions of chromatic adaptation. Best known in this respect is Stiles' work on two-color increment thresholds (Stiles, 1961, 1978). Using this technique, that is, different wavelengths for test and background light, wave-band selective adaptation processes have been revealed, the well-known but still poorly understood π mechanisms (see Boynton, 1979). These mechanisms give rise to multibranched t.v.i. functions, the branches reflecting the separate activation of the mechanisms in question.

An example of Stiles' (1961) data is shown in Fig. 7. The lower branch of the t.v.i. function reflects the activity of the green sensitive mechanism (π_4), which has a lower threshold for the 475 nm test flash than the other, blue sensitive, mechanism involved (π_1). At high light levels, however, π_4 becomes so insensitive (due to the green background), that the next most sensitive mechanism (π_1), which is less sensitive to the adapting effect of the green background, takes over the detection of the test flash.

Stiles π mechanisms have spectral sensitivities that are slightly broader than those of the cones, thus suggesting weighted inputs from more than one cone type (Ingling & Tsou, 1977). The π mechanisms may nevertheless be involved in controlling the von Kries coefficients that describe the sensitivity adjustment of cones (Walraven, 1981; Werner & Walraven, 1982). However, the nature of the π mechanisms is still far from clear, in particular those systems associated with short-wave sensitivity control (π_1, π_2, and π_3). Complex interactions, partly at the level of opponent processing (see Chapter 6) have been revealed in quite a few studies (Pugh, 1976; Stromeyer, Kranda &

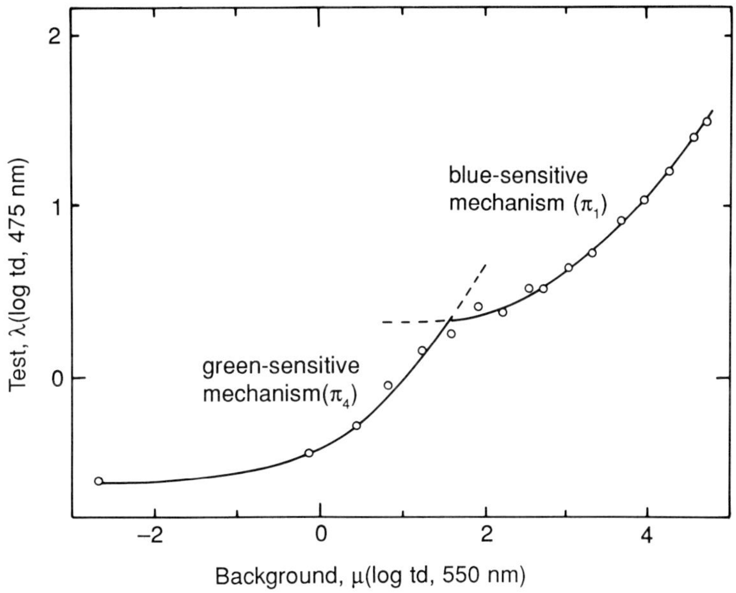

Fig. 7 Two-color increment-threshold function obtained with a blue (475 nm) test field, λ, flashed on a green (550 nm) background, μm. The two branches are thought to represent detection by different π-mechanisms. After Stiles (1961).

Sternheim, 1978; Mollon & Polden, 1979; Pugh & Mollon, 1979; Sternheim, Stromeyer & Khoo, 1979; Haegerstrom-Portnoy, Verdon & Adams, 1988).

4. Color Constancy

We already discussed that perfect color constancy cannot exist. Still, depending on the stimulus conditions, the degree of color constancy the visual system can achieve is quite impressive. Figure 8 shows an example from a study by Walraven et al. (1989).

The data shown in Fig. 8 were obtained in an experiment in which the stimulus pattern was generated on a computer-driven color monitor. The display simulated reflected light of an array of 35 Munsell color samples, arranged in a 5 × 7 matrix (see inset Fig. 8). The samples were shown on an achromatic surface that could be either a standard white (100% reflectance) or black (no reflectance). A selection of these samples, consisting of 10 chromatic (25% reflectance) and 3 achromatic ones (50, 70, and 90% reflectance), was used as test stimuli. The other samples only served to provide a picture with sufficient color variety. The chromaticities of the test samples, expressed in CIE x,y units, were so chosen that they formed an approximately uniform color circle centered around the achromatic standard used (D65). The open circles represent the chromaticities of the set of test colors under white illumination. The cross in the center of the set, coinciding with the chromaticity of the achromatic samples, indicates the chromaticity of the white light source. The squares relate to the same set, but now under green illumination. These show how the colors are shifted in the direction of the chromaticity of the green light source, which is indicated again by the cross. The solid arrow shows this shift for one of the samples. The size and direction of the shifts were computed (using standard colorimetric methods) from the spectral reflectances of the samples and the spectral emittance of the light source to be simulated. What the two sets of open symbols represent has nothing to do with perception. They only show the physical change in color that results from changing the illumination.

In order to measure how the perceived color of the samples is affected by the color of the light source, the samples in colored light (the test stimulus) were presented to the left eye, whereas the samples illumi-

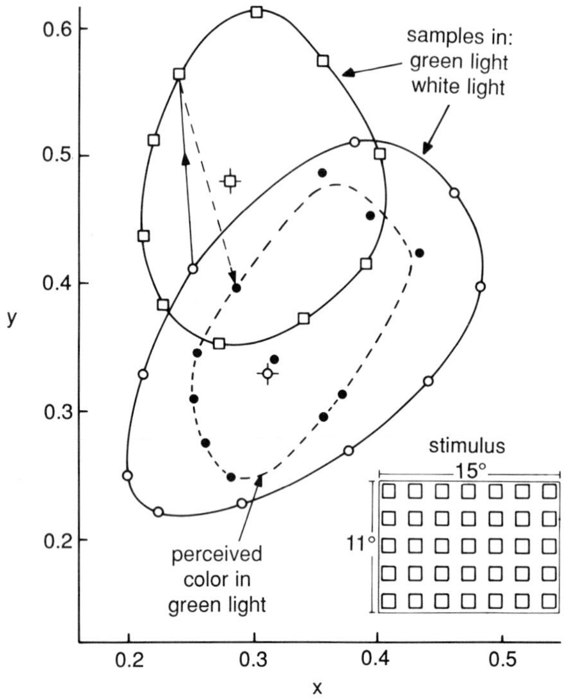

Fig. 8 Data showing the effect of color constancy, as obtained in the experiment discussed in the text. Open symbols: chromaticities of test colors illuminated by either white light (circles) or green light (squares). Filled symbols: chromaticities of samples in white light (seen by the left eye) that match the same samples in green light (seen by the right eye). The solid arrow shows, for one sample, the physical color shift due to the change in illumination. The dashed arrow shows how the colors are shifted back, perceptually, due to the action of color constancy mechanisms. After Walraven et al. (1989).

nated by white light (matching stimulus) were shown, one at a time, to the right eye. The test and matching stimuli were presented alternately. The observer's task was to match the samples illuminated by white light to the corresponding samples seen under green light. Thus, the observer used one, neutrally adapted eye to register the colors seen with the other, color adapted eye.

As is shown by the filled circles, the matching colors that were selected were close to the sample colors as seen under white rather than under green illumination. So, apparently the physical color shift produced by the green illuminant was counteracted by an opposite shift (see the dashed arrow) produced by chromatic gain control. This corrective action did not fully restore the perception under white light, the remaining differences indicating that the colors appeared slightly desaturated under green light. It is of interest that this result was actually found to be consistent with predictions based on a von Kries transformation (Walraven et al., 1989). The idea behind this transformation, which is also implied in the well-known Retinex theory (e.g., McCann, McKee & Taylor, 1976; Land, 1986), is that the sensitivities of the three types of cones are adjusted in such a way that their response ratio when adapted to colored light is the same as that produced by white light. This implies an operation consistent with that producing Weber's law.

When, in the above experiment, the white background was replaced by a dark background, thus making the color samples appear like light sources (self-luminous colors), color constancy was found to be almost absent. That is, the chromaticities the subjects selected for matching the test samples matched the chromaticities of the samples under green rather than under white light. Results from experiments by Arend and Reeves (1986) point in the same direction. Apparently, color constancy, like lightness constancy, is a phenomenon that relates to the perception of matter (surface colors) rather than light (self-luminous colors). How the visual system is able to make the matter versus light distinction is still one of the basic problems in visual perception (Marr, 1982; Rubin & Richards, 1982). The study of color constancy may well be one of the more promising roads to the solution of that problem.

C. Recovery of Sensitivity

> Everyone is familiar with visual adaptation in two different aspects, one very convenient and one very inconvenient. The convenient aspect is the eye's automatic adjustment to the general level of illumination so as to keep contrast and indeed nearly all aspects of appearance unchanged though the actual light energies may alter some thousand-fold. The inconvenient aspect is experienced when, after ad-

> aptation to strong light, we go into very dim surrounding, e.g. from sunlight into a darkened lecture theatre. At first we are nearly blind and we only recover full sensitivity after 15–30 min. [Rushton, 1969, p. 544]

These are the words of William Rushton, who himself has contributed much to this field, in particular to the "inconvenient" aspect of the slow recovery of visual sensitivity, called dark adaptation. Being more concerned here with the convenient aspect of visual adaptation, we briefly discuss only some of the major findings pertaining to dark adaptation.

After a full bleach of the rods, which is easily achieved during a sunny day on the beach, dark adaptation may take more than 30 min for its (near) completion. This is not advantageous from a functional point of view, of course. The fact that evolution has nevertheless permitted such a slow system to survive may be due to the fact that, under natural conditions, one rarely has to plunge from bright light into total darkness.

The slowness of dark adaptation can be related to the slow rate of photopigment regeneration. The proportion of regenerated pigment (P) as a function of recovery time(t) can be roughly approximated by a first-order chemical reaction (Rushton, 1958, 1972),

$$p(t) = 1 - (1 - p_0)\, e^{-t/t_0} \qquad (9)$$

where p_0 is the fraction unbleached pigment at $t = 0$, and t_0 is the time constant. Actually, t_0 is not truly constant, as it may depend on experimental conditions. However, for not too short bleaches, $t_0 = 400$ sec seems to be a reasonable estimate of the average value found for rods (Alpern, 1971), whereas 120 sec will do for cones (Hollins & Alpern, 1973). For cones, in particular, t_0 seems to decrease with shortening of the bleaching time, which means that Eq. (9) is not a complete description for pigment regeneration (e.g., Smith, Pokorny & Van Norren, 1983). As has been shown by Coolen and van Norren (1988), a more refined account for (in situ) pigment regeneration can be obtained by assuming a store of 11-*cis*-retinal (a building block of the photopigment molecule), as was also proposed by Rushton and Henry (1968).

The recovery of visual sensitivity during dark adaptation is only to a slight degree attributable to the restoration of the quantum catching power (optical density) of the photopigments. Figure 9 illustrates this point, and also reveals what the actual relation between sensitivity and pigment content may look like. In this figure, the left ordinate refers to the change in visual threshold (circles), whereas the ordinate on the right indicates the proportion of cone pigment in the bleached state (triangles), as measured with a reflection densitometer. That information can be used to calculate the threshold elevation to be expected if loss of pigment were the only factor involved. Recovery of sensitivity would be described, then, by the dashed curve, which clearly does not fit the data at all. The discrepancy is even more pronounced for rods, where bleaching of 10% of the pigment already produces a hundredfold increase in threshold. Because of this and because of the kinetics of the rod pigment, about 12–13 min must elapse before the bleached rods begin to surpass the sensitivity of the, by then fully recovered, cones. This initiates the rod phase of dark adaptation during which a hundred- to thousandfold increase of sensitivity occurs over a period of about

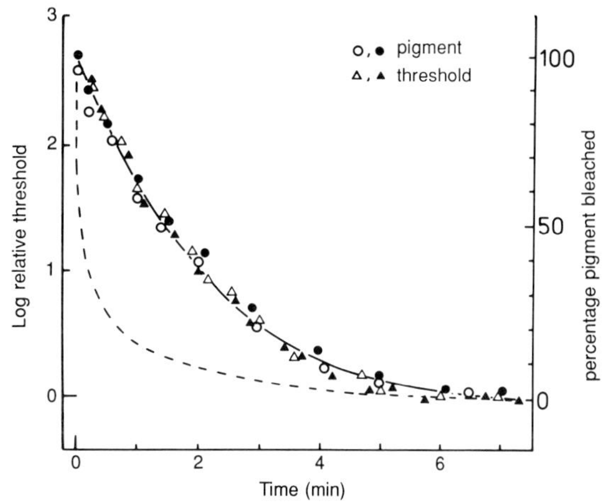

Fig. 9 Recovery of sensitivity (circles) and regeneration of cone pigment (triangles) during dark adaptation. Open and closed symbols relate to different experiments. The dashed line indicates the expected threshold elevation due to pigment depletion only. The increase in sensitivity (or decrease in relative threshold) is shown as a function of time (t) after extinguishing of the bleaching light at $t = 0$. After Rushton (1965).

30 min. Overall, then, the recovery of sensitivity in the dark amounts to a factor of about a million.

The fact that in Fig. 9 the recovery of threshold and the regeneration of pigment follow the same time course indicates that they are linked. However, there appears to be a logarithmic rather than a linear relationship between threshold and fraction of bleached pigment, or

$$\log(T/T_0) = c(1 - p) \tag{10}$$

where T/T_0 is the threshold relative to absolute threshold (T_0), and p represents the fraction of unbleached pigment. The relation given by Eq. (10) was first obtained for rods, in the eye of the rat by Dowling (1960) and in the human eye by Rushton (1961), and is known, therefore, as the Dowling–Rushton relation.

Unfortunately, the pretty picture shown in Fig. 9 does not apply to all experimental conditions, especially not when relatively weak bleaches are involved (Rushton & Powell, 1972), which is actually the normal condition for the visual system. Moreover, there is, as yet, no rational basis for Eq. (9). An attractive alternative proposal by Lamb (1981) gives a good account of dark adaptation, for all bleaching levels, using the simple assumption that threshold is linearly related to the concentration of bleaching products. The fact that recovery of log threshold is fast at first and then slows down (Fig. 9) is explained in Lamb's model by assuming different intermediate products with different kinetics. Matters are complicated, however, because of conflicting data on the relation between threshold and pigment concentration. Data obtained from a rod monochromat (Nordby, Stabell & Stabell, 1984) suggests a log–log relationship between threshold and fraction of bleached rhodopsin, rather than the log–linear relation indicated by Eq. (10).

One of the problems in the understanding of dark adaptation is to identify the separate contributions of "dark" light (i.e., aftereffects related to photochemistry), and the more direct effects evoked in the presence of real light (Gouras, 1972). There is good evidence that dark adaptation can be described in terms of increment thresholds measured on a slowly decaying background of "dark light" (i.e., the afterimage), that behaves in the same way as (stabilized) real light (Barlow & Sparrock, 1964; Blakemore & Rushton, 1965b; Spillmann, Wolf & Nowlan, 1971; Rushton & MacLeod, 1986). This is the important concept of the equivalent background, first discussed by Stiles and Crawford (1932). According to the Crawford transform, each threshold obtained during dark adaptation can be expressed in terms of the steady background that raises the increment threshold to the same value. The intensity of this (real light) background is assumed to have an effect equivalent to the process underlying the dark threshold; it is by substituting one for the other that the equivalent background versus time curve is derived. However, there are many cases in which the equivalent-background concept has been found to fail (Hood & Finkelstein, 1986). Such failures may be due, perhaps, to the fact that during the presence of real light, neural mechanisms are activated that are no longer employed when the light is extinguished (Westheimer, 1968; Teller & Gestrin, 1969; Buss, Hayhoe & Stromeyer, 1982).

The equivalent background principle still provides an important link in the study of dark and light adaptation. Apparently, the absorption of light produces certain products that play a role in the control of visual sensitivity, even for some time after the light has been extinguished. However, as has been shown by Pugh (1975), the concentration of bleached photopigment is not necessarily indicative of the concentration of those other, as yet unidentified, products.

D. Failure of Sensitivity Control

Compared to the slow recovery of sensitivity in the dark, the time course of light adaptation is extremely rapid. Still, adjustments of sensitivity following the onset of a light stimulus are not instantaneous. Flashed fields are more effective, therefore, in passing the sensitivity control unscathed. The incomplete sensitivity control for flashed as compared to steady fields is accompanied by relatively high increment thresholds at the onset of an adaptation field (Crawford, 1947; Boynton & Kandell, 1957). Figure 10 allows comparison of the different t.v.i. functions ob-

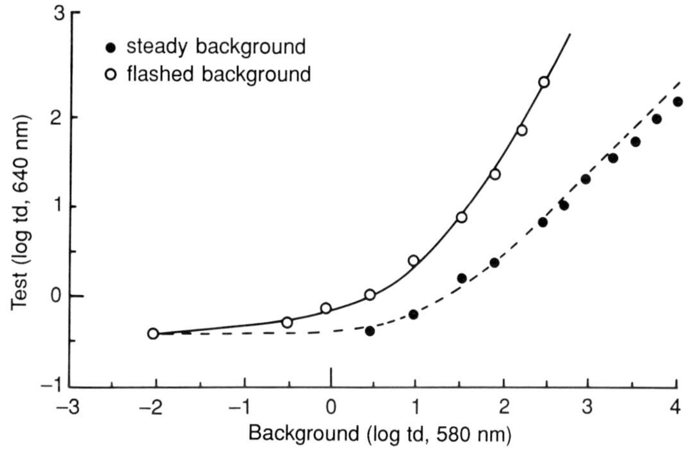

Fig. 10 Foveal threshold-versus-intensity functions (t.v.i.) measured on steady and flashed backgrounds. The 1° test field (40 msec, 640 nm) was presented in the center of a 2° (580 nm) background. The field was presented either continuously or for 500 msec. The solid curve is the fit of a response compression model (see text). The dashed curve is the best fit of a model (incorporating the same parameters) schematized in Fig. 15. After Finkelstein, Harrison, and Hood (1988).

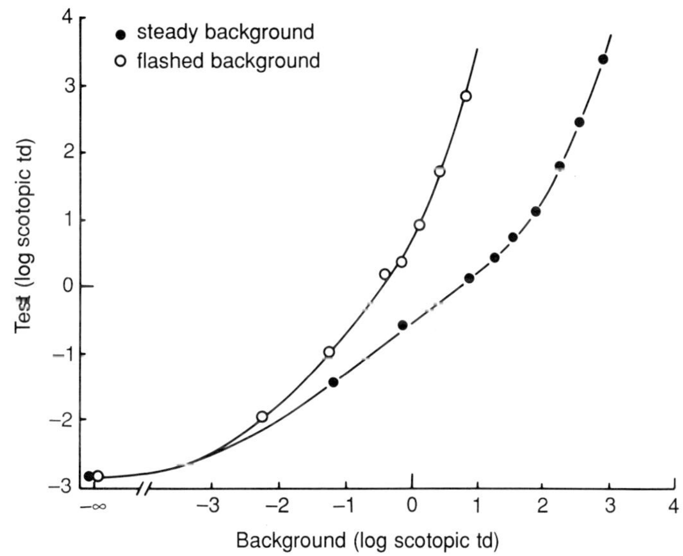

Fig. 11 Rod system increment thresholds measured on steady adapting fields (filled circles) and flashed (400 msec) adapting fields (open circles). The curves were fitted by eye. From Adelson (1982).

tained with steady and flashed backgrounds for the foveal cone system. The test light was presented either against a steady field or at the onset of a 500 msec flash. Notice the striking effect of field duration on the shape of the increment threshold function. At moderate to high adapting intensities, the t.v.i. function for the steady field follows a slope of 1.0, whereas thresholds on a flashed field increase in accordance with an accelerating slope greater than 1. The sharp loss in sensitivity caused by brief lights is reminiscent of the rod saturation seen in the presence of steady fields. In fact, this finding has been called "cone saturation" (Alpern, Rushton & Torii, 1970; Shevell, 1977). It is likely, though, that the saturation takes place at a stage of processing beyond the receptors (Stromeyer, Kronauer & Madsen, 1979; Finkelstein and Hood, 1981), so this phenomenon might be better labeled "cone system saturation."

As can be seen in Fig. 11, which shows a comparison of rod system t.v.i. functions for flashed and steady fields, flashed fields are also more effective than steady fields in elevating threshold in rod vision (Geisler, 1979; Adelson, 1982). The rod system can be shown to exhibit saturation to brief fields that are 30 to 100 times weaker than the steady fields producing saturation.

E. Mechanisms of Sensitivity Control

The saturating t.v.i. functions obtained with flashed backgrounds show what happens when the visual system's sensitivity control is not given sufficient time to take action. It is unable, then, to protect the photoreceptors and/or subsequent neurons from being driven to their response ceiling. In the following we discuss how such failures of sensitivity control provide information about the nature of the various mechanisms involved.

1. Response Compression

Figure 12A illustrates an intensity–response function for a hypothetical neuron. The magnitude of the response is plotted as a function of the intensity of a brief flash of light. The response first increases roughly proportional with flash intensity but ultimately reaches a maximum or saturation level. This kind of stimulus–response function was first used by Naka and Rushton (1966) to describe intensity–response functions of neurons in the fish retina. It has since been recorded from cells in the retinas of many other animal species and can be described by

$$r/r_{\mathrm{m}} = i^n/(i^n + \sigma^n) \qquad (11)$$

where i is the stimulus strength (expressed in photons/unit area/unit time, or equivalent units), and r/r_{m} is the electrical response (r) normalized relative to the maximum response (r_{m}). The constant σ, the semisaturation constant, represents the stimulus intensity for which $r/r_{\mathrm{m}} = 0.5$, and n is an exponent whose value is usually in the range of 0.7 to 1. Measurements of the membrane current of single rods and cones in the primate retina are better described by an exponential function, as discussed below (Section IV,A,3). The difference between the two descriptions is small however, and of no concern for what follows.

The psychophysical data obtained from a wide variety of experiments employing brief adapting fields suggest that the stimulus–response characteristics of our dark-adapted rod and cone systems can be described by a function similar to that shown in Fig. 12A (Alpern et al., 1970; Geisler, 1978; Hood & Finkelstein, 1979; Hood, Finkelstein & Buckingham, 1979; Walraven, 1980; Adelson, 1982). For example, the solid curve in Fig. 10 is the fit of a model based on that function. The model, based on response compression only (see below), assumes that the incremental light becomes visible when the response to the increment plus the flashed field exceeds the response to the flashed field by a criterion amount.

To appreciate the need for adaptation mechanisms consider the consequences of a system without adaptation. In other words, suppose that the visual system were to respond to steady lights in the same way it responds to brief lights. Under this assumption, the response function in Fig. 12A would describe the visual system's response to both steady and flashed lights. The filled circles in Fig. 12A indicate the response to adapting fields at five different intensities. Note that higher adapting intensities leave little of the response range available to incremental lights. This decrease in responsiveness is referred to as response compression.

The effects of response compression are better illustrated in Fig. 12B, where the incremental response above the response to the steady field is shown as a function of the intensity of the incremental light, for each of the five steady fields in Fig. 12A. Notice that the fields of low intensity have little effect on the size of the incremental response, but that the higher field intensities leave the system virtually without response range to spare for incremental lights. If the (flashed) adaptation field does not modify the stimulus–response function, then ambient lights of moderate intensity would essentially "blind" the visual system. This is what we see reflected in the steep upswing of the t.v.i. functions shown in Figs. 10 and 11.

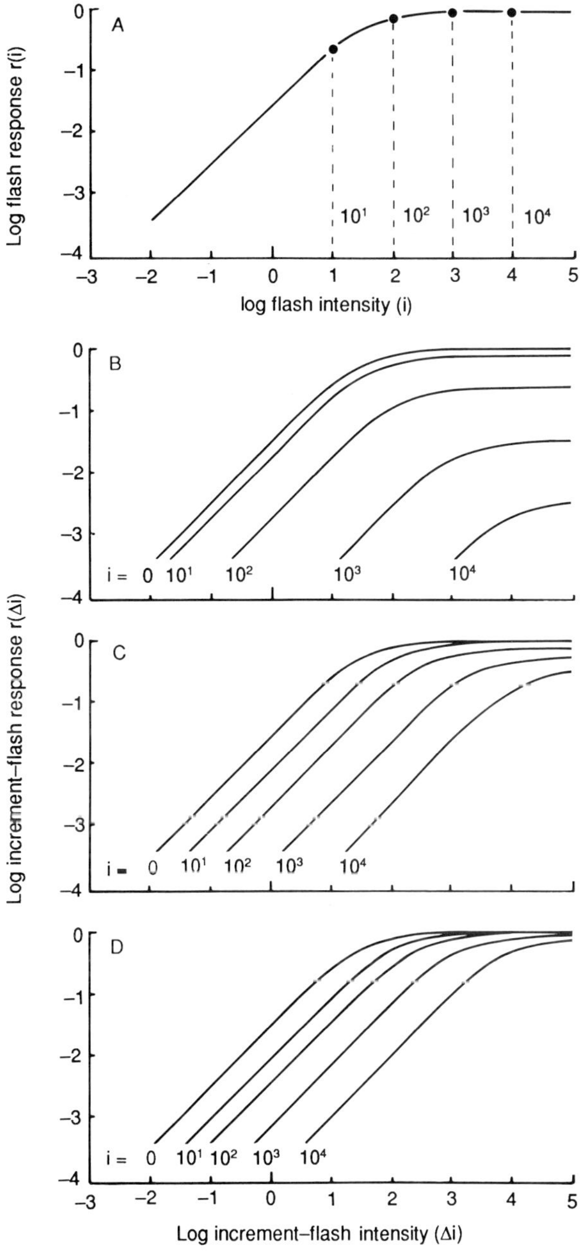

Fig. 12 Effects of mechanisms of adaptation on stimulus–response functions. The stimulus can be a single flash (i) or an incremental flash (Δi) on a background. (A) Intensity–response function for the dark-adapted visual system. The graph shows response amplitude as a function of the intensity of a single flash (i) and illustrates response compression. The saturating function shown here was calculated from Eq. (11). The filled circles mark the response of the system to five potential adapting intensities. (B) Effect of response compression on the incremental intensity–response function of the light-adapted eye. The curves show the response to incremental flashes of light (Δi) presented on adapting fields of five intensities (i) and in the dark. The curves are of the form $r(\Delta i) = r(i + \Delta i) - r(i)$, where r varies with i or Δi in accordance with Eq. (11). (C) Combined effects of multiplicative adaptation and response compression on the incremental intensity–response function. (D) Same as C, but now with the added effect of subtractive adaptation. Subtractive mechanisms discount or subtract out much of the response of the adapting field, thus restoring some of the sensitivity lost to response compression. After Hood and Finkelstein (1986); © Wiley.

Some investigators define mechanisms of adaptation as those that decrease the sensitivity of the visual system to ambient lights. By this definition, response compression would be a mechanism of adaptation. But if by adaptation we mean keeping the visual system responsive to small changes in contrast over a large range of adapting lights, then mechanisms of adaptation are best thought of as those modifying the intensity–response function and thereby protect the system from response compression. Here we categorize such mechanisms as multiplicative or subtractive (Adelson, 1982). It is the action of these mechanisms, or the absence thereof, that is reflected in the different t.v.i. functions obtained with steady and flashed adaptation fields, respectively.

2. Multiplicative Adaptation

To protect itself from response compression, the visual system employs a number of physiological mechanisms that have the same effect as decreasing the effective light intensity by a multiplicative constant ("dark-glasses" adaptation). Figure 12C illustrates how a multiplicative decrease in light intensity modifies the intensity–response function. The modification consists of a lateral shift of the entire stimulus–response function along the log intensity axis. Notice that the system is less sensitive to low light levels after multiplicative adaptation, but it has recovered much of its response range. One example of a multiplicative mechanism is pigment depletion. Light breaks down visual pigment molecules and thereby decreases the number of molecules available to catch the photons. It is actually this mechanism that enables the cones to continue operating at high ambient light levels. At low light intensities, where the effect of pigment depletion is still negligible, neurons in the visual system have nevertheless been shown to modify their gain in a way that mimics pigment depletion. In lower vertebrates this adaptation mechanism has been observed at both the receptoral and postreceptoral level (e.g., Normann & Werblin, 1974; Werblin, 1974; Green et al., 1975; Kleinschmidt & Dowling, 1975). For mammals, the evidence supports postreceptoral gain changes at the level of horizontal, bipolar, and ganglion cells. However, there appears to be little multiplicative gain control in the rods. The extent to which mammalian cones exhibit multiplicative gain control is still not quite clear.

The combined effects of response compression and multiplicative adaptation on the t.v.i. function are illustrated in Fig. 13. The solid curves are the empirical t.v.i. functions for steady lights and the predicted t.v.i. functions based on response compression. Without adaptation, response compression produces the threshold elevations described by the curve labeled response compression. Remember from Fig. 10 (solid curve) that a model assuming only response compression fits the flashed cone t.v.i. data for brief fields. The dashed curves in Fig. 13 show the predicted t.v.i. functions for steady backgrounds if the rod and cone systems have available only multiplicative adaptation (to forestall response compression). Notice that saturation is avoided by the cone system and delayed in the rod system. However, the predicted t.v.i. functions still deviate from the empirical t.v.i. functions; multiplicative mechanisms alone are not sufficient to account for the t.v.i. functions. Apparently, another adaptation mechanism must be involved. In order to describe the data, we must assume that this additional mechanism has the same effect as subtracting a fixed percentage of the signal from the adapting field.

3. Subtractive Adaptation

The need for a mechanism to subtract (or discount) the effects of a steady field is well accepted in the literature on color appearance (Hurvich & Jameson, 1958; Walraven, 1976; Shevell, 1978). Physiologically, the biphasic impulse response function for cone receptors (see Section IV, A, 7) implies one possible mechanism by which the response to a steady light is substantially decreased. Lateral inhibitory mechanisms provide another method. Subtractive mechanisms that remove most (80–90%) of the effects of the steady field can account for the difference between the dashed curves and the empirical t.v.i. functions in Fig. 13 (Geisler, 1981; Adelson, 1982; Wal-

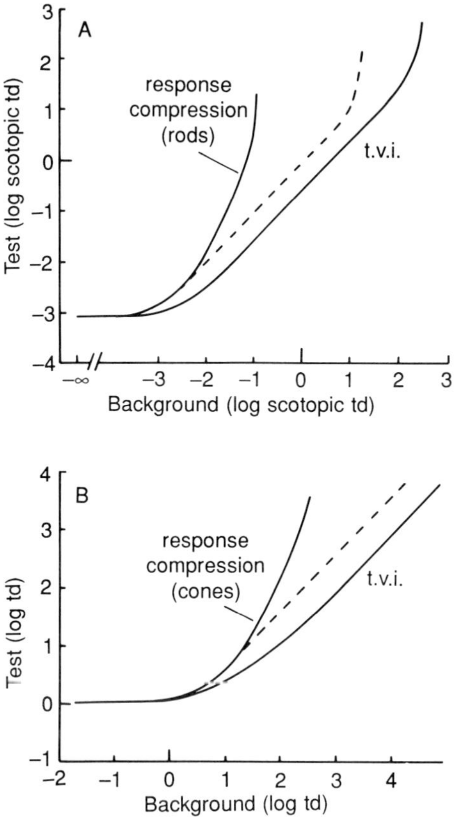

Fig. 13 Increment-threshold curves derived from models of response compression and multiplicative adaptation are compared with empirically determined t.v.i. curves. A and B relate to the rod and cone systems, respectively. The solid curves labeled "t.v.i." are the empirical steady background functions. The curves labeled "response compression" are the increment-threshold functions predicted from the compressive response function of Fig. 12D. Combining multiplicative adaptation with response compression (as in Fig. 12C) yields the increment-threshold functions given by the dashed curves. To bring these thresholds into line with those actually obtained requires a third mechanism, namely, response subtraction. From Hood and Finkelstein (1986); © Wiley.

raven & Valeton, 1984; Hayhoe, Benimoff & Hood, 1987). Figure 12D shows the effects on the intensity–response function of subtracting 80% of the signal of the steady field. The subtractive mechanism restores most of the response range lost to response compression.

4. Time Course of Adaptation

Although the neural adjustments in visual sensitivity that are attributable to multiplicative and subtractive mechanisms are not instantaneous, they are nevertheless very rapid. Figure 14 is from Crawford's (1947) classic study of early light adaptation. Much of the adjustment to an adapting field takes place very rapidly, within the first second of the onset of an adapting field. Although, at higher adapting intensities, small changes in sensitivity can require over 10 min for completion (Baker, 1949), these very slow changes are probably due to pigment bleaching (Geisler, 1981).

If we restrict ourselves to adapting lights that bleach little visual pigment, the multiplicative changes in the human cone system are extremely rapid and can be complete within 50 msec (e.g., Hayhoe et al., 1987). The subtractive changes, also in part rapid, can take seconds to run their complete course. The changes in sensitivity measured by Crawford (1947) and Baker (1953), immediately after the onset of an adapting field (see Fig. 14), can be explained by a very rapid multiplicative change followed by a slower

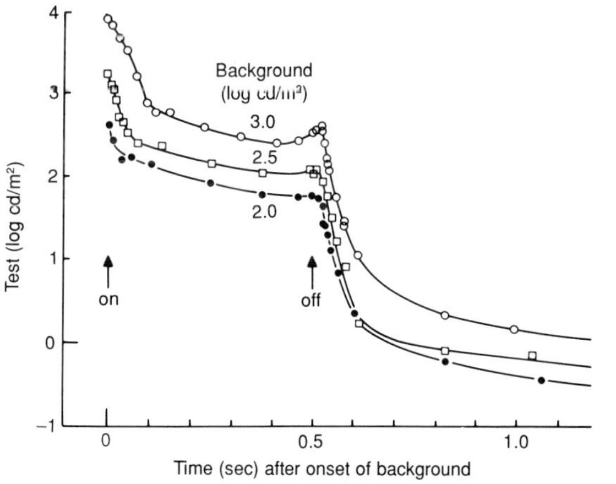

Fig. 14 Change in increment threshold at the onset of a flashed background (0.5 sec) for three luminance levels. The log luminance of a test flash is shown as a function of the time after the onset of the background adapting field. The test flash was 30′ in diameter and 10 msec in duration. The background flash was 12° in diameter and 524 msec in duration. After Crawford (1947).

buildup of a subtractive process. For the rod system, much of the sensitivity change is probably complete within 100 msec after the onset of the adapting field, although 30 sec or more are required for completion of the subtractive process (Adelson, 1982).

F. Models

A two-site model of sensitivity control is summarized in Fig. 15. The first site is assumed to have the properties of the receptors. The second site represents postreceptoral processes of sensitivity change. Both sites have a compressive, nonlinear response function (f_1 and f_2) and sources of noise. The mechanisms labeled m and s are multiplicative and subtractive adaptation mechanisms, respectively. The initial linear function is the site of photon absorption.

The model for the human rod system assumes no multiplicative or subtractive adaptation for the rod receptors (the dashed circles in Fig. 15 only apply to cones). The postreceptoral response function (f_2) saturates at intensities considerably below the intensities that saturate the rod receptors. The time-dependent adaptation changes are effected by mechanisms labeled m_2 and s_2. The psychophysical evidence for a multiplicative mechanism (m_2) at the second site is very strong (Geisler, 1979; Adelson, 1982). Physiologically this mechanism is identified with the gain control of the inner nuclear layer of the retina (Shapley & Enroth-Cugell, 1984). Psychophysical evidence for the existence of a subtractive mechanism (s_2) in the rod system is less conclusive (see, e.g., Geisler, 1979, versus Adelson, 1982). In this model, changes in the sensitivity of the rod receptors play little role in sensitivity control until adapting field intensities between 1.0 and 2.3 log scotopic td are reached. For small, brief test lights and relatively low adapting field intensities, photon noise (n_1) and receptor noise (n_2) are thought to determine sensitivity.

Different models have been proposed to predict rod t.v.i. functions (as in Fig. 13) for relatively large, long test lights (Treisman, 1964; Barlow, 1965; Shapley & Enroth-Cugell, 1984; Walraven & Valeton, 1984; Hood & Greenstein, 1988). These models differ in the assumptions they make about the sites and nature of the different sources of noise, the different (time-dependent) adaptation mechanisms, and the detector. Most of these models have two features in common. One, the models explicitly or implicitly assume that receptoral and photon noise are unimportant at all but the lowest adapting intensities. Two, they require either a multiplicative mechanism (m_2), or a noise source (n_2) to produce the Weber law behavior observed for steady fields.

The multiplicative gain control at the second site

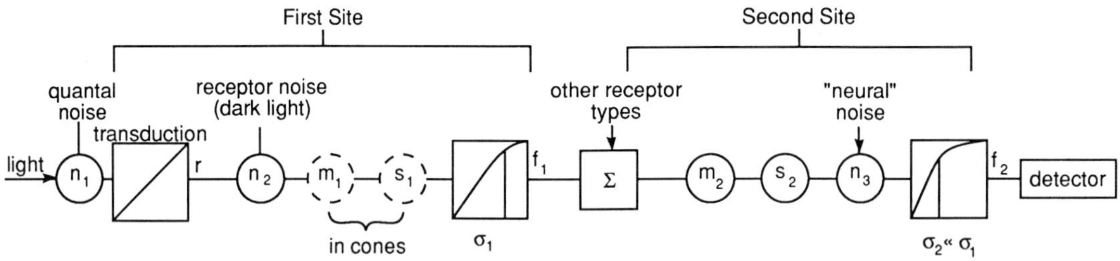

Fig. 15 Schematic to illustrate a two-site model of the rod and cone system. The model includes three noise sources: quantal noise, n_1; receptor noise, n_2 (often assumed to be equivalent to the psychophysically determined "dark light"); and postreceptoral noise, n_3. Both sites have instantaneous nonlinear intensity–response functions, f_1 and f_2. The circles labeled m_1, m_2, s_1, and s_2 indicate time-dependent adaptation mechanisms, thought to act as if they scale the intensity of all lights by a multiplicative constant (mechanisms m_1 and m_2) or decrease the intensity of the background by an additive constant (mechanisms s_1, and s_2). The sites indicated by dashed circles (m_1, s_1) are assumed to be lacking in the rod system.

(m_2) implies signal reduction at the input to that stage. Since that input corresponds to the output from the first site, that is, the receptor signal, the action of m_2 can be described as a scaling of the receptor response. If this is a rapid mechanism that aims at keeping the output constant (i.e., proportional gain adjustment), the second site might serve as the contrast processor, or "Weber machine," mentioned in Section II, A, 4. However, this is just one of the possible interpretations, which should not detract from the more obvious function of m_2, namely, protecting the second site from response saturation.

The model shown in Fig. 15, but now with the dashed parts included, also applies to the human cone system. It assumes that receptors saturate at intensities considerably above the postreceptoral site (cf. f_1 and f_2). The most recent physiological data suggest receptor semisaturation constants of the order of 4 log td (see Section IV). Many of the psychophysical data (see Fig. 13) are fitted with semisaturation constants 100 to 1000 times smaller (e.g., Geisler, 1981; Hayhoe et al., 1987; Hood & Greenstein, 1987), thus suggesting that the second site response function, f_2, is largely responsible for the elevation of threshold in the presence of brief fields as in Fig. 10 (see also Stromeyer et al., 1979; Finkelstein & Hood, 1981).

Psychophysical and physiological evidence can be found for multiplicative and subtractive mechanisms at both the receptor and postreceptor sites of the cone system. The need for a second site with a multiplicative mechanism is well established, both psychophysically and physiologically. Postreceptoral subtractive mechanisms are also based on reasonably firm psychophysical and physiological evidence (e.g., Hayhoe, 1986). For the receptors it is not clear how much weight to give to multiplicative as opposed to subtractive changes in modifying cone receptor sensitivity at higher adapting intensities (although pigment depletion takes care of all adaptation at retinal illuminances above 4 log td). Likewise, the role of photon and receptor noise, although likely to be involved only at low adapting intensities and/or for small, brief test lights, is still debated.

IV. PHYSIOLOGICAL FINDINGS

A. Photoreceptors

The first step in the transformation from light to sight is the absorption of quanta in the photoreceptors and the resultant generation of an electrical signal. In the dark, positively charged sodium ions flow steadily into the outer segment of a rod or cone. (The outer segment is that portion of the cell that contains the photopigment.) The entry of sodium is blocked by the action of light and thus provides the interface by which the retinal image is translated into electrical signals.

When a photon is absorbed in a photopigment molecule it may cause, with about 67% chance, a configuration change in that molecule (isomerization), thus making the pigment molecule enzymatically active. The activated pigment triggers a series of chemical reactions that culminates in the closure of some of the ion channels through which the sodium enters (Baylor, 1987). The reduced influx of sodium results in a hyperpolarization of the cell membrane, that is, the inside of the cell becomes more negative relative to the outside. The hyperpolarization is conducted passively from the outer segment to the synaptic ending, where it reduces the rate of release of transmitter molecules from the synapse. This reduction provides the signal to bipolar cells and horizontal cells that light has been absorbed (Fig. 16).

The membrane current of single rods and cones has been measured by drawing an outer segment into a closely fitting glass electrode. The electrode collects the membrane current of the outer segment and thus registers the change in the current elicited by light absorption. An example of this kind of experimental preparation is given in Fig. 17, which shows a photomicrograph of a piece of retina from the toad, *Bufo marinus,* with a rod sucked into the electrode. The same technique has also been used to measure the membrane current of single rod and cone outer segments in isolated retinas of humans and the monkey,

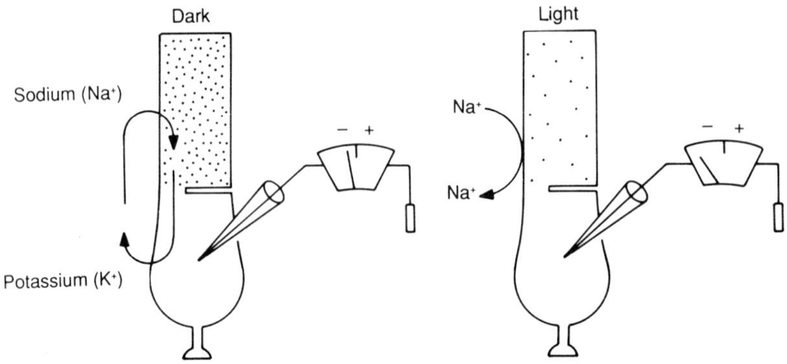

Fig. 16 Schematic of a vertebrate rod. In the dark there is a steady flux of sodium ions into the outer segment. (This inward current is balanced by an efflux of potassium from the rest of the cell.) Upon illumination, channels through which the sodium flows are closed, causing a reduction in sodium influx and hyperpolarization of the membrane. From Schnapf and Baylor (1987).

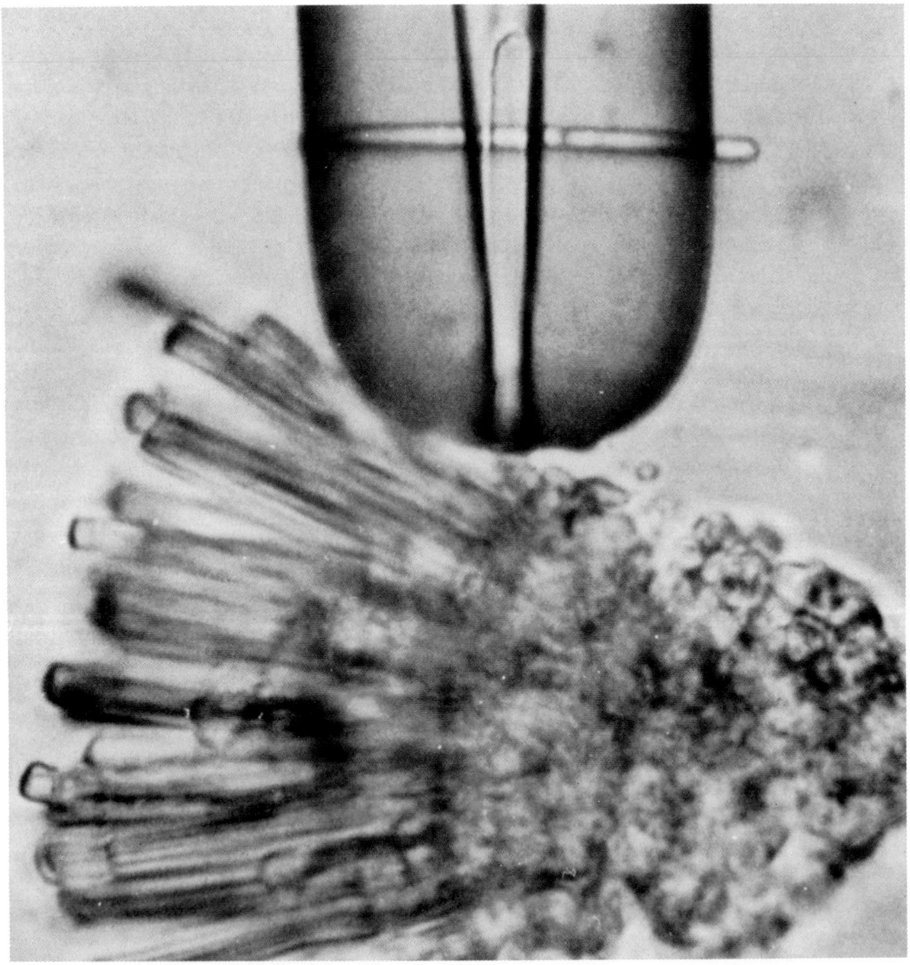

Fig. 17 Photomicrograph of a piece of retina from the toad (*Bufo marinus*). Outer segments of the rods can be seen protruding from the piece. A single outer segment has been drawn into the glass suction electrode for measurement of the membrane current. The narrow beam of light that traverses the outer segment is used for eliciting the rod response.

Macaca fascicularis (Baylor et al., 1984; Baylor, Nunn & Schnapf, 1987; Schnapf, Kraft & Baylor, 1987). Both the results from these physiological measurements and those from behavioral studies (DeValois et al., 1974) indicate that the photoreceptors of this species are functionally similar to those of man.

1. Single Photon Detection

From the elegant psychophysical experiments of Hecht, Shlaer, and Pirenne, (1942), it has been known for some time that our rods are capable of signaling the absorption of single photons. Electrical responses elicited by single photons can now also be recorded directly from rods (Baylor, Lamb & Yau, 1979; Baylor et al., 1984). In such experiments, the outer segment is stimulated with light which is so dim that only about one isomerization per flash is evoked on average. Because of the particle and stochastic nature of light itself, the rod's response is not constant from flash to flash, but shows a characteristic fluctuation in amplitude. With some flashes the peak amplitude of the response is about 1 pA (10^{-12} amperes), with others it is about 2 or 3 pA, and often no detectable response is elicited at all (Fig. 18). A quantitative analysis of the variation in response size is consistent with the idea that the fluctuations are mainly due to fluctuations in the number of photons absorbed per flash, and the amplitude of the response to a single photon is about 1 pA. That is, the frequency at which responses of about 1 pA are observed is just the frequency at which one would expect (on the basis of Poisson statistics) that one photon elicits one and only one isomerization. Likewise, the frequency at which 2 pA responses are seen is equal to the frequency at which one would expect that, on the average, two photons are absorbed, etc. Further analysis contradicts the idea that two or more photon absorptions are needed to elicit an electrical response.

The response to a single photon in a cone is difficult to observe directly because its amplitude is small compared to the noise. However, the single photon response can be derived from the response to flashes eliciting multiple absorptions (for stimuli which are sufficiently weak to ensure that the response amplitude scales linearly with stimulus strength). From the amplitude of the flash response and estimates of the number of isomerizations elicited per flash, it is cal-

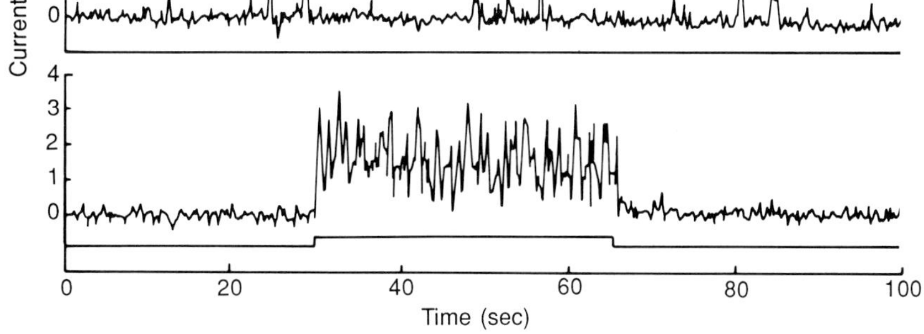

Fig. 18 Single photon responses in a monkey rod. The change in membrane current is plotted as a function of time. The stimulus trace is shown below the current traces. The top two traces show responses to brief flashes of light. Each flash elicited, on average, about one isomerization. Note the variability in response size from flash to flash. The bottom trace shows the response to a dim step of light that elicited about 10 isomerizations/sec. From Schnapf and Baylor (1987). Copyright © April 1987 by *Scientific American*. All rights reserved

culated that the amplitude of the photon response in a cone is about 10^{-2} pA, a hundred times smaller than that of the rod.

Photons are, of course, not all alike. Each has a characteristic energy or wavelength. What is the effect of wavelength on the electrical response in a rod or cone? Measurements of membrane current show that once a photon is absorbed, the electrical response it elicits is independent of the wavelength of the photon. Wavelength influences only the probability of absorption. In macaque rods, the probability is maximal when the wavelength of the light is about 490 nm; photons of shorter and longer wavelengths are less likely to be absorbed. The wavelength dependence of photon absorption, as measured in single macaque rods, corresponds closely to the wavelength dependence of human scotopic vision (Crawford, 1949; Baylor et al., 1984). The same correspondence is found for the spectral sensitivities of the cones. The action spectra obtained by direct physiological recording (Baylor et al., 1987; Schnapf et al., 1987; Baylor, 1987) match those estimated from psychophysics (e.g., Vos, 1978).

2. Dark Light

While isomerization of only a single rhodopsin molecule is required to elicit an electrical response in a rod, coincident isomerizations in roughly 5 to 10 rods are needed to detect a dim flash reliably (Hecht et al., 1942). This limitation can at least partly be explained by the instability of rhodopsin in darkness. The greater the number of extraneous signals a rod generates in the dark, the more difficult it is to distinguish light-evoked responses from spontaneous events. Measurements in complete darkness show that, at random, about once every 160 sec, rods spontaneously produce a signal that is indistinguishable from a photon-elicited event (Baylor et al., 1984). This estimate of the "dark light" equivalent of receptor noise confirms the surprisingly accurate estimates from psychophysical data (Barlow, 1957). Experiments measuring dark light in rods of the toad as a function of temperature support the hypothesis that these signals arise from thermally activated isomerization of rhodopsin (Baylor, Matthews & Yau, 1983). From the rate of these events in monkey rods and the number of rhodopsin molecules per rod (about 100 million) it is estimated that spontaneous isomerization of a rhodopsin molecule takes place, on the average, about once every 600 years. So, while rhodopsin can be "triggered" by only a single photon, it is also incredibly stable, just what is required for reliable detection of dim light.

This low rate of false signals, nonetheless, appears to be detected by our visual system. The "dark light" level that can be derived from psychophysical experiments is about -2.6 log scotopic td, or roughly one isomerization per rod every 100 sec. This value is close to the dark light measured in the monkey rod. It should be noted, however, that the dark light values measured psychophysically in different subjects vary by as much as a factor of 16 (Aguilar & Stiles, 1954; Barlow, 1957). Moreover, there is also some uncertainty about the quantitative assumptions required to relate photons incident on the cornea to isomerizations per rod. This makes it difficult to determine the extent to which other sources of noise in the visual system may also contribute to the psychophysical estimates. It is clear, though, that spontaneous isomerizations play an important role. For example, experiments by Copenhagen, Donner, and Reuter (1987) indicate that threshold responses in ganglion cells of the toad are limited by spontaneous isomerizations in the rods. Furthermore, behavioral experiments (Aho, Donner, Hyden, Larsen & Reuter, 1988) show that toads are more successful in detecting prey (under dim light conditions) when their body temperature, and hence the noise level, was lowered. This suggests that dark light may well be the limiting factor determining the dark-adapted contrast threshold.

Dark light in cones has not received much attention, neither in physiological nor in psychophysical studies (but see Barlow, 1958a). One of the reasons for this might be that cones operate at light levels where noise (at least photon noise) is less relevant than in scotopic vision. However, in visual discrimination tasks involving stimuli bordering on the spatial and/or temporal resolution of the visual system, the signal-to-noise ratio becomes just as relevant as in dark adaptation. It is estimated, although this is no more than an educated guess, that the dark light of the cones is of the order of 1 to 10 photopic td, or 10 to 100 isomerizations per cone per second. However, a comparison with physiological estimates from single cone responses is not yet available.

3. Stimulus–Response Characteristic

The waveform of the photon response can be visualized by averaging a large number of responses to dim flashes. The rod response rises slowly to a peak in about 200 msec and then decays back to baseline. Responses from the three kinds of cones are different from that of the rods but are similar to one another; they all rise to a peak in about 55 msec. The cone response is further distinguished from that of the rod by a prominent undershoot in the current before return to the dark level (Fig. 19). This undershoot gives the response a characteristic "resonance" of about 5 Hz. In other words if a cone were stimulated by sinusoidally modulated light, the amplitude of the modulation of the cone's response would be maximal for a frequency of the modulation of about 5 Hz; frequencies greater or less than this would be less effective. The rod, on the other hand, would respond maximally to all frequencies less than about 3 Hz, while higher frequencies would be progressively less effective. This would be consistent, then, with temporal characteristics of scotopic and photopic vision derived from measurements of the sensitivity of the human observer to sinusoidally flickering lights (e.g., Kelly, 1972b).

As the strength of a flash of light increases, the size of the photoreceptor response increases monotonically to some maximal value; further increases in flash strength produce no further increases in peak amplitude but do increase the duration of the response (Fig. 20A). For brief flashes of light, the relationship between photon density, i (in photons μm^{-2}), and the

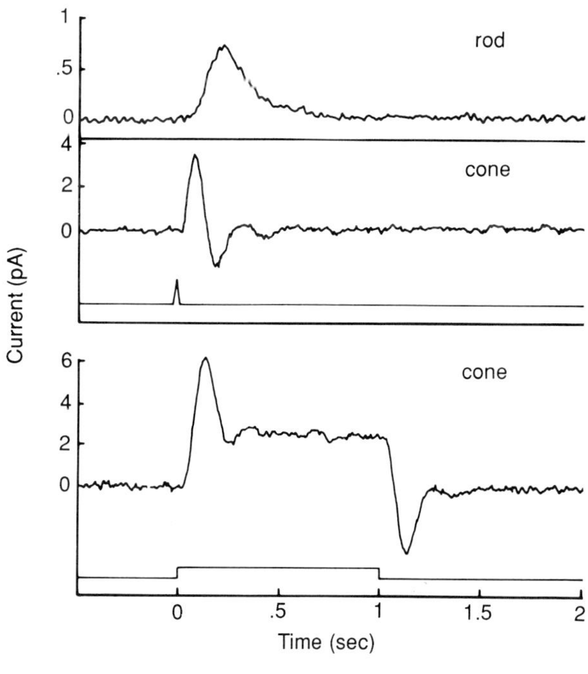

Fig. 19 Waveform of the single photon response in a monkey rod (top) and cone (middle). The average change in membrane current is plotted as a function of time after a brief flash. Flashes isomerized, on average, 1 pigment molecule in the rod and 200 in the cone. The responses are scaled versions of the single photon effects in the two cells. The bottom trace is the cone's response to a 1 sec pulse of light evoking roughly 5000 isomerizations/sec. This response corresponds to the time integral of the response to a flash. From Schnapf and Baylor (1987). Copyright © April 1987 by *Scientific American*. All rights reserved

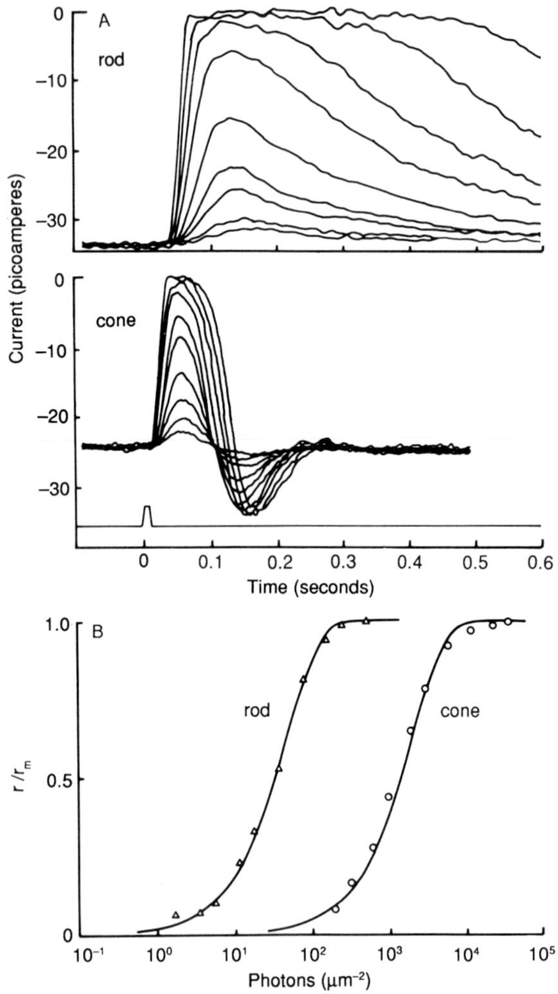

Fig. 20 Flash responses in a rod and a cone of the monkey retina. (A) Families of superimposed responses to flashes of increasing strength. In each successive trace the flash strength has been increased by a factor of about 2. From Schnapf and Baylor (1987). (B) Peak amplitude of the flash response as a function of photon density for light of 490 nm (rod) and 560 nm (cone). The smooth curves are generated by Eq. (12).

amplitude of the response at the peak, r (in pA), is given by

$$r/r_m = 1 - \exp(-ki) \qquad (12)$$

where r_m is the amplitude of the maximal response and k is a scalar. The value of r_m is about 35 pA. The value of k determines the range of photon densities over which the photoreceptor can signal; it varies from cell to cell and is also a function of wavelength. When plotted on a log photon density scale, functions with differing k values are simply slid along the abscissa while retaining their shape. Figure 20B shows such stimulus–response functions, respectively, for a ("red") cone and a rod in the macaque retina. The photon densities are given for light striking the outer segment perpendicular to its long axis (see Fig. 17) and at wavelengths to which each cell was found to be maximally sensitive (560 nm for the cone and 490 nm for the rod). Note that when the flash is brief relative to the duration of the response, the input may be considered an impulse. When the system is behaving linearly, the response to the impulse (containing all possible frequencies) may be used to calculate the response to any input by convolution of the response with the input waveform. For long duration steps of light this is simply the time integral of the flash response.

While the ability of rods and cones to absorb incident light at their respective optimal wavelengths is approximately equal, more light is needed to elicit a response of a given size in a cone than in a rod. In Fig. 20B the rod requires roughly 40 times less light than the cone to elicit a criterion response; averaged over a large number of rods and cones this factor was about 70. This is close to the ratio of the amplitudes of the photon responses in rods and cones, indicating that the difference in the range of light intensities over which the rods and cones respond is a function of the photon response amplitude. The number of isomerizations (in a short flash) required to elicit a response of half-maximal size is about 30 in a rod and 2000 in a cone, or roughly 25 scotopic td sec and 200 photopic td sec. The observed differences in the flash response of single rods and cones constitute a large part of the difference in the intensity ranges over which the scotopic and photopic systems operate.

4. Rod Light Adaptation

In the presence of a steady background light the sensitivity of the visual system to flashes of light declines with increasing intensity of the background. To examine the effects of light adaptation in single rods, responses to brief flashes of light are measured both in the presence and absence of a steady background. When the background is on, a brighter test flash is required to elicit a response of criterion size; the greater the background intensity, the greater the strength of the flash needed to elicit the criterion flash response. The points in the right portion of Fig. 21 plot the results of the physiological experiments. The background intensity (L) is expressed in photometric units. The ordinate gives the amount of light (ΔL) in the test flash needed to elicit the criterion response, relative to the amount needed in the absence of the background (ΔL_0). For comparison, the curve to the left shows a psychophysically measured t.v.i. function. It is clear that the two t.v.i. functions are quite different from each other.

In the physiological experiments, the test flashes were so dim that the flash responses scaled linearly with flash strength. As a result, the value $\Delta L/\Delta L_0$ is a measure of the reduction in the size of the rod's response to single photons. For example, at a background of 25 scotopic td, $\Delta L/\Delta L_0 = 2$, indicating that the photon response was half its dark-adapted size. This reduction in response size can be largely accounted for by response compression. Response compression (see Fig. 12B) is simply a consequence of the limited number of ion channels in the outer segment that may be closed by light. Photons from the background close some fraction of these channels, making fewer available to be closed by photons from the test flash. Consequently, the size of the quantal response shows diminishing returns; if only 5% of the available channels remain open when the background light is on, then the quantal response amplitude will be reduced by a factor of 20 (Baylor et al., 1984).

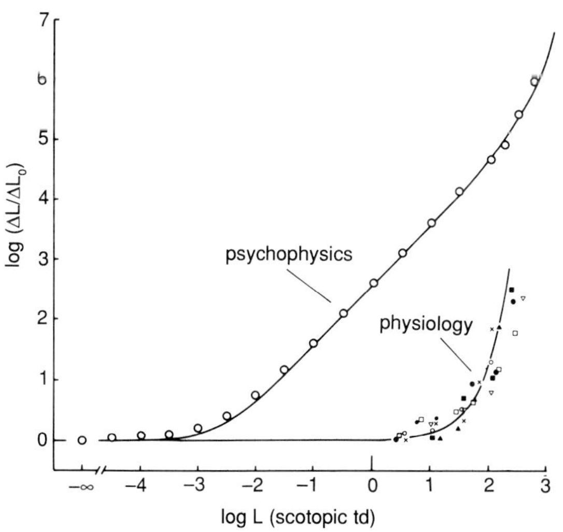

Fig. 21 Psychophysically measured threshold-versus-intensity (t.v.i.) function for the rod *system* and the physiologically derived t.v.i. function for a *single* rod. The physiological data are described by a function based on response compression only (Baylor, Nunn & Schnapf, 1984). The psychophysical t.v.i. function is the same function as shown in Fig. 5.

The smooth curve drawn through the data points plots the desensitization calculated on the basis of response compression. This function starts to rise steeply to infinity when the background drives the rod to its maximum response. It is of interest that this saturation effect occurs in the range of 2–3 log scotopic td, that is, in about the same range where the psychophysical t.v.i. function starts to saturate. It seems very likely, therefore, that the phenomenon of rod saturation reflects response compression at the level of the rods themselves.

While the increment saturation phenomenon exhibited by the psychophysical t.v.i. function may originate in the rods, the overall function clearly does not parallel the size reduction in the rod's photon response. For example, a background of 1 log scotopic td has virtually no effect on the rod response, yet it produces a dramatic elevation in psychophysical threshold. Part of the difference in the two functions may be accounted for by rod noise. Backgrounds that are too dim to affect the size of the rod's photon response nonetheless elicit large fluctuations in the steady level of the membrane current (Fig. 18). The noise is due to the random superposition of responses to photons in the background. This elevation in noise must have a deleterious effect on the visual system's ability to detect small changes in the membrane current evoked by the test flash. Indeed, with certain stimulus configurations, the elevation in rod noise appears to account completely for the elevation in psychophysical threshold (Barlow, 1957). With different stimuli, a gain control mechanism central to the rod outer segment is suggested, but this mechanism may be driven by noise (Barlow, 1964a; Copenhagen et al., 1987).

Although changes in the amplitude of the photon response of the individual rod are not in evidence over most of the range covered by the psychophysical t.v.i. function, both the lower and upper limit of sensitivity control in the rod system may be largely determined by rod "constants," that is, the absolute threshold, determined by spontaneous isomerizations, and the onset of saturation, as a consequence of response compression.

5. Cone Light Adaptation

Preliminary experiments measuring membrane current in macaque cones (Baylor, Nunn & J. Schnapf, unpublished observations) indicate that desensitization of the photopic system occurs at background lights roughly 200 times dimmer than that required to produce comparable reductions in the photon responses of the cones themselves. The exact relationship between cone receptor and cone system sensitivity has yet to be characterized. It is clear, though, that additional postreceptoral mechanisms exist and that cones, as opposed to rods, cannot be saturated by steady backgrounds. Photopigment bleaching, which conveniently stops further increases in light absorption at light levels in excess of about 4 log td (at which the cones still have half their response range left), enables the cones to operate up to the light-damage limit.

In addition to bleaching adaptation, primate cones might also be equipped with other means of multiplicative gain control. But the evidence for such a cellular adaptation mechanism in primates is based only on mass (voltage) responses and appears to be conflicting. It is virtually absent in the earliest recordings (Boynton & Whitten, 1970), but it does show up in the results of Valeton and Van Norren (1983), where it accounts for about 1 log unit in gain.

6. Voltage Recordings

Measurements of outer segment current are useful because they essentially reflect processes occurring only in that single outer segment. It is the membrane potential, however, that controls the rate of release of transmitter molecules signaling second-order cells. The membrane potential of photoreceptors is regulated not only by the light-sensitive conductance in the outer segment, but also by voltage-controlled conductances in the inner segment and synaptic ending, and by synaptic inputs from other cells. Recordings of membrane current made in the manner described above are by and large insensitive to these other factors.

While membrane potentials have not been recorded in single primate photoreceptors, extensive recordings have been made from photoreceptors in lower vertebrates by inserting a fine microelectrode into the interior of the cell and recording the potential difference between the inside and outside. A review of these results (Green, 1986) may provide insights into possible mechanisms that are operating in the primate retina. It should be kept in mind, though, that both quantitative and qualitative interspecies differences exist.

Both rods and cones hyperpolarize to light. The duration of these responses are briefer than the light-evoked changes in outer segment current. The difference is due in part to voltage-dependent conductances, which, when activated by the hyperpolarization, bring the membrane potential back toward the resting dark level (Fain, Quandt, Bastian & Gershenfeld, 1978; Torre & Owen, 1981; Attwell, Werblin & Wilson, 1982; Baden, Bertrand & Schwartz, 1982).

7. Horizontal Cell Feedback

In cones, voltage responses to light are influenced by an additional source of "negative feedback" derived from synaptic input from horizontal cells. Reciprocal chemical synapses link horizontal cells and cones; both cell types act as pre- and postsynaptic elements. The horizontal cell receives synaptic input from hundreds of cones. The light-elicited hyperpolarization of these cones causes the horizontal cell to hyperpolarize. Hyperpolarization of the horizontal cell antagonizes the light response in the cone by eliciting (with a delay) a depolarization in the cones. Since absorption of light in only a few cones is a rather ineffective stimulus for the horizontal cell, the inhibitory action of the horizontal cell on the light response of a cone is only evident when the stimulus is large enough to elicit isomerizations in many adjacent cones (Baylor, Fuortes & O'Bryan, 1971). As a consequence, when the light stimulus is diffuse, the flash response of a cone is briefer, and the steady-state response to a step of light smaller, than that evoked by a small spot of light. The effect of horizontal cell feedback, then, is to emphasize changes in illumination over space and time. Spatially discrete stimuli are more effective than diffuse, and steady-state responses are reduced. So, at the level of the photoreceptors there is already evident a primitive code for spatial and temporal contrast.

8. Receptor Coupling

Photoreceptors are linked directly to one another at their synaptic endings through electrical junctions. Ions are free to move across these junctions so that changes in the membrane potential of one photoreceptor are seen in all the photoreceptors linked into the network. The coupling of signals (as studied in lower vertebrate species) is greatest for cells that are nearest neighbors; the farther two cells are from each other, the less the membrane potential in one cell will influence that of the other. Cones are effectively coupled to each other over a distance of about 50 μm (Detwiler and Hodgkin, 1979); rods are coupled over about 100–200 μm (Copenhagen & Owen, 1980). One effect of rod coupling is that the change in membrane potential in any one rod elicited by a single photoisomerization is reduced because the photocurrent is distributed over 10 or more rods in the network. The photon signal is not lost, however. Neurons postsynaptic to the collection of rods will be able to "regain" the signal by summing synaptic outputs of neighboring rods.

It is not quite clear what advantages, if any, are gained by electrical coupling. One possibility is suggested by the observation, in the toad retina, that the transmission of signals across the rod synapse is nearly saturated when each rod absorbs only one or two photons (Belgum & Copenhagen, 1988). Thus, by distributing the photon response of one rod into many rods in a coupled network, saturation of any one synapse can be avoided at low light levels when on average less than one photon is absorbed per rod. The disadvantage of coupling is clear: loss of fine spatial resolution.

Photoreceptors of like kind couple strongly to each other: red cones to red cones, rods to rods, etc. (Baylor & Hodgkin, 1973; Detwiler & Hodgkin, 1979). However, rods and cones may be coupled together as well (Schwartz, 1975; Nelson, 1977; Attwell, Wilson & Wu, 1984). It is not known if photoreceptors in the primate retina are functionally coupled to one another or receive horizontal cell feedback; anatomical similarities in the synapses of primates and lower vertebrates would suggest that they probably do. Furthermore, the psychophysical evidence, particularly from studies slowing color-specific spatial interactions (e.g., Alpern & Rushton, 1965; DuCroz & Rushton, 1966), suggests a retinal architecture in which cones with the same spectral tuning are electrically coupled.

B. Retinal Interneurons

The receptor signals discussed in the previous section are transmitted to at least two kinds of retinal interneurons, bipolar and horizontal cells. These cells respond to inputs with graded membrane potential changes. Common to all vertebrates is that the main flow of retinal information is directed inward, from receptors in the outer retina, via the bipolar cells, toward ganglion cells in the inner retina. Horizontal cells, situated closely to the receptors, and a third kind of interneuron, the amacrine cell, close to the ganglion cells, provide pathways for lateral interactions in the outer and inner plexiform layers, respec-

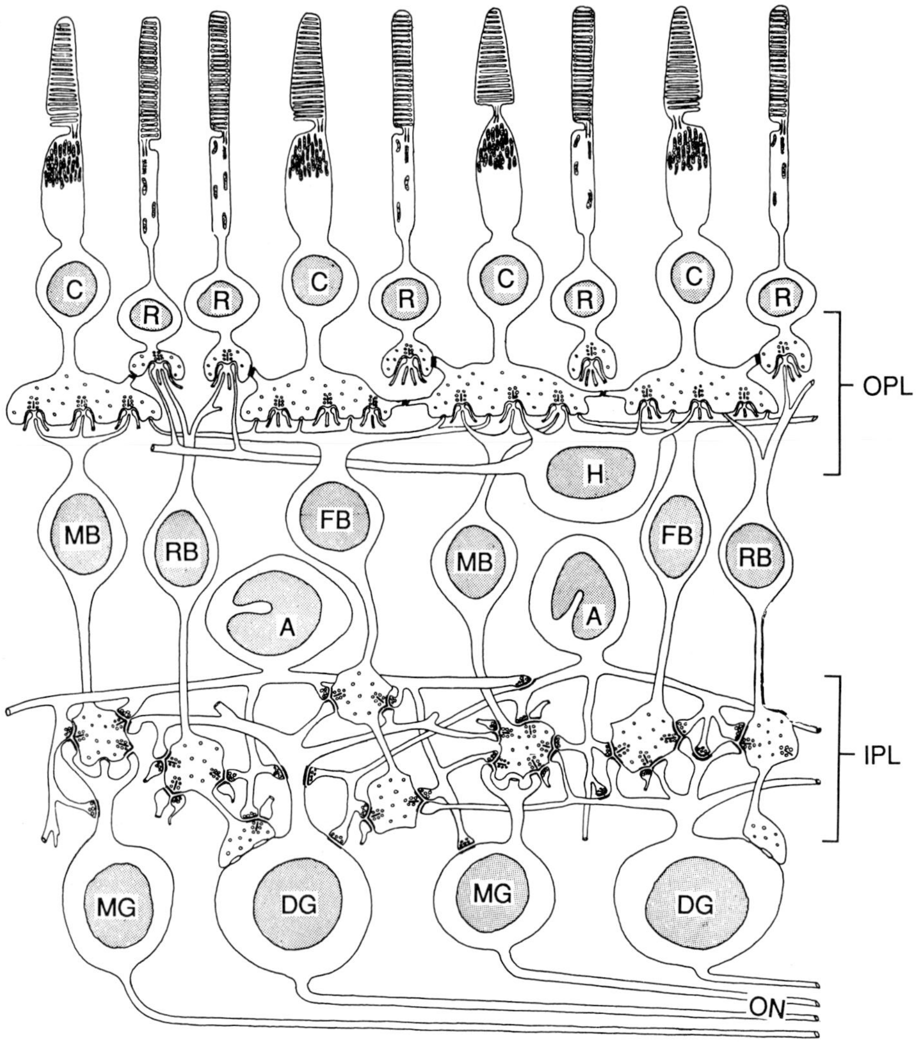

Fig. 22 Diagram of the principal elements in the primate retina. R, Rod; C, cone; MB, midget bipolar; FB, flat bipolar; H, horizontal cell; A, amacrine cell; MG, midget ganglion cell; DG, diffuse ganglion cell; ON, optic nerve fibers; OPL, outer plexiform layer; IPL, inner plexiform layer. From Dowling and Boycott (1966), with slight revision by Professor Boycott.

tively. Figure 22 shows a diagram of the primate retinal architecture.

Of all the vertebrate retinal neurons only the ganglion cells transmit information by means of classical "all-or-none" action potentials or spikes. Most ganglion cells, at least in the cat and in primates, also produce action potentials, at a more or less irregular rate, in complete darkness. Interestingly, maintained firing also occurs when the retina is illuminated uniformly by steady light. So, in most cells, a stimulus that does not vary in time or space will elicit only a maintained ganglion cell discharge. Under natural conditions this usually does not occur, because eye movements cause the retinal image to sweep over the receptor mosaic. However, in the physiological preparation, in which the eye is usually immobilized, modulation of the retinal illumination is used to elicit ganglion cell *responses*, as manifested by *changes* (increase *or* decrease) in the frequency of the maintained firing.

In order to understand retinal mechanisms of (human) visual adaptation, it would be best to have reliable information about the adaptive properties of interneurons in the eye of mammals, preferably primates. Unfortunately, all we have is scant information from the cat. The major problem is that mammalian interneurons in general are quite small. This makes it difficult to obtain stable intracellular recordings from intact mammals for the prolonged times required to collect reliable data on adaptive behavior.

One investigator, Steinberg (1971), did succeed early in doing this. His data on cat horizontal cells are still the best available on the adaptive behavior of any cat interneurons. In experiments with stimulus conditions so chosen that the horizontal cells were driven exclusively by rods, Steinberg showed that the decline in incremental gain followed Weber's law over roughly 2 log units. However, this Weber-type behavior started at backgrounds 2–4 log units higher than those at which the rod-driven retinal ganglion cells entered their Weber region. Steinberg's results suggest that cat rods behave differently from primate rods (see previous Section IV, A, 4) in that cat rods may not be entirely without gain control. Sakmann and Filion (1972) reached a similar conclusion by comparing the adaptive behavior of cat retinal ganglion cells and late rod receptor potentials.

Since the introduction of the perfused isolated cat eye preparation (Gouras & Hoff, 1970; Niemeyer & Gouras, 1973), intracellular recordings also have been obtained from bipolar cells and from several of the more than 20 morphologically different kinds of amacrine cells which have been described in the cat (Kolb & Nelson, 1984). Intracellular recordings from retinal interneurons have also been obtained from the isolated eye cup of primates (Dacheux & Raviola, 1988). However, with the exception of Steinberg's horizontal cell results, there is hardly any quantitative information about how stimulus–response relationships in cat or primate interneurons change with mean retinal illumination. It is therefore necessary to look for such information in data from cold-blooded vertebrates, many of which have large interneurons. Moreover, the cold-blooded eye cup preparation is relatively easy to maintain for prolonged periods of time in acceptable functional condition. This preparation has been used by many investigators as a rich source for quantitative information about adaptive behavior of retinal interneurons (Dowling, 1987). However, linking the adaptive behavior of retinal neurons in species like mud puppy, skate, and frog, perhaps "via" the cat and subhuman primates, to psychophysical phenomena in humans has its problems. In the following some examples of such difficulties are discussed.

In both cold- and warm-blooded species, bipolar cells come in two varieties: they either depolarize or hyperpolarize when the light is increased in the center of their receptive fields (Werblin & Dowling, 1969; Kaneko, 1970; Matsumoto & Naka, 1972; Schwartz, 1974; Dacheux & Miller, 1981; Kolb & Nelson, 1984). In mud puppy it is well established (Werblin & Dowling, 1969) that both kinds of bipolars have surrounds which, in response to a flash, antagonize the center's response. Burkhardt (1974) and Thibos and Werblin (1978a, b) determined stimulus–response relationships for small flashes delivered to the center of the receptive fields of mud puppy bipolar cells, while exposing more peripheral portions of their fields to increasing amounts of steady light. Thibos and Werblin found a shift of the stimulus–response curves to the right along the log intensity axis, consistent with a decrease in retinal gain (multiplicative adaptation) at the bipolar cell level. This study differed somewhat from that of Burkhardt with regard to the spatial distribution and the intensities of the steady lights that were employed. Even so, it is surprising that Burkhardt found the opposite effect, namely, "sensitization" rather than a decrease in gain. In the cat, although bipolar cells are known to be either of the depolarizing or hyperpolarizing kind, only one (depolarizing) bipolar cell type, one which is contacted by cones only, has been shown to possess an antagonizing surround (Kolb & Nelson, 1984); experiments with steady adapting lights do not appear to have been done on cat bipolars.

Thus, not only are some data on stimulus–response relationships during exposure of the surround to steady lights in one particular cold-blooded species inherently puzzling, but we do not even know whether the receptive fields of the presumably corresponding bipolars in the cat have an antagonistic surround that responds to steady light. These kinds of problems (which are not restricted to the consideration of bipolar cells) should be kept in mind when discussing the retinal mechanisms which may underlie visual adaptation. It is important to realize that although the general principles of retinal circuitry are much the same in all cold- and warm-blooded vertebrates, the anatomical and physiological details are not.

Detailed descriptions of receptor, bipolar, horizontal, amacrine, and ganglion cells go back to Cajal (1892) and Polyak (1941). Not until considerably later did anatomists and physiologists become interested in yet another type of retinal interneuron, the interplexiform cell (not shown in Fig. 22). It was described and named in the cat by Gallego (1971), but interplexiform cells are found in both cold- and warm-blooded species, including man (Linberg & Fisher, 1986). At first, these cells were considered to be very scarce, an opinion which many authors no longer hold. (For a brief history see Boycott, Dowling, Fisher, Kolb & Laties, 1975; Linberg and Fisher, 1986). The common "trademark" of interplexiform cells is that they are postsynaptic in the inner plexiform layer, presynaptic in the outer plexiform layer, and may be both pre- and postsynaptic in both plexiform layers. They should thus be particularly well suited to participate in the regulation of retinal gain, since they can provide pathways for feedback signals between retinal layers (see Fig. 22). However, their exact role in retinal adaptation is presently even less well known than the role of other interneurons in mammalian retinas.

C. Retinal Ganglion Cells

Whatever the role of the retinal interneurons, the information extracted from the retinal image has to travel to the brain via the ganglion cells, the output neurons of the retina. The rest of this section is primarily devoted to the adaptive behavior of center–surround organized on- and off-center cells of the kind Kuffler described (1952, 1953) and which, on the basis of different spatial summation properties, later were divided into X- and Y-cells (Enroth-Cugell & Robson, 1966) or "brisk sustained" and "brisk transient" cells in the terminology of Cleland and Levick (1974a). Only adaptation with lights too weak to bleach a significant amount of photopigment is dealt with. These Kuffler cells, which have mutually antagonistic center and surround regions, may help us establish some correlations between retinal neurophysiology in the cat and perception in man. However, there is the complication that (in both cat and primate) the Kuffler cells constitute only a portion of all the existing functional retinal ganglion cell types. In the cat, X- and Y-cells constitute roughly 60% of all the retinal ganglion cells. The adaptive properties of all the other types are almost entirely unknown, but it is likely, in view of their central connections, that they play a less prominent role in conscious visual perception.

1. Sensitivity and Gain Control

Barlow and Levick (1969) studied how the sensitivity of cat retinal ganglion cells varied as a function of background illumination with the specific aim of determining the importance of three factors: (1) noise, that is, the irregularity of the maintained firing, (2) temporal integration, and (3) gain. Their conclusion was that gain was the most important factor in determining a cell's increment sensitivity over many log units of adapting backgrounds. One may expect, therefore, a strong link between physiologically measured gain and psychophysically measured sensitivity, even if sensitivity may reflect the effects of both noise and gain (cf. Section III).

In electrophysiological experiments analogous to Crawford's (1947) psychophysical experiments (see Fig. 14, Section III, E, 4), Enroth-Cugell and Shapley (1973a) determined the time course of the gain change of rod-driven (presumed) Y-cells. They found that the gain decreased approximately by a factor of two during the first 100 msec after the onset of an adapting background. Saito and Fukada (1986), who carried out very similar experiments on X- and Y-cells under both scotopic and mesopic conditions, reported a similar time course. These retinal ganglion cell results agree rather well with results from psychophysical experiments in which, under comparable conditions, 90% of the inferred gain change was established within 200 msec (e.g., Adelson, 1982; Shapley, 1986).

How vital for the cat's retinal ganglion cells their gain changing ability is becomes evident when realizing that, as the cat goes about his or her nightly and daily business, the retinal illumination changes over at least a 7 log unit range (see also Fig. 1). How is a ganglion cell, that can alter its firing rate by only little more than 2 log units, going to signal changes in illumination over that kind of a range? The solution to the problem is shown in Fig. 23. A multiplicative gain mechanism moves the cell's entire stimulus–response curve, parallel and to the right, along the stimulus axis. This mechanism of range adjustment, which may also be observed beyond the ganglion cell level (Jacobs, 1965; Virsu & Lee, 1983), may explain at least part of the sensitivity change traced by the psychophysical t.v.i. function.

If the amount (in log units) by which the stimulus–response curve in Fig. 23 shifts to the right were to exactly correspond to the amount by which the background luminance was increased (proportional gain adjustment), then the cell would obey Weber's law. Actually, the shifts shown in Fig. 23 are somewhat less than demanded by Weber's law, that is, about 0.7 (instead of 1) log unit per log unit change of background luminance. If, on the basis of these results, one were to describe how the gain determines the increment threshold, one would arrive at t.v.i. function with a slope of 0.7. In fact, it has been shown that the t.v.i. function, as measured under (mesopic) conditions comparable to those applying to the data of Fig. 23, indeed has a slope of 0.7 (Mansfield, 1976). Why Weber's law fails under these conditions and holds under others is still subject to speculation. Psychophysical data obtained in cat horizontal cell data

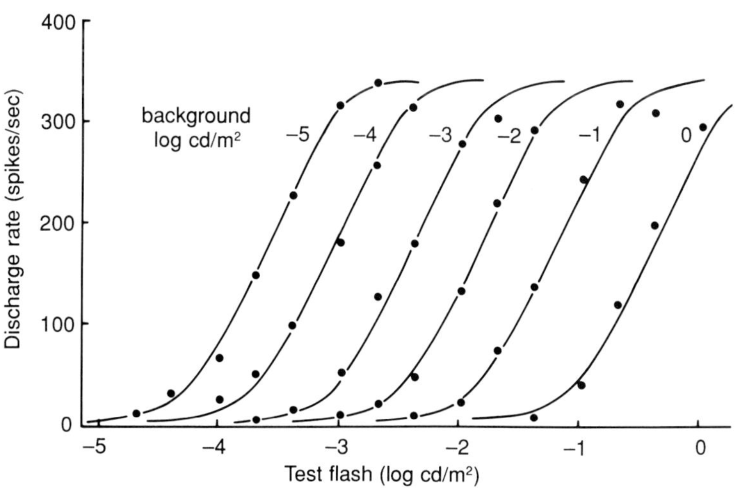

Fig. 23 Stimulus–response curves from a cat on-center cell obtained against various steady backgrounds. From Sakmann and Creutzfeldt (1969).

(Steinberg, 1971), and cat retinal ganglion cell data (Enroth-Cugell & Shapley, 1973a) all follow Weber's law over some range when employing the conventional rod isolation technique (Aguilar & Stiles, 1954), i.e. red backgrounds and a blue–green test stimulus. In view of the results of Sharpe *et al.* (1989), as discussed above (Section IIIA, 1), it would be interesting to see whether Weber's law would still be in evidence when backgrounds are used that produce relatively less cone stimulation.

2. Importance of Flux

What aspect of the light that falls on the retina determines the ganglion cell's response magnitude and gain? Hartline (1940), who was the first to record from single vertebrate retinal ganglion cells, provided the data to answer the first part of that question. That is, as Barlow (1953) phrased it: "Hartline found that the discharge of an optic nerve fiber was determined by the quantity of light falling in its receptive field (Ricco's law). It made little difference if the light was concentrated on one or two receptor cells or if it was spread out over many!" In other words, it is not illumination as such, but flux, the product of illumination and area, that determines the cell's response. It is now generally accepted that for cat retinal ganglion cells the same holds true with regard to steady lights (Cleland & Enroth-Cugell, 1968; Enroth-Cugell & Shapley, 1973b; Enroth-Cugell, Lennie & Shapley, 1975).

The importance of flux leads to a number of testable predictions. One prediction is that area and retinal illumination should (within limits) be interchangeable if the illumination is weighted by the spatial distribution of the gain within the region covered by the adapting field. (For spatial distribution of gain, see below.) It has been shown that cat retinal ganglion cells behave as predicted in this respect (see Shapley & Enroth-Cugell, 1984). Another consequence of the "flux-rule" is that at any one level of uniform adapting illumination, cells with large centers should become more light adapted than cells with small centers. Enroth-Cugell and Shapley (1973b), working in the scotopic range and using small flashing spots in the middle of the receptive field, found that this was indeed the case. More recently Linsenmeier, Frishman, Jakiela, and Enroth-Cugell (1982) deduced the gain for a large population of X- and Y-cells using sinusoidal grating patterns and mesopic retinal illumination. Their results and those of others (Fischer & May, 1970; Cleland, Levick & Sanderson, 1973) support the notion that at any one ambient illumination level, large receptive field centers are more light adapted than small centers. However, Cleland (1983) has since raised doubts that the gain of X-cell centers depends on center size.

Another question regarding the receptive field properties of cat retinal ganglion cells is whether or not center and surround mechanisms adapt independently of each other. There is fairly robust evidence, summarized by Shapley and Enroth-Cugell (1984), that the surround is not involved in regulating the gain of Y-cell centers, and this applies also to X-cells under scotopic and mesopic conditions (see also Saito & Fukada, 1986). That is, neither "desensitization" nor "sensitization" of the center mechanism has been observed as a result of subjecting the surround to steady lights. Less is known about the surround's effect, or lack thereof, on the center mechanism of cone-driven X-cells. There is evidence from one X-cell (Lennie, Hertz & Enroth-Cugell, published in Shapley & Enroth-Cugell, 1984) that when a steady background field of fixed retinal illumination is increased in size beyond the summing area of the center mechanism, there is a small increase in the gain of the center. Since intracellular recordings from cat bipolar cells have demonstrated an antagonistic surround in one type of cone bipolar cell, although not in any rod bipolars, one might speculate that in X-cells, driven by cones, gain is influenced by bipolars with an antagonistic surround.

3. Contrast Processing

It has long been understood that the luminance of a surface is meaningless when not placed in the context of illumination (Helmholtz, 1867). The implication that contrast should be the main determinant of (constant) lightness perception (See Section IIC and IIIA, 4, 5) has also been recognized for some time (e.g., Hering, 1920, quoted from Heinemann, 1955), even if the explicit formulation and testing of this notion is of rather recent date (Wallach, 1948). Yet, it was not until the mid-1980s that ganglion cell responses were measured over an adequate range of both contrasts and overall light levels, using stimuli which, like most stimuli in the natural visual world, involve the entire receptive field of ganglion cells. The last part of this section describes the results of such experiments, in relation to Rodieck's (1965) model for the center–surround organization of the ganglion cell's receptive field.

To learn what role the retinal signal plays in various aspects of vision one needs to know how ganglion cells respond, not only to one particular stimulus, such as a small flashing spot in the center of the cell's receptive field, but to any arbitrary stimulus. If we know how the cell's response to small spots varies as a function of stimulus position within the receptive field, and if the signals elicited at different positions combine linearly, then it is possible to predict the cell's response to any arbitrary spatiotemporal pattern. Rodieck and Stone (1965), following the work of Wagner, MacNichol, and Wolbarsht (1963) on goldfish, used small flashing light spots to map the spatial distribution of responsiveness within the receptive fields of Kuffler cells in the cat. Based on these and other results, they proposed the first model for cat ganglion cell receptive fields (see also Chapters 6, 7, and 8). They suggested that one can treat the center and the surround of a Kuffler cell as two distinct response mechanisms, each having its own summing area and generating its own response component or signal, and that these two signals combine linearly to determine the cell's response. They suggested that the form of spatial distribution of gain within each mechanism could be approximated by a Gaussian surface and that the volume under each surface represents that mechanism's total integrated gain. The difference between the two Gaussians (sometimes referred to as a "Mexican hat") was taken to describe the gain distribution within the cell's receptive field. According to this model (Rodieck, 1965) the spatial distribution of gain within a receptive field can be roughly estimated by recording responses to spot stimuli in different positions. However, accurately measuring the amplitude of small responses to many spots in a population of cells is a near-impossible task.

Sinusoidal gratings (see Fig. 24) lend themselves better than arrays of small spots to the experimental determination of the spatial distribution of gain within receptive fields. Another useful feature of grating stimuli is that, to a certain extent, one can use them to "tease apart" the contributions of the center and the surround to the cell's response (Enroth-Cugell & Robson, 1984). To elicit a response from ganglion cells the grating stimulus has to be temporally modulated (see the discussion in Section IV, B on maintained discharge). One way of doing this is to reverse the contrast of the grating according to a sinusoidal time course, as indicated in Fig. 24B.

The upper two tracings in Fig. 24C show vertical sections (along one receptive field axis) through the center's tall and narrow and the surround's low and wide Gaussian gain distribution surfaces. The solid curve is the difference between the upper two and thus represents the distribution of gain within the cell's receptive field, as a function of distance along one axis. Considering these gain profiles together with the three luminance profiles of sinusoidal gratings (1, 2, and 3) leads to the following insight: at low spatial frequency (1), each bar of the grating is wide enough to span the entire summing area of center and surround alike, and, thus, as the contrast is reversed (Fig. 24B) each mechanism generates a large signal. However, because the light increases and decreases over both the center and the surround in synchrony, and the two mechanisms antagonize each other, the cell's response will be small. That is, the cell's gain can be expected to be low at low spatial frequencies. As spatial frequency is increased (gratings 2 and 3), a frequency will be reached such that contrast reversal will cause receptors under neighboring grating bars to generate signals of opposite sign. These signals will thus, within each individual response mechanism, partially

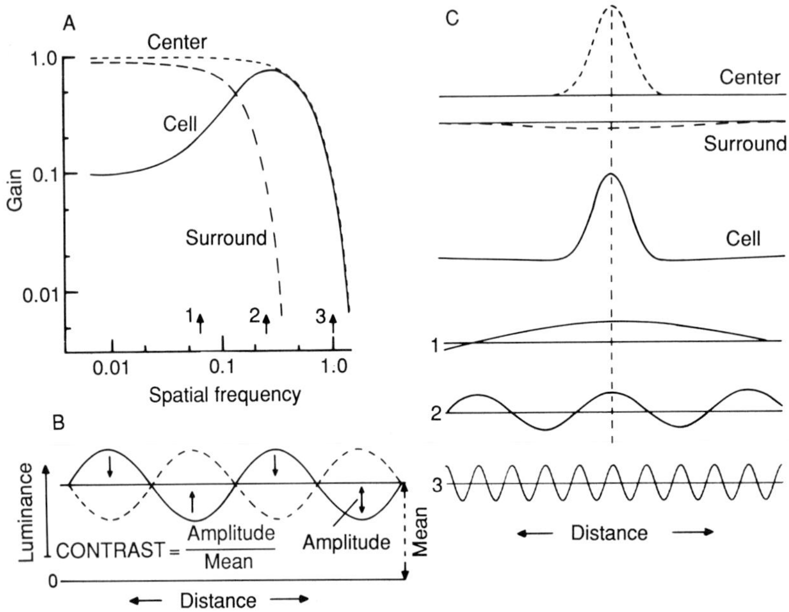

Fig. 24 Receptive field model (after Rodieck, 1965) of retinal ganglion cells with a mutually antagonistic center–surround organization. In C the two uppermost (dashed) profiles represent the distribution of the center's and the surround's gain, as a function of distance, along one receptive field diameter. Their difference, the solid curve, is the cell's gain profile. In A the solid curve represents the cell's relative gain (responsivity) as a function of spatial frequency and corresponds to the difference between the center's and the surround's relative gains. In the lower part of C are shown luminance profiles of sinusoidal grating stimuli of low (1), medium (2), and high (3) spatial frequency. Note that the peak of the cell's gain profile and the peaks of one grating cycle are lined up. In experiments these gratings are temporally modulated by contrast reversal, as illustrated in B.

cancel each other. Because the surround's summing area is so much larger than that of the center, cancellation will become complete within the surround at a lower spatial frequency than within the center. At that frequency, the surround will cease generating an antagonizing input to the cell.

Turning to Fig. 24A, notice that each dashed curve is half the Fourier transform (Weisstein, 1980) of the corresponding gain profile in C. That is, in A we are looking at gain (integrated over center and surround), not as a function of distance as in C but as a function of spatial frequency. Again, the solid curve in A is the difference between the two broken curves. Figure 24A and C actually show the same profile, but in different ways. That is, for a sinusoidal grating of low spatial frequency, which is not much different from a uniform field (as seen in C), the gains of both the center and the surround mechanisms are high and almost equal. As spatial frequency increases, the surround's gain begins to fall off earlier than that of the center, resulting in a lower cutoff frequency for the surround. The overall gain is low at spatial frequencies where the gains of the two mechanisms are almost equal, because the center and surround oppose each other as far as their effect on the cell's firing rate is concerned. At the highest spatial frequencies the cell's response is almost entirely determined by the center (e.g., at the frequency labeled 3), because now the surround's gain has fallen to almost zero.

Kuffler cells respond better to contrast at some spatial frequencies than at others. If the model in Fig. 24 holds, then this spatial selectivity is a consequence of center–surround antagonism at low spatial frequencies, and the cells high-frequency cutoff must be set by the diameter of the center's summing area. An example of this spatial selectivity is shown for a Y-cell in the insets of Fig. 25. For X-cells the general shape of such spatial tuning curves is similar. However, at any one retinal location, the diameters of the central summing area of Y-cells are larger than those of X-cells (e.g., Peichl & Wässle, 1979). The latter are able, therefore, to resolve higher spatial frequencies than Y-cells in that same location. Another important aspect of the spatial selectivity of X- and Y-cells is

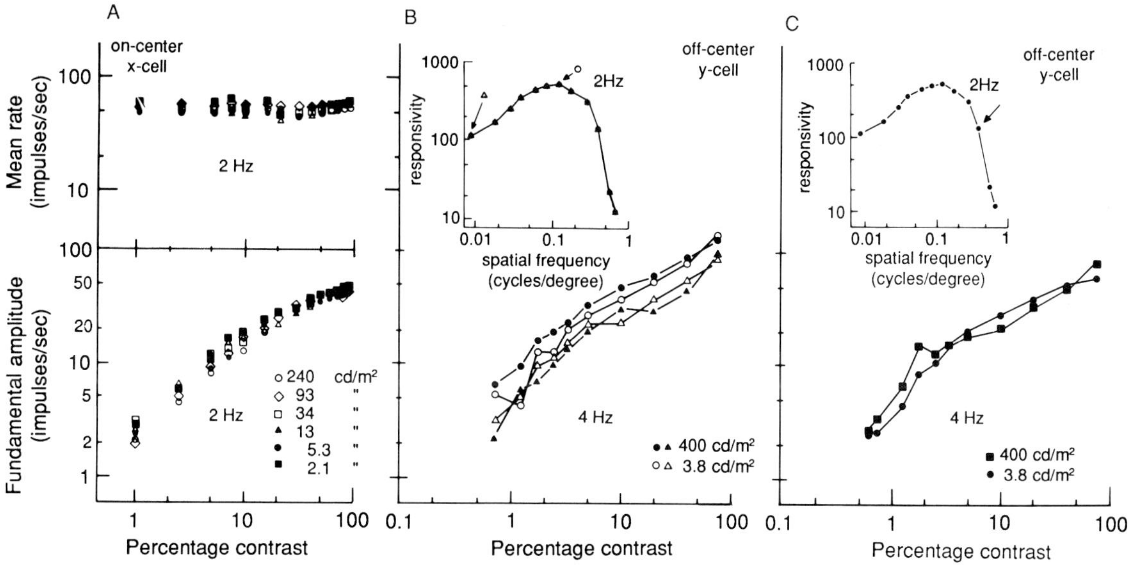

Fig. 25 Recordings from single fibers in the optic nerve of two cat retinal ganglion cells stimulated with sinusoidal grating patterns. Data shown in B and C are from the same cell. The grating stimuli were sinusoidally modulated in time at the rates indicated. The cells responded by modulating their discharge in synchrony with the stimulus. On the vertical axis of the insets in B and C, "responsivity" represents the slope of the stimulus (contrast)–response curve in the region of low contrast. In the lower half of A the vertical axis gives the cell's mean firing rate during stimulation at the same mean luminances and contrasts as in the upper half of A. In A the spatial frequency at which the cell's responsivity was at a maximum was used. In B and C the insets show gain (or responsivity) as a function of spatial frequency. The arrows indicate the spatial frequencies used to determine the response versus contrast curves. The luminances shown in the figure refer to the mean luminance of the grating. From Troy et al., (1987); © 1987 IEEE.

the interdependence of the spatial and temporal properties of these cells (Derrington & Lennie, 1982; Enroth-Cugell, Robson, Schweitzer-Tong & Watson, 1983; Frishman, Freeman, Troy, Schweitzer-Tong & Enroth-Cugell, 1987). As the cat moves around in his or her natural habitat, and the ambient illumination changes, neither the maximum sensitivity to contrast of X- and Y-cells nor the character of their spatial selectivity changes significantly until the retinal illumination falls to scotopic levels and/or a change occurs in the temporal frequency at which the visual scene stimulates the cat's retina (Derrington & Lennie, 1982).

From Fig. 24 it should be clear that, by using grating stimili which cover the entire receptive field, the experimenter can choose whether to drive the cell with the center mechanism alone or with both mechanisms. Yet another advantage of using grating stimuli is that it is easy to vary the mean luminance (which changes the level of adaptation) over a wide range while the contrast remains constant. Inserting neutral filters of different densities in front of the stimulator will do just that, because such filters reduce the amplitude and the mean of the sinusoidal pattern by the same factor. From the discussion in Section III, it follows that such changes in overall illumination should not much affect the cell's response, because multiplicative gain control (i.e., "dark-glasses") adaptation, will compensate for variations in illumination.

Next, some experiments are described in which sinusoidal grating stimuli were used at different levels of adaptation over a contrast range of 0 to 100% (Troy, Enroth-Cugell & Robson, 1987). Figure 25 shows the response of one X- and one Y-cell to gratings of fixed spatial and temporal frequencies, but varying mean luminance levels was measured.

The cells were tested with frequencies that mainly stimulated the center or both the center and the surround. The major message of these data is as follows: whether the ganglion cell is driven predominantly by the center (Fig. 25, A and open and filled circles in B), by the center alone (C), or nearly equally by the center and surround (filled and open triangles in B), it is contrast, not absolute changes in retinal illumination, that primarily determines the response amplitude. For example, note that for the open circles in A the absolute value of the modulation of the retinal illumination is more than 100 times larger than for the filled squares, yet the two curves coincide over almost the entire contrast range. Very similar results were obtained from 9 additional X-cells and 7 Y-cells. It is also worth noting that over the whole 2 log units of mean retinal illumination used in this experiment, the mean firing rate (Fig. 25A) of the cell remained virtually unchanged. This held for all X-cells tested. This is the expected result of a (multiplicative) gain control that responds to changes in illumination level with commensurate changes in the gain factor.

As discussed in foregoing sections, the visual system should respond to luminance relations (i.e., contrast), rather than absolute levels of illumination, in order to register an invariant world. It is clear from Fig. 25, which shows the ganglion cell response to vary only with contrast, that this is indeed what happens. The observed invariance of the contrast response, over a wide range of illumination, represents a physiological correlate of lightness constancy. So far, the retinal ganglion cell data allow only conclusions with respect to the mesopic and photopic range. However, Pasternak and Merigan (1981), who measured cat contrast sensitivity as a function of spatial frequency with behavioral methods, used mean luminances in the mid-mesopic to scotopic range. Their behavioral results were qualitatively very similar to what is found in man under comparable conditions, that is, a progressive decrease in contrast sensitivity with decreasing scotopic luminance levels. The only difference between the two species is that, at all levels, the cat's contrast sensitivity is lower than that of man and shifted toward lower spatial frequencies. There are thus some basic similarities between the dependence of human and cat contrast sensitivity on state of adaptation. The ongoing work by Purpura, Kaplan, and Shapley (1988) on contrast gain of retinal ganglion cells in our closer relative, the macaque monkey, holds further promise for the interfacing of animal neurophysiology and human psychophysics.

V. THE SITES OF VISUAL ADAPTATION: INTEGRATING PSYCHOPHYSICAL AND PHYSIOLOGICAL FINDINGS

In Section III we saw how psychophysical experiments provide information on some of the basic characteristics of the mechanisms subserving the visual system's sensitivity control and, also, how this information can be used to model the action of these mechanisms and indicate their sequential arrangement. Then, in Section IV, we used electrophysiological and anatomical findings to trace the visual signal through the retina. Clearly, these two approaches to visual adaptation—the physiological and the purely psychophysical approach—should generate mutually consistent accounts of the visual system. It is as if we were mapping the same piece of terrain using two different methods, one, say, using measurements from the ground, and the other, from the air. In such an enterprise it is essential to keep relating the two sets of data to each other. This permits consistency checks, but also, and more important, it allows us to transfer knowledge from one domain to the other by using as reference points landmarks that have been identified in both domains. Accordingly, in this section we try to bring the psychophysical and the physiological–anatomical maps into register by noting the structural implications of the psychophysically documented characteristics of the adaptation process. As in previous sections, though, this structural focus will provide a framework for discussing the visual costs and benefits of the inferred processes.

A. Pathways of Sensitivity Control

1. Rod–Cone In(ter)dependence

The issue of the site of visual adaptation has been addressed in psychophysical experiments of many kinds, but most of them share a common logical framework: they ask whether an adapting field that excites one set of receptors can modify sensitivity for a test stimulus that excites another set. If it can, then the relevant adaptation process must be located at a site in the visual pathway where signals from both sets of receptors converge. If it cannot, then any modification of sensitivity must be introduced at a stage of processing where the signals from the different sets of receptors remain segregated.

Suppose, for example, that an adapting field excites only rods while the test stimulus excites only cones. In this case physiological and anatomical observations make it clear that the two sets of receptors share a common path from the ganglion cells to the brain. If adaptive changes take place in that common path, then an adapting light exciting the cones will be able to change an observer's sensitivity for test lights stimulating the rods. But if the rod and cone receptors are equipped with separate sensitivity regulating mechanisms, operating independently, no such rod–cone interaction in adaptation would be expected. Experiments to examine this point are slightly complicated by the fact that any light which stimulates the cones will also stimulate the rods to some degree (and vice versa). To get around this problem, one can compare two adapting lights that differ for the cones but have been matched for the rods. For example, a photopically dim green adapting light can be compared with an about hundredfold brighter red one of equal scotopic luminance. Rushton (1968) and Hayhoe, MacLeod, and Bruch (1976) found that after preexposure to two such lights, at intensities high enough to bleach a substantial proportion of the visual pigments, the time course of recovery of rod sensitivity in the dark was similar in the two cases. Under these conditions cones were bleached strongly by the red light and only weakly by the green, yet this had no measurable differential effect on rod sensitivity. This could mean either that adaptation occurs independently in the rod and cone receptors themselves or else that the rod system adapts at a postreceptoral site, but one to which cone signals have no access.

In these experiments the sensitivity of the rod system could be measured without intrusion from cones by using test stimuli to which rods are much more sensitive than cones. To test whether bleaching the rods affects cone sensitivity requires a stimulus invisible to rods. Such a stimulus can be produced by abruptly substituting one of two scotopically equated lights for the other (e.g., a dim green for a bright red). Using this method of "silent substitution" (Rushton, Powell & White, 1973), MacLeod and Hayhoe (1974) and Hayhoe et al. (1976) were able to show that under the conditions of that experiment, bleaching the rods does not affect the sensitivity of the cones.

Under other conditions, though, clear failures of rod–cone independence in adaptation have been demonstrated. For example, although the rod threshold is raised to about the same extent by scotopically equated backgrounds that differ for cones (Flamant & Stiles, 1948), cone excitation by the background tends to cause an additional elevation of rod threshold (Makous & Boothe, 1974), especially when the background luminance is high (Makous & Peeples, 1979). This could mean either that the primary rod system sensitivity regulating mechanism has some relatively minor cone input or that, despite rod–cone independence at the earliest adaptation process, later mechanisms mediate the interaction.

Cone–cone interactions, between different classes of cone, have been investigated similarly, and with similar results, although in this case the bipolar cells as well as the ganglion cells may be expected to combine signals from the different classes of cone (in lower vertebrates at least). Williams and MacLeod

(1979) found that an afterimage formed by selectively bleaching only one class of cones was not revived by background substitutions that stimulated only another class of cones. But again (two-color) increment threshold measurements, using the paradigm described in Section III, indicate slight deviations from complete cone–cone independence. In the case of the short-wavelength sensitive ("blue") cones a "multiple site" interpretation of the interaction has good experimental support. Signals from these cones pass through two successive sites, one receiving predominantly or entirely short-wavelength cone ("blue") input, and the other receiving a strong antagonistic influence from the other classes of cone. Part of the evidence for this is that the sensitivity losses imposed at the two stages combine multiplicatively, a result inconsistent with a single stage model (Pugh & Mollon, 1979). It is tempting to identify the second site with a chromatically opponent postreceptoral cell, but if cones receive feedback from horizontal cells, both sites could conceivably be receptoral.

2. Diffuse Rod and Punctate Cone Sensitivity Control

Rushton and Westheimer (1962) found that rod stimuli delivered to nearby retinal areas interact in adaptation. A bleach confined to one region of the visual field caused a subsequent loss of sensitivity in neighboring regions. Sensitivity was, in fact, no different if the test light fell outside that region but close to its boundary. From this it follows that the sensitivity loss is not implemented in the rods themselves. It must all be imposed at a neural "pool" that averages the signals from a group of neighboring rods, which send signals to the pool to reduce sensitivity in the area subserved by that pool.

This conclusion is supported by observations using a refined technique to test for strictly local processes in adaptation (MacLeod, Chen & Crognale, 1989). Here the bleaching flash and the subsequently exposed test stimulus are gratings that differ slightly in spatial frequency (Fig. 26). If sensitivity were regulated independently in different rods, the strips of retina illuminated by the light bars of the bleaching grating should have their sensitivity reduced, whereas sensitivity in the intervening strips where the dark bars fell should be unchanged. Thus, a sensitivity profile can be generated as shown by the top curve in Fig. 26. In that case, the observer would be viewing the test grating with alternating sensitive and insensitive strips of retina, somewhat as if it were being observed through a grid. In some regions, where the test grating is in register with the sensitive strips (Fig. 26, middle) it will be able to stimulate effectively, generating a spatial excitation profile with relatively high peaks (Fig. 26, bottom). But in neighboring areas (left and right, Fig. 26) the test grating will fall on insensitive strips and will not produce much excitation. Since the "in register" regions, where stimulation is effective, occur at a spatial frequency equal to the difference between the test and bleaching grating frequencies, the excitation profile contains a prominent Fourier component at that frequency, just as a Moiré pattern does (dashed line, Fig. 26). However, if the rod adaptation mechanism is not localized within the rods but in the rod pool, the bleaching grating might not be resolved at the adapting site, and the sensitivity loss would be more or less uniform. In that case no Fourier component at the difference frequency would be generated. The visibility of the difference-frequency grating can therefore be used to verify whether the sensitivity regulating mechanism is able to resolve the much finer bleaching grating. An advantage of this approach is that resolution losses in the visual system at stages following the sensitivity regulation cannot affect the outcome; these later stages of the system need only resolve the relatively coarse difference-frequency grating. By using test and bleach gratings of similar frequencies the difference-frequency grating can be made arbitrarily large in scale (to ensure that the later stages do resolve it) even if the test and bleaching gratings themselves are far above the resolution limit of rod vision.

MacLeod et al. (1989) looked for difference-frequency gratings in rod vision. They could observe them only if the test and bleach gratings were both quite low in spatial frequency—less than 7 cycles per degree of visual angle subtended at the eye. Since this is roughly the resolution limit for rod vision, it ap-

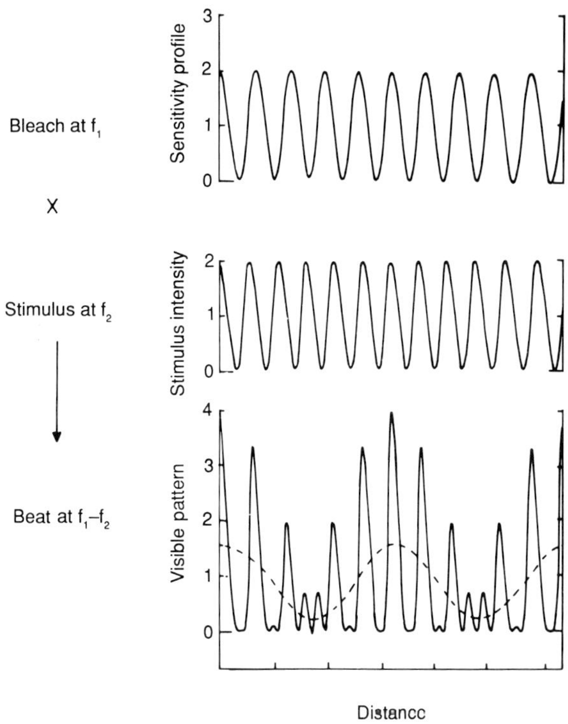

Fig. 26 Difference-frequency grating (bottom) generated by combining a test grating (middle) with a sensitivity profile (top), generated by bleaching with a grating differing slightly in frequency from that of the test stimulus.

pears that practically the entire loss of resolution associated with rod vision occurs before rod sensitivity is set. This negative result strongly supports Rushton's proposal that rods do not independently regulate their own sensitivity, since even a modest local variation of sensitivity would have generated a visible difference-frequency grating. However, the extent of the pooling appears to be more restricted than the 1–2 cycle per degree claimed by Rushton and Westheimer (1962), a conclusion corroborated by the results of Barlow and Andrews (1973).

In cone vision the situation is completely different. Here MacLeod, Williams, and Makous, (1985) and Burton (1973) found for steady-state adaptation that difference-frequency gratings could be observed using test and bleach gratings as high as 130 cycles per degree, far above the limit of visual resolution. This implies that the cone system does have a powerful, and strictly local, sensitivity regulating mechanism, perhaps in the cones themselves. The quantitative results suggested that the only resolution losses affecting cone sensitivity are those due to spatial integration of absorbed energy within individual cones.

The conclusion that rod adaptation is pooled, but cone adaptation is not, is consistent with most of the mammalian electrophysiological evidence reviewed in Section IV. In particular the absence of gain control in monkey rods is a case in point. One major discrepancy is the finding of cone adaptation pools in cat ganglion cells. Another is that the psychophysical evidence for strictly local sensitivity control (i.e., within the cones) is not corroborated by measurements of the photocurrent in primate cones.

B. Why More Light Means Better Sight

It is obvious that at high light levels we can see texture and detail that we cannot see when the illumination is dim (e.g., Hecht, 1928; Craik, 1939). Yet the reasons for this are not fully understood. The rod–cone transition is not the whole explanation since the phenomenon can be observed within the photopic range. Photon noise becomes relatively insignificant at higher light levels, but this by itself does not explain the improvement: variability in ganglion cell firing rates is almost independent of illumination (Barlow & Levick, 1969), and, moreover, it has not been demonstrated that photon noise contributes appreciably to that variability at photopic levels. An attractive view is that the improvement occurs because adaptation changes the spatial organization of the retina. Barlow, Fitzhugh, and Kuffler (1957) found in cat retinal ganglion cells, and Ramoa, Freeman, and Macy (1985) in cat cortical cells, that light adaptation increases the prominence of the antagonistic surround relative to the center, thereby reducing the effective size of the central summing area of each cell. As Barlow (1972a) noted, the effect is rather like reducing the grain size in a photographic film. Like the photographic analog it could provide an efficient way of regulating sensitivity, because the system gains a useful improvement in resolution by sacrificing sensitivity that is no longer needed or even desired. According to this idea, then, visual sensitivity would be regulated in part by changes in spatial organization.

There are various lines of psychophysical evidence supporting this attractive idea (Bouman, 1950; Barlow, 1958b), in particular the different t.v.i. functions that are obtained with small and large test fields. This is illustrated in Fig. 27. The important feature in Fig. 27 is the convergence of the two t.v.i. functions with increasing adaptation level. The greater sensitivity (lower thresholds) observed with the larger test field is due to spatial integration. The fact that this difference diminishes with increasing background intensity has been taken as evidence that adaptation reduces the area over which light is integrated. However, this interpretation is difficult to reconcile with the proposal made above, that photopic sensitivity is strictly locally regulated. Also the experimentally observed modulation of surround effectiveness is quite incapable of accounting for it.

A possible way out has been offered by Chen, MacLeod, and Stockman (1987) who propose an explanation based on local adaptation processes, without any change of spatial integration. They pointed out that thresholds for small stimuli are of higher intensity than those measured with large stimuli, and that this by itself might already cause the observed convergence of t.v.i. functions with increasing adaptation level. Indeed, suprathreshold t.v.i. functions (constant brightness curves) measured by Whittle and Challands (1969) and similar data on chromatic adaptation from Walraven (1976) show the same kind of picture as in Fig. 27. Since in these studies the effect cannot be linked to spatial integration (the size of the test field was not varied), the sensitivity regulating mechanism involved must be locally active. Chen et al. (1987) were able to show that all, or nearly all, the difference in threshold elevation for large and small flashes can be explained on the basis of purely local factors.

The t.v.i. functions shown in Fig. 27 indicate that increasing the adaptation level causes a less steep rise in threshold for bright (small) fields than for dim (large) fields. What remains to be explained is the nature of the mechanism that reacts to the intensity (rather than size) of the test stimulus. Apparently, strong stimuli are relatively less attenuated by the mechanisms that regulate sensitivity control. This can be implemented, or at least described, in various ways. One possibility, as proposed by Chen et al. (1987), is a steepening of the (incremental) stimulus–response function (the kind of function shown in Fig. 12); that is, an increase in the exponent relating incremental response to incremental intensity. Such an effect has been demonstrated by Barlow and Levick (1976) in cat ganglion cells, but they attributed this to a change in spatial organization rather than a strictly local sensitivity change. As noted in Section III, Weber's law implies that changes in illumination are exactly compensated by a reciprocal adjustment of sensitivity, thus making the signals dependent only on contrast and not on illumination. A visual system that would exactly implement Weber's law in that way would not give us better vision in bright light. In fact, however, the change in sensitivity is generally less

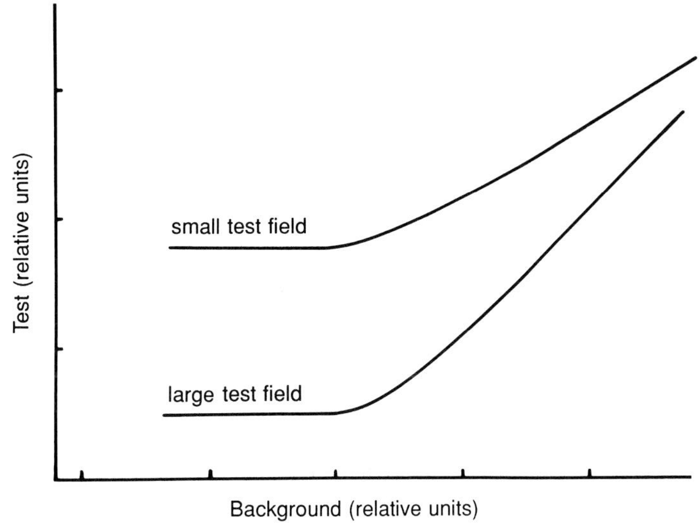

Fig. 27 Generalized threshold-versus-intensity (t.v.i.) functions, showing the characteristic difference in result when employing a test field with small (about 5′) or large (about 1°) diameter.

than dictated by Weber's law, and hence less than is needed to compensate fully for a change in light level. The shortfall from Weber's law is especially pronounced with small or finely detailed test objects, due to their greater local effects at threshold. Strictly local processes can therefore explain why we see better in bright light: not because the grain of the neural response is finer, but because the signals are bigger.

C. Overloading by Spatial Contrast

So far, this section has been concerned with the effects of relatively large uniform adapting fields. With such fields the possible loci of sensitivity change are confined to the early stages of the visual system, because large homogeneous fields are of limited effectiveness in exciting neurons at the later stages. One mechanism for filtering out uniform input is the center–surround antagonism of retinal ganglion cells and cells at later stages (Section IV, B, 3B). Another is the more or less transient response of such cells, subjectively reflected in the fading of stabilized images (Cornsweet, 1970; Arend, 1973). Since vision is maintained only by the temporal transients generated by small involuntary eye movements near the border of a field, it follows that the interior of a uniform background field does not carry any ultimately effective visual signal. Such a background can modify sensitivity only at stages where it has not yet been "discounted" (Section III, B, 2) or otherwise made physiologically ineffective. However, edge signals from all backgrounds that provide spatial and temporal transients in the vicinity of the border of the test stimulus can penetrate more effectively to central stages and may thus have the opportunity to modify sensitivity there.

In the human cone system, a dramatic loss of sensitivity, amounting to functional blindness, is demonstrable at the center of small background fields of even moderate intensity, of the order of 10 td (Buss et al., 1982). This is what would be expected if the background overloads a spatially opponent neuron that is required for transmission of the signal elicited by the test flash (Westheimer, 1965; see also Chapters 6 and 13). The optimal background diameter for reducing sensitivity increases from a few minutes of arc at the central fovea to about 30 min of arc in the near periphery, following approximately the center sizes of receptive fields of macaque retinal ganglion cells

(Spillmann et al., 1987). Sensitivity can be restored by enlarging the background up to a diameter comparable with the receptive field surround. As mentioned in Section IV,B, the few relevant mammalian ganglion cell recordings (on cats) show little or no effect of this sort (Enroth-Cugell et al., 1977), although it has been found in X-cells in the dorsal lateral geniculate nucleus of the cat (Essock, Lehmkuhle, Fracella & Enoch, 1985).

However, there are arguments that would place the overloading at a stage prior to the ganglion cell. The main consideration is that the ganglion cell's response is of a transient nature, whereas the effect discussed here relates to a sustained (tonic) response, which may even persist after bleaching (Hayhoe, 1979a) or during stabilization (Hayhoe & Smith, 1989). A second argument for an early locus of the overloading effect is that the loss of sensitivity is so complete and abrupt (Hayhoe, 1979a; Buss et al., 1982) that it probably occurs before the visual pathways bifurcate into on- and off-channels (see Chapter 7, this volume). On- and off-bipolar or ganglion cells would probably not go into overload simultaneously as background intensity increases, or be relieved from overload at the same instant during recovery from bleaching. If we reject the ganglion cell as a candidate site because of its preference for transient input, the bipolar cell appears to be the most plausible locus for overloading by small photopic adapting fields. Another possible locus, prior to the on–off bifurcation, might be the cone synaptic membrane, with resolution losses created by cone–cone cross talk.

Curiously enough the rod system shows only a weak effect of overloading by spatial contrast, although small backgrounds do elevate the rod threshold more than large ones, the so-called Westheimer effect (Westheimer, 1965). However, the extra loss of sensitivity produced by small backgrounds does not develop strongly with increasing background intensity (Lennie & MacLeod, 1973) as in the way found with cones. Moreover the rod system's reduced sensitivity when the background is small is mainly, or perhaps entirely, due to temporal transients generated by eye movements. Barlow and Sakitt (1973) reported that the Westheimer effect is nearly abolished by stabilizing the retinal image. Experiments using small and large bleaching fields (which do not generate transients during eye movements) consistently indicate no extra sensitivity loss at all after the small bleach (Westheimer, 1968; Teller & Gestrin, 1969; Hayhoe, 1979a). These results are in sharp contrast to those obtained for the cone system. Moreover the reduced sensitivity to rod stimuli on small backgrounds depends largely or mainly on cone input from the background (Lennie & MacLeod, 1973; Latch & Lennie, 1977; Blick & MacLeod, 1978). These studies suggest, therefore, that there is little or no overloading by spatial contrast within the rod system itself.

The scotopic adaptation mechanism, when activated by large adapting fields, shows relatively little influence of cone input, as discussed above, and is practically indifferent to image stabilization (Sparrock, 1969; Tulunay-Keesey & Jones, 1977). The second site selectively probed by small backgrounds may be central, since the insensitivity to rod stimuli produced by small backgrounds persists for a long time following removal of the background stimulus, in a way that is reminiscent of pattern adaptation associated with the fatigue of cortical neurons (Latch & Lennie, 1977; Hayhoe, 1979b). There is strong physiological evidence against retinal involvement: cat retinal ganglion cells show no improvement in sensitivity to rod stimuli as the adapting field is increased in size (Section IV, B).

VI. CONCLUSIONS

Rod regulation of visual system sensitivity does not occur at a spatially opponent site. This is quite surprising in the light of the physiological and psychophysical evidence for adaptation pooling in the rod system. It is difficult to pinpoint a retinal site that would exhibit pooling without also showing spatial opponency. Spatial opponency is found already at the bipolar level, and although it has yet to be demonstrated for the mammalian rod bipolar, the lateral inhibitory action of horizontal cells probably makes it universal. Electroretinographic evidence also indicates an adaptation locus earlier than the bipolar (see the review by Green, 1986). Sensitivity control by feed-forward inhibition from horizontal cells could provide pooling without opponency in the control of sensitivity (MacLeod, 1978). The pool could be larger than the spread of horizontal cell processes since these cells are connected by gap junctions. Another possibility consistent with the psychophysical evidence is that rod adaptation is based on a compressive nonlinearity of synaptic transmission at the rod synapse (Belgium & Copenhagen, 1988). A synaptic mechanism like this would be consistent with the lack of adaptation in photocurrent recording of the rod outer segment (Section IV, A). Connections between rods, mediated by gap junctions, could then provide the substrate for the adaptation pool, and also for an influence of cones on rod sensitivity. But the apparent lack of gap junctions directly coupling rods with rods (Raviola & Gilulua, 1973) argues against this alternative.

In the case of the cone system, the lack of pooling puts a strong psychophysical constraint on the possible site of adaptation. Cone photocurrent recordings in primates do not show cone receptor adaptation at low intensities; extracellular voltage recordings (Valeton & Van Norren, 1983) are more consistent with the psychophysics. Once again, a sensitivity regulating mechanism at the presynaptic membrane could affect psychophysical sensitivity without influencing the outer segment photocurrent recordings. However, a difficulty with this proposal is that gap junctions between the cones would then be expected to lead to some pooling, and this has not been observed.

Thus, although there is some uncertainty as to the precise site of adaptation, it is probably no later than the first synaptic stage for both rod and cone systems. This makes functional sense. An early adaptation locus is needed to protect early stages of the system from overload. In view of this, it may seem rather puzzling that rods do not have an independent internal adaptation mechanism. Why would regulating sensitivity in the rod system be postponed until the neural interaction required for adaptation pooling has occurred? A possible answer is to be found in the stochastic nature of the light stimulus. At light intensities below the cone threshold, where vision is mediated only by rods, the incident photon flux is so sparse that, on average, isometizations occur in individual rods less than once a second. Under these conditions individual rods cannot represent the fluctuating light intensity with useful precision, so a rapid and appropriate adjustment of sensitivity is impossible on physical grounds, unless the signals from different rods are averaged. In the intensity range of cone vision this problem does not arise, and pooling is not necessary.

This selective review of the sites of adaptation has shown that while our present theoretical framework will not always accommodate both psychophysical and physiological data without stress, approximate and tentative statements can be made consistent with evidence from both sources. The parallels between structure and function are close enough to show that it is indeed the same territory that is being mapped by the functional geography of psychophysical experiments, on the one hand, and by physiology and anatomy on the other.

ACKNOWLEDGMENTS

Preparation of this chapter was supported by the following research grants from the National Institutes of Health: EY 00206 and EY 06669 (C. E. C.), EY 02115 (D. C. H.), EY 01711 (D. I. A. M.), EY 07642 (J. L. S.); and a Stein Professorship from Research to Prevent Blindness, Inc. (J. L. S.)

6

PARALLEL PROCESSING OF VISUAL INFORMATION

Peter Lennie, Colwyn Trevarthen, David Van Essen, and Heinz Wässle

I. INTRODUCTION

Parallel processing is usually understood to mean that different properties of the visual scene are analyzed concurrently, and to some degree independently. Several different lines of thought have shaped our present ideas about the parallel organization of vision. A particularly influential one originated in a symposium comprised of papers by Ingle (1967), Schneider (1967), Trevarthen (1968), and Held (1968). These authors distinguished two roles of vision. One involved orienting the animal in space and guiding its larger movements. This *ambient* vision is sensitive to motion and is very dependent on the peripheral visual field. *Focal* vision is used for the detailed examination and identification of objects, is associated with the fovea and exploratory eye movements, and is perhaps especially well developed in primates. These two forms of vision, often characterized as "where" and "what" vision, were linked to two major projections of optic nerve fibers to the midbrain and to the thalamus. Although the functional distinction drawn by Ingle, Schneider, Trevarthen, and Held survives in much current thinking about parallel pathways, it is less tied to the two major central projections of the optic nerve. More recent work has emphasized two other features of the parallel organization of the visual system: first, that each of the major central projections from the retina contains several classes of neurons that differ in their visual properties and probably in their roles; second, that there are multiple representations of the visual field on the cortex that to some degree are manifestations of parallel analyses of the retinal image.

Anatomical and physiological investigations are rapidly revealing how these different forms of parallelism are related, and a great deal of related psychophysical work complements this by attempting to isolate individual pathways for study. This chapter focuses principally on the anatomical and physiological work, although we review a number of psychophysical findings. We begin by considering the value of parallel processing. We then discuss the characteristics of the major pathways, distinguishing two fundamental types: one containing neurons that are specialized detectors of visual stimuli, the other containing neurons that transmit a largely untransformed copy of the retinal image to cortex. We argue that the latter type of pathway is the foundation of any highly developed visual system and permits the development of specialized analyses in cortex. We then look at the different kinds of analysis that are undertaken in visual cortex.

A. Parallel representations?

1. Time Constraints

Complex perceptual decisions are arrived at quickly, often within a few hundred milliseconds. Since these decisions depend on neurons whose operational speed is of the order of a few milliseconds, the calculation cannot involve more than about one hundred serial stages. These "hundred time steps" (Feldman & Ballard, 1982) are to be contrasted with the millions of (rapidly executed) steps made by sophisticated computer programs that recognize visual objects, and we therefore have to consider what design permits slow computing elements to perform extremely complex tasks rapidly.

One feature that distinguishes the brain from a conventional computer is that the brain can undertake many operations in parallel, while conventional computers cannot. Consider the representation of a visual scene in the optic nerve: each fiber represents a small part of the visual field, and few fibers represent the same place. Information about a large region of space is therefore delivered concurrently to central mechanisms. Contrast this with the representation of a scene provided by a television camera: the signal from any point is transmitted very rapidly, but the image on the tube is scanned point by point, so the whole representation is transmitted slowly. Because the visual system's parallel representation of points in space is so obviously faster, we are led naturally to ask whether the parallel representations of the image should be regarded as adaptations to the problem of slow computing elements.

2. Modularity of Perception

Work in computer science (e.g., Ballard, Hinton & Sejnowski, 1983) suggests that breaking up a task into components that can be computed separately is a practicable means of coping with slow computing elements. Moreover, the idea that percepts consist of separable components is well established in the psychological literature and powerfully reinforced by intuition: we can articulate the components of most visual objects that we recognize, and we can "detach" certain properties from complex percepts. For example, we can readily imagine how a normal scene would look devoid of color, or at a different spatial scale. Clinical neurologists occasionally encounter patients who have relatively specific perceptual deficits that result from cortical lesions. These deficits include *achromatopsia*, a loss of color vision without attendant loss of other perceptual functions, *prosopagnosia* (named for an inability to recognize faces, although the deficit extends to identifying members of other complex categories), and other rare conditions, such as that reported by Zihl, von Cramon, and Mai (1983) which resulted in grossly impaired perception of movement. Although cases like these are too rare and too idiosyncratic to provide more than informal pointers to perceptual organization, they are important because, together with the (generally milder) congenital/developmental abnormalities of color vision and stereopsis, they bolster the case that normal percepts depend on relatively autonomous mechanisms that each contribute distinctive components.

Given the broad consensus about what Marr (1982) called the "principle of modular design," the important question to examine is, how should perceptual tasks be segmented? Visual scientists have devised several techniques to show how perceptual tasks might be decomposed into component problems that are solved relatively independently. Treisman (1988) discusses a number of these, as do Chapters 7, 8, and 11 in this volume. Work on computer vision (Marr, 1982) also provides explicit demonstrations of how certain visual tasks (e.g., the identification of position in depth from stereopsis) can be divided into subtasks that are solved in parallel. This work has provided modest hints about the kinds of decomposition that might be involved, but remarkably little of it touches upon the fundamental question of how the task *ought* to be divided for efficient computation. We need to specify the task precisely before we can establish how it is best devolved.

The goals of human vision are complex and difficult to define, although we can confidently specify some minimal ones: the visual system should be able to articulate and identify objects in the face of changes in their orientation and position in relation to other objects and to the observer, and it should be able to cope with changes in the amount or composition or position of the illumination in which the objects are viewed. This problem is commonly cast as one of perceptual constancy: the organism has to abstract the stable properties of the world from the variable retinal image. Because some such tasks have been precisely specified it has been possible to formulate solutions for them—the problem of identifying objects under changing conditions of illumination (color constancy) has become one of the more tractable ones—but most of the problems of visual perception have not been articulated precisely enough for efficient solutions to be found. Thus, the visual physiologist is encouraged to believe that parallel pathways are a good thing, but receives modest guidance from perceptual psychology and computer science about the properties that these pathways should possess.

II. THE FORMATION OF PARALLEL PATHWAYS

Different representations of the image begin at the very earliest stages of visual analysis: the rods and the different classes of cone in the retina are connected in different ways to bipolar cells, and in some cases are connected to different bipolar cells, which in turn are connected to different ganglion cells, whose axons form the optic nerve. Although we are now beginning to learn a good deal about the earliest stages in the formation of parallel pathways (e.g., Sterling, Freed & Smith, 1988), the bulk of what we know about them comes from work on ganglion cells, which, because they generate axon potentials that can be recorded with extracellular electrodes, have always been more accessible to the electrophysiologist.

The axons of retinal ganglion cells project to several central sites, of which in mammals the superior colliculus and lateral geniculate nucleus of the thalamus (LGN) are the most prominent. The collicular pathway is phylogenetically older and is the more prominent in lower mammals. In higher mammals, particularly primates, the thalamic pathway predominates. These major fiber tracts contain distinct subpathways; some arise from bifurcating fibers and carry the information from a single neuron to different central sites, but in most cases it seems that quite different classes of ganglion cell give rise to the different projections.

A. Classification of Cells

How do we recognize distinct classes of ganglion cell? In the late 1970s this was the subject of acrimonious debate, but it is no longer contentious. Rodieck and Brening (1983) make clear in their analysis of the problem that we identify classes of cells by the clustering of their physiological and/or anatomical properties: when we measure the physiological/anatomical properties on some number of dimensions, and plot the location of a cell in this N-dimensional space, the cells fall into clear groups.

Cajal (1893) recognized the morphological diversity of ganglion cells in the retina. He classified cells by their size and by the type and level of branching of their dendrites; Polyak (1941) later classified ganglion cells by the size of the cell body and by the size and shape of the dendritic tree. Neither of these classification schemes fully captures the discreteness of cell classes, but that becomes clear from more recent analyses of flat-mounted retinas, which very clearly

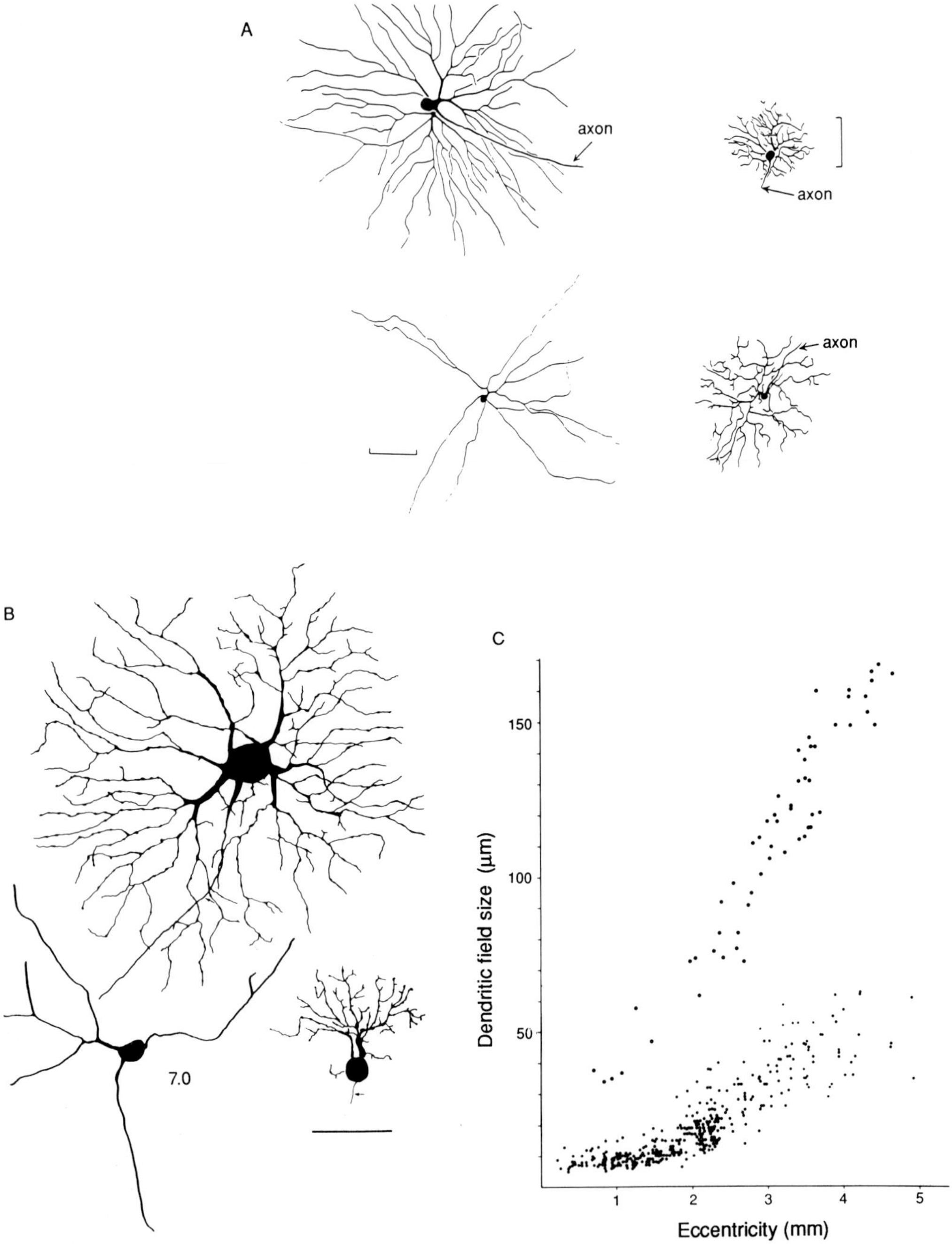

FIG. 1 (A) Examples of four morphological types of ganglion cell in the cat's eye, identified in a flat-mounted retina. All lie at similar eccentricities. Upper left, α cell; upper right, β cell; lower left, γ cell; lower right, δ cell. From Boycott and Wässle (1974). (B) Three morphological varieties of ganglion cell in the retina of the monkey, all lying at similar eccentricities. Top, M or P_α cell; lower right, P or P_β cell; lower left, Pγ cell. From Perry et al. (1984) and Perry and Cowey (1984). (C) Variation with eccentricity in the diameters of dendritic fields of P_α (M) cells (larger points) and P_β (P) cells (smaller points). At all eccentricities where diameters are measured, those of M-cells are about 3 times larger than those of P-cells. From Perry et al. (1984).

reveal the dendritic morphologies of cells. Figure 1A shows some examples of cells from the cat, taken from the work of Boycott and Wässle (1974), and Fig. 1B shows examples obtained from monkey by Perry, Oehler, and Cowey (1984).

We may not need a large number of dimensions to identify distinct types, especially if along any one dimension cells fall into discrete groups. Figure 1C shows the distribution of diameters of the dendritic fields of ganglion cells in the retina of the monkey *Macaca fascicularis*, plotted as a function of distance from the fovea. Figure 1C reveals distinct populations of cells, but it is clear that had we not also known the eccentricity at which a cell lay we could not have discerned two groups. Even this plot may disguise further groups that could be identified by measuring some other property of the cells. For example, we know that within the group having smaller dendritic fields there are two *physiologically* distinct types of cell (about which we say more later) although they have not yet been distinguished anatomically.

Bishop and O'Leary (1938) discovered distinct physiological classes of neurons by recording the compound action potential in the cat's optic tract following electrical stimulation of the optic nerve. This potential contained two (sometimes three) modes, implying the existence of distinct groups of fibers that had different conduction velocities. Figure 2A shows an example from Stone and Freeman (1971) and Fig. 2B the results of an equivalent analysis undertaken on the monkey by Ogden and Miller (1966).

Although the *functional* heterogeneity of ganglion cells was emphasized by Granit and by Barlow in their early work on cat and frog retinas, parallel pathways aroused little interest until Enroth-Cugell and Robson (1966) characterized the X- and Y-cells of the cat. This work showed very firmly that the visual characteristics of mammalian ganglion cells place them in *discrete* physiological classes, and it led to a burgeoning of interest in the field.

1. Plain and Elaborate Receptive Fields

It is useful to distinguish informally two broad physiological groupings of ganglion cells: one containing

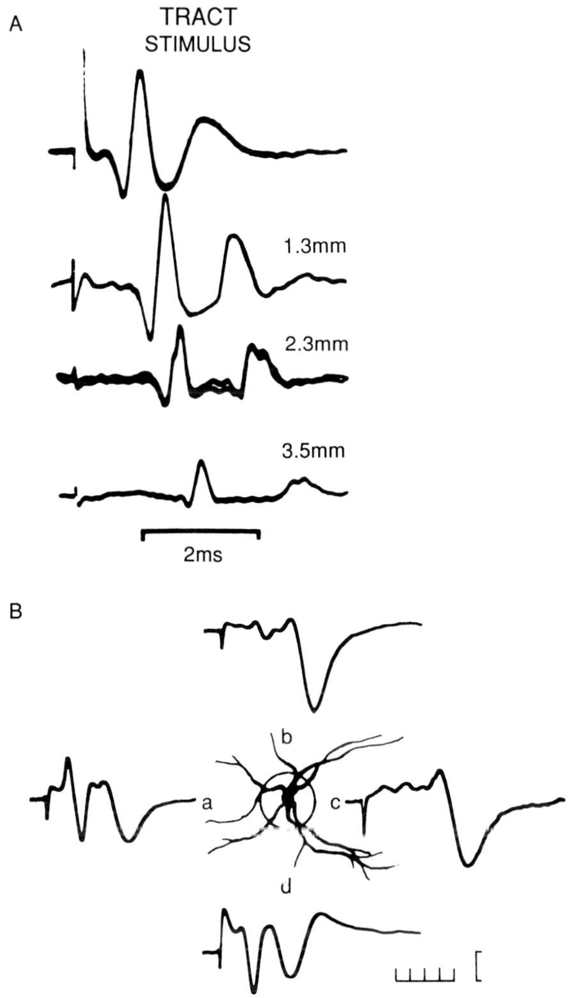

FIG. 2 (A) Compound action potential evoked by an electrical stimulus to the optic tract, recorded in cat from the optic disk and at three points in the retina increasingly distant from it. The sharp pulse at the beginning of each trace marks the delivery of the electrical stimulus; each of the following upward-going waves (better separated in the lower traces) represents the massed action potential generated by it. The earlier wave represents a fast-conducting group of fibers (α cells), the later a slower group (β cells). Within the retina the difference in conduction velocities is revealed as a progressive separation of the two waves. From Stone and Freeman (1971). (B) Compound action potential recorded at points around the margin of the optic disk in the monkey. The sharp pulse at the beginning of each trace marks the electrical stimulus; downward-going waves show two distinct conduction groups that represent M- and P-cells at points on the nasal and inferior margins of the optic disk (a, d) but only one (slower conducting) group at points on the temporal and superior margins, (c, b) over which pass the fibers from the fovea. From Ogden and Miller (1966).

types of cells that have relatively plain receptive fields, the other containing cells that have more elaborate receptive fields. The prototypical plain receptive field is that of the cat's X-cell; cells with properties like it are the most common type found in higher mammals. The receptive field can be thought of as plain because it transforms the image very little. We know from the earliest investigations (Kuffler, 1953) that plain receptive fields are approximately circularly symmetric, with two concentric antagonistic regions. Following Rodieck (1965), the receptive fields of such cells are represented by two distinct but overlapping mechanisms whose spatial distributions of sensitivity can be described as Gaussian surfaces of different scale. Figure 3A shows a three-dimensional representation of the resulting distribution of sensitivity within the receptive field of an X-cell. Each mechanism sums the weighted signals received from photoreceptors, and the response of the cell reflects the difference between the signals accumulated by center and surround.

Two forms of X-cell are recognized: in one the discharge is raised by increasing illumination of the center ("on-center" cell); in the other the discharge is lowered by increasing illumination of the center ("off-center" cell). An important feature of this model, which accounts well for the behavior of X-cells (Enroth-Cugell & Robson, 1966), is that the cell combines signals linearly: its response to any stimulus that is the sum of some number of component stimuli is the same as the sum of the responses to each of the component stimuli presented separately. Cells of this sort are sensitive to local contrast in the image and respond poorly to uniform illumination of the receptive field, but they do not otherwise discard much information about the distribution of light in the retinal image. Because such cells filter the image so little, a single cell communicates little about the nature of the visual stimulus. For example, a spot moving in any direction across the receptive field of an X-cell will generally give rise to the same response; a large dim spot on the receptive field will generally evoke the same response as a smaller, brighter one; and a coarse grating pattern moving across the receptive field will generally be indistinguishable from a fine grating pattern.

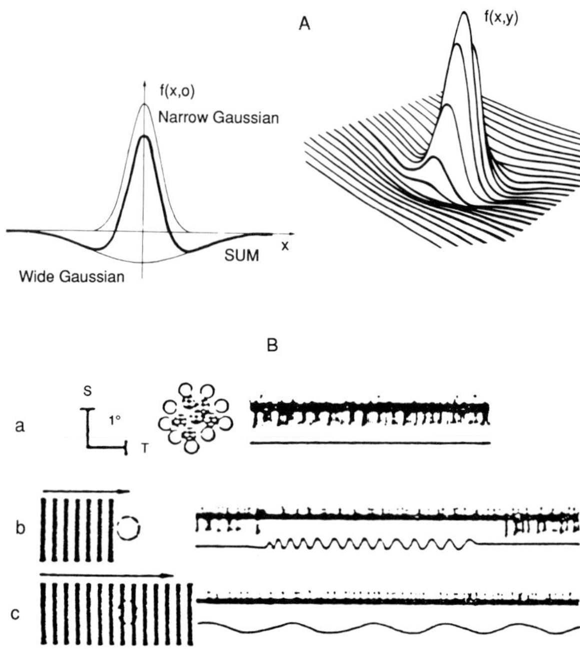

FIG. 3 (A) Distribution of sensitivity within the receptive field of a ganglion cell with a plain receptive field. The center and surround are considered distinct mechanisms, each of which has a Gaussian distribution of sensitivity in two dimensions. Because the surround is larger, the overall distribution of sensitivity of the cell follows the heavy line (left-hand graph) and is represented by the "top-hat" three-dimensional profile at right (from Rodieck, 1965), which shows the distribution of sensitivity within the receptive field of an X-cell in the cat's retina. (B) Responses of the cat's "suppressed by contrast" cell to various stimuli. In all segments of the figure the upper trace shows a train of action potentials discharged as a stimulus passed across the receptive field. The lower trace shows the luminance variation at the center of the receptive field. (a) No stimulus; (b) rapidly moving grating; (c) slowly moving grating. Adapted from Cleland and Levick (1974b).

Consider now the cat's "suppressed by contrast" ganglion cell, first described by Rodieck (1967). Within a relatively large receptive field, in which the spatial distribution of sensitivity cannot be simply represented, the presence of luminance contrast (a spot or a grating) suppresses a healthy maintained discharge. The cell is insensitive to the polarity of contrast; its discharge is most heavily depressed by the slow movement of the contrast pattern through the receptive field and may remain depressed for seconds after the stimulus is removed. Such cells are manifestly nonlinear: their responses to stimuli made of several components are not the sums of their responses to the components presented separately. The peculiarities of their behavior are clearly expressed in their responses to grating patterns (Fig. 3B). A suppressed by contrast cell is evidently well suited to signaling the presence of a salient object moving in the receptive field, but it preserves very little information about the light distribution in the image and is consequently ill suited to represent the local spatial structure of an object that excites it.

Cells that have elaborate receptive fields (often referred to as W-cells) are common in the cat, where, despite small axons and cell bodies, they have been extensively studied (Stone, 1983). They appear to be relatively rare in the monkey, and their small size makes them relatively inaccessible (Schiller & Malpeli, 1977).

III. IMPORTANCE OF EARLY FILTERING

To some degree all the pathways from the retina discard information (the different classes of cell would not be distinguishable otherwise). Neurons in cortex are very selective for certain features of the stimulus, and in that context the existence of specialized pathways is perhaps not surprising—the properties of higher mechanisms might reflect the special properties of their inputs. However, information discarded early can never be recovered, so it might be presumed better to transmit from the eye a representation that is as little transformed as possible (via some mechanism like the X-cell) and allow later stages the flexibility to create any specialized transformations that they need. Thus, a substantial question we have to deal with is, why are specialized representations formed early in the visual pathway? The next section discusses some possibilities.

A. Limitations Imposed Centrally

There is much more information in the retinal image than is used by the nervous system. This is made obvious by the demonstrated limitations of color vision and of spatial vision: normal color vision provides only a three-dimensional representation of lights and surfaces, adequate for most natural visual environments but insufficient to represent all lights and surfaces unambiguously; the spatial resolving power of foveal vision is well matched to the quality of the image, but in the peripheral visual field resolving power is much poorer than can be explained by the loss of image quality. Part of the loss arises in receptors, which are too widely spaced to sample the image fully, but a large part of the loss must be due to postreceptoral mechanisms, because beyond the parafovea visual acuity falls much more rapidly than does the density of cones. In fact, the decline in visual acuity rather closely follows the declining density of retinal ganglion cells, a point we expand on later.

If for some reason mechanisms beyond the retina had limited capacity for transmitting or analyzing information it would make sense to minimize the information load at an early stage. One way to do this is to send information only about the restricted domains of the image that are important to the organism. By introducing selectivity early, and thereby creating distinct classes of neuron that sample the stimulus domain selectively, we reduce the demands on central mechanisms. Different species with different visual requirements might have rather different specializations. What central limitations might provoke this kind of organization?

It is popularly supposed that the optic nerve is a substantial bottleneck in the transmission of information. The argument is that the larger the optic nerve the less mobile the eye and the larger the blind spot, so there must be strong pressure for the visual system to be as economical as possible with optic nerve fibers. There may be strong pressure to limit the number of fibers in the optic nerve, but there is very little reason to believe that the mechanical properties of the optic nerve constrain the number of fibers in it. The cat's eye is almost exactly the same size as that of *M. fascicularis* and usually less mobile, yet it contains about one sixth as many optic nerve fibers. Birds with mobile eyes have almost as many optic nerve fibers as macaques (Bruesch & Arey, 1942).

If there is pressure to minimize the number of fibers in the optic nerve it is much more likely to reflect central limitations: animals lack the central apparatus to handle the information that would be transmitted by more fibers. By recent estimates (Van Essen & Maunsell, 1980) about half the total cortical area of the macaque monkey contains topographically organized representations of the visual field. Were we to double the size of the optic nerve and maintain the same innervation density in cortex, the macaque would require 50% more cortex than it has now. One could thus argue that imposing selectivity early in the visual pathway (and thereby encouraging the development of parallel representations) limits the load on central mechanisms. An implied corollary is that the greater the central capacity of an organism the less the need for parallel pathways.

In higher mammals with optic nerves that contain large numbers of fibers, most fibers have plain receptive fields that transform the image little, although there are still classes of cell that have elaborate receptive fields. Indeed, R. W. Rodieck (personal communication) has drawn attention to the fact that when one excludes ganglion cells with plain receptive fields, there is little to choose between different mammals in the number (100,000–200,000) and variety of more specialized optic nerve fibers. Thus, although limited central capacity may well constrain the number of optic nerve fibers, it does not seem to have much to do with the variety of pathways.

B. Piecemeal Accretion

An alternative account of the early formation of parallel pathways is that they have developed piecemeal and represent adaptations to new demands placed on the evolving visual system. If an animal has simple visual requirements—finding a limited range of prey and avoiding a limited range of predators—it makes sense for it to have pathways specialized for the detection of particular stimuli. It needs little central capacity, and it can economize on optic nerve fibers. The most celebrated simple visual system is that of the frog, and it provides a useful illustration of the selectivities of different classes of ganglion cells. Lettvin, Maturana, Pitts, and McCulloch (1961) identified five types of ganglion cell (which they thought might be tied to five morphological types of ganglion cell distinguished by Cajal), some properties of which are summarized below. Boundary detectors respond to any contrast boundary in the receptive field, providing it is sharp. Large changes in uniform illumination of the receptive field evoke no response from the cell. Movement-gated, dark convex boundary detectors respond to a contrast border in the receptive field, but only if it is sharp and curved, with the darker area convex, and moves through the receptive field. Moving or changing contrast detectors respond well to rapid movement of a contrasty stimulus within the receptive field. Dimming detectors have poor resolution, respond to any dimming in the whole receptive field, and are unconcerned with boundaries. Unclassified cells have no well-defined receptive field but have a maintained discharge that varies inversely with the mean level of illumination.

In naming cells as they did, Lettvin et al. unashamedly tied the physiological properties of ganglion cells to presumed perceptual functions. The important implication is that these cells may provide as full a representation of the world as the frog needs. Barlow (1953) emphasized this point in discussing "on–off" cells (Lettvin et al.'s changing contrast detectors):

> . . . an optic nerve fibre is the final common path for activity aroused over a considerable region of retina, and if some purposive integration has taken place it should be possible to relate this to the visual behaviour of the frog. According to Yerkes (1903), the frog uses its eyes mainly for feeding; it also escapes from large moving objects, but it does not use visual cues in orienting itself in its habitat. When feeding, its attention is attracted by its prey, which it will approach, and finally strike at and swallow. Any small moving object will evoke this behaviour, and

> there is no indication of any form discrimination. In fact, 'on–off' units seem to possess the whole of the discriminatory mechanism needed to account for this rather simple behaviour. [Barlow, 1953, p. 86]

Although specialized visual pathways equip the frog to catch flies and avoid large predators, they provide a poor foundation for any future expansion of the frog's visual capabilities because their selectivity is produced by discarding information that can never be recovered. The animal has to evolve a new pathway to cope with any new demands. As more general capabilities are required of the visual system, piecemeal accretion of pathways becomes a progressively less efficient means of handling information. If an animal has the central machinery to handle the information, it makes sense to invest in pathways that transmit a representation of the image that is little filtered, allowing higher mechanisms to analyze different aspects of the image in whatever ways are appropriate. This is very much what we see in the organization of the visual systems of higher mammals: the greater the degree of encephalization, the greater the proportion of the afferent pathway occupied by neurons that have plain receptive fields. A crude index of this is provided by the proportion of optic nerve fibers that project to the thalamus, for in all mammals so far studied the overwhelming bulk of cells that project to the LGN have plain (linear, isotropic, and not sharply tuned for spatial frequency) receptive fields. By contrast, relatively few of the fibers that project to the midbrain and other diencephalic sites appear to have plain receptive fields.

The preceding argument suggests that at least some of the parallel pathways arose in response to changing requirements for the visual system; the interesting question is what is their continued value in higher vertebrates with well-developed thalamic pathways in which the cells have plain receptive fields? One possibility is that they transmit information that cannot be transmitted by the cells with plain receptive fields. For example, mechanisms of light and dark adaptation compress information efficiently to cope with the limited dynamic range of optic nerve fibers, and the discharges of most ganglion cells contain no information about the absolute level of illumination. However, this information is needed for the control of the pupil, and it may be provided by a particular class of ganglion cell (the so-called "luminance unit" or "sluggish-sustained" cell) that has a conspicuously regular maintained discharge that follows the absolute level of illumination.

Other kinds of cells may persist in higher vertebrates because they support specialized functions. The optokinetic reflex (OKR) helps stabilize the visual scene on the retina. It is elicited by coherent movement of a large region of the visual field. Two brain stem nuclei (the nucleus of the optic tract, NOT, and the dorsal terminal nucleus, DTN) seem to be critically involved in its generation (see Chapter 13, this volume). In cat a distinctive group of neurons in the NOT (called retinal slip neurons by Ballas and Hoffmann, 1985), which are driven primarily by the contralateral eye, have pronounced selectivity for movements in a temporal–nasal direction (Hoffmann & Schoppmann, 1975). Although their retinal inputs have not been characterized precisely, we do know that they have slow-conducting axons and have a distinctive morphology (Ballas, Hoffmann & Wagner, 1981). Pathways like this presumably survive because they are economical and fast.

IV. GENERAL PURPOSE PATHWAYS

Our discussion so far has concentrated on the specialized ganglion cells, and a plausible case can be made that these have well-defined but circumscribed roles. We now need to consider the pathways that in higher mammals convey a relatively faithful copy of the light distribution in the retinal image, and probably carry the bulk of the information that leaves the retina. Our thesis is that any general purpose visual system requires mechanisms of the kind represented by X- and Y-cells (cat) and P- and M-cells (monkey), but we have not so far characterized these classes of cells.

Cells with plain, concentrically organized receptive fields have been most extensively studied in cat and monkey, and more is known about them than about any other kinds of ganglion cells, principally because they have the largest cell bodies and largest, fastest conducting axons. They project mostly, but not exclusively, to the LGN. In the cat, but not in the monkey, some cells with slow-conducting axons (and possibly elaborate receptive fields) also project to the LGN (Wässle, 1982); however, they are seldom encountered with microelectrodes, and little is known about their visual sensitivities.

A. Cat

We have already described the major properties of X-cells. All X-cells project to the LGN, although some send collateral axons to the midbrain (Wässle, 1982). In the work that first characterized the properties of X-cells, Enroth-Cugell and Robson (1966) identified a second class of ganglion cell (Y-cells) that also had concentrically organized receptive fields and occurred in both on- and off-center forms. Y-cells and X-cells are distinguished by several properties, but receptive field size and linearity of spatial summation are especially notable: at any one eccentricity the centers of receptive fields of Y-cells are about 3 times larger than those of X-cells. X-cells and Y-cells also differ in the temporal characteristics of their responses, a point emphasized by Cleland, Dubin, and Levick (1971), who called them "sustained" and "transient" cells respectively. Y-cells show a pronounced nonlinearity in the summation of signals from photoreceptors lying within the receptive field. This nonlinearity gives rise to a distinct rectified ("on–off") component in the response of a Y-cell so that the cell discharges a burst of impulses at both presentation and removal of a contrast pattern.

The authoritative account of the Y-cell's receptive field (Hochstein & Shapley, 1976) represents it as linear center and surround mechanisms with Gaussian distributions of sensitivity (like an X-cell) with, in addition, "subunits" that generate rectified responses and are distributed throughout the linear receptive field and a substantial region beyond it (Fig. 4). The subunits have finer spatial resolution than center and surround, and are less sensitive, so contribute most to the discharge of a Y-cell when it is stimulated by contrast patterns that contain high spatial frequencies. Under most conditions, Y-cells behave like sensitive X-cells with large receptive fields.

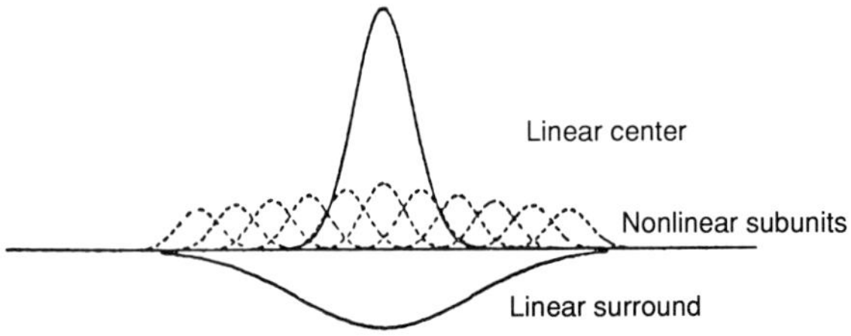

FIG. 4 Distribution of sensitivity within the receptive field of a Y-cell in cat, showing both the linear mechanisms (center and surround) and the rectifying subunits. The linear receptive field can be represented as in Fig. 3A; the rectifying (nonlinear) mechanisms act to increase the discharge of the cell at both light onset and offset. These are selective for stimuli that are small in relation to the center of the linear receptive field, so contribute distinctively to the behavior of Y-cells principally when patterns of high spatial frequency fall on the receptive field. From Hochstein and Shapley (1976).

The physiologically identified X- and Y-cells have recognized anatomical substrates in the β and α ganglion cells first characterized by Boycott and Wässle (1974). Wässle, Levick, and Cleland (1975) identified α cells as the substrates of Y-cells by recording from every Y-cell in a small patch of retina and then showing how the positions of receptive field centers matched the locations of α cells. Peichl and Wässle (1981) extended this work by showing that the dendritic morphology of a particular α cell determines the size and shape of the center of the receptive field. Peichl and Wässle also showed that the dendrites of on- and off-center cells were stratified in distinctly different parts of the inner nuclear layer. The identity of β cells and X-cells, made initially on circumstantial evidence, was firmly established by Saito (1983) and Fukuda, Hsiao, and Watanabe (1985), who filled physiologically identified cells with the anatomical marker horseradish peroxidase (HRP). Like α cells, the on- and off-center β cells have dendrites that branch at different depths within the inner nuclear layer (Nelson, Famiglietti & Kolb, 1978). From anatomical work we also know that α cells constitute 3–5% of ganglion cells at all eccentricities; β cells constitute close to 55% (Wässle, Boycott & Illing, 1981).

B. Monkey

The visual systems of the macaque monkey and human appear to be very much alike, and for this reason a great deal of the more recent work on parallel pathways has concentrated on the macaque. Two major classes of ganglion cell have concentrically organized receptive fields. They were first identified by Gouras (1968), who called them "tonic" and "phasic" cells because of differences between the temporal characteristics of their responses, but are now more widely known as P- and M-cells because of their different projections to the parvocellular (P) and magnocellular (M) laminae of the LGN. Because the connection between the two classes of ganglion cell and their counterparts in the LGN is very well established, and the neurons in LGN seem to have properties almost indistinguishable from those of the ganglion cell that drive them, our account of the physiology draws heavily on work undertaken on the LGN, where cells are more easily studied.

The centers and surrounds of receptive fields of P-cells can be represented by Gaussian functions (Derrington & Lennie, 1984), and in several respects (particularly linearity of spatial summation) these neurons behave like X-cells in cat (Kaplan & Shapley, 1982; Derrington & Lennie, 1984). However, the receptive fields have a color-opponent organization superimposed on the spatial organization: center and surround have different spectral sensitivities. There are clearly two distinct subgroups of P-cells: those that have a "red–green" chromatic opponency and those that have a "yellow–blue" chromatic opponency (DeValois, Abramov & Jacobs, 1966; Wiesel & Hubel, 1966; Derrington, Krauskopf & Lennie, 1984). In the latter, the center–surround arrangement of the chromatically opponent mechanisms is less pronounced (Fig. 5a; see also Chapter 8, this volume). Near the fovea receptive fields of P-cells (especially those with red–green opponency) are very small, and centers are probably driven by single cones (Wiesel & Hubel, 1966). The upshot of this arrangement is that P-cells (particularly the red–green opponent ones) respond well to achromatic spatial contrast except at low spatial frequencies; when the spatial frequency is low they respond well to chromatic patterns modulated in time (Fig. 5B).

M-cells have in common with P-cells the center–surround arrangement of receptive fields, although the center of the receptive field has 2–3 times larger diameter and the chromatic opponency is weak at best. A few M-cells show nonlinearities of spatial summation like those seen in the cat's Y-cells (Kaplan & Shapley, 1982), but the bulk of them behave strikingly like X-cells (Derrington & Lennie, 1984). Within the range of spatial frequencies to which both respond, M-cells are substantially more sensitive than P-cells to achromatic contrast, and this advantage is more pronounced at higher temporal frequencies.

The morphological substrates of P- and M-cells in the retina are now well established, at least for the cells in and near the fovea (Leventhal, Rodieck & Dreher, 1981; Perry et al., 1984). Although several different terminologies have been used to describe these neurons, an emerging consensus supports the use of the names given to their physiological counterparts. P-cells have small cell bodies and small dendritic fields and are very numerous, constituting perhaps 80% or more of ganglion cells. M-cells have large cell bodies and large dendritic fields and are much less numerous than P-cells, constituting perhaps 10% of ganglion cells. Figure 1C shows the distribution of the dendritic field diameters of M- and P-cells in the macaque retina. These morphological types have also been found in the human retina (Rodieck, Binmoeller & Dineen, 1985). As would be expected from their larger cell bodies, M-cells have

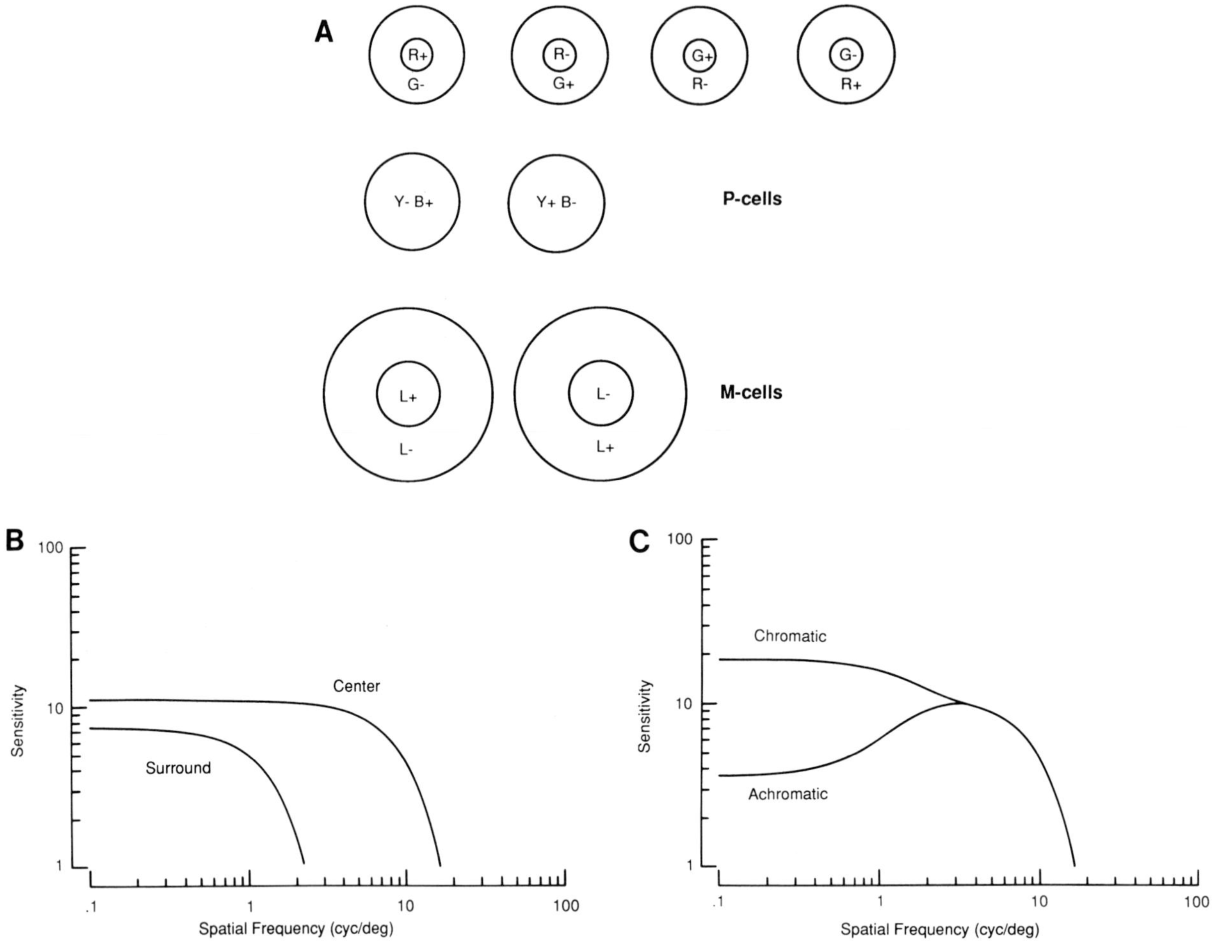

FIG. 5 (A) Diagrammatic representation of the types of receptive fields found in parvocellular and magnocellular divisions of the lateral geniculate nucleus of the macaque. The parvocellular division contains two quite distinct classes of cells (P-cells), one receiving inputs from only L and M cones (by various estimates, about 90% of the total), the other receiving an additional input from S cones. In those that receive inputs from only L and M cones (top row), the two classes of cone contribute with unequal weight to center and surround, so that the receptive field is chromatically as well as spatially opponent. In and near the fovea, the centers of most such receptive fields probably receive signals from a single cone. Receptive fields of cells that receive inputs from S cones (second row) usually have much less pronounced center–surround organization, and the chromatically opponent mechanisms may be coextensive. The contributions of the three classes of cones to these mechanisms are not firmly established. In most cells it appears that one mechanism is driven by signals from S cones, the other by signals from both L and M cones. Neurons in the magnocellular division (M-cells) appear to form a single class (bottom row). Receptive fields have center-surround organization, are larger than those of P-cells, and lack or show very weak chromatic opponency. (B) Illustration of spatial contrast sensitivities of a P-cell for chromatically modulated gratings and achromatically modulated gratings. The left graph shows separately the sensitivities of the center and surround; the right graph shows the sensitivity of the cell to chromatically modulated gratings and achromatically modulated ones. When stimulated by chromatically modulated gratings, center and surround respond in phase, so the overall sensitivity of the cell is represented by the sum of the two curves in the top graph. When stimulated by achromatic gratings, center and surround respond in antiphase, so the overall sensitivity of the cell is represented by the difference of the curves.

larger and faster conducting axons and make a distinctive contribution to the compound action potential recorded at the optic disk (Fig. 2).

C. Multiple General Purpose Pathways

Our earlier discussion suggested why in animals with sophisticated visual systems many ganglion cells have plain receptive fields of the kind represented by X- and Y-cells (cat) and M- and P-cells (monkey), but it leaves unanswered the question of why higher mammals have two (or more) classes of them. It has proved difficult to isolate the different classes through perceptual experiments, although several lines of evidence point to particular roles. In the following we consider this perceptual evidence, together with information from physiological and anatomical investigations.

1. Univariance of Single Neurons

Most analyses of the behavior of neurons assume that information is conveyed by the rate at which action potentials are discharged. Moreover, since the steady rate of discharge is not propagated well from one level of the visual pathway to the next it is widely supposed that *changes* in discharge rate are informative, and most attention is paid to rates measured over periods of tens of milliseconds to a few seconds. Although lip service is paid to the possibility that information is conveyed by the temporal fine structure of the discharge, neurons in the visual pathway are generally treated as though only the local average discharge rate carried information. This supposed one-dimensionality or univariance of response is important when considering the roles of parallel pathways because several dimensions of the retinal image must be sampled at a point. If optic nerve fibers are univariant, we ought to need as many classes of fiber as there are dimensions of the image to be represented at a point in the visual field. We do not know how many are needed for the cat (perhaps two), but for human vision we know that there are at least three dimensions (those required for the perception of color), and this might lead one to suppose that we need three classes of fiber. Since we understand this aspect of primate vision much better than we understand the cat's, the following analysis deals mostly with primates, although the principle should apply equally to the cat.

By three-dimensionality we mean not that three values are required to specify the position of an object in space, but that for human beings three values are required to specify the color and lightness of its surface. The three-dimensionality is demonstrated rigorously by color matching experiments, but it can be represented quite simply in diagrams like Fig. 6, which have their origin in perceptual analyses undertaken in the ninteenth century (see Chapter 8, this volume).

The three dimensions of this space are lightness, hue, and saturation, and most colors can be represented somewhere in the diagram. Our trichromatic vision depends on three classes of cone photoreceptors, but it also depends on postreceptoral pathways preserving three signals. A wealth of psychophysical

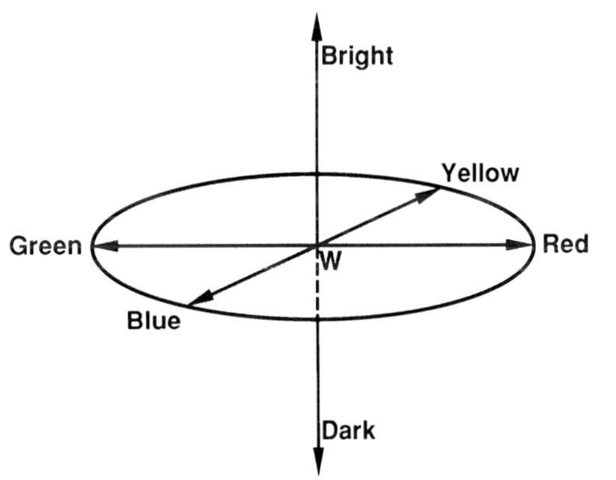

FIG. 6 Three-dimensional color space in which we can represent color and lightness. The three orthogonal axes are one of red–green variation, one of yellow–blue variation, and one of light–dark variation. These intersect at a white point. Movements within the plane that contains the red–green and yellow–blue axes change hue and saturation, but not lightness. Movements orthogonal to this plane change only brightness. Within the constant-lightness plane, saturation increases with distance from the white point.

evidence (Chapter 8; see also Lennie & D'Zmura, 1988) points to the existence of three postreceptoral mechanisms that carry transformations of the signals that arise in cones. One mechanism carries the difference between the signals that arise in long-wavelength sensitive (L) and middle-wavelength sensitive (M) cones (a red–green opponent signal), one carries the difference between the signal in short-wavelength sensitive (S) cones and a combined signal from L and M cones (a yellow–blue opponent signal), and the third carries a combined signal from L and M cones, with perhaps some input also from S cones (a lightness or achromatic signal). We know also from psychophysical work that the spatial properties of the achromatic mechanism differ from those of the red–green and yellow–blue mechanisms: the achromatic mechanism has higher spatial resolution than either of the opponent mechanisms, but it also is markedly less sensitive to low spatial frequencies than it is to intermediate spatial frequencies, while the opponent mechanisms are most sensitive to low spatial frequencies. Figure 7 shows, on a uniform scale, how the sensitivities of these mechanisms vary with spatial frequency. The temporal resolution of the achromatic mechanism appears to exceed that of the opponent mechanisms (Wisowaty, 1981).

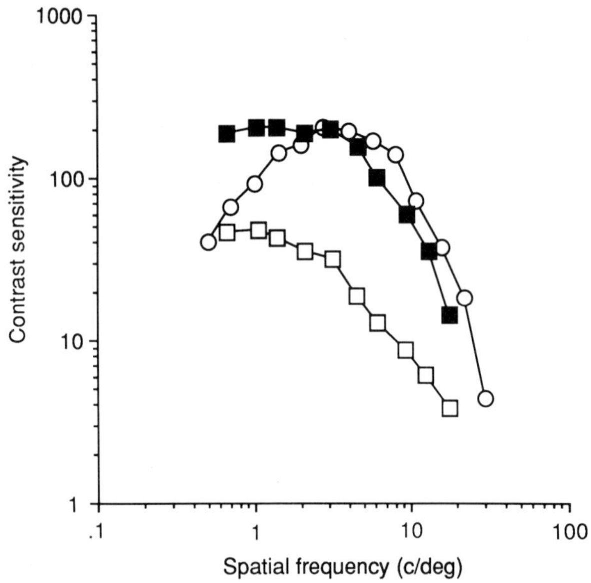

FIG. 7 Spatial contrast sensitivities of the putative postreceptoral mechanisms. Sensitivity is calculated as the reciprocal of the greatest modulation of any class of cone at threshold. Results redrawn from Robson (1966) for achromatic gratings (open circles) and from Van der Horst and Bouman (1969) for gratings modulated along axes that isolate the putative "red–green" mechanism (filled squares) and "yellow–blue" mechanism (open squares).

The properties of the three postreceptoral pathways inferred from psychophysical experiments resemble in a number of respects the properties of the M-cells and two classes of P-cells studied physiologically. P-cells might be the embodiment of the two sorts of opponent mechanism, and M-cells the embodiment of the achromatic mechanism. However, several attributes of P- and M-cells are inconsistent with their proposed roles. We discuss these in the following paragraphs, dealing first with the putative achromatic pathway, which is presumed to support high spatial and temporal resolution.

2. Sampling of the Retinal Image

The retinal image is sampled discretely by photoreceptors, and the density of this sampling sets an upper limit to the spatial frequencies that can be represented faithfully in the nervous system (for review, see Williams, 1986; Chapter 10, this volume). Figure 8 shows diagrammatically how this occurs. Above the sampling limit the mosaic can still transmit information about the image, but this will be ambiguous, so while visual stimuli may be *detected* reliably, they cannot be *identified* reliably. The so-called sampling aperture or effective diameter of an individual photoreceptor sets the upper limit to the spatial frequency that can be resolved by a single photoreceptor, and thus sets a limit to the highest detectable spatial frequency. If the aperture is large this limit may be lower than the sampling limit imposed by the mosaic. Such evidence as we have (Miller & Bernard, 1983) suggests that the sampling aperture of receptors never limits the performance of the visual system.

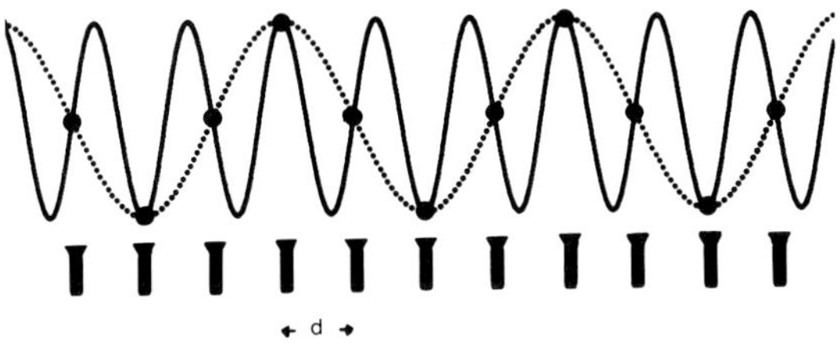

FIG. 8 Diagram showing how a regularly spaced array of cones can provide identical representations of a pattern of low spatial frequency (dotted line) and a pattern of higher spatial frequncy (solid line). These two patterns are members of a set of *aliases* (patterns that have identical effects on the mosaic). The highest spatial frequency that can be represented unambiguously is $\frac{1}{2}d$, where d is the distance between cones. From Williams (1986).

The sampling considerations that apply to photoreceptors apply equally to postreceptoral neurons, so the mosaics of bipolar and ganglion cells impose resolution limits, as do the sampling apertures of individual neurons. For both cat and monkey, anatomical work has revealed the distributions of photoreceptors and of the major classes of ganglion cell that have plain receptive fields. We can therefore deduce, with some assumptions about the fine structure of the mosaics, what spatial frequencies can be resolved by the different classes of cells. Physiological work tells us about the sampling apertures of individual neurons and what spatial frequencies they can resolve. We can therefore calculate which classes of cells could, and which could not, underpin the performance measured in psychophysical experiments. We deal first with the cat, for which we have very precise information about the arrangement of ganglion cells, then consider the monkey.

The mosaic of cones in the cat can resolve higher spatial frequencies than can the mosaics of α and β cells, which therefore probably limit visual performance. In calculating the limit imposed by a class of ganglion cells we have to decide whether the functional mosaic consists of all ganglion cells of that type, or half of them, since the on- and off-center cells have distinct lattices. There are good reasons to suppose that the on- and off-center mosaics should be considered separately. First, they extract different information from the image (see Chapter 7, this volume). Since most neurons have low rates of resting discharge and signal information more efficiently by increases in discharge than by decreases (Levick, 1973), on-center cells better represent luminance increments and off-center cells luminance decrements. Second, and more important in the present context, the mosaics of on- and off-center cells tend to be regularly related (Wässle, Peichl & Boycott, 1983). Irregular spacing of sampling elements reduces the reliability of sampling (Yellott, 1982). If we therefore assume that we are dealing with separate mosaics, and further assume that each is a regular triangular lattice, the highest spatial frequency that can be reliably identified is given by

$$F = (2\sqrt{3}/D)^{1/2}$$

where D is the sampling density. α cells in the cat's area centralis can resolve about 2 cycles/degree (although for the nonlinear mechanism the limit is higher); for the β cells the limit is 6 7 cycles/degree. Individual α and β cells can resolve spatial frequencies at least as high as those that are reliably transmitted by their respective mosaics. Since the behaving cat can resolve between 4 and 5 cycles/degree—a performance unsupportable by α cells—we can conclude that its acute spatial vision must depend on β cells (Horn & Pasternak, 1988).

A similar analysis can be undertaken for the monkey. The average densities of P- and M-cells outside the fovea have been measured by Perry et al. (1984) and Perry and Cowey (1985); close to the fovea the ganglion cells are layered, and displaced from the cones to which they are connected, so their effective density is less easily deduced from the distribution of their cell bodies. The argument that we made for treating the lattices of the cat's on- and off-center cells as separate mosaics applies equally to monkey, and it is bolstered by recent estimates (Schein, 1988; Perry & Cowey, 1988) that in and near the fovea there are at least two P-cells per cone. The density of M cells outside the fovea is uniformly about 10% of the density of P-cells; indirect evidence suggests that their density may be relatively lower in the fovea. For example, Ogden and Miller (1966) measured the compound action potential at points around the margin of the optic disk following delivery of an electric shock to the optic tract (see Fig. 2B) and found no evidence for the existence of a fast-conducting group of fibers (M-cells) in the bundle coming from the fovea. This might just mean that M-cells in the fovea have small axons, but when taken in conjunction with evidence that the magnocellular division of the macaque's LGN occupies a smaller proportion of the part of the nucleus receiving a foveal projection than it does the part receiving peripheral projections (Malpeli & Baker, 1975), it suggests a reduced M cell representation of the fovea.

Nevertheless, if we assume that M cells constitute a constant 10% of ganglion cells and that in the central retina there are two P-cells per cone, we can (ignoring for the moment differences between classes of cone) use reliable measures of cone density in the central retina (Perry & Cowey, 1985) to estimate the resolving power of the mosaics of ganglion cells. If again we assume triangular lattices, the mosaic of P-cells in the fovea has a resolution limit of 50–60 cycles/degree; that of M-cells could resolve approximately 20 cycles/degree. The resolution limit of *individual* foveal P-cells, which ought to be determined by the sampling aperture of cones, has been measured at up to 40 cycles/degree (Blakemore & Vital-Durand, 1986), but for a variety of technical reasons this and lower estimates (e.g., Crook, Lange-Malecki, Lee & Valberg, 1988) probably underestimate the true limit. The measured resolution limit of *individual* M-cells is only slightly lower than that of P-cells (Blakemore & Vital-Durand, 1986; Crook et al., 1988).

The conventional resolution limit of macaque vision is near 40 cycles/degree (De Valois, Morgan & Snodderly, 1974), and therefore requires a mosaic of P-cells. Outside the fovea the densities of ganglion cells are known more certainly, although their mosaics are probably less regular. Figure 9 shows (using assumptions described in the caption to the figure) how human visual acuity and the resolution limits of the mosaics of P- and M-cells vary with eccentricity. The mosaic of P-cells, but not that of M-cells, is adequate for the task.

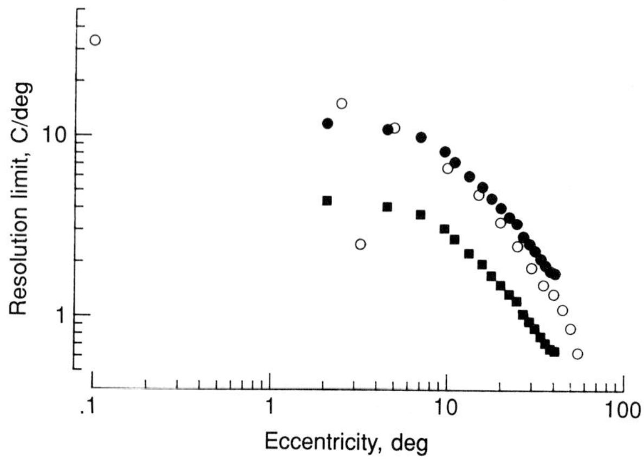

FIG. 9 Variation of resolution acuity with eccentricity. Open circles show measurements of acuity obtained by Wertheim (1894). Observers viewed a small patch (5 cycles) of a square-wave grating whose distance was increased until its orientation (vertical or horizontal) could no longer be identified correctly. Filled symbols show for P-cells (circles) and M-cells (squares) the highest spatial frequency that could be indentified by the mosaic, assuming that the mosaic is regular and triangularly packed, that the mosaics of on- and off-center cells are independent, and that the human eye has the same number of ganglion cells as the macaque, distributed on a larger retina. Ganglion cell numbers are from Perry et al. (1984).

The achromatic pathway is widely assumed to be responsible for our acute spatial vision, so the fact that the mosaic of M-cells cannot sample the image densely enough to support our high visual acuity invalidates the notion that M-cells are the major substrate of the achromatic pathway. Although the mosaic of P-cells samples the image adequately, some physiological properties of P-cells (color opponency) are apparently inconsistent with their carrying the achromatic signal. However, when we recall the spatial organization of the receptive field, it becomes clear (especially for the very numerous red–green class) that most P-cells respond well to achromatic contrast in stimuli that contain high spatial frequences. There is in fact a strong case to be made, both from their numbers and from the analysis of their receptive fields, that the red–green subgroup of P-cells carries both the red–green opponent signal and the achromatic one. These signals are probably confounded in the discharge of a single neuron, although relatively simple schemes (e.g., that of D'Zmura & Lennie, 1986) can be devised to segregate them at a later stage in the visual pathway. We examine this issue further when we consider multiple representations in cortex.

The upshot of our analysis of image sampling is that M-cells are probably not the substrate of the high-acuity achromatic pathway, although we have not excluded their involvement in other aspects of spatial vision. Merigan and Eskin (1986) and Merigan (1989) investigated their functions in experiments that used the neurotoxin acrylamide to destroy the P ganglion cells in macaque without apparently damaging the M cells. As might be expected from the foregoing discussion of receptive field properties, color discrimination was grossly impaired, as was sensitivity to spatiotemporal contrast over most of the range of spatial and temporal frequencies to which macaques are normally sensitive. However, sensitivity to stimuli of low spatial and high temporal frequency was relatively unimpaired.

3. Special Advantages of Large Receptive Fields

We have concentrated so far on the disadvantages of sparse mosaics and large receptive fields, but large receptive fields also have some advantages. We examine some of these in the following paragraphs.

Larger receptive fields permit higher sensitivity. Inevitable fluctuations in the quantum catch from a nominally steady visual stimulus (together with quantumlike events that arise spontaneously in the photoreceptors) produce noise that sets a fundamental (and calculable) limit to the sensitivity of a cell to changes in illumination (see Chapter 5, this volume). This quantum noise is Poisson distributed about the mean (n), so has a standard deviation $\sqrt{n}$, which sets the limit to the detectability of changes in illumination. Other factors being equal, the sensitivity of a linear cell that sums signals from all the photoreceptors in its receptive field will depend straightforwardly on the area A of the receptive field. The noise that limits detectability is proportional to $\sqrt{A}$, so the signal-to-noise ratio, which determines the detectability of a stimulus, therefore grows as $\sqrt{A}$. Larger receptive fields thus permit the detection of stimuli at lower levels of illumination. [At the very lowest levels of illumination the surround of the receptive field is relatively ineffective (Barlow, Fitzhugh & Kuffler, 1957; Enroth-Cugell & Lennie, 1975) and can be neglected for the moment.] Of course, one might at some central site be able to achieve the benefits of a large receptive field by combining the signals from cells with many small receptive fields, but only if this combination could be undertaken without introducing noise.

The situation becomes more complicated when we consider the behavior of cells at high levels of illumination. Mechanisms of light adaptation (discussed in Chapter 5), which act separately in center and surround, adjust the sensitivities of cells according to the prevailing level of illumination. Some of the advantage of having a large receptive field center is lost because the mechanisms of light adaptation are driven by the quantum flux accumulated from the whole of the receptive field center, so absolute sensitivities of cells with larger receptive fields decline at lower levels of illumination than do the sensitivities of cells with small receptive fields (Enroth-Cugell & Shapley, 1973a; Linsenmeier, Frishman, Jakiela & Enroth-Cugell, 1982). Against this has to be set the fact that at high levels of illumination the receptive field surround acts to reduce sensitivity to low spatial frequencies, so cells with large receptive field centers will be better equipped to detect stimuli of low spatial frequency. The result of these forces seems to be that Y-cells have a definite advantage in detecting stimuli of low and intermediate spatial frequency (Troy, Robson & Enroth-Cugell, 1986; Troy, 1987).

At high levels of illumination, the peak contrast sensitivities of M- and P-cells in macaque differ by perhaps 5-fold or more (Kaplan & Shapley, 1982; Derrington & Lennie, 1984), and an individual M-cell therefore should have a substantial advantage in detecting low spatial frequencies. Purpura, Kaplan, and Shapley (1988a) found that at low levels of illumination the contrast sensitivities of P-cells fell much more rapidly than did the contrast sensitivities of M-cells, and they suggested that P-cells are little involved in rod (scotopic) vision. This conclusion needs some qualification in view of Fairchild and Lennie's (1988) finding that scotopic acuity over a range of eccentricities is much better than can be predicted by the mosaic of M-cells. Nonetheless, under many conditions an M-cell could detect stimuli that a P-cell could not. Part of this advantage is due to the larger receptive field of the M-cell having an improved signal-to-noise ratio, and would be diminished if a higher mechanism summed the signals from a group of adjacent P-cells. Were we to assume noiseless summation of signals from nine P-cells (approximately the number needed to create a receptive field center to match that of an M-cell) this higher mechanism would be at most 3 times more sensitive than an individual P-cell. It therefore seems likely that factors in addition to quantum noise are involved in making P-cells so much less sensitive than M-cells.

Shapley and Perry (1986) have drawn attention to one possibly beneficial side effect of the low contrast sensitivity of P-cells: over the whole of the range of contrasts to which P-cells respond the amplitude of response is proportional or very nearly proportional to contrast. The higher sensitivity of M-cells results in their more often giving saturated responses to high-contrast stimuli and hence becoming insensitive to differences in contrast (Sclar, Maunsell & Lennie, 1989).

4. Speed of Signal Transmission

The relatively large axons of Y-cells and M-cells give them a conduction advantage over X- and P-cells, respectively. For M- versus P-cells the advantage from retina to V1 is about 4 msec; for Y- versus X-cells the advantage is 2–3 msec. More important are the comparative latencies of responses to visual stimuli. No such comparison exists for the monkey, but Bolz, Rosner, and Wässle (1982) compared the latencies of responses of X- and Y-cells in cat, and found that Y-cells had shorter latencies to stimuli of any given contrast. This results from Y-cells being more sensitive to contrast, for the difference between classes disappears when responses of equal size are evoked (Troy & Lennie, 1987). Thus, under many circumstances, Y-cells will respond reliably faster than X-cells. This may be perceptually significant. Several psychophysical results (e.g., Breitmeyer, 1975, 1984; Harwerth & Levi, 1978) show that simple reaction time to the onset of a grating pattern of high spatial frequency exceeds that to the onset of a grating of low spatial frequency. Although these results implicate distinct fast and slow mechanisms, they are open to alternative interpretations that associate responses of different time-course with gratings of high and low spatial frequencies (Lennie, 1981).

5. Temporal Characteristics of Response

M- and P-cells (and also X- and Y-cells) differ in their temporal characteristics: M-cells respond well at temporal frequencies to which P-cells are quite unresponsive, but they show relatively greater loss of responsiveness as temporal frequency falls below about 10 Hz (Derrington & Lennie, 1984). They therefore respond more transiently than P-cells to step changes in contrast. These characteristics of M-cells, coupled with their high contrast sensitivity and large receptive fields, equip them well for the detection of fast-moving objects that produce only small changes in spatiotemporal contrast within the receptive field. P-cells, on the other hand, will be relatively insensitive to such patterns, but will respond well to slower moving patterns of higher spatial frequency.

A psychophysically based distinction between movement- and pattern-sensitive mechanisms was first clearly drawn by Tolhurst (1973), who found that the temporal requirements for contrast adaptation depended on the spatial frequency range being used in the the measurement: adaptation to patterns of low spatial frequency required flickering or moving stimuli. Tolhurst suggested the the mechanisms revealed by his experiments might correspond to X- and Y-cells (M- and P-cells in primates). His distinction between movement and form mechanisms, and the association with M and P pathways, has found considerable support in more recent work that has traced these pathways in cortex. We review this in Section V.

D. Conclusions

In transmitting information efficiently the visual system has to reconcile conflicting demands for sensitivity and spatial resolution, and perhaps the two classes of cells with plain, isotropic receptive fields have evolved to cope with this: cells with large receptive fields (M, Y) are inherently more sensitive than cells with small receptive fields (P, X) and are much more capable of signaling the low spatiotemporal contrasts produced by fast-moving stimuli. However, they are likely to be saturated by stimuli of high contrast and in general cannot resolve high spatial frequencies. On the other hand, cells with small receptive fields signal high frequencies in the image, but at the expense of sensitivity.

We have not yet come to grips with the analysis undertaken by cortex: if we adopt the position that the signals arriving at cortex via the thalamic pathway provide a relatively faithful copy of the retinal image, then the arguments we reviewed earlier lead us to expect that multiple parallel analyses will be undertaken in cortex. We also might be able more firmly to establish the roles of the different pathways from LGN were we able to trace them to regions whose function we can confidently infer from the specialized properties of the cells within them, or from the specific effects on behavior of damage to them. We examine these topics next in Section V.

V. ANALYSIS OF SIGNALS IN CORTEX

In both cat and monkey the principal projection from the LGN is to striate cortex (V1), but while the cat also has direct projections to areas 18 and 19 and to the lateral suprasylvian region, the monkey appears to have no other projection of any substance. V1 in cat thus appears to be one of several parallel representations of the visual field (a good deal of work shows that, despite removal of V1, the cat can make reasonably fine visual discriminations), while in monkey V1 appears to be yet one more stage in the serial elaboration of visual signals, and removal of it leaves the monkey essentially blind (see also Chapter 14, this volume, for a discussion of human cortical blindness). Because the organization of cortex differs so greatly in cat and monkey, and because we know a great deal more about the organization in monkey, the remainder of this chapter deals almost exclusively with the latter species.

A. Organization of V1

Like the LGN, V1 in macaque contains a representation that preserves the retinal topography. Striate cortex has distinctive cytoarchitecture—the striation for which it is named is a prominent feature of layer 4—and physiological recordings show that the area contains a single representation of the visual field, disproportionately weighted toward the fovea. The representation of 1 degree at the fovea extends over about 15 mm cortex, but at 10° eccentricity 1 degree is represented by about 1 mm (Van Essen, Newsome & Maunsell, 1984). Figure 10 shows diagrammatically the major projections from LGN to V1. Parvocellular neurons project principally to cortical layers 4Cβ and 4A, with a smaller projection to both layer 1 and the upper part of of layer 6 (Hubel & Wiesel, 1972; Hendricksen, Wilson & Ogren, 1978). The different projections appear to arise in different neurons (Blasdel & Lund, 1983). Magnocellular neurons project almost exclusively to layer 4Ca (Hubel & Wiesel, 1972; Hendricksen et al., 1978). Despite the strict segregation of afferents, the signals from M and P streams may be mixed from the outset of cortical processing, since dendrites from cells in one component of layer 4C extend into the other.

Receptive fields in the subdivisions of layer 4 are in many respects much like those found in LGN. Al-

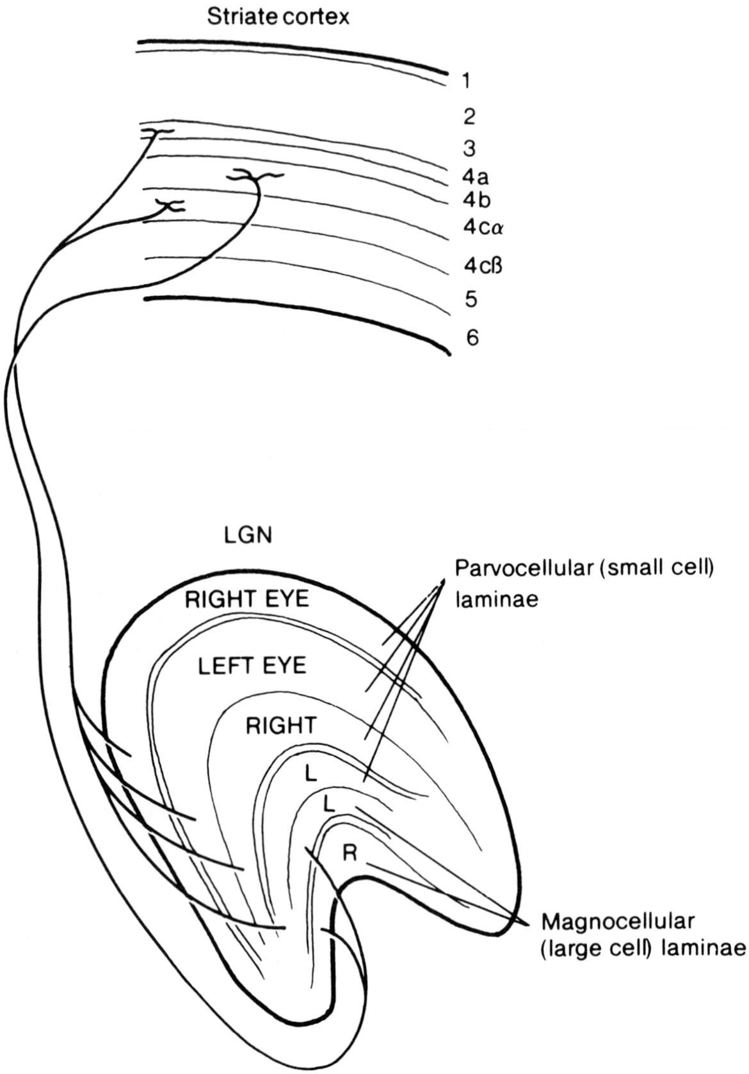

FIG. 10 Principal projections of P- and M-cells in LGN to striate cortex. The drawing shows a coronal section through the left LGN of the macaque. P-cells project principally to layers 4Cβ and 4A, but there are also minor projections to layers 1 and 6. M-cells project principally to layer 4Cα.

most all are monocularly driven, and many are concentrically organized. Inputs from the two eyes are sharply segregated into long strips running parallel to the surface of V1. These ocular dominance slabs are readily demonstrated anatomically (LeVay, Hubel & Wiesel, 1975) and physiologically (Hubel & Wiesel, 1968). Beyond the recipient zones of layer 4 the M and P streams are not strictly segregated anatomically, although they project predominantly to different places. M neurons in layer 4Cα project principally to layer 4B, which in turn sends substantial projections out of striate cortex to the second visual area (V2), the third visual area (V3) and the middle temporal area (MT); layer 4Cα also has lesser projections to parts of layer 2/3 within striate cortex (Fitzpatrick, Lund & Blasdel, 1985). P neurons in layer 4Cβ project principally to layer 4A and to the lower part of layer 3. The strict segregation of the eyes is lost outside layer 4, and in the layers above and below it many neurons are driven by signals from both eyes. Here too receptive fields are more elaborate, and orientation-selective simple and complex cells are common (Hubel & Wiesel, 1968). Across the width of a single ocular dominance slab the preferred orientations of neurons progress through about 180° (Hubel & Wiesel, 1968).

Although M and P streams are brought into close anatomical proximity in the upper cortical layers, their physiological convergence has been little studied. No established properties of cortical receptive fields seem to demand inputs from both classes of afferent, and we have to rely on experiments in which the M or P pathways are selectively disabled, or selectively excited, to provide information about convergence. Malpeli, Schiller, and Colby (1981) injected the local anesthetic lidocaine separately into parvocellular and magnocellular layers of LGN and found signs that about half the simple and complex cells received inputs from both types of afferent. This is a remarkable finding in view of the anatomical segregation of M and P inputs to cortex.

The high contrast sensitivities of M-cells in the LGN are reflected in the sensitivities of cells in layers 4Cα and 4B (Hawken & Parker, 1984), and this, coupled with their relatively large receptive fields, their responsiveness to high temporal frequencies, and sometimes pronounced direction selectivity (Hawken, Parker & Lund, 1988), equips them well for the detection of fast-moving objects that produce rather low spatiotemporal contrasts during passage across the receptive field. These properties suggest the beginnings of a pathway for the analysis of motion. We return to this later, when we examine the properties of neurons in regions to which layer 4B projects.

Earlier we drew attention to the fact that the P-cells in LGN probably carry most of the information about both the chromatic and the spatial structure of objects. Livingstone and Hubel (1984, 1987b) have suggested that within V1 the spatial and chromatic signals are analyzed separately, resulting in the formation of distinct "color" and "form" pathways. This two-pathway scheme is founded principally on a correlation between the visual sensitivities of neurons and a distinctive anatomical feature of striate cortex. Tangential sections through the upper layers of striate cortex reveal a mosaic of roughly circular patches ("blobs") that stain densely for the mitochondrial enzyme cytochrome oxidase. High concentrations of this enzyme are associated with high metabolic activity. The blobs lose their identity in layer 4 (which stains uniformly for cytochrome oxidase) but are visible in layers 5 and 6. The source of their inputs is unknown but in the upper layers is widely assumed to arise mainly from P-cells. Livingstone and Hubel (1984) found in the blobs a preponderance of neurons that had concentrically organized receptive fields with relatively poor spatial resolving power and relatively high sensitivity to chromatic contrast; neurons in the intervening spaces had spatially more elaborate receptive fields and showed little chromatic opponency. Livingstone and Hubel suggest that neurons in the blobs are the substrate of a specialized pathway for chromatic information, while neurons in the intervening regions support the analysis of form.

These conclusions receive mixed support from other work. Tootell, Silverman, Hamilton, DeValois and Switkes (1988) found that following exposure to spatially-diffuse isoluminant chromatic modulation there was preferential uptake in the blobs of radiolabeled 2-deoxyglucose, and Ts'o and Gilbert (1988) found that chromatically opponent neurons were common in blobs. However, Tootell, Hamilton and Switkes (1988; Tootell, Silverman, Hamilton, Switkes & DeValois, 1988) also found that achromatic patterns of low spatial frequency preferentially labeled blobs, and Lennie, Krauskopf, and Sclar (unpublished) found no *preferential* distribution of chromatically opponent neurons in blobs in the upper layers. We thus have some evidence for the existence of distinct "form" and "color" pathways in V1, and although the distinction is not a sharp one, much has been made of it in work that has analyzed the progress of visual signals beyond VI.

B. Dispersion to Specialized Representations

V1 sends major projections to (and receives reciprocal projections from) three regions of extrastriate cortex. These regions, known as the second visual area (V2), the third visual area (V3), and the middle temporal area (MT), are marked on the exploded views of Fig. 11 and the unfolded cortical surface in Fig. 12. V1 also sends minor or inconsistent projections to areas V3A, V4 and PO. All these areas (and the others indicated in Figs. 11 and 12) are recognized as distinct regions by virtue of their connections, myeloarchitecture, topographic organization, physiological properties, or some combination of these. V2, V3, and MT each receive a topographically organized projection from V1 (although in V3 this represents only the lower visual field) and contain, at least crudely, a topographic map of the visual field (Van Essen, Newsome, Maunsell & Bixby, 1986; Maunsell & Van Essen, 1983). [Receptive fields of neurons in extrastriate cortex are larger than those of neurons in V1; receptive fields of neurons in MT are so much larger (100 times by area) that the precision of the topography is correspondingly hard to discern.] V2, V3, and MT receive projections from different parts of V1, and appear to be associated in different ways with the information carried by the P- and M-streams.

We remarked at the beginning of this chapter that although parallel representations were probably essential for speedy perceptual analysis, little was known about how perceptual tasks ought to be decomposed. In considering the function of extrastriate visual areas, physiologists and anatomists have therefore relied very heavily on hints offered by the properties of receptive fields of neurons, and on information about the properties of neurons in the parts of V1 from which a particular projection is derived. We know rather little about the visual characteristics of neurons in most extrastriate areas, or about the interconnections of different visual areas, and what follows is therefore a mostly circumstantial and tentative account of some of the visual analyses undertaken by extrastriate cortex.

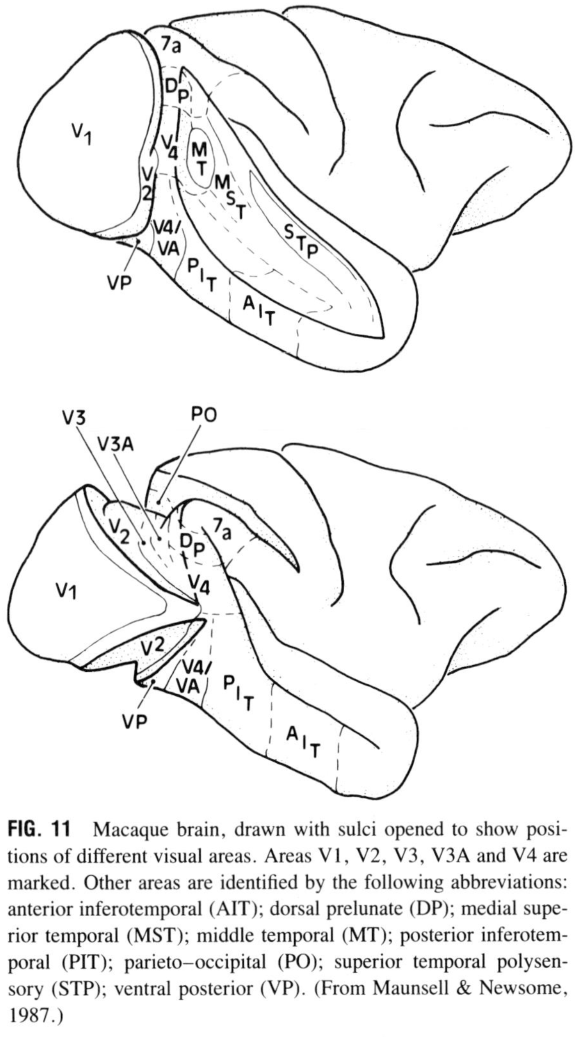

FIG. 11 Macaque brain, drawn with sulci opened to show positions of different visual areas. Areas V1, V2, V3, V3A and V4 are marked. Other areas are identified by the following abbreviations: anterior inferotemporal (AIT); dorsal prelunate (DP); medial superior temporal (MST); middle temporal (MT); posterior inferotemporal (PIT); parieto–occipital (PO); superior temporal polysensory (STP); ventral posterior (VP). (From Maunsell & Newsome, 1987.)

1. The Second Visual Area (V2)

The anatomy and physiology of V2 have received considerable attention, and this work offers us some hints about the roles of the M and P pathways. When

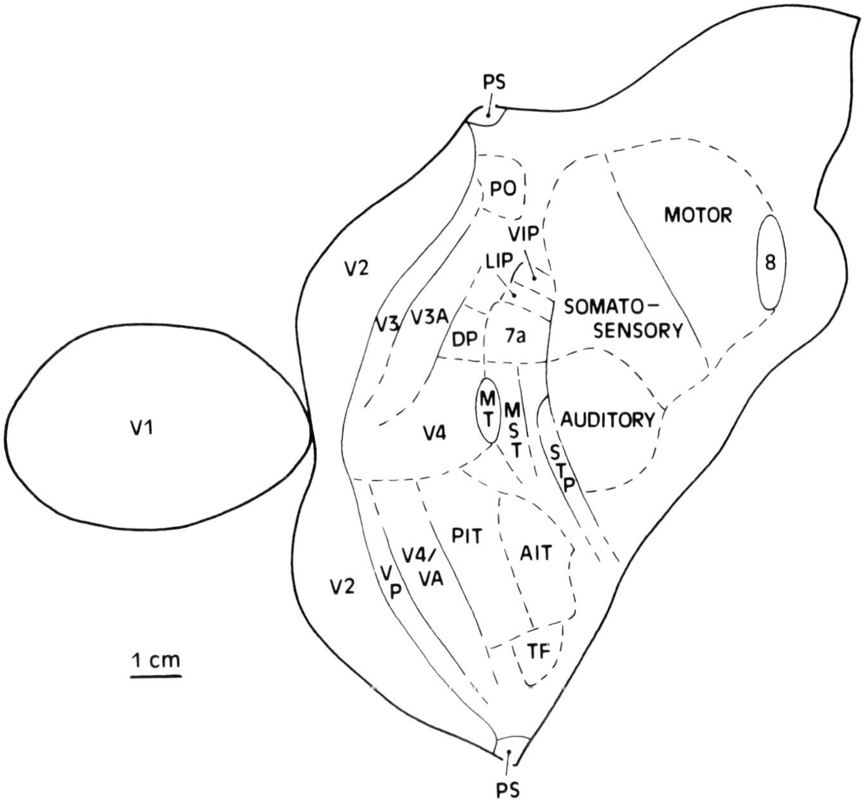

FIG. 12 Whole macaque cortex from the right hemisphere, unfolded to show the relative sizes and positions of different visual areas. Areas are identified by the abbreviations used in Fig. 11. (From Maunsell & Newsome, 1987.)

stained for cytochrome oxidase, tangential sections of V2 appear striped, dense-staining regions alternating with pale ones (Tootell, Silverman, DeValois & Jacobs, 1983; Livingstone & Hubel, 1984). In the squirrel monkey, the dense-staining stripes appear alternately thick and thin, but in macaque, with which we are particularly concerned, this distinction is sometimes hard to draw (Hubel & Livingstone, 1987), although the thick stripes can be identified independently by their immunoreactivity to the antibody CAT 301 (DeYoe & Van Essen, 1985).

Livingstone and Hubel (1984) showed that the blobs in V1 projected to the stripes in V2 and that the interblob regions in V1 projected to the interstripe regions of V2. In the squirrel monkey only the thin stripes receive input from blobs; the thick stripes receive input principally from layer 4B (Livingstone & Hubel, 1987a). The picture is similar in macaque: two sorts of stripes can be distinguished by their inputs from V1 (Livingstone & Hubel, 1984, 1987a), by the sites to which they project (DeYoe & Van Essen, 1985; Shipp & Zeki, 1985), and by the visual sensitivities of neurons contained in them (DeYoe & Van Essen, 1985; Hubel & Livingstone, 1987). The most complete description so far available comes from Hubel and Livingstone (1987), who observed that the thick stripes in squirrel monkey (and one set of stripes in macaque), which are presumptively associated with the M pathway, contained a preponderance of complex cells that showed pronounced selectivity for binocular disparity; the thin stripes (and the other set of stripes in macaque), which are presumed associated with the P pathway, contained a preponderance of cells that lacked orientation selectivity and in the macaque were chromatically opponent; the inter-stripe regions contained many neurons that had "end-stopped" receptive fields.

V2 appears to be an early stage in the formation of specialized representations that develop from the P and M streams. Since we know rather little about the properties of its neurons, however, it would be unwise to depend on that conclusion.

2. The Third Visual Area (V3)

Only the lower part of the visual field is represented in V3; a corresponding area (the ventral posterior area, VP) that contains a representation of the upper part of the visual field is no longer considered to be a part of V3 because of differences in cytoarchitecture, projections from V1, and the visual characteristics of the cells (Felleman & Van Essen, 1987). V3 receives inputs from layer 4B of striate cortex and from the thick stripes of V2 (Felleman et al., 1988). The visual properties of cells within V3 have provided few clues about its visual function: most cells are strongly orientation selective, and many are strongly directionally selective and sensitive to binocular disparity. Relatively few are chromatically selective. The most distinctive cells, which are rarely encountered, are narrowly tuned for several orientations or directions of motion of a simple stimulus (Felleman & Van Essen, 1987).

The visual properties of neurons in V3 provide no clear suggestion that it is organized to represent any particular dimension of the visual image or support any specialized perceptual task. We learn a little more about its possible role by considering its projections to more specialized areas.

3. A Motion-Selective Pathway?

The middle temporal area has been implicated in the analysis of movement since Dubner and Zeki's (1971) discovery that the bulk of the neurons in it were strongly directionally selective. MT receives major direct projections from V1, arising in layer 4B (Maunsell & Van Essen, 1983) and layer 6 (Fries, Keizer & Kuypers, 1985); and indirect input via the cytochrome-oxidase thick stripes in V2 (DeYoe & Van Essen, 1985; Shipp & Zeki, 1985). MT also receives input from V3 (Maunsell & Van Essen, 1983; Ungerleider & Desimone, 1986). These projections are intimately linked to the M pathway from the LGN, which projects via layer 4Cα largely to layer 4B of V1.

The strongest evidence tying MT to the analysis of movement comes from experiments that show neurons in it responding distinctively to the movement of complex patterns, from experiments to examine the effects of small chemical lesions on oculomotor behavior, and from experiments that link perceptual thresholds directly to the responses of neurons in MT. Movshon, Adelson, Gizzi, and Newsome (1986) found that when two sinusoidal grating patterns of different orientation were superimposed and moved as a whole across the receptive field in different directions, orientation-selective neurons in V1 responded as if to the component patterns presented separately, and not to the whole, giving a first peak response when one component of the pattern was aligned with the preferred orientation and another when the other component of the pattern was aligned with the preferred orientation. Most neurons in MT behaved similarly, but about 20% of them responded best to the complex when as a unit it moved in the direction preferred for a single component, rather than along a trajectory that aligned one of the components with this preferred direction. Newsome, Wurtz, Dursteler, and Mikami (1985) made small chemical lesions in MT and found that monkeys were temporarily less able to capture and pursue targets moving through the affected portion of the visual field. Newsome and Pare (1988) have also shown that the behaving monkey and individual neurons in MT can detect moving dynamic texture patterns under the same conditions.

Although this work strongly implicates MT in the analysis of movement, we do not yet know much about how it contributes to the *perception* of movement or about the mechanisms that endow it with its distinctive properties. Nor is it clear how signals from V2 and V3 shape the properties of its neurons. V3 and the thick stripes in V2 contain relatively few cells that are directionally selective, but both areas contain many neurons with high sensitivity to binocular disparity, which is not a conspicuous attribute of neurons in MT.

4. A Pathway for Color?

Zeki (1973) identified in macaque an area that runs from the anterior bank of the lunate sulcus on to the prelunate gyrus and contains many neurons that have pronounced chromatic selectivities. He called this V4 (Figs. 11 and 12) or the V4 complex (Zeki, 1977). There is wide agreement that at least parts of the V4 complex contain large numbers of neurons that are chromatically selective (e.g., Schein, Marrocco & DeMonasterio, 1982; Desimone, Schein, Moran & Ungerleider, 1985). V4 receives a small direct projection from V1; the bulk of its input arises in V2 and V3. The projection from V2 arises in one set of cytochrome-oxidase stripes (thin in the squirrel monkey) and in the interstripe regions (DeYoe & Van Essen, 1985; Shipp & Zeki, 1985), the former by implication being the source of the chromatically opponent signals. The origin of the projection from V3 is unknown.

Although V4 is widely acknowledged to have an important role in the analysis of color, the details of the analysis are unclear. Many neurons are no more chromatically selective than are those in V1 (DeMonasterio & Schein, 1982). Receptive fields, despite being large (4–6 times the linear dimensions of receptive fields at comparable eccentricities in V1), have spatial and orientational selectivities much like those of neurons in V1 (Desimone et al., 1985). This fine spatial selectivity within a large receptive field is reminiscent of a complex cell, but other properties of the receptive fields make it clear that neurons in V4 are unlike complex cells in V1. For many cells the part of the receptive field from which an overt response can be elicited is small, but this region is surrounded by a much larger region within which illumination generally suppresses the response.

One major function we might expect of higher level chromatic mechanisms is that they would contribute to color constancy, the perceived stability of the colors of objects despite variations in the spectral composition of the illumination falling on them (e.g., in moving from daylight to tungsten light). The formal requirements for color constancy have been thoroughly studied (see Lennie & D'Zmura, 1988, for further discussion of these), but it is not easy to see what should be the embodiment of mechanisms to achieve it. Some of the properties of neurons in V4 are relevant here: large receptive fields with chromatically opponent organization could help discount changes in the spectral composition of the illumination falling on a scene, and thereby contribute to the stable appearance of colored objects. Zeki (1983a) found that the responses of cells in V4 (to a physically constant stimulus in the middle of the receptive field) varied with the color of surrounding regions in a way that was correlated with the appearance of the central stimulus to a human observer.

These observations suggest that V4 forms a stage in some higher level chromatic analysis, but it must do other things as well, since it receives input from the interstripe regions of V2, which appear to have spatially elaborate receptive fields, and from V3, which contains relatively few neurons that show overt color opponency. Its involvement in spatial vision was demonstrated clearly by Heywood and Cowey (1987) who showed that bilateral damage to V4 in macaque impaired chromatic discriminations and left pattern and orientation discriminations grossly disturbed. Moreover, V4 provides the major input to posterior inferotemporal cortex (PIT) and anterior inferotemporal cortex (AIT), regions in which damage greatly impairs monkeys' capacities to recognize and distinguish objects (Mishkin, 1982). The ambiguous role of V4 is also emphasized by the observation that in human patients who have a relatively specific impairment of color vision (achromatopsia) as a result of a cerebral accident, the damage is commonly confined to regions of ventral occipitoparietal cortex that are unlikely to be homologous to V4 (see Chapter 8, this volume).

C. Higher Level Representations

We have discussed only 5 of the more than 20 identified visual areas in the macaque's cortex, and have only touched on the complexity of their interconnections. The hierarchical arrangement of the different visual areas is to some degree established by anatomical work, but little is known about the kinds of representations they contain. There is some suggestion, from both clinical neurology and experimental physiology, that higher visual areas fall into two groups, one particularly concerned with locating objects and the other with identifying them (Ungerleider & Mishkin, 1982; Mishkin, Ungerleider & Macko, 1983; Maunsell & Newsome, 1987). These constellations of areas seem to diverge beyond V2 and V3, with one (apparently involving MT) running toward superior parietal cortex, a region that from clinical neurology we know is involved in disturbances of space perception (Ungerleider & Mishkin, 1982). The other group of areas (apparently involving V4) leads into inferior temporal cortex, a region in which damage disrupts the capacity to recognize objects (Mishkin, et al., 1983; Damasio, 1985).

A general feature of the organization of extrastriate cortex is that the farther removed an area is from V1, the larger are its receptive fields. This raises the question of whether in regions such as inferior temporal cortex, in which receptive fields can be very large (up to 1000 degree^2), the visual areas actually contain topographically organized representations. Some visual representations must be freed from the retinal map, because our percepts are not tied to retinal coordinates, but we do not yet have well-developed principles for recognizing them.

VI. GENERAL CONCLUSIONS

Our discussion makes very clear that the visual system is organized for parallel analyses of the image. The early stages of these analyses are well characterized by anatomical and physiological work, although that work provides only modest hints about the dimensions along which the image is analyzed. Work on cortex reveals the richness of the parallel representations, but single-unit recording, which has been the principal means of discerning the properties of the representations in different areas, provides mixed information about them. For some areas (notably MT) the physiological work seems to provide clear pointers to function, but for others (e.g., V3 and V4) the picture is much less clear. One potential weakness of single-unit physiology is that unless the visual requirements of a neuron are relatively simple or are already known, no stimulus presented to it may excite it optimally. We should expect to encounter this problem often in extrastriate cortex, and we should draw on information from other sources (e.g., evidence on the perceptual consequences of identified cerebral lesions; evidence from perceptual experiments on the dimensions along which parallel analyses of the image are undertaken) in guiding our physiological explorations.

The parallel analysis of the image is valuable because it enables the rapid assembly of percepts, but it does introduce problems: How is the information contained in the separate representations brought together to yield unified experience of the visual world? We can expect this question to be a major target of future research.

ACKNOWLEDGMENTS

The National Institutes of Health supported Peter Lennie (through grants EY 04440 and EY 01319) and David Van Essen (through grant EY 02091).

7

THE PERCEPTION OF BRIGHTNESS AND DARKNESS
RELATIONS TO NEURONAL RECEPTIVE FIELDS

Adriana Fiorentini, Günter Baumgartner, Svein Magnussen, Peter H. Schiller, and James P. Thomas

I. INTRODUCTION

This chapter deals with one of the fundamental phenomena of vision, the perception of brightness and darkness. The problem has attracted the attention of many scientists, notably the founders of modern visual science: Helmholtz (1867), Hering (1878), and Mach (1897). These early students of vision were well aware of the discrepancies between the distribution of perceived brightness in the visual world and the physical distribution of light in the retinal image, and they offered possible explanations in terms of neural processes taking place in the retina and in the brain. Their interpretations, based on detailed psychophysical experiments, were essentially correct. However, they were largely speculative as to the real nature of the underlying neural processes, because of the lack of knowledge at the time. The subsequent advances in knowledge of the physiological properties of the retina and the higher visual centers, as well as the development of psychophysical methods that supply detailed quantitative data on brightness perception and related phenomena, now permit more informed interpretation of perceptual phenomena in terms of neural functions. One theme that has emerged over the years is that brightness and darkness are qualitatively different, rather than points on a single continuum of perceived intensity. Jung (1961) was among the first to suggest that the perception of brightness and darkness may be subserved by two different populations of cells with opposing responses, namely, the ON- and OFF-cells.

The discussion is divided into four sections. Section II briefly introduces the basic perceptual phenomena of brightness and darkness perception and of simultaneous and successive contrast. Section III deals with neurophysiological findings on the properties of the ON- and OFF-cells that are believed to underlie these phenomena. Section IV reports psychophysical evidence for the perceptual correlates of the ON- and OFF-channels. Section V discusses some of the models for the interpretation of border contrast effects. The chapter concludes with a general review of the present state of knowledge about the topics of the previous sections.

For the sake of clarity, some of the terms that frequently recur in the following sections are defined here (also see Wyszecki & Stiles, 1982). Vision is said to be *photopic* at high levels of ambient illumination, as in daylight or bright artificial lighting. Night vision, that is, vision at low levels of illumination, is called *scotopic*. Twilight vision is called *mesopic*. The photometric quantity most relevant to our topic is *luminance*, defined as the light flux emitted per unit of solid angle from the unit area of the object surface projected perpendicular to viewing direction. *Reflectance* of a matte diffusing surface is the ratio between the light flux reflected by the surface and the incident flux, both relative to the unit area. The luminance of a homogeneously illuminated diffusing surface is proportional to its reflectance.

Brightness and darkness are attributes of visual sensation and perception. Brightness is the attribute according to which an area of the visual field appears to emit more or less light than surrounding areas. Usually it refers to self-luminous stimuli. Darkness generally refers to the opposite of brightness. When several reflecting objects are simultaneously present in the visual field, and are illuminated by daylight, some of them may appear *white* (objects with very high reflectance), while others may appear *black* (objects with very low reflectance). *Lightness* is the attribute of visual sensation according to which an object appears to reflect more or less light in comparison with an object that appears white. Thus, lightness is an attribute of apparent reflectance and is related to the perception of the object surface.

In this chapter, we mainly deal with brightness and darkness as attributes of the perception either of self-luminous objects surrounded by other areas of different luminance or of objects with matte diffusing surfaces of various reflectances. In the latter case, it might be more appropriate to speak of "lightness" rather than "brightness." However, for the most part we use the terms interchangeably on the grounds that the neural mechanisms discussed in this chapter affect brightness and lightness in similar fashion.

We also assume that the flux reaching our eyes from the various points in the visual field is largely independent of wavelength. Thus we deal only with achromatic sensations. Separating achromatic brightness perception from the perception of chromatic aspects of a visual stimulus is in line with the Hering (1878) theory of opponent processes mentioned below (Section II,B,2). This theory assumes the existence of separate mechanisms for the processing of the achromatic and chromatic components of a visual stimulus. Consistent with this theory is the finding by Werner, Cicerone, Kliegl, and DellaRosa (1984) suggesting that the blackness (darkness) of a color is inversely related to its luminance and is independent of hue. Recent anatomical and neurophysiological data also support the existence of separate neural pathways for the processing of achromatic and chromatic stimulus components (Hubel & Livingstone, 1987).

II. BASIC PERCEPTUAL PHENOMENA

A. Brightness and Darkness

The terms brightness and darkness usually describe the sensation of light, or its converse (Helmholtz, 1867). It is important to point out, however, that brightness and darkness perceptions depend on the spatial (and temporal) distribution of light in the visual field. A single illuminated object, in a completely dark surround, always appears bright. Even a piece of coal appears bright if illuminated in isolation under these conditions. However, when two objects of different reflectances are presented next to one another, the previous sensations are modified. For instance, a piece of chalk placed against the piece of coal turns the latter into "black" (Gelb, 1929). The chalk appears "white." Thus, the first problem we face when dealing with brightness sensation is its dependence on spatial and temporal changes in the physical distribution of light flux reaching our eyes from the various portions of the visual field.

The Gelb effect described above is but an extreme

case of a large class of phenomena that are traditionally referred to as simultaneous or successive contrast effects. The sections which follow consider four classes of contrast effects: simultaneous contrast, successive contrast, border contrast and area contrast. An additional section summarizes the literature on short-range brightness induction as a means of measuring the size of human perceptive fields.

B. Simultaneous Contrast

In a normal visual environment, illuminated by daylight, neutral objects appear brighter or darker according to whether they reflect a higher or lower percentage of the incident light. However, an object of moderate reflectance appears relatively brighter or darker according to whether spatially adjacent regions are considerably darker or brighter than the object itself. This dependence of the brightness of one region on the relative brightnesses of adjacent regions is called *simultaneous contrast*. An important property is that the contrast effect is not necessarily limited to areas immediately adjacent to the borders. If the borders enclose a large homogeneous region, the change in brightness produced by the contrast effect spreads uniformly over the entire enclosed region. This widely spreading effect is called *area contrast* to distinguish it from more localized contrast effects. Figure 1 illustrates simultaneous contrast, including area contrast.

1. Brightness Constancy

It is a common experience that the perceived brightness of real objects in a natural environment is largely independent of changes in the overall level of illumination. For example, the pages of this book appear white and the printed letters black, no matter whether illuminated by bright sunshine or by the much weaker light of a desk lamp. This phenomenon is known as *brightness constancy*. It tends to keep constant the brightness attributes of objects despite variations in the overall level of illumination. "Without this approximate constancy, a piece of chalk on a cloudy day would manifest the same color as a piece of coal does on a sunny day, and in the course of a single day it would have to assume all possible colors that lie between black and white" (Hering, 1878).

Experiments have shown that the perceptual constancy of objects in complex scenes, viewed at different illumination levels, holds more for *light-*

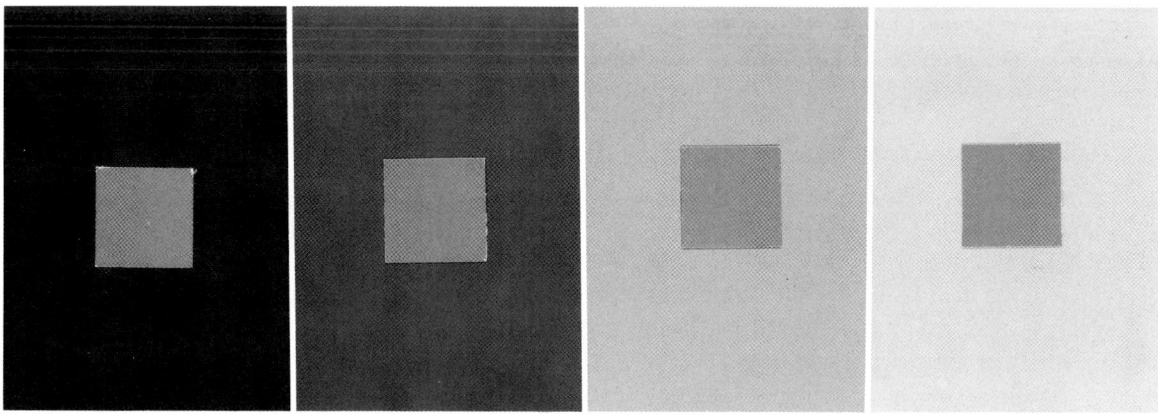

FIG. 1 Classical example of simultaneous contrast (area contrast). The inner squares all have the same luminance, but they appear different: the darker the surround, the brighter the inner square. After Hering (1920).

ness (i.e., the surface attribute related to reflectance) than for brightness. As illumination is increased (or decreased) and object luminance increases (or decreases), the object appears brighter (or darker). However, the change is perceived as resulting from (approximately) constant surface properties and varying illumination, rather than from changing reflectance (Arend & Goldstein, 1987). For this particular situation, the term *lightness constancy* might be more appropriate than *brightness constancy*. However, in the discussion which follows, the latter term will be used to indicate subjective constancy because it is more widely used, even in contemporary literature.

The effects of simultaneous contrast and brightness constancy can be better understood if a quantity is defined that expresses the relative luminance of the object surface with respect to the background. This *objective* contrast, C, can be defined as

$$C = (L_o - L)/L = \Delta L/L$$

where L_o and L are the luminances of the object and the background, respectively. The difference ($\Delta L = L_o - L$) is the incremental (if positive) or decremental (if negative) luminance of the object with respect to the background. For uniformly illuminated diffusing surfaces, the luminance is proportional to the surface reflectance. Thus the objective contrast, or relative luminance of an object with respect to its background, depends only on the reflectances of the object and background and is invariant with respect to overall illumination changes (Shapley & Enroth-Cugell, 1984).

2. Brightness and Darkness Processes

To the extent that brightness constancy holds, it can be said that brightness is determined solely by objective contrast. However, there are limits to brightness constancy. If the light level is very low, the range of apparent brightnesses is very restricted. As noted by Hering (1878), in complete darkness one perceives no brightness differences, but merely a sensation of intrinsic gray (Eigengrau). At twilight, one can perceive at least vague differences of gray levels among different regions of the visual field. At day break, the range of brightness levels increases considerably: bright objects appear increasingly bright, and dark objects appear increasingly dark. The fact that some objects grow darker under increasing illumination was the cornerstone of Hering's theory of opponent processes. Hering (1878, 1905) claimed that the perceptual scale of brightness from black to white does not result from the increasing excitation of a single perceptual mechanism, but from the antagonistic responses of two opponent mechanisms, one responsible for brightness and the other for darkness.

The observation that, when illumination is raised from low to high levels, objects of high reflectance grow in brightness and objects of low reflectance increase in darkness was experimentally verified by Jameson and Hurvich (1964). The result (which is now considered controversial, however) was taken as evidence that darkness is a real sensation, qualitatively different from a mere decrease in brightness. Accordingly, brightness and darkness have been considered the products of two opponent processes. Jung (1961, 1973) proposed that the antagonistic mechanisms responsible for brightness and darkness perception be identified with populations of ON-center and OFF-center neurons in the visual system. This proposition is discussed in Section III, and psychophysical evidence consistent with the opponent theory is presented in Section IV.

3. Spatial Factors in Brightness Perception

There are further exceptions to brightness constancy. In other words, even in photopic conditions brightness is not always determined merely by objective contrast. Other factors may come into play.

The lightness resulting from effects of simultaneous contrast can also vary considerably according to whether the edges between regions of different luminance in the background (e.g., the edges of the large squares in Fig. 1) are attributed to differences in reflectance of the adjoining surfaces or to steps of illumination on an otherwise uniform surface (Gilchrist, Delman & Jacobsen, 1983). For example, brightness depends on the sharpness of the boundary which separates two regions. So far, we have assumed tacitly that the various objects were separated from their background by sharp edges, that is, by luminance steps. This is certainly a common occurrence in our visual environment. However, there may be gradual changes of luminance from one point to another in our visual field, either because of nonuniform illumination or because the illuminated surfaces are not flat or not uniformly diffusing. These gradual changes in luminance (which are transformed into low spatial frequency components in the Fourier domain) are not effective stimuli for our visual system, and are largely neglected (see Chapters 10 and 15, this volume).

In some cases, area contrast interacts with form perception (Koffka, 1935). For instance, an annulus of uniform reflectance superimposed on a bipartite field (two areas, separated by a sharp edge, with reflectances higher and lower than the annulus) appears uniformly bright. Thus, the area contrast is not perceived if the annulus appears as a solid figure in front of the background. However, if the annulus is divided into two parts by a black line aligned with the edge in the background, the two halves of the annulus appear to have different brightnesses.

Another phenomenon, which appears paradoxical when compared with the simultaneous contrast effects demonstrated in Fig. 1, is assimilation. It was first described by von Bezold (1874), who noticed that some arabesque patterns used for decoration had a striking effect on the perceived brightness of their background. A neutral background of intermediate luminance appears brighter if the superimposed pattern is made of white lines (lines of higher luminance than the background). On the other hand, the same background appears darker if the pattern consists of black (low luminance) lines (see Fig. 2). Thus, the pattern alters the brightness of the underlying surface in a sense opposite to that of simultaneous contrast. Assimilation is particularly evident with patterns of thin and finely spaced lines (Helson, 1963; Hurvich & Jameson, 1966) and may thus depend on spatial integration within retinal receptive fields (Hurvich & Jameson, 1974).

C. Border Contrast Effects (Short-Range Effects)

Border contrast effects constitute another important class of contrast phenomena. They are localized subjective changes in brightness and darkness which are

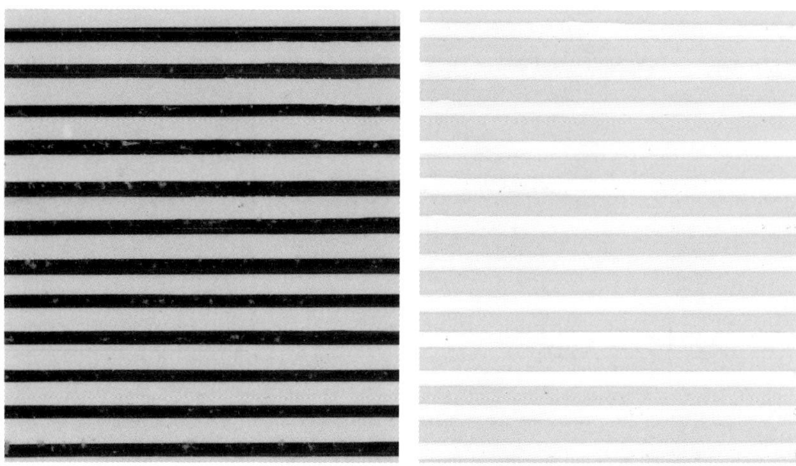

FIG. 2 Example of assimilation. The gray background has the same reflectance in both parts of the figure. However, where the black lines are superimposed, the background appears darker; where white lines are superimposed, it appears lighter.

perceived near the transition from a region of high luminance to a region of low luminance. They cause the perceived brightness distribution to deviate substantially from the physical luminance distribution.

Impressive examples of a border contrast effect are the Mach bands, first described by the Austrian physicist and philosopher Ernst Mach (1865). Mach bands are bright and dark lines that appear near the brighter and darker border, respectively, of a blurred edge between two uniform regions of different luminance (Fig. 3). These subjective lines enhance the border between the two regions, as real lines would do. The luminance ramp must be neither too shallow nor too steep if the Mach bands are to be visible. Periodic patterns with triangular or trapezoidal luminance profiles also exhibit Mach bands, provided their spatial frequency (number of stimulus periods per degree of visual angle) is not too high (Ross, Holt & Johnstone, 1981) and their mean luminance not too low (Fiorentini & Maffei, 1973; Ross et al., 1981).

These subjective border contrast effects must result from neural processing of the luminance distribution in the retinal image. Mach (1866a,b) offered an explanation in terms of lateral inhibition in the retina. He proposed that each functional unit in the retinal network has an excitatory component adjacent to an inhibitory component. The strength of the latter decreases with distance from the center of the unit.

A network composed of neural units of this kind accounts, at least qualitatively, for the Mach bands produced by various types of luminance distributions (see Ratliff & Hartline, 1959). Figure 4 shows how the spike activity of single ganglion cells of the cat retina vary in response to a contrast edge (Baumgartner, 1964; Enroth-Cugell & Robson, 1966). The response profiles contain minima and maxima which are analogous to Mach bands. (For a review of early models of retinal networks proposed to explain Mach bands in terms of lateral inhibition, see Ratliff, 1965.)

However, the analogy between perception and single

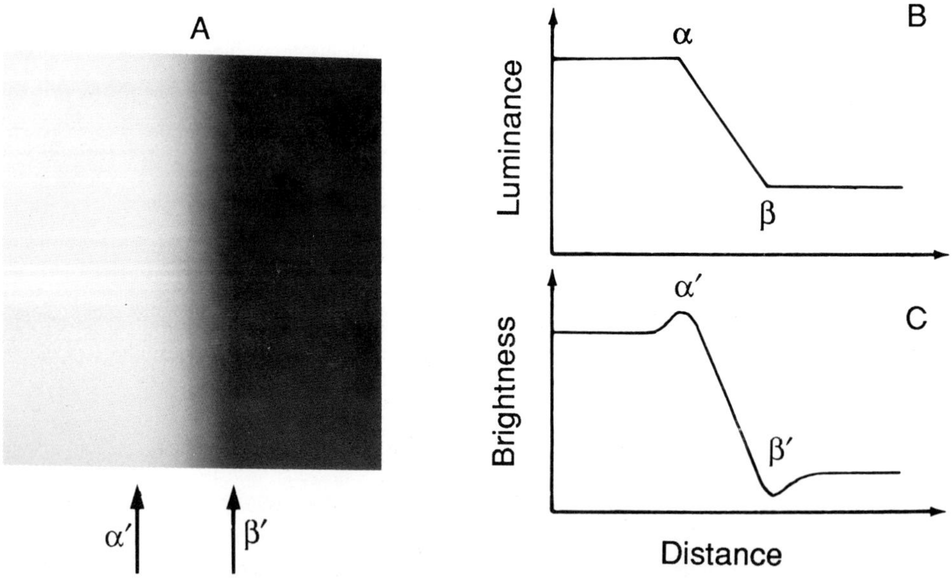

FIG. 3 Mach bands. In A there are two uniform zones of different luminance separated by a luminance ramp, as indicated in B. We perceive bright and dark bands (α', β') near the transitions (α, β) from the ramp to the uniform regions, as illustrated in C. From Fiorentini (1972).

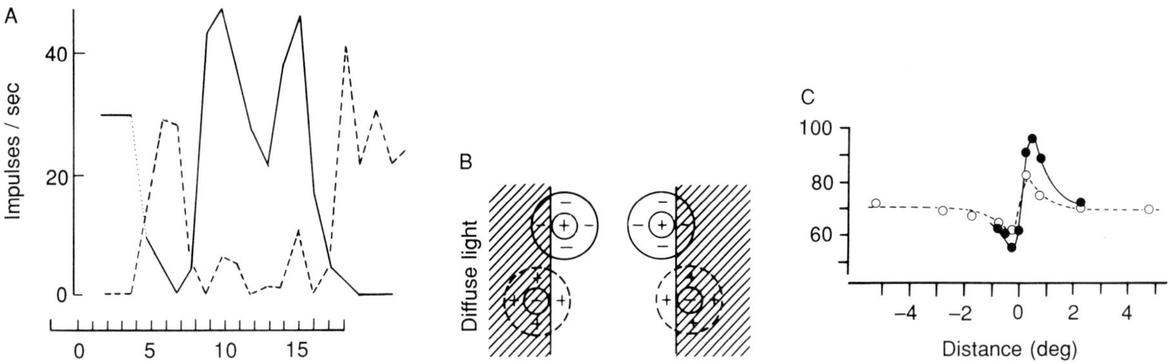

FIG. 4 (A) Responses of an ON-center neuron (solid line) and an OFF-center neuron (dashed line) in the cat retina to diffuse light (initial part of the curves) or to the contrast pattern shown in B (a bright bar of 5.5 degree width, between two dark regions). The curves indicate the responses of the two types of neuron to successive presentations of the contrast pattern imaged at various positions with respect to the neurons' receptive fields, as indicated on the abscissa. (Each step corresponds to 42 arc min.) The strongest responses are obtained when the edges of the rectangular bright bar are tangential to a receptive field center, as indicated in B. The receptive field is represented by concentric circles; + indicates ON-responses, and − indicates OFF-responses. Redrawn from Baumgartner (1961b). (C) Responses of a cat retinal ganglion cell (ON-center, X cell) to a contrast edge separating a dark region (to the left of the edge) from a light region. The vertical edge was held stationary at different distances from the receptive field center (indicated on the abscissa), and the stimulus contrast was alternately turned on and off. The ordinate indicates for each edge position the average spike frequency recorded during the first 20 sec after the introduction of the edge. Two different contrast levels were used: filled circles, 0.4; open circles, 0.2. From Enroth-Cugell and Robson (1966). Note that although the border is enhanced in the neural signals, the difference between the dark and light regions is not preserved.

cell response is not complete. Lateral inhibition within circularly symmetric neural units predicts that Mach bands are present and prominent on either side of a sharp edge. Yet, this seems not to be the case: most observers fail to perceive Mach bands at a sharp edge (Fiorentini, 1972; Tolhurst, 1972; Ross et al., 1981; Ratliff, 1984). Explanations have been proposed which address this problem (Tolhurst, 1972; Ratliff, 1984; Morrone, Ross, Burr & Owens, 1986). For instance, Tolhurst (1972) suggested that the neural mechanisms responsible for the detection of edges (edge detectors) and bars (bar detectors) inhibit each other when the corresponding stimuli are at a small distance from each other. At larger distances this particular type of inhibition is not active. Thus, Mach bands are seen on either side of a luminance ramp because the optimally excited edge detector is centered on the ramp, while the optimally excited bar detectors are aligned along the borders of the ramp. If the ramp is wide enough, the bar and edge detectors do not inhibit each other, and the Mach bands are seen. However, if the two borders of the ramp are close enough for the bar and edge detectors to inhibit each other, then no Mach bands are perceived. Ratliff (1984) has provided experimental evidence of the lack of Mach bands at sharp edges which is consistent with this explanation. Recent models of neural networks that may account for Mach bands are discussed in Section V.

Chevreul, in 1839, described another contrast effect, one that is generated by a series of parallel stripes of different luminances. Luminance is constant within each stripe, but increases from one stripe to another in staircase fashion. When looking at this staircase of luminances, one perceives a sawtooth brightness distribution. Despite its uniform luminance, each stripe looks brighter near the border with the lower luminance and looks darker near the border with the higher luminance (see Ratliff, 1965, for illustrations).

The Chevreul illusion was described by Hering

(1878) as an example of a border contrast effect. More recently, it has been investigated by von Békésy (1968) and Ross et al. (1981). According to von Békésy, the illusion can be explained in terms of lateral inhibition in the retina, as originally suggested by Hering. However, the lateral extent of the inhibitory interactions required to account for the illusion is greater than that required to explain Mach bands. Ross et al. also pointed out important differences between the two phenomena. In particular, the Chevreul or staircase illusion is unaffected by dark adaptation and is present both at low and high spatial frequencies

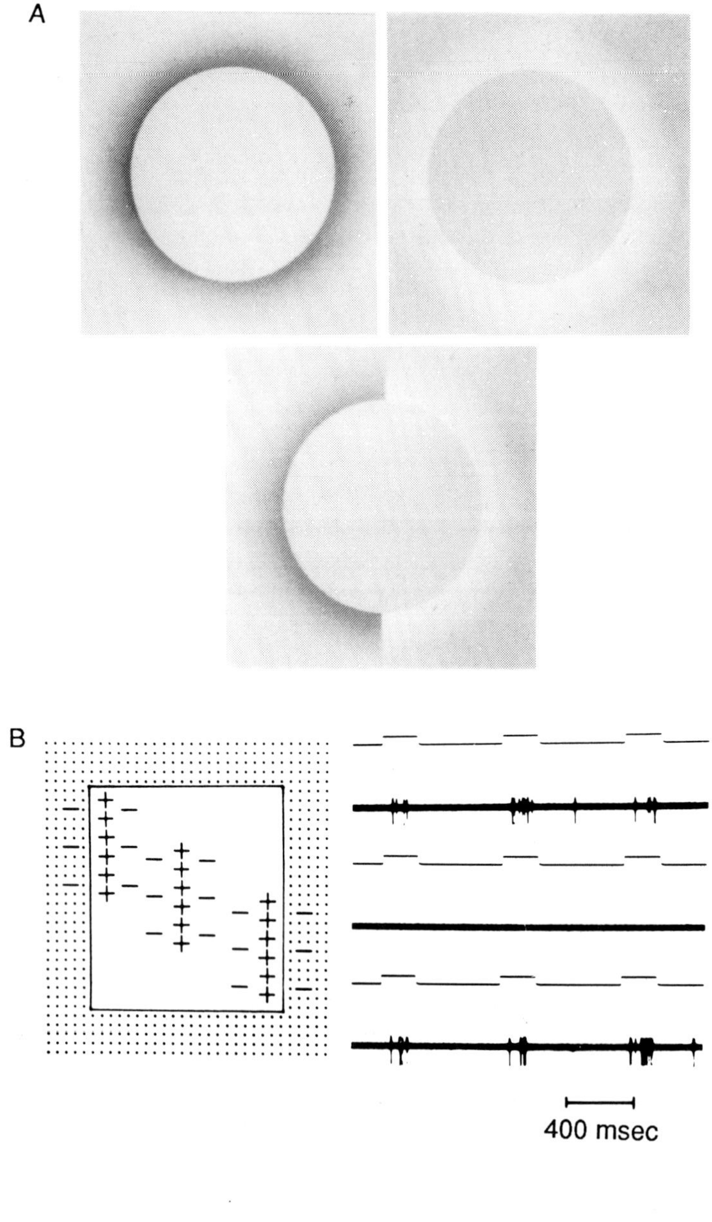

FIG. 5 (A) Craik–O'Brien–Cornsweet illusion of border induced area contrast. The disks are all of equal luminance, as can be checked by covering their surrounds. However, the top two disks appear different in lightness, because of local luminance modulations of opposite signs near their edges. Inverting the contrast gradients from one half of the disk to the other weakens the illusion (lower disk). (B) Responses of a single neuron in Area 17 of the monkey to a rectangular surface of homogeneous luminance when the receptive field of the neuron is located either at the borders (first and third trace from top) or within (second trace) the homogeneous surface (+ and − indicate excitatory and inhibitory regions of the receptive field, respectively). The line above the neuronal responses is the photocell recording. Upward deflections indicate light on. From Baumgartner (1986).

(up to 15 stripes per degree), that is, it occurs under conditions in which no Mach bands are perceived. These findings are consistent with von Békésy's assumption of different neurophysiological mechanisms for the two phenomena.

Mach bands are local subjective overshoots and undershoots of brightness that are perceived where there are no corresponding luminance modulations. Interestingly, a local modulation of luminance in an otherwise uniform surface can generate an illusory perception of different brightnesses. The modulation simulates an edge between areas of different luminances, but in fact the luminance is constant except for the localized modulation. As a result, the viewer perceives two regions of different brightnesses, separated by an edge (Fig. 5A). The effect is known as the Craik–O'Brien–Cornsweet illusion (Craik, 1966; O'Brien, 1958; Cornsweet, 1970). The interesting fact is that the illusory difference in brightness extends for a long distance to either side of the simulated edge. How this local contrast manipulation generates a global brightness difference, namely, area contrast, challenges any model of contrast perception based on neurophysiological findings. Recording from single neurons of the monkey striate cortex has failed to reveal a correlate of the illusion (Fig. 5B).

There are limits to the ability of local contrast to generate area contrast (Burr, 1987). The Craik–O'Brien–Cornsweet illusion is relatively strong when the contrast of the localized luminance modulation is low or moderate. However, when the peak-to-peak amplitude of the local luminance profile exceeds a critical value, the illusion diminishes. The illusion disappears completely at high local contrasts, probably because the local luminance modulation is perceived as a pair of adjacent, contrasting lines. On the other hand, the illusion persists despite great changes in the spatial parameters of the stimulus (Burr, 1987).

D. Illusory Contours

Certain combinations of incomplete figures generate edges that are clearly visible even though no corresponding luminance steps are present in the stimulus (Kanizsa, 1955). In one sense, these illusory contours recall the contrast border effects described above. However, in the Kanizsa figure, the most compelling aspect of the illusion is the surface outlined by the illusory contour: the surface appears uniformly lighter than the surround (see Fig. 10 in Chapter 11, this volume). Similarly, in the Ehrenstein (1954) illusion, the black radial lines with their terminal points generate the illusory contour of a circle which appears brighter than the surround (see Fig. 15 in Chapter 11). The illusory figures appear dark if the contrast of the inducing pattern is reversed in polarity, for example, white lines on a black background.

Illusory contours have a neurophysiological correlate in the responses of single neurons in the prestriate Area V2 of the monkey visual cortex (Von der Heydt, Peterhans & Baumgartner, 1984; Peterhans, Von der Heydt & Baumgartner, 1986; see Fig. 11 in Chapter 11). It is interesting to note that the perception of an edge, even an illusory edge, is sometimes accompanied by the perception of area contrast.

E. Area Contrast

We can now summarize the various factors that are likely to determine brightness perception in a complex visual scene under stationary conditions. (1) Brightness of an enclosed area is determined primarily by the average local contrast at the edges of the area. (2) An edge (luminance step) between two areas influences their brightness, but the strength of its contribution decreases with increasing distance. (3) A local modulation in luminance which simulates an edge can generate area contrast. (4) Gradual changes in luminance from one spatial region to another (as well as uniform stimulation from homogeneous areas) are not very effective in determining local brightness. These shallow gradients are mostly filtered out by the visual system.

In his book *Zur Lehre vom Lichtsinn [Theory of the Light Sense]*, Hering (1878) distinguishes between brightness contrast (which we have called area contrast) and boundary contrast (which we have called edge or border contrast). He ascribes both to reciprocal interactions between elements of the visual system. At present, we have a fairly good knowledge of how local contrast is processed by single neurons in the visual system. However, the way in which local contrast at edges produces area contrast and determines the brightness of extended surfaces is still largely unknown. No neurophysiological correlate of area contrast has been found, at least in the response properties of single neurons. Our knowledge about area contrast has not improved much since the time of Hering.

Spatial interactions within a cooperative network are needed to carry the signal from the border across the enclosed area. This process has been called filling-in by Gerrits and Vendrik (1970) and is based on the assumption that the perceived brightness or darkness of an area is determined by the contrast at the edge. As long as this contrast does not change, the perceived brightness of the area will remain the same. However, when the luminance step is increased or decreased, area brightness will instantaneously shift in the opposite direction. This mechanism requires that the border signal be constantly refreshed by small eye movements to sustain the retinal image and to prevent local adaptation. Thus, without eye movements the percept is equivalent to that experienced in a Ganzfeld (an unstructured void).

F. Successive Contrast

In addition to the simultaneous contrast effects described above, temporal changes in luminance also influence brightness perception. These *successive contrast* effects make a surface of a given luminance appear brighter or darker according to whether the preceding luminance was lower or higher. Prolonged viewing of a given luminance produces local adaptation in the region exposed and may cause long lasting aftereffects in brightness perception (afterimages) when luminance is changed.

When stimulus contrast is not too large, a prolonged exposure results in a reduction of apparent contrast and even in stimulus fading (Troxler, 1804). This effect is only observed with steady fixation and in peripheral vision, suggesting that fading depends on sustained stimulation within visual perceptive fields (Gerrits, Stassen & van Erning, 1984). Eye movements and blinks will revive the faded image, although not for long. Without continued temporal modulation, fading may reoccur. Even continuous motion or flicker of the stimulus may not be sufficient to prevent fading (Hunzelmann & Spillmann, 1984; Schieting & Spillmann, 1987). Analogous results have been observed with stabilization of the retinal image (Riggs, Ratliff, Cornsweet & Cornsweet, 1953; Yarbus, 1967; Ditchburn, 1973). Here, even the perception of foveal stimuli will fade provided there is no residual image slip (Barlow, 1963; Gerrits, 1978). Afterimages are thought to be largely retinal (Brindley, 1970), whereas fading of moving and flickering stimuli transfers interocularly and therefore must involve higher levels as well. This conclusion is supported by experiments in which cortical processes have been shown to be effective in prolonging afterimages on modulated background (Gerling and Spillmann, 1987).

Afterimages can be considered "dark light" and are associated with increased noise in the photoreceptors when photopigments are bleached (Barlow & Sparrock, 1964; see also Chapter 5, this volume). The dark light remaining after recovery from a bleach is call Eigengrau (intrinsic gray). It probably corresponds to random activity of cells in complete darkness. Electrophysiological correlates of afterimages in humans have been reported (Burr, Fiorentini & Morrone, 1987).

Gerrits, van Erning, and Eijkman (1988) distinguish the early fluctuations in brightness following a strong flash and observable in darkness (what they call the true afterimage) from the longer lasting contrast phenomenon, observable against both a dark or a bright background (what we called an afterimage above). The former have been correlated with oscillatory responses of ON- and OFF-units in the visual system (Jung, 1961, 1973).

There are also transient effects of successive contrast that probably have a nonretinal component. When a field of high luminance is suddenly presented next to another field of moderate luminance, the latter appears transiently darker. This effect occurs even with dichoptic stimulation, in which one field is presented to the right eye and the second to the left eye (Fiorentini, 1961). Thus, the phenomenon must be subserved, at least in part, by a cortical mechanism.

G. Short-Range Brightness Induction: Perceptive Field

The Hermann grid illusion (Hermann, 1870) is an interesting phenomenon that is classified as a brightness illusion because the distribution of perceived brightness is not easily predicted from the physical distribution of luminance. The stimulus is a grid of white bars on a black background. Dark spots are perceived at the intersections of the white bars. If the bars are black and the background white, light spots are seen at the intersections (Fig 6).

The strength of the illusion depends on the dimensions of the bars: their width and length, namely, the distances that the bars extend from a given intersection before being truncated (Baumgartner, 1960; Spillmann, 1971). Quantitative analysis of the relationship between these parameters and the strength of the illusion has provided estimates of the spatial ranges of the excitatory and inhibitory interactions which generate the illusion. These ranges have been interpreted as representing the diameters of the center and antagonistic surround of the perceptive field, a perceptual correlate of neuronal receptive fields (Baumgartner, 1960). This assumption is supported by a neurophysiological demonstration obtained by recording from single cells of the cat striate cortex. The diameter of the perceptive field center, as estimated from Hermann grid data, increases as a function of retinal eccentricity (Jung & Spillmann, 1970). Thus, the perceptive field has been defined in terms of a local brightness contrast effect (see Section IV for perceptive field estimates based on spatial summation of brightness and darkness).

Two other psychophysical methods were introduced in the late 1960s to investigate short-range spatial interactions. Both are based on measurements of the increment threshold for a small test probe (a spot or a thin line) in the presence of an interacting stimu-

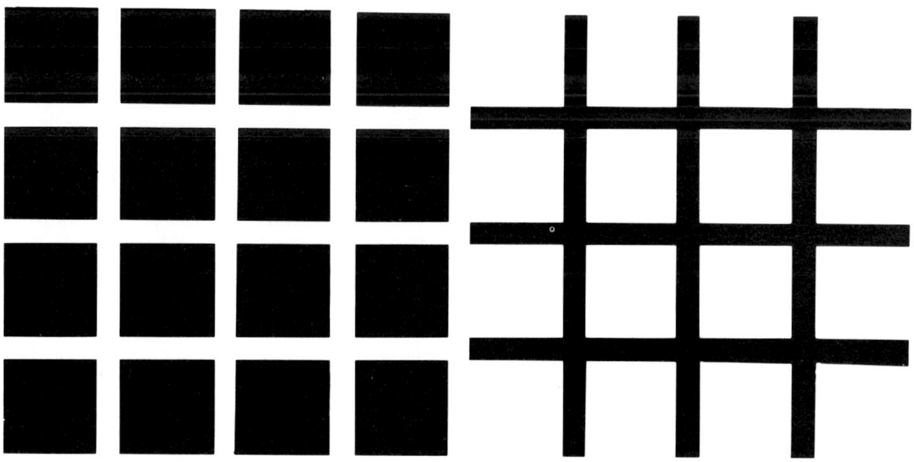

FIG. 6 Hermann grid illusion. Dark (or bright) blobs appear at the intersections except where viewed foveally. If the angular subtense of the intersecting lines is sharply reduced, the illusion can also be perceived in central vision indicating that the receptive fields assumed to mediate the effect are very small in the fovea.

lus. In one procedure (Fiorentini & Mazzantini, 1966; Fiorentini & Maffei, 1968; Fiorentini, 1972), the interactions occur between two stimuli of subthreshold contrast: two parallel lines, or a spot and an annulus. The distance between the subthreshold stimuli is varied in order to estimate how the strength of the interaction varies as a function of distance (Fig. 7). The function relating changes in increment threshold of the probe to the distance between the probe and the interacting, subthreshold stimulus is interpreted as the perceptive field profile. This procedure has been widely applied to the evaluation of psychophysical channels (see Chapter 10, this volume).

In the second procedure (Westheimer, 1967), the test probe is a small spot of light superimposed on the center of a disk of light of suprathreshold luminance and variable diameter. The increment threshold for the probe is measured as a function of the disk diameter. The resulting function, sometimes called a Westheimer function (Fig. 8), can be interpreted in terms of a perceptive field profile. The function represents the *integral* of the perceptive field, integrated over different diameters. As disk size increases, the threshold first increases to a peak and then decreases. The disk diameter at which the change in threshold reverses sign (from an increase to a decrease) represents the range of excitatory interactions and corresponds to the diameter of the perceptive field center. Beyond this range, an increase in background size causes a decrease in threshold, which has been interpreted as resulting from activation of the inhibitory surround of the perceptive field. As the size of the disk is increased further, a diameter is reached at which the threshold levels off at a value identical to that obtained on a uniform background. This diameter is taken as an estimate of the outer diameter of the inhibitory surround of the perceptive field (Spillmann, Ransom-Hogg & Oehler, 1987).

Obviously, perceptive field estimates based on different visual phenomena do not necessarily coincide. However, there is general agreement that the field

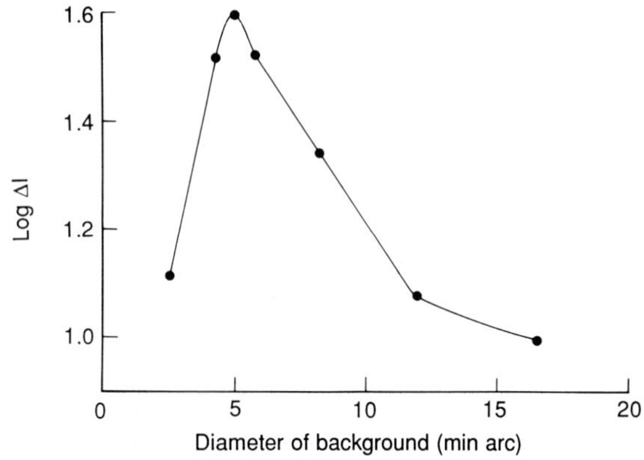

FIG. 8 Incremental threshold (Log Δ I in millilamberts) for a 10-ms test flash, 1 min arc diameter, viewed foveally against a circular background of varying diameter (abscissa). Background luminance: 2.5 millilamberts. (Replotted from Westheimer, 1967).

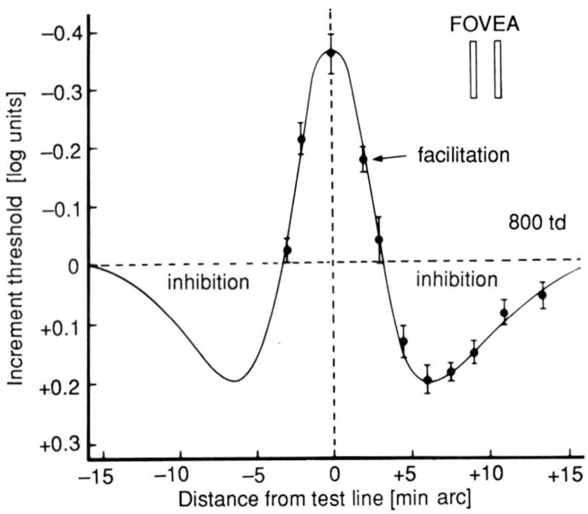

FIG. 7 Distribution of facilitatory and inhibitory subthreshold interactions between two incremental thin lines. The ordinate indicates the log threshold for the test line, measured in the presence of a second line of subliminal luminance, at various spatial separations between the two lines. Zero on the ordinate represents the log threshold of the test line measured in the absence of the subliminal line. Decrements in the threshold (plotted above the dotted line) represent facilitatory interactions between the two lines, and increments (plotted below the dotted line), inhibitory interactions. Replotted from Rentschler and Fiorentini (1974).

center is very small (4–5 arc min) in the fovea under photopic conditions. The size of the perceptive field increases (up to 2 degrees) rapidly with increasing eccentricity and is larger under scotopic than photopic conditions (Ransom-Hogg & Spillmann, 1980). When the stimuli are lines, the profile of the perceptive field depends on orientation, suggesting a cortical origin (Rentschler & Fiorentini, 1974).

These findings are stimulating in view of our attempt to correlate properties of human visual perception with the neurophysiological and neuroanatomical data from other animal species. Several investigators have compared psychophysical estimates of the perceptive field in humans and monkeys with anatomical and electrophysiological findings (Ransom-Hogg & Spillmann, 1980; Oehler, 1985; Spillmann et al., 1987). The size of the perceptive field center, as estimated from the Westheimer function, increases with retinal eccentricity in a similar fashion for humans and monkeys (Fig. 9). Furthermore, in the monkey the size of the perceptive field center at each eccentricity corresponds well with the average size of the receptive field center in phasic, broadband cells (M-cells), a class of retinal ganglion cells (DeMonasterio & Gouras, 1975).

There is also good agreement in the monkey between perceptive field sizes, on the one hand, and anatomical measurements of dendritic field size (Perry, Oehler & Cowey, 1984) on the other. This good correspondence in the monkey suggests that in humans, as well, the perceptive field centers estimated from Westheimer functions may indicate how the average size of single receptive field centers varies with distance from the fovea. It should be borne in mind, however, that in humans one cannot specify with certainty the level (or levels) in the visual system where the interactions occur which are described as "perceptive field." Also, these interactions may represent the integrated activity of several, partially overlapping receptive fields.

The next section describes properties of single neurons in the visual systems of cats and monkeys which are relevant to the processing of light increments and decrements.

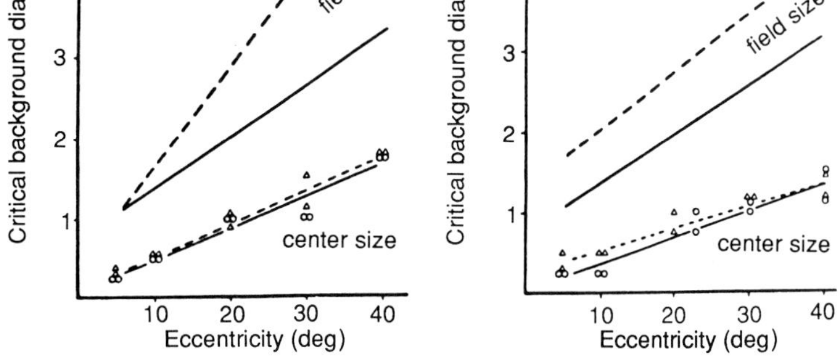

FIG. 9 Comparison of perceptive fields and field centers for monkey and human observers. Critical background diameters, derived from Westheimer functions, are plotted as a function of retinal eccentricity along the temporal (left) and nasal (right) horizontal meridians. For the center sizes, the values for two monkeys and two human observers are given together with the corresponding regression lines. For the total field sizes, variability was large, and only the regression lines are given. From Spillmann, Ransom-Hogg and Oehler (1987).

III. THE ON- AND OFF-CHANNELS OF THE VISUAL SYSTEM

A. ON-Center and OFF-Center Retinal Ganglion Cells

Recording from the retina of the optically intact cat eye in the late 1940s, Kuffler (1953) discerned two kinds of retinal ganglion cells: ON-center cells, which increased their activity when light increments were presented in their receptive fields (bright stimuli), and OFF-center cells, which were excited by light decrements (dark stimuli). Kuffler also found that the circular center of the receptive field of ganglion cells is surrounded by an antagonistic region which responds with opposite polarity. As a result of the arrangement of the receptive field in two concentric antagonistic regions, ganglion cells respond more vigorously to small spots of light confined to the center of the receptive field than to large spots or uniform illumination. ON-center cells respond best to a spot brighter than the background, OFF-center cells, to a spot darker than the background (Fig. 10).

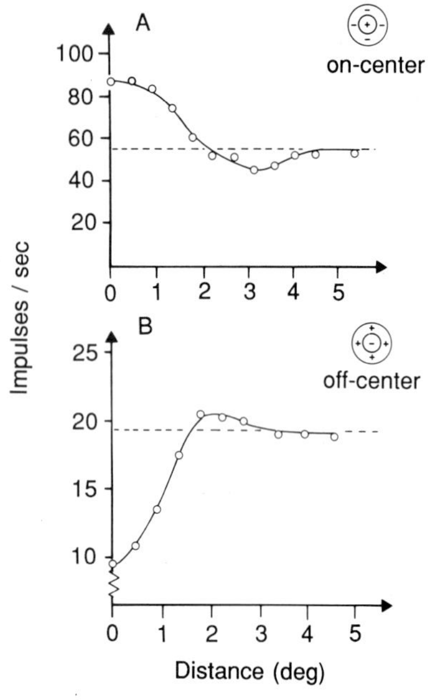

FIG. 10 Average rate of discharge an ON-center (A) and of an OFF-center ganglion cell (B) of the cat retina as a function of the distance from the receptive field center to a spot of light of 52 (A) or 34 (B) min arc diameter, luminance 2 cd/m², superimposed on a homogeneous background of 0.1 cd/m². The dashed lines indicate the average discharge in the absence of the spot. The receptive field type is schematically indicated at the top of each graph (+ indicates activation, − indicates inhibition by light stimuli). From Maffei (1968).

B. The ON- and OFF-Channels in the Retina

In the 1960s, it became possible to record from the various types of cells of the retina and to identify these cells histologically by injecting them with dyes after the recording. This kind of work established that all vertebrate receptors are hyperpolarized by light and that the ON- and OFF-systems are first present at the level of the bipolar cells (Werblin & Dowling, 1969). Sign conserving synapses made on these cells formed OFF-bipolars, whereas sign inverting synapses formed ON-bipolar cells. It appears therefore that from the single ended system of the receptors, nature has created a double system at the bipolar cell level. It is likely that significant gains in visual information processing are obtained from this arrangement.

In the cat retina, the ganglion cells belong to three morphological classes: the α, β and γ cells (Boycott & Wässle, 1974; see also Chapter 6, this volume). The α cells have large cell bodies, large dendritic trees, and thick axons. The β cells have medium-size cell bodies and small dendritic trees. The γ cells are a heterogeneous class of cells.

All the ganglion cells with a receptive field concentrically organized in two antagonistic regions present the ON–OFF dichotomy: their receptive field is either ON-center or OFF-center. The ganglion cells classified as brisk-transient cells or Y cells on the basis of their physiological properties (cells with transient response characteristics and nonlinear spatial summation within their receptive field) correspond to the α class. The cells classified as brisk-sustained or X cells (with sustained response properties and linear spatial summation) correspond to the β class. For all these cells the physiological subdivision in ON-center and OFF-center cells has an anatomical counterpart: the dendritic trees of ON-center and OFF-center ganglion cells branch at different depths in the inner plexiform layer (IPL). OFF-center cells have dendrites branching in the outer portion of the IPL, while the dendrites of ON-center cells branch in the inner portion of the IPL (Nelson, Famiglietti & Kolb, 1978; Peichl & Wässle, 1981).

In either morphological class of cells (α and β cells) the two subpopulations of ON-center and OFF-center cells form a regular mosaic (Fig. 11) and, although superimposed, are independent of each other (Wässle, Peichl & Boycott, 1983). This anatomical segregation of ON and OFF ganglion cells is striking. It suggests that the retinal images can be sampled independently by the ON- and OFF-systems.

A similar segregation is also likely to take place in the primate retina (Perry & Silveira, 1988). Interestingly, in the most central region of the monkey fovea, the number of ganglion cells is more than twice the number of cones. This means that, in principle, the ON- and the OFF-systems can use independently the full sampling capacity of the cone array (Wässle, 1988). Thus, the retina seems to have all the machinery required to process in parallel the visual message by a dual system, characterized by the opposite polarity of responses to light transients. In what follows we refer to the population of ON-center and OFF-center neurons and to the corresponding neural pathways as the ON- and OFF-channel, respectively.

C. Effects of Blocking the ON-Channel: Electrophysiological Findings

Several hypotheses have been advanced in an attempt to explain why the ON- and OFF-systems have evolved. An important discovery has made it possible to test some of these hypotheses. Slaughter and Miller (1981) found that when they applied the glutamate neurotransmitter analog 2-amino-4-phosphonobutyrate (APB) to the mud puppy retina, the ON bipolars, ON amacrines, and ON ganglion cells became unresponsive to light, whereas the OFF-cells of the retina essentially maintained their response properties.

Subsequent to this discovery a number of laboratories applied APB to the mammalian retina. The studies by Schiller (1982, 1984) and Schiller, Sandell, and Maunsell (1986) concentrated on the monkey. This work began by developing a way of infusing APB into the retina so that the activity of single cells could be studied in various parts of the visual system before, during, and after APB application. The physiological studies showed the following (Schiller, 1982): (1) APB blocks the responses of ON-center ganglion cells and ON-center lateral geniculate nucleus (LGN) cells while leaving the responses of OFF-center cells largely unaffected. (2) The center–surround antagonism of OFF-center retinal ganglion cells and of OFF-center LGN cells is not significantly altered by APB administration. These findings suggest, therefore, that the center–surround antagonism of retinal ganglion cells and LGN cells is not a product of the interaction between the ON- and OFF-systems. It appears that these two systems remain segregated up to the cortex, a finding also supported by several other kinds of data (Cleland, Dubin & Levick, 1971). (3) In the visual cortex, administration of APB blocks the responses of single cells to a light edge but has little effect on the responses to a dark edge. Other receptive field attributes, such as orientation and direction specificities, are unaffected by APB. Similar results have been obtained in the cat (Horton & Sherk, 1984; Sherk & Horton, 1984). These findings suggest that the ON- and OFF-systems converge on single cells in the cortex but that this convergence does not play a vital role in producing orientation and direction selectivity of cortical cells. The ON- and OFF-systems must serve other purposes.

D. Effects of Blocking the ON-Channel: Behavioral Findings

In order to gain further insight into the functions of the ON- and OFF-systems, psychophysical studies

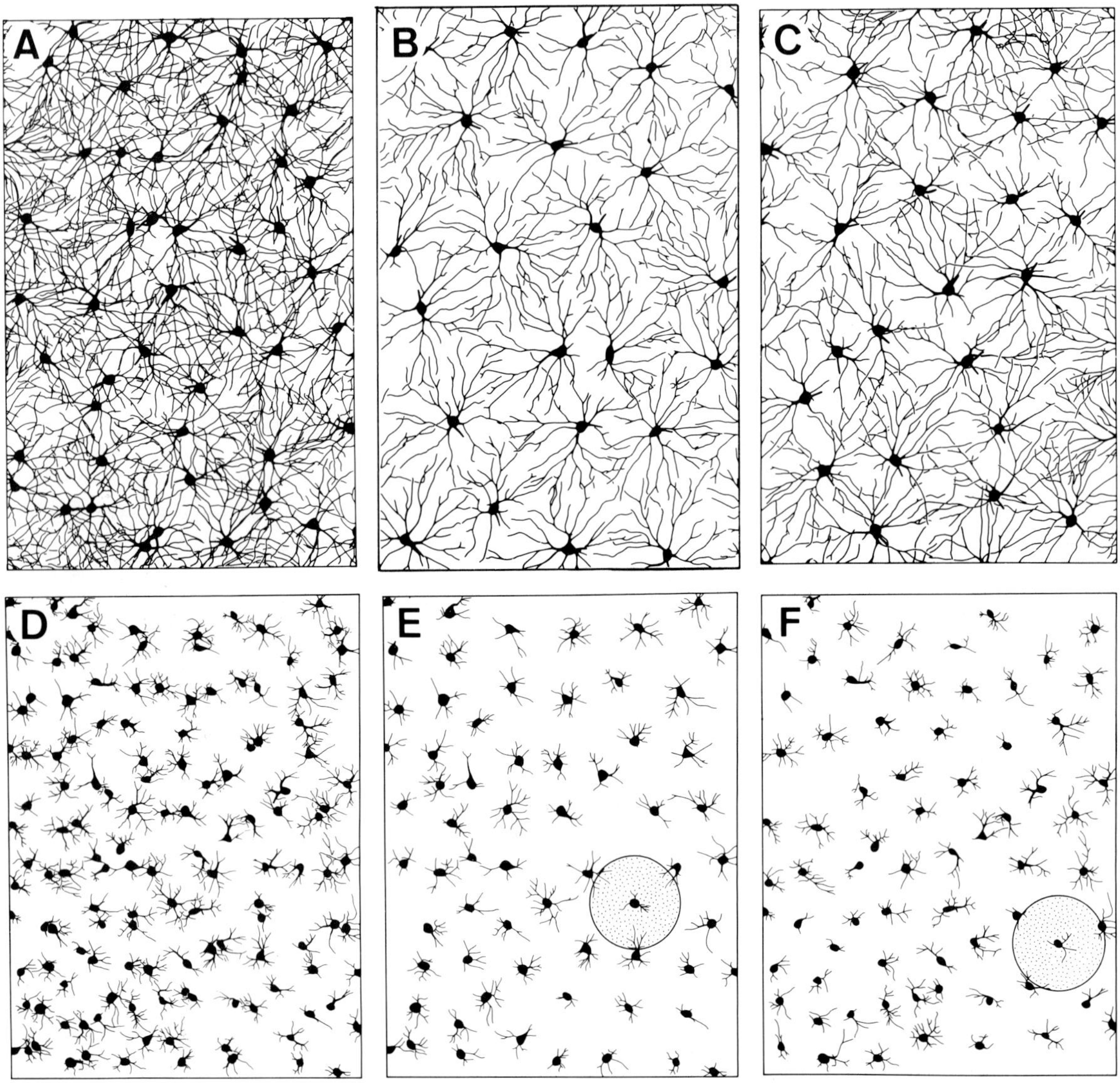

FIG. 11 All α (A–C) and β (D–F) cells stained in a small field of a cat retina. The dendritic trees form an irregular mosaic in A and in D. B and C are obtained from A, selecting only the ON-cells (B) or only the OFF-cells (C). Similarly, E and F represent the populations of ON- (E) and OFF-cells (F), selected from D. Note the regular mosaics formed by the selected ON and OFF populations. The β cells are shown at twice the magnification of the α cells. From Wässle, Peichl, and Boycott (1983).

were undertaken in which the visual capacities of monkeys were examined before, during, and after the ON-channel was blocked with APB (Schiller et al., 1986). To accomplish this monkeys were trained on a variety of detection and discrimination tasks involving eye movements, which were recorded with the scleral coil method (Fuchs & Robinson, 1966). Visual targets were presented to the animal either in isolation (detection task) or together with nontarget stimuli (discrimination task). The animal's task was to make a saccade to the correct target. For the detection task, the animal had to fixate a small central spot of light as soon as it appeared. After a variable time interval, a target was presented in one of several possible locations with respect to the central spot, and the animal's task was to make saccades to it. If the saccade brought the fovea to within 2 degrees from the target center, the trial was considered to be successful and the animal rewarded. Otherwise the trial was interrupted. For the discrimination task several targets were presented simultaneously after the central spot was fixated. One of these targets was different from the rest, and the task of the animal was to fixate the "different" target.

With this method it was possible to obtain not only percent correct responses, but also response latencies. A number of visual capacities were examined which included the detection of light increments and decrements, movement perception, critical flicker fusion, stereopsis, color vision, and contrast sensitivity. Visual capacities were studied under both scotopic and photopic conditions.

The results may be summarized as follows (Schiller et al., 1986): (1) There was a dramatic loss in the ability to detect light increments of relatively high contrast, but not light decrements. Reaction times for saccades to increments were doubled, after APB injections, and the proportion of correct responses dropped from 100% to chance levels. The responses to decrements were not affected. (2) There was a 25% (3 decibel) loss in contrast sensitivity for patterned stimuli. (3) In agreement with data according to which all rod bipolars are of the ON type (Müller, Wässle & Voigt, 1988), it was found that perception was severely impaired for all stimuli in the dark-adapted animal. (4) There was little loss for the perception of movement, pattern, flicker, and stereopsis, but reaction times were increased by 30–60 msec.

The results of these behavioral studies suggest two possible reasons for the emergence of the ON- and OFF-channels in vision. One is to provide a means of transmitting to the central nervous system all cone-mediated information by an excitatory process, namely, by an increase in the rate of discharge. This assures a rapid transfer of information about visual stimuli, no matter whether these consist of light increments or light decrements. The second reason may be to improve contrast perception.

IV. PERCEPTUAL CORRELATES OF ON- AND OFF-CHANNELS

The functional roles of the ON- and OFF-channels are still a matter of debate. It has been proposed that ON- and OFF-center cells form independent and antagonistic neural subsystems for signaling brightness and darkness in response to luminance changes of opposite sign (Grüsser & Creutzfeldt, 1957; Baumgartner, 1961a,b; Jung, 1961, 1973, 1978). This proposal was supported by experiments conducted in Freiburg in the early 1960s. It was found that in the retina, LGN, and striate cortex of the cat, stimuli containing a luminance step (contrast border) produced a change in the spike discharge of individual cells that could be interpreted as brightness enhancement, in the case of ON-center neurons, or darkness enhancement, in the case of OFF-center neurons (Baumgartner & Hakas, 1962).

The Freiburg experiments also established a correlation between electrophysiological effects described by Gernandt & Granit (1947) and the sensory effects, observed by Helmholtz (1867), of electrical polarization of the human eye. Helmholtz produced light sensations by placing one electrode on the eye and another on the neck and applying a galvanic current. Changing the direction of current flow produced opposite effects on the Eigengrau sensation: a brightness enhancement when the polarization was cathodic and a darkness enhancement when the polarization was anodic. Gernandt and Granit reported that cat ganglion cells which respond to light increments with an increase in their rate of discharge (ON-cells) were also activated by cathodic galvanic polarization. Cells which respond to light decrements (OFF-cells) with an increase in spike discharge were activated by anodic galvanic polarization. Comparing these results with the subjective effects of galvanic currents supports the proposition that the ON- and OFF-systems subserve brightness and darkness sensations, respectively.

This section reviews evidence from human psychophysics for a dual pathway theory of brightness perception and discusses the relationship of the psychophysical data to the neurophysiological findings. Two types of psychophysical studies are particularly relevant: (1) experiments which show that manipulations of the spatial and temporal parameters of suprathreshold stimuli produce perceptual changes of opposite polarity, depending on whether the stimuli are luminance increments or decrements; and (2) experiments which demonstrate selective adaptation to increments and decrements. Unless otherwise stated, the terms "increments" and "decrements" denote targets which are either brighter or darker than the background.

A. The Perception of Luminance Increments and Decrements

1. Spatial Summation of Brightness and Darkness

When the brightness or darkness of suprathreshold, disk-shaped increment or decrement flashes is measured as a function of stimulus area, typical area–sensation curves are obtained (Fig. 12A). As area is increased from zero, the strength of the brightness/darkness sensation first increases with stimulus area. This range of increased strength of sensation is followed by a second range in which the strength of sensation decreases. Finally, there is a third range in which brightness and darkness are independent of stimulus area. Figure 12A illustrates these relationships for both increments and decrements. The data are replotted from experiments by Higgins and Rinalducci (1975) and Bjørklund and Magnussen (1979). In these experiments, a test disk of variable size was matched in brightness to a comparison disk of fixed area, either by varying the luminance of the test disk (curve at top) or the comparison disk (curve at bottom). To facilitate comparison of the two sets of data, the ordinate scale in the upper part of Fig. 12A has been inverted. Note the polarity of the results: increasing the stimulus area increases both the brightness of an increment as well as the darkness of a decrement.

Although psychophysical data are likely to reflect the responses of many neurons, an analogy may be drawn with the functional properties of single neurons. The shapes of the curves suggest the area–response profiles of ON-center and OFF-center cells. That is, maximal response is observed when the stimulus of appropriate sign fills the receptive field center. For larger stimuli the antagonistic surround depresses the response, and a plateau is reached when stimulus area extends beyond the receptive field. Thus, the size-dependent variations in brightness and darkness reveal areas of excitation and inhibition that may be interpreted in terms of antagonistic responses within concentric areas of ON- or OFF-center perceptive fields. Notice the resemblance to the analysis of the Hermann grid illusion and Westheimer paradigms (Section II).

The results for increments and decrements presented in Fig. 12A come from two separate experiments and are thus not strictly comparable. For one thing, the stronger inhibitory effect of increment stimuli may be due to a larger flash amplitude (2.0 log unit increment, compared to 0.3 log unit decrement; see Higgins & Rinalducci, 1975; du Buf & Roufs, 1986). The most obvious difference between the top and bottom curves, however, is the difference in position of the inflection point on the abscissa. This misalignment could be due to different retinal locations tested in the two experiments. However, experiments with foveal stimuli (du Buf & Roufs, 1986) also show

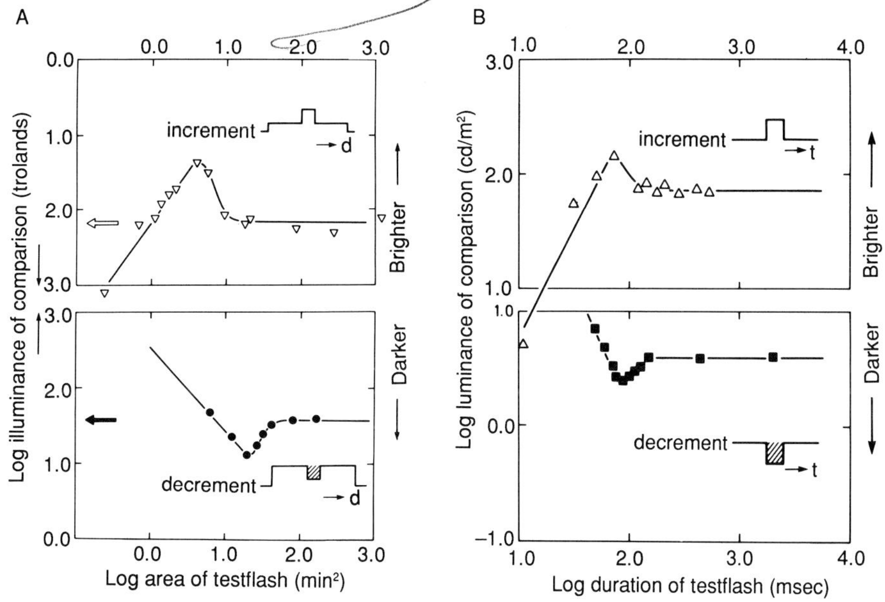

FIG. 12 Spatial and temporal Broca–Sulzer effects for luminance increments and decrements. (A) Area–brightness relationships for luminance increments (top) and decrements (bottom). Note the inverted ordinate in the upper graph: brightness enhancement is indicated by a lower test luminance required to match the brightness of a comparison field of fixed luminance. Results are replotted from Higgins and Rinalducci (1975) and Bjørklund and Magnussen (1979, Fig. 2). (B) Time–brightness relationships for increments (top) and decrements (bottom). Results are replotted from Corwin and Giambalvo (1974) and Bjørklund and Magnussen (1979), (© The American Academy of Optometry, 1974).

that the inflection point of the decrement curves is systematically shifted to a larger spatial value as compared with the increment curves. According to the perceptive-field model, this might indicate that OFF-center cells subserving human central vision have larger perceptive fields than ON-center cells. However, there are so far no neurophysiological data to support this conclusion. Findings obtained from human visual evoked potentials in response to positive- and negative-contrast stimuli suggest possible asymmetries in ON- and OFF-subsystems (Zemon, Gordon & Welch, 1988), but the asymmetries suggest that the OFF-system may have finer spatial resolution than the ON-system. This result, if anything, would indicate smaller receptive field centers for the OFF-system. Obviously, the question is open.

Apart from these small discrepancies, the estimates of foveal and parafoveal perceptive field sizes obtained with brightness matches are consistent with psychophysical estimates derived from Hermann grids and Westheimer functions in both humans and monkeys. They also compare favorably with neurophysiological measurements of single-cell receptive fields in the monkey retina (Spillmann et al., 1987; Crook, Lange-Malecki, Lee & Valberg, 1988).

2. Broca–Sulzer Effect: Brightness and Darkness Enhancement for Stimuli of Short Duration

An enhancement of brightness/darkness is also found in the time domain, stimuli of short duration evoking stronger sensations than long duration stimuli. This enhancement is called the Broca–Sulzer effect. Brewster (1834) noted that "the intensity of a given light may be increased physiologically by causing it to act upon the retina by successive impulses of a given duration." Exner (1868) observed that short single flashes may be more effective than longer ones. Broca and Sulzer (e.g., 1902, 1904) extended these observations. They showed that, for very brief increment flashes, brightness increased with flash duration to a peak at 50–150 msec. However, as stimulus duration increased further, brightness decreased until it became independent of stimulus duration. Bartley (1938) repeated the experiment with flickering lights and confirmed that stimuli of medium flicker frequencies were perceived as brighter than those of low and high flicker frequencies.

The top graph of Fig. 12B shows the results from a typical Broca–Sulzer experiment (Corwin & Giambalvo, 1974). It shows how the brightness of an increment changes as a function of the duration of the flash. Brightness was measured by adjusting the luminance of a comparison flash of constant duration. Analogous effects for decrements were reported by Glad and Magnussen (1972) for flicker stimuli and by Bjørklund and Magnussen (1979) for single flashes. Results from the latter experiment are shown in the lower graph of Fig. 12B.

The flicker and single flash effects are closely related. When square-wave flicker stimuli are used, the perceived brightness peaks are observed between 2 and 10 Hz, depending on stimulus luminance (Magnussen & Glad, 1975a). These frequencies correspond to durations of 250–50 msec for individual flashes in the flicker train, which is similar to the range of durations at which maximal brightness enhancement for single flash stimuli is found (Aiba & Stevens, 1964).

In the present chapter, the term Broca–Sulzer effect is applied to the whole family of related phenomena caused by flicker or single flash stimuli. These phenomena include the enhancement of apparent contrast in flashed sinusoidal gratings (Kitterle & Corwin, 1979). This latter effect may be thought of as a combined increment and decrement Broca–Sulzer effect enhancing the light and dark bars of the grating simultaneoulsy.

Magnussen and Glad (1975a) found that the psychophysical functions relating brightness and darkness to flicker frequency were basically similar: under the conditions tested, brightness and darkness enhancement occurred over the same frequency range and shared a common peak frequency. Single flash experiments (White, Irwin & Williams, 1980), on the other hand, suggest slightly longer optimal flash durations for decrements than for increments (Fig. 12B). This might indicate an asymmetry between ON- and OFF-channels in the time domain parallel to the asymmetry found in the space domain.

3. Brightness and Darkness Enhancement Induced by Simultaneous Contrast

Another member of the Broca–Sulzer family is the induction of temporal brightness and darkness enhancement through simultaneous contrast (Magnussen & Glad, 1975b; Magnussen, 1987). In these experiments the stimulus pattern was a small test field of steady luminance surrounded by a larger inducing field whose luminance was modulated, in square-wave fashion, symmetrically about the test field luminance. The perceptual result of such a manipulation is a vivid impression of a test field whose brightness is modulated in counterphase: when the surround becomes brighter, the test field appears to become darker and vice versa. Magnussen and Glad (1975b) measured the bright and dark contrast effects by matching the test field to a comparison field flashed briefly at various phases of the inducing field modulation. Matches were obtained for various temporal frequencies of the inducing field. Representative results are presented in Fig. 13. They are similar to results describing the modulation in brightness during the light and dark phases of real flicker. However, in comparison with other Broca–Sulzer effects, the induced change is smaller, and the peaks and the high-frequency cutoff occur at lower flicker frequencies (Magnussen & Glad, 1975b; DeValois, Webster, DeValois & Lingelbach, 1986).

4. Neurophysiological Interpretation of Broca–Sulzer Effects

The coexistence of distinct increment and decrement Broca–Sulzer effects offers strong circumstantial evidence for independent channels signaling brightness and darkness, respectively. Grüsser and Creutzfeldt (1957) were the first to point out the striking similarity between the brightness enhancement of a flickering light and the enhanced flicker responses of ON-center retinal ganglion cells in the cat for certain tem-

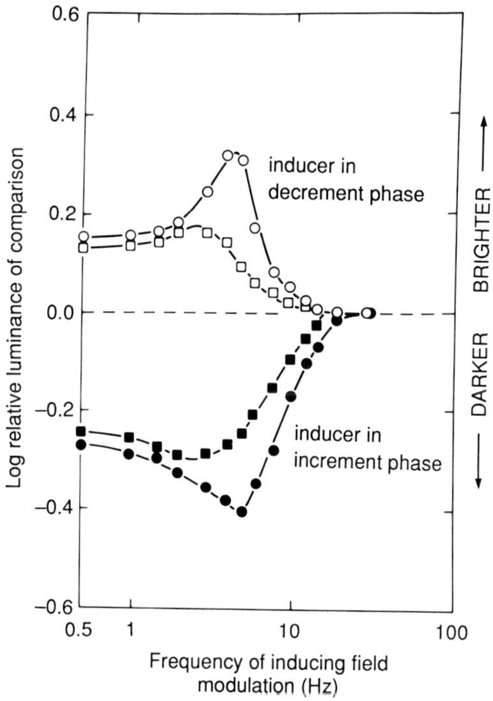

FIG. 13 Simultaneous contrast with a time-modulated inducing field. Ordinate: relative comparison luminance required to match the test field during the decrement (upper curves) and increment (lower curves) phases of the inducing field. Zero stands for the comparison luminance required to match the brightness of the test field at modulations above the critical fusion frequency. Abscissa: frequency of modulation of the inducing field. Results are shown for two mean luminances: 1.0 (squares) and 4000 cd/m² (circles). Replotted from Magnussen and Glad (1975b).

poral frequencies. On the basis of neurophysiological results obtained from OFF-center neurons, they also predicted the phenomenon of darkness enhancement, which was later confirmed by psychophysical experiments. These comparisons between single units and perception were elaborated and further strengthened in a number of subsequent papers (for review see van de Grind, Grüsser & Lunkenheimer, 1973; Magnussen & Glad, 1975a). By including the antagonistic receptive field surround, Magnussen and Glad (1975b) extended the neuronal model to the induced Broca–Sulzer effect.

The receptive field model is simple. It accounts for, and actually predicted, many of the perceptual phenomena discussed. Indeed, there are several striking parallels between psychophysical and single-unit stimulus–response relationships. But these correlations may be misleading. A closer analysis reveals that the psychophysical results cannot be derived from either the behavior of single cells or from population averages. Rather, the psychophysical results are composite functions, to which various subpopulations of neurons probably contribute to different degrees, and which involve processing at several levels of the visual system. For instance, it is important to consider the relative contribution to brightness perception of neural mechanisms with transient or sustained responses. Transient mechanisms are likely to contribute predominantly to the brightness (darkness) of stimuli of short duration or of rapid changes of luminance (Cavanagh & Anstis, 1986), whereas sustained mechanisms are likely to contribute predominantly to the brightness of long flashes. This transient–sustained dichotomy is supported, for instance, by the fact that adapting to a 6 Hz sinusoidal flicker stimulus abolishes the Broca–Sulzer effect, that is, it reduces the perceived brightness for stimuli of that duration (40–150 msec), but leaves the perception of longer flashes unaffected (Kitterle & Beard, 1983).

Some spatial and temporal properties of brightness and darkness induction, however, are difficult to explain with a receptive-field model. Brightness and darkness changes can be induced in fields much larger than the size of receptive fields of single neurons (Maffei & Fiorentini, 1972; Magnussen & Glad, 1975b; DeValois et al., 1986). Brightness and darkness induction through simultaneous contrast must therefore involve lateral pathways which extend beyond the single-unit receptive field. Several authors have proposed hypothetical filling-in processes at central stages to account for such long-distance brightness interactions (Gerrits & Vendrik, 1970; Grossberg, 1983; Hamada, 1985). But, as noted in Section II, when dealing with area contrast, neurophysiological correlates of these long-range processes of brightness and darkness induction are still lacking.

B. Selective Adaptation of ON- and OFF-Pathways

One direct way to test hypotheses about the function of subclasses of neurons is to inactivate selected classes of neurons and observe the consequences on visual functions. Pressure blocking of Y fibers (Burke, 1986) and APB blocking of ON-center neurons (Section III) are examples of methods that can be applied in behavioral experiments with animal subjects. In human psychophysics the technique that comes closest to neural blocking is selective perceptual adaptation, which has proved useful in mapping stimulus-selective mechanisms in the spatial and temporal domains (Sekuler & Blake, 1985).

The logic of selective adaptation is illustrated by the following experimental scheme. The observer inspects a high-contrast adapting stimulus for a few minutes. The adapting stimulus is then removed, and the contrast threshold for detecting test stimuli of similar spatial and/or temporal characteristics is determined. If thresholds are raised above the pre-adaptation values, we may infer that the sensitivity of the underlying neural mechanism mediating detection is temporarily reduced (by fatigue or inhibition). The range of test stimuli affected by adaptation serves as an indication of the stimulus specificity of the detecting mechanisms.

1. Polarity Specific Temporal Aftereffects

Using selective adaptation, Krauskopf (1980) and Hanly and MacKay (1979) provided psychophysical evidence that transient increments and decrements of luminance were independently processed. In one experiment, Hanly and MacKay adapted their subjects to a low frequency (1–2 Hz) sawtooth modulation of the luminance of a large homogeneous stimulus field. The sawtooth modulation could either be a slow increase in luminance followed by a rapid decrease or vice versa. The depth of modulation was the same in both cases. Following adaptation to each of these ramp stimuli, the threshold (minimum modulation depth detectable) was determined for ramps of either polarity. At all conditions tested, thresholds were raised after adaptation. However, the threshold elevations were greater when adapting and test ramps had the same polarity than when they had opposite polarity. These polarity specific adaptation effects support the hypothesis that separate neural mechanisms signal brightening and darkening in the human visual system. Moreover, since a sawtooth stimulus combines a slow change with a rapid one of the opposite polarity, the results show that the polarity sensitive channels are sensitive to the rate of amplitude change.

A change of threshold is but one consequence of adaptation. Another consequence is a change in the appearance of suprathreshold "neutral" stimuli. Anstis (1967, 1986) reported a suprathreshold version of polarity selective adaptation. He found that after adaptation to sawtooth luminance modulation at 1 Hz, a uniform test field of steady luminance appeared to change its brightness over time in a direction opposite to the slow phase of the adapting modulation. Thus, when the adapting stimulus was a slowly increasing luminance ramp, the observed aftereffect was a slow darkening of the field, similar to that produced by a slowly decreasing luminance ramp.

Anstis (1979, 1986) further found that this aftereffect could be induced through lateral pathways. A physically steady central field embedded in a ramp-modulated surround appears to be ramp modulated with the opposite polarity (compare with the induced Broca–Sulzer effect). In turn, this simultaneous contrast effect causes an aftereffect in the steady central field, and this aftereffect has the same polarity as the adapting ramp. So the induced aftereffect is also polarity specific. The aftereffects studied by Anstis did not survive the interocular transfer test: they disappeared when adapting and test stimuli were viewed by separate eyes. In contrast, Hanly and MacKay (1979) found some interocular transfer in their experiments, but the transfer was not polarity specific. Thus, the polarity selectivity of the temporal adaptation to luminance ramps would seem to arise in monocular pathways. Whether these effects occur subcortically, that is, prior to the convergence of the pathways from the two eyes, or in monocular cortical structures cannot be inferred from these results.

2. Polarity Specific Spatial Aftereffects

Psychophysical evidence for contrast polarity selective adaptation at the level of the visual cortex comes from experiments on spatial aftereffects, related to the aftereffect originally reported by Blakemore and Sutton (1969). They found that adaptation to a high-contrast grating may shift the perceived spatial frequency of subsequently viewed test gratings: no change is observed at the adapting frequency itself, but gratings of higher spatial frequencies appear even finer and gratings of lower spatial frequencies appear coarser than before adaptation. DeValois (1977) and Burton, Nagshineh, and Ruddock (1977) modified the original experiment using gratings with rectangular luminance profiles for both adaptation and testing. In the adapting gratings, the black bars were broader than the white bars or vice versa; in the test gratings, the black and white bars were equal in width. The results showed that the black and white bars of the gratings were independently size adapted and that their perceived widths changed in opposite directions.

Figure 14A demonstrates this phenomenon. Note first that the right-hand pair of gratings has black and white bars of equal width. The left-hand pair consists of one grating with broad black and narrow white bars (light–dark ratio 1:2) and one with broad white and narrow black bars (light–dark ratio 2:1). To demonstrate the shift in perceived duty cycle, let your eyes scan the black line on the left for about 30 sec and then transfer your gaze to the right fixation line. Notice that the light–dark ratio of the bar widths no longer appears to be unity, but is shifted in opposite directions in the upper and lower gratings.

This aftereffect is not confined to grating stimuli. DeValois (1977) also studied size adaptation with single black and white bars slowly drifting back and forth across the visual field. The results are shown in Fig. 14B. The data illustrate the difference between

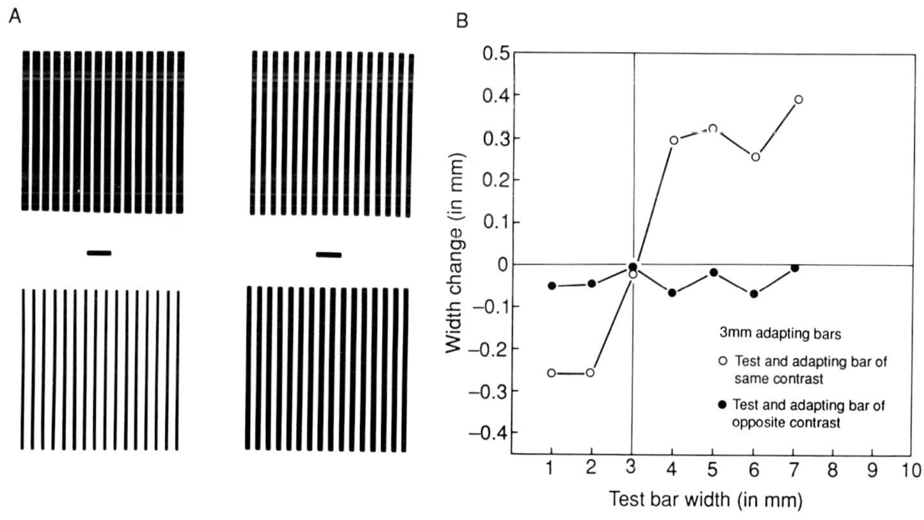

FIG. 14 (A) Demonstration of contrast-polarity selective size adaptation. Adaptation to the pair of gratings on the left changes the apparent width of the black and white bars in the gratings on the right. (B) Changes in the apparent width of single black or white lines following adaptation to a 3 mm (4.2 min visual angle) line of the same or opposite contrast. Results are from two observers and are taken from DeValois (1977).

pairs of adapting and test lines having the same contrast or opposite contrast. The change in apparent width of the test bars is small (less than 10%) but consistent, and it is only observed when the contrast of the adapting and test bars have the same sign (black–black or white–white).

Two properties of polarity specific size adaptation point to a cortical origin of this aftereffect. First, it is orientation specific. As the relative orientation difference between the adapting and test grating increases, the aftereffect decreases (Burton et al., 1977). Second, the effect transfers interocularly. The transfer can be demonstrated by repeating the informal experiment of Fig. 14A, covering one eye during adaptation and switching to the other eye when viewing the test pattern. Notice that the effect still occurs, although it is perhaps less intense. In subjects with normal binocular vision the interocular transfer of the spatial aftereffect is of the order of 50–70% of the monocular effect (Bjørklund & Magnussen, 1981; Blake, Overton & Lema-Stern, 1981).

On the basis of these findings, it has been suggested that black and white size-specific information is handled independently by the visual system. This seems to be the most plausible interpretation for the aftereffects of single bars. [For the aftereffects obtained with gratings, an alternative explanation in terms of mechanisms sensitive to spatial-phase relationships between the harmonic components of the grating may better account for the results (Cavanagh, Brussell & Stober, 1981)].

In conclusion, there seems to be evidence to support the existence in the human visual system of cortical mechanisms selective for size and orientation, but responding preferentially either to white or black bars. This, of course, is consistent with the properties of single neurons in the striate cortex of cats and monkeys.

Whether or not the ON- and OFF-pathways in humans are kept separate through all stages of processing is not clear. Some psychophysical findings in humans seem to imply a convergence of ON- and OFF-pathways on cortical units. For example, the fact that the tilt aftereffect does not show selectivity to the polarity of luminance contrast (Magnussen & Kurtenbach, 1979) and the finding that the polarity selectivity of temporal ramp modulation is lost in interocular transfer (Hanly & MacKay, 1979) suggest a convergence of ON- and OFF- pathways on binocular cortical units. Obviously, there are many pieces missing in the puzzle, and the literature may even contain a few odd ones. However, taken as a whole, the psychophysical evidence suggests some parallel processing of brightness and darkness in the cortex.

V. SINGLE CHANNEL AND MULTICHANNEL MODELS OF BORDER CONTRAST EFFECTS

Illusions of darkness and lightness (i.e., the lack of monotonic correspondence between luminance and lightness) are often thought to provide cues to the manner in which the visual system encodes spatial patterns. Consequently, these illusions have been the subject of much scientific thought and experimentation. This section briefly describes some of the models which have been applied to the illusions. In particular, it will concentrate on Mach band phenomena. As we have seen in Section II, Mach bands are subjective overshoots and undershoots in a lightness distribution which do not have a counterpart in the physical distribution of luminance. It is in this sense that we classify Mach bands as illusions.

A. Some Basic Concepts

1. Receptive Fields as Linear Filters

In nearly all models, the receptive field itself is treated as a linear filter whose momentary output is a weighted sum of the light intensities falling at different points in the field. Specifically:

$$F = \iint_{-\infty}^{+\infty} L(x,y)\ S(x,y)\ dx\ dy$$

where F is the momentary response of the receptive field; x and y are the two spatial dimensions; $L(x,y)$

is the luminance distribution on the receptive field; and $S(x,y)$ is the weighting function. $S(x,y)$ is also called the sensitivity function because it describes the responsiveness of the receptive field to illumination at each point in space. A positive weight indicates that illumination at that point excites the receptive field unit; a negative weight indicates an inhibitory effect.

The form of the sensitivity function varies, depending on the type of neuron or pathway. However, in nearly all cases the receptive field is divided into two or more antagonistic subregions. In the cells of the retina and lateral geniculate nucleus, the receptive fields have a central circular region and an opposing annular surround (Barlow, 1953; Kuffler, 1953). This form of organization is commonly modeled as a difference of Gaussians (Rodieck, 1965) or as a Laplacian operator (Marr, 1982). The receptive fields of cortical cells are organized as oriented, parallel antagonistic bands. This organization has been modeled, as illustrated in Fig. 15, as a difference of Gaussians (Wilson & Bergen, 1979; Wilson & Gelb, 1984) or as a Gabor function (Daugman, 1980; Webster & DeValois, 1985; Watson, 1983).

The receptive field can also be described in the Fourier domain by indicating the sensitivity to different Fourier components as a function of their orientation and spatial frequency. To the extent that the receptive field is linear, the sensitivity to different Fourier components is given by the Fourier transform of the sensitivity function $S(x,y)$.

Although this linear concept of the receptive field is widely used in psychophysical models, and will be used in the present discussion, the reader should note that it is an idealized description which ignores some

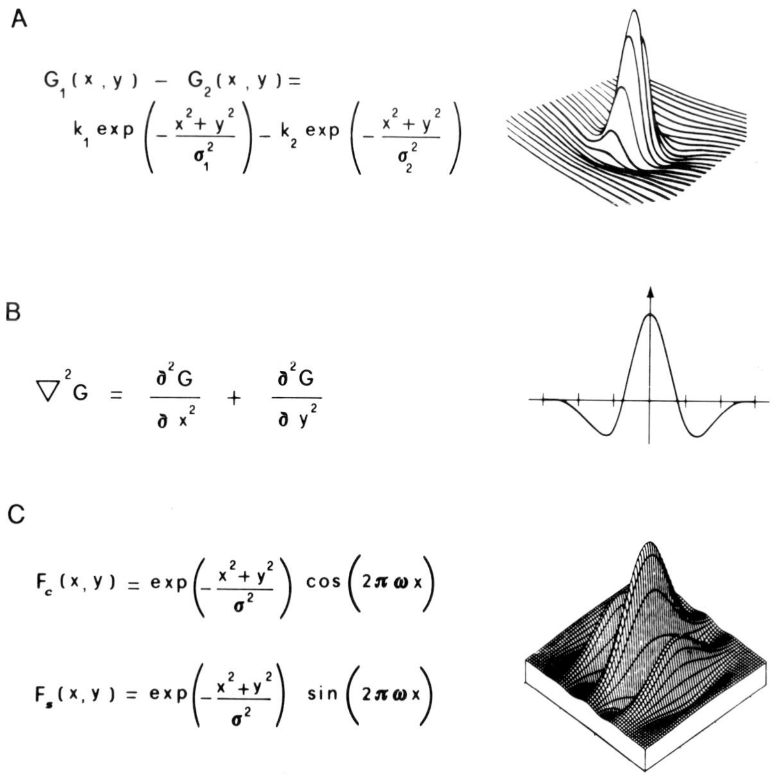

FIG. 15 Functions describing possible receptive field profiles. (A) Difference of two two-dimensional Gaussians and their profile (Rodieck, 1965). (B) Laplacian of Gaussians, where G represents the two-dimensional Gaussian distribution. The curve on the right represents the one-dimensional profile (Marr, 1982). (C) Cosine and sine Gabor functions and a two-dimensional profile of a cortical simple cell receptive field described by a cosine Gabor function (Daugman, 1980).

established facts. For one thing, as discussed in Section III, visual pathways are divided into separate ON- and OFF-responding units, and this division is a form of nonlinearity. A second fact is that there are many receptive fields, both in the retina and in the cortex, which are highly nonlinear in other ways as well (Robson, 1975). For instance, spatial summation within the receptive field is highly nonlinear in some populations of neurons, like the Y ganglion cells in the cat retina. Presumably, these receptive fields contribute to our percepts, but their role is not well understood and is largely ignored by current psychophysical models.

Each receptive field drives a neuron or visual pathway. While the receptive fields are modeled as linear, the subsequent pathways are often treated as introducing a nonlinear transform. That is, the response of each pathway is treated as a nonlinear function of the momentary response, F, of its receptive field. For a further discussion on this point, see Olzak and Thomas (1986).

2. Channels

Each receptive field samples only a small part of the visual scene. In order to see the full scene, it is necessary to have many receptive fields, each sampling a somewhat different patch. Such a mosaic of receptive fields is called a channel (Sachs, Nachmias & Robson, 1971). As we see in Section V,C, it is possible to have several channels, each differing from the other channels with respect to some property of its receptive fields. For example, the sizes of the receptive fields might vary from one channel to another (Thomas, 1970; Marr, 1982).

3. Channel Response Profile

When a visual pattern is presented, the receptive fields in each channel encode that pattern. The first level of encoding consists of the responses of the receptive fields. The channel response profile is a plot of these responses as a function of the spatial position of each receptive field. Examples of response profiles are shown in Figs. 16–18. When all of the receptive fields in a channel have the same sensitivity function (except for location), the response profile is given by the convolution of the sensitivity function with the luminance function of the stimulus:

$$R(x,y) = \iint_{-\infty}^{+\infty} L(x',y')\, S(x - x', y - y')\, dx'\, dy'$$

where $S(x - x', y - y')$ is the common sensitivity function defined in terms of distances from the center of the receptive field at x,y.

4. Decoding Rules

The channel response profile incorporates the filtering or "image processing" effects of the receptive fields which are thought to generate many illusions of lightness and darkness (e.g., Mach bands). However, the profile is only the first of many steps which lead to the conscious percept. Later steps link the profile and the ultimate percept, and hypotheses or assumptions about these steps can be thought of as decoding rules. The hypotheses range from assuming a simple isomorphism between channel profile and percept to rather complex computations which extract basic visual features.

B. Single Channel Models

Most of the commonly encountered explanations of Mach bands, Hermann grids, and similar illusions of lightness and darkness are based on a single-channel model of the visual system. In this type of model, all receptive fields are of the same form, usually consisting of a central excitatory area and an inhibitory surround. The size or scale of the receptive fields increases as a function of eccentricity (Glezer, 1965; Ransom-Hogg & Spillman, 1980), but each point in the visual field is served by only one size.

Figure 16A shows a receptive field sensitivity function which is typical of the functions used with this type of model. The area under the positive portion of the function is greater than the two negative areas combined. Consequently, the receptive field responds to regions of uniform luminance. However, because of the lateral interactions represented by the positive and negative areas, there is greater responsiveness to

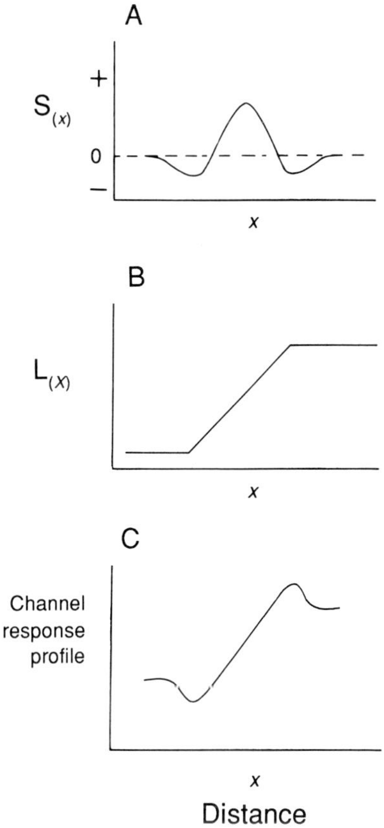

FIG. 16 Single-channel explanation of Mach bands. (A) receptive field sensitivity function. (B) Luminance profile of the Mach band stimulus. (C) Channel response profile obtained by convoluting the sensitivity function with the luminance profile. The localized minimum and maximum in the response profile are perceived as the dark and bright Mach bands, respectively.

regions in which the luminance changes at a nonuniform rate. Parts B and C of Fig. 16 illustrate this latter point. Figure 16B is the luminance profile of a stimulus which generates Mach bands. Figure 16C is the channel response profile generated by convoluting the sensitivity profile shown in A with the luminance profile shown in B. Note the "undershoot" and "overshoot" that occur in the response profile at the points corresponding to the discontinuities in the luminance profile.

The most common decoding rule used with single-channel models is simple isomorphism between the channel response profile and the percept. That is, the perceived brightness or lightness at a given point is assumed to be a monotonic function of the magnitude of the response profile at that point. Dips in the profile are perceived as darker areas and peaks are perceived as lighter areas. Applying this interpretation to the response profile shown in Fig. 16C, the gradual transition from a dark area, seen on the left, to a light area on the right is bounded by a narrow dark region, or dark Mach band, and a narrow light region, or light Mach band.

The single-channel model provides a qualitative explanation for a large number of phenomena involving perceived brightness or lightness, including Mach bands (von Békésy, 1960; Ratliff, 1965; Fiorentini, 1972); Hermann grids (Spillmann, 1971); the Craik–O'Brien–Cornsweet effect (Cornsweet, 1970); the "staircase" or Chevreul illusion (Cornsweet, 1970); and the manner in which the brightness of an object is affected by the sharpness of its contours (Thomas & Kovar, 1965; Thomas, 1966). The model can also be used as a partial explanation of contrast and constancy phenomena (Cornsweet, 1970). Presumably, the qualitative success of the model occurs because these phenomena all depend, at least in part, on a basic property of visual receptive fields: the division into antagonistic regions.

Quantitative applications of the model, on the other hand, have not been totally satisfactory. Given some reasonable auxiliary decoding rules, the sensitivity profiles of the receptive fields can be estimated psychophysically (von Békésy, 1960; Fiorentini & Mazzantini, 1966; Patel, 1966; Thomas, 1968), and the estimates used to generate quantitative predictions about perceived lightness and darkness. These efforts have been moderately successful when the visual features used to estimate the sensitivity functions and to test the predictions were similar in scale (von Békésy, 1960) but markedly less successful when features differed in scale (Thomas, 1966; Thomas, Rourke & Wilder, 1968).

Finally, it should be noted that, even on a qualitative level, single-channel models fail to account for one property of Mach bands. Single-channel models predict that the bands will be most prominent when the edge between dark and light areas is a step. In fact, the phenomenon is greatly reduced, if not totally abolished, at step edges.

C. Multiple-Channel Models

At the cortical level, each patch of the visual field is served by cells with widely differing receptive fields (Hubel & Wiesel, 1974). Each individual cell responds to only a limited range of orientations and spatial frequencies, but the ranges vary from cell to cell so that all orientations and a wide range of spatial frequencies are represented (see Chapter 10, this volume). There is also much psychophysical evidence that each patch of the visual field is served by pathways with many different types of tuning characteristics. The psychophysical evidence indicates that when the task of the observer is to detect the presence of a visual pattern, the different pathways are treated as independent sources of information. For further detail, see Graham (1985) and Olzak and Thomas (1986).

Each cell can be considered to be part of a mosaic of cells, with similar sensitivity and receptive field properties, that samples all parts of the visual field. That is, the cell is part of a channel which responds to only a limited range of stimulus components. Cells with different sensitivity characteristics constitute different channels with different sensitivity ranges. Because each channel responds to a different set of stimulus components, the response profiles will differ from channel to channel.

The visual scene is represented at this stage by the set of differing response profiles. The question to be addressed here is how these multiple profiles are interpreted and translated into a conscious percept of lightness and darkness. Under what conditions are the different profiles combined and how? What decoding rules are applied and are they applied to individual profiles or to composites? The discussion which follows examines two of the answers which have been proposed. The treatment is limited to channels which differ from one another only with respect to scale, this is, only with respect to the bands of spatial frequencies to which they respond. The discussion is also limited to stimuli in which luminance varies along only a single spatial dimension.

1. Watt and Morgan's MIRAGE Model

The essential features of this model (Watt & Morgan, 1985) are that each response profile is divided into positive- and negative-going parts; the profiles are combined across channels to form two composite profiles, one positive- and one negative-going; and the composite profiles are interpreted to locate bars and edges. Published versions of the model are one-dimensional, that is, stimulus luminance, receptive field sensitivity, and channel response profiles vary along only a single spatial dimension.

The model assumes that each receptive field is divided into three parts as shown in the upper-right part of Fig. 17, a central area flanked by two opposing regions. Watt and Morgan make the central region inhibitory and the flanks excitatory, but the opposite arrangement could be used just as well. The integral of the sensitivity function is zero, that is, positive and negative regions are equally balanced. Consequently, the receptive fields respond to edges and bars but make no response to parts of the stimulus in which luminance is either constant or changes at a constant rate.

The response profile generated in each channel is not simply isomorphic with the luminance profile. Consequently, decoding rules must be applied to identify the features. The response to a very narrow bright bar is a replica of the receptive field profile and contains three active regions: a region of negative response flanked by regions of positive response (see Fig. 17A). The response to a narrow dark bar is the mirror image, of course. The response to an edge is the integral of the receptive field profile and contains only two active regions, a region of positive response followed by a region of negative response in the case of a left-facing edge (Fig. 17B). The response to a right-facing edge is the opposite sequence. Generally

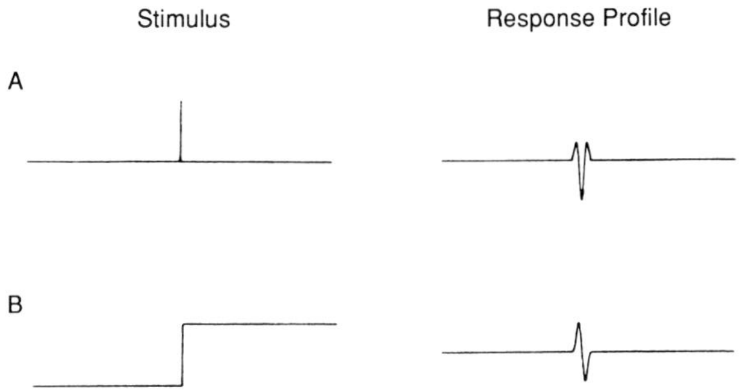

FIG. 17 Response profiles from the MIRAGE model. On the left are the luminance profiles of two stimuli: a narrow bright line (A) and an edge (B). On the right are shown the channel response profiles obtained by convolution with the MIRAGE sensitivity function. Note that the response profile is not isomorphic with the stimulus that produces it. Decoding rules are required to identify the stimulus which produced the response.

each feature generates a unique sequence of positive- and negative-going responses, bounded by regions of no response. The decoding process consists of looking for and identifying these sequences.

As indicated earlier, the decoding process is not applied to each channel response separately, but to composite positive-going and negative-going responses formed by combining the rectified profiles of the individual channels. Separating the positive- and negative-going portions of the profiles can be justified on the basis of the evidence for separate ON- and OFF-pathways which is discussed in the previous sections. However, Watt and Morgan (1985) adopt the procedure for another reason: the procedure prevents the detail resolved by small-scale channels from being lost when the small-scale profiles are combined with the profiles of large-scale channels. Information about the detail is provided by the sequence of transitions between positive- and negative-going responses in the profiles of the small-scale channels. The profiles of the large-scale channels, having low resolution, lack corresponding transitions. Thus, simple averaging of the profiles would tend to average out or lose the critical transitions. This loss does not occur when the positive- and negative-going portions of the profiles are combined separately.

2. Marr Model

Marr and colleagues (Marr, 1982) have proposed a quite different scheme in which the response profile of each channel is analyzed separately and the results of the analyses compared across channels. The rationale for this approach is that perceptual information is carried by intensity changes which can occur at different scales and are best detected by analyzing each channel response separately.

Marr and colleagues also have used a tripartite receptive field or filter function (Marr & Hildreth, 1980). Specifically, it is the Laplacian of a two-dimensional Gaussian (Fig. 15B). The filter has band-pass sensitivity in the frequency domain. The scale of the filter, that is, the range of spatial frequencies to which it responds, is set by manipulating the standard deviation of the Gaussian.

The premise of Marr's approach is that intensity changes or edges carry a wealth of perceptual information. Thus, the first step in Marr's decoding process is to locate the edges in the visual scene. Given the filter function used by Marr, an edge is represented in the channel response profile as adjacent positive- and negative-going responses. The spatial location at which the response changes from positive to negative, that is, the zero-crossing, corresponds to the position of the edge. Thus, the initial step is to locate the zero-crossings in the response profile of each channel.

Most physical edges contain a broad spectrum of spatial frequency components and produce characteristic zero-crossings in several channels at once. Therefore, a second step is to compare the locations of zero-crossings across channels to identify those which occur at a common location and signal a single edge. In the case of a low contrast or noisy visual scene, this step provides a type of averaging which increases the signal-to-noise ratio. Witkin (1983, 1984) has described a procedure for making these comparisons across channels.

Many visual features will not be represented in all channels, however. For example, small-scale channels are insensitive to gradual changes in illumination from one spatial position to another, while large-scale channels are insensitive to fine detail, such as narrow lines and fine texture. Thus, the overall percept may be a composite of features which are seen and processed separately at different scales, as well as features which activate channels in common.

3. Multichannel Interpretations of Mach Bands

The approach advocated by Marr leads to a possible explanation of the classical Mach band illusion. Basically, the notion is that the large-scale channels respond to the stimulus just as they would to an edge and signal a luminance change from dark to light. The small-scale channels are insensitive to the linear change in luminance that which constitutes the ramp portion of the stimulus, but they respond to the discontinuities at the bottom and top of the ramp in the same way that they would respond to a dark bar and a bright bar, respectively. Thus, the small-scale channels signal the presence of a dark and a bright bar at the boundaries of the luminance ramp. The overall percept is the composite of the luminance change, which the large channels signal, and the flanking bars, which the small channels signal.

Figure 18 illustrates this explanation. In this example, Gabor functions (Fig. 15C) are used to describe the receptive field sensitivity functions. The reason for this choice is that they are probably physiologically more realistic than tripartite functions. As Webster and DeValois (1985) have argued, Gabor functions more adequately describe cortical receptive fields than do simple tripartite functions.

Figure 18 shows the responses of two channels which differ in tuning with respect to scale by a factor of 6. The top row shows the response profiles to a delta function (i.e., a function having value 1 at the origin and 0 elsewhere); these profiles are identical to the sensitivity functions of single receptive fields in the channels. As can be seen by comparing the first and third rows for the large-scale channel, the difference between the response to a line and an edge is one of phase. The response to a line is odd symmetric [i.e., $R(x) = -R(-x)$] while the response to an edge is even symmetric [i.e., $R(x) = R(-x)$]. Although not illustrated in Fig. 18, the same difference characterizes the responses of the small channel to lines and edges. Thus, the decoding rules for these two features may involve phase sensitive mechanisms of the type described by Field and Nachmias (1984).

The second row of Fig. 18 shows the response of each channel to a luminance ramp. The third row shows the response of the large channel to an edge and the response of the small channel to appropriately located dark and bright bars. These latter responses are so similar to the responses which the respective channels give to the luminance ramp that they support the explanation offered, even in the absence of explicit decoding rules.

Mach bands can be explained using tripartite receptive field functions if the MIRAGE decoding rules are applied to the responses of each channel separately. When each channel is decoded separately the small-

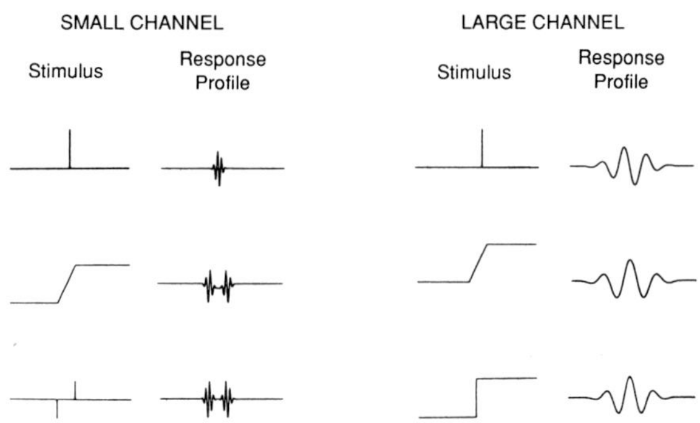

FIG. 18 Multichannel explanation of Mach bands. At left are the response profiles generated in a small-scale channel by three stimuli: a bright bar (top), a luminance ramp (middle), and spatially separated dark and bright bars (bottom). Note that the response to the ramp is almost identical to the response to the dark–bright bar pair. Thus, this channel responds to the ramp by signaling the presence of dark and bright bars. On the right are response profiles generated in a large-scale channel by three stimuli: a bright bar (top), a luminance ramp (middle), and an edge or luminance step (bottom). In the case of the large-scale channel, the response to the ramp is almost identical to the response to the luminance step. Thus, this channel signals a luminance step while, at the same time, the small-scale channel signals flanking dark and bright bars.

scale channels signal dark and bright bars and the large-scale channels signal an edge or luminance step. However, if the channel responses are combined before decoding, only the dark and bright bars are signaled (Watt & Morgan, 1985). If the stimulus is a luminance step, instead of a ramp, channels of all scales respond to the step as an edge at a common location. In this case, the composite percept is of a single edge, and no Mach band illusion is perceived.

VI. CONCLUSION

A. What Have We Learned about Brightness Perception, and What Is Open to Future Research?

We may now try to draw some conclusions from what has been illustrated in the previous sections. Some experimental facts are sufficiently well established, both psychophysically and neurophysiologically, to justify an interpretation of the perceptual findings in terms of neural functions. For other phenomena or findings, the interpretation in terms of known properties of neural channels is still a matter of debate. Let us discuss the various findings in detail.

1. The Role of ON- and OFF-Channels in the Perception of Brightness and Darkness

Experimental results on the spatial and temporal aspects of brightening and darkening effects are consistent with the early notions that brightness and darkness perception may be subserved by two independent channels. The behavioral experiments on monkeys treated with APB, described in Section III, strongly support the proposition that ON- and OFF-channels provide independent processing of localized light increments and decrements, respectively. The behavioral responses to light increments, but not decrements, are impaired by APB, which blocks activity in ON-center neurons, but not OFF-center neurons.

But why have two channels? If we were interested merely in the perception of small luminance steps (either spatial or temporal) above or below a mean photopic luminance level, there would be no need for a dual mechanism to signal these small luminance changes. One mechanism could transmit small modulations of the light input quite efficiently. And indeed, in APB-treated monkeys, thresholds for increments and decrements of light seem to be equally (and slightly) affected under photopic conditions (Merigan & Pasternak, 1983). However, a dual system is much more efficient in extending the range of discriminable input steps both above and below the mean luminance of the visual stimulus by reducing the effects of saturation of neuronal discharges (Bayly, Cervetto, Fiorentini & Maffei, 1971). This extended range can be achieved more economically without requiring a high maintained discharge in single cells. To keep a cell firing at a high rate in the absence of a stimulus is costly in terms of sustained metabolic activity.

In conclusion, the role of the ON- and OFF-channels in the suprathreshold perception of light increments and decrements, respectively, seems to be well established. However, the way in which the two systems contribute to the perception of brightness and darkness under more general conditions of illumination and objective contrast remains to be assessed.

B. Spatiotemporal Contrast Effects in Relation to the Properties of Neuronal Receptive Fields

The qualitative analogy between local contrast effects (resulting from short-range interactions between stimuli of different luminances) and the spatial distribution of excitation and inhibition in the receptive fields of single neurons is certainly striking. However, as pointed out in Sections IV and V, this analogy does not permit the conclusion that the psychophysical perceptive field directly represents the activity of single neurons. If anything, the perceptive field may reflect the combined activity of a number of neurons. Moreover, we know from neurophysiology that populations of neurons with different functional properties may contribute to different extents to the processing of visual stimuli. For instance, neurons with a sustained or a transient type of response, or neurons with different contrast sensitivity and contrast gain (Shapley & Perry, 1986), may contribute differently to produce contrast effects, depending on the temporal and spatial parameters of the stimulus (see Sections II,C, II,F, and IV).

When considering the response of populations of neurons and their effects on local brightness and contrast, it is important to take into account not only the amplitude but also the phase of the response. Receptive fields with perfectly symmetric profiles (i.e., having equal proportions of antagonistic flanks on either side of the central excitatory or inhibitory region) do not alter the spatial phase of a stimulus with sinusoidal luminance distribution. The phase response of these even-symmetric receptive fields is 0 degrees (or cosine). Neurons with odd-symmetric receptive fields (i.e., with one antagonistic flank of equal weight to the excitatory flank) produce a 90 degree shift in the phase of a sinusoidal input (sine phase). Morrone and Burr (1988) have proposed a model whereby the responses of the even- and odd-symmetric fields (both ON and OFF) are combined in a nonlinear manner to signal the position of key features in an image. If the response is predominantly from the even-symmetric fields, the feature will appear as a line, as in the case of Mach bands (Morrone et al., 1986). If the response is from the odd-symmetric fields, the feature will appear as an edge and cause a change in brightness, as in the case of the Craik–O'Brien–Cornsweet illusion (Burr, 1987). This model predicts the perception and position of Mach bands more satisfactorily than other models and also explains their absence at sharp edges.

Neurophysiological findings in the striate cortex of the cat indicate that simple cells with even-symmetric receptive fields often are paired with adjacent cells having odd-symmetric receptive fields, with both members of the pair having the same size and orientation tuning (Pollen & Ronner, 1981). The receptive fields of complex cells, on the other hand, contain subunits of both odd- and even-symmetry (Gaska, Pollen & Cavanagh, 1987). Both sets of findings may offer support for the above model.

C. Border Contrast versus Area Contrast: The Role of Various Cortical Areas

The crucial question of whether and how local contrast at edges may help produce brightness contrast over large stimulus areas has not yet been answered. Retinal ganglion cells seem capable of processing local contrast, possibly for brightness constancy (see Chapter 5, this volume). But so far we know of no neurophysiological correlate of area contrast, either in the retina or in the LGN. Possibly, area contrast is subserved by cortical mechanisms, which would be consistent with the fact that some of these effects occur under dichoptic conditions (Section II,F).

Even in the cortex, there is no easily identified neural correlate of area contrast. Individual neurons provide no simple answer, since neurons whose receptive fields fall within a homogeneous area are not active at all. However, oriented neurons not only encode orientation, disparity, and size, but may also be selective either for white or for dark bars. One could argue that area contrast is produced because oriented neurons code the direction of contrast gradients at each border and that this information is somehow propagated from one border to another across space. Thus, the brightness of an area of homogeneous luminance would be extrapolated from the directions of the contrast gradients at the border. Therefore, reversing the gradients on either side of a contrast area should alter the brightness perception in between, as is indeed the case.

If this were true, area contrast would be an example of the economy of cortical activity in modeling the visual scene with a minimum of active cells. It would also explain why cortical scotomas after occipital lesions are not perceived. Indeed, to the extent that neurons under area contrast conditions are silent, higher processing levels should not be able to discriminate whether the lack of information from these neurons is physiological or due to a localized lesion.

But where is neuronal activity bound directly to the perception of light and dark? And how does this occur? In Area V1 there are neurons coding for a dark bar or a bright one. In Area V2, neurons code for a real bright bar or a real dark bar, but they may also respond to an apparent bar, and induce corresponding anomalous contours. One has to assume, therefore, that the perception of brightness and darkness is carried out in several cortical areas (at least V1 and V2) by processes which become more and more selective, and which involve fewer and fewer but increasingly specific neurons. At the same time that these neurons increase in specificity, they become invariant for the features for which they are selective. But where in this process the actual percepts of brightness and darkness are generated is still not known.

8

COLOR PERCEPTION
Retina to Cortex

Eberhart Zrenner, Israel Abramov, Munehira Akita, Alan Cowey, Margaret Livingstone, and Arne Valberg

I. INTRODUCTION

Color exists only within neuronal networks that mediate perception. The outer physical world provides a mixture of light quanta, the energy and frequency of which have little resemblance to the colors perceived. The first step in perception involves illumination of the photoreceptors in the retina which hyperpolarizes the outer segments so that phototransduction leads to a receptor potential. Since a single cone contains only one type of pigment, it cannot signal specific information about the frequency of a light quantum. Therefore the signals of different cone types in subsequent neurons must be compared to extract information about color. For many decades, it has been a challenge to physiologists, psychologists, and physicists to find the link between the physical properties of visible light and its perceptual qualities. In this chapter, this link is approached from two sides: neurophysiology and psychophysics. The underlying mechanisms in the different levels of the visual system, from photoreceptors via the lateral geniculate nucleus (LGN) to cortical centers, are described and correlated with visual perception where possible.

The historic color-matching experiments of Maxwell (1856) and Helmholtz (1867), which were quantified by Grassmann's laws, clearly established the principle of trichromatic color vision. More recently, the techniques of molecular genetics (Nathans, Piantanida, Eddy, Shows & Hogness, 1986; Nathans, Thomas & Hogness, 1986) provided the ultimate proof of trichromacy determined in the human genome. There is also considerable physiological insight into the interaction of spectrally different cones as expressed in the principle of color opponency, introduced by Hering (1878), proven neurophysiologically by DeValois, Smith, Kitai, and Karoly (1958) and Svaetichin and MacNichol (1958), and quantitatively assessed by psychophysical techniques by Jameson and Hurvich (1955).

Starting with these fundamental findings, numerous psychophysicists, physiologists, and morphologists have established many details about the processing of chromatic information in the visual system. However, there are many problems that still remain to be solved. How is spectral, temporal, and spatial information interlaced in various areas of the visual field? How is information about brightness and hue, separated in the initial stages of the visual system, reintegrated in the perception of color? Are there different qualities of brightness signals processed in opponent and nonopponent pathways? How is color segregated from form, movement, and depth processing in the visual system? These and many more questions are addressed in this chapter as the signals that code color are followed up from the cone outer segment through retinal opponent neurons to the LGN and the visual cortex, always with the goal of demonstrating how neurophysiological results can be linked to perceptual phenomena. Additional insight into processing of color is provided in Section VII of this chapter, where physiological and psychophysical findings from patients and animals with brain damage are presented. Many answers engender still other questions to be addressed by color scientists of the next generation.

II. COLOR APPEARANCE

A. Spectral Colors

By the middle of the nineteenth century, it was apparent that three variables (three receptor types) were required to account for the color mixture experiments of Maxwell (1856) and Helmholtz (1867). As we shall see in the following, this view was verified nearly 100 years later by microspectrophotometry and electrophysiology that established the existence of three univariant classes of cone photoreceptor, with peak absorbances at short, middle, and long wavelengths, therefore called S, M, and L cones. These observations explain why some wavelength distributions are indistinguishable from others, but they do not explain the hues that we experience.

To account for the appearance of the spectrum, Helmholtz proposed that each receptor type directly signals a particular hue. For this reason, he called the short, middle, and long wave cones the "blue," "green," and "red" receptors. Helmholtz did not choose these labels merely because the receptors are maximally sensitive in the regions of the spectrum that normally look blue, green, and red. Rather, he believed that there was a direct correspondence between activity in the "blue" receptor, for example, and the perception of blueness. Of course, he realized that the receptors must overlap in spectral sensitivity so that each wavelength would stimulate different ratios of receptor activity to signal the many hues of the spectrum.

Hering (1878) objected to Helmholtz's theory of color appearance although, contrary to some historical accounts, he did not object to Helmholtz's three-receptor explanation for color mixture. Hering's arguments were based on careful observations and introspection about the nature of color experience. He pointed out, for example, that according to the Helmholz theory, blue–green hues were due to the combined activity of a "blue" receptor and a "green" receptor. Consistent with common experience, one can distinguish the elemental components of blue and green in such hues, as implied by Helmholtz. But according to Helmholtz, yellow is a hue that is a perceptual mixture of red and green, and this, Hering argued, is contrary to our experience. The sensation of yellow is elemental and cannot be reduced to a red–green perceptual mixture. In fact, the notion of reddish green or greenish red violates our experience, since these hue mixtures are never experienced. Red and green sensations cancel, or oppose, each other, as do the sensations of blue and yellow. Thus, Hering proposed that there are four elemental hue sensations that code our perceptions by paired, opponent processes. Red–green and yellow–blue opponent processes, according to Hering, account for the hues of spectral lights.

The squares in Fig. 1 show results of a hue-scaling experiment in which observers, naive about color vision theory, were asked to describe the appearance of monochromatic lights from 400 to 700 nm by assigning percentages to the terms, red, green, yellow, and blue. For example, a light at 600 nm would ordinarily

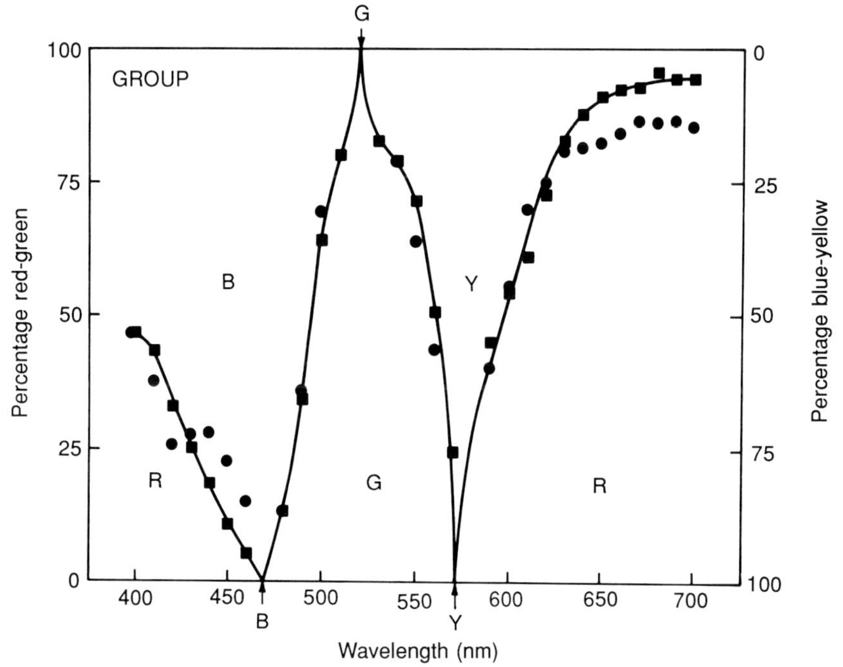

FIG. 1 Average hue-naming data (squares) and average predicted hue naming (circles) based on opponent-cancellation functions for three observers. Red–green is plotted from 0 to 100% on the left ordinates; blue–yellow is plotted from 100 to 0% on the right ordinates. The smooth curves were drawn by eye through the obtained hue-naming data. The arrows indicate the loci of unique blue, unique green, and unique yellow as determined by separate measurements. Reprinted from Werner and Wooten (1979).

be described as orange, but the observers in this experiment described it, on average, as about 50% yellow and 50% red. Similarly, when describing the violet appearance of a 400 nm light they reported 60% blue and 40% red. Observers can do this quite reliably, as originally shown by Boynton and Gordon (1965). Figure 1, therefore, represents the appearance of the spectrum plotted in terms of percentage redness or greenness from 0 to 100 on the left-hand ordinates, percentage blueness or yellowness from 100 to 0 on the right-hand ordinates. The data could be plotted in this way because the subjects almost never used the terms red and green simultaneously, nor did they use the terms yellow and blue simultaneously, as expected from Hering's opponent-colors theory.

Hering proposed that four hue terms were both necessary and sufficient to describe the hues of the spectrum in normal observers. The data in Fig. 1 are consistent with this view, but one might wonder whether the observers were simply assigning color terms that were allowed even if they did not completely describe their experience. For example, perhaps the term orange would be better than 50% red, 50% yellow. Sternheim and Boynton (1966) tested this hypothesis by asking observers to describe the hues of lights between 530 and 620 nm, but in different sessions, different color names were permitted. Their results showed that lights which appeared orange could be described just as well by the terms red and yellow, but the terms red and yellow could not similarly be disallowed in describing these monochromatic lights. The same conclusion was reached by Fuld, Wooten, and Whalen (1981) about the appearance of lights that can be described as violet or purple. These terms are not necessary; the color names for the elemental hues blue and red are adequate to describe their appearance. Thus, these experiments are consistent with Hering's proposal that there are four, and only four, fundamental hues.

The data described so far have not included a complete description of the appearance of spectral lights because in addition to the four hue variables, one must consider the blackness or whiteness components in a color. For example, the term maroon (a dark brownish red) has a red hue component as well as a blackness component, while pink has a red hue component with a whiteness component. To account for the achromatic dimensions of color experience, Hering postulated the existence of a black–white opponent process. Thus, in the Hering theory there are six fundamental colors, coded by three opponent processes, red–green, yellow–blue and white–black.

B. Contrast Colors

We experience many colors in everyday life that we do not see when monochromatic lights are viewed as a uniform test spot. For example, the color brown would never be reported under the conditions in which the data of Fig. 1 were collected. If, however, a 580 nm light is presented in the center of a bright, white annulus, it will appear brown, as described by Hering (1878). Brown is a nonspectral color, and it is also called a contrast color because it is experienced only under conditions in which there are two or more (contrasting) colors in the field of view. By varying the contrast ratio (changing the intensity of the white annulus from low to high values), it is possible to produce a series of contrast colors that vary from yellow, to tan or beige, light brown, brown, dark brown, and black.

Hering accounted for contrast colors in terms of reciprocal inhibitory connections across the retina between paired, opponent processes. Thus, a white annulus will induce its opposite, black, in the center. If the spot in the center is yellow, the presence of the annulus will produce a blackish yellow, or brown. Indeed, by using various wavelengths of center and surround, it is possible to produce any color imaginable. Hering believed that contrast colors involved spatial interactions between red–green, yellow–blue and white–black opponent processes. He also acknowledged, though, that these colors sometimes lose their independent qualities, which may be why some observers have difficulty describing brown as a blackish-yellow (Fuld, Werner & Wooten, 1983) with the same ease that they describe orange as reddish–yellow. Changes in the appearance of a color will also occur as a result of preceding stimulation, an effect called successive color contrast. Helmholtz and Hering provide many detailed examples of the conditions under which this occurs and the physiological processes that might make it possible. Wooten (1984) has obtained hue scaling data to quantify successive color contrast effects and he argues that they must involve physiological changes that alter the signals at both receptoral and opponent-neural levels. His interpretation of successive color contrast results is consistent with the Jameson and Hurvich (1968) model to be presented in Section II,D.

C. Psychophysical Measurement of Opponent Processes

Hering (1920) proposed that "corresponding to the four hue variables . . . there are four physiological variables" (trans. by Hurvich & Jameson, 1964, pp. 47–48). This idea was criticized by followers of Helmholtz because opponent processes imply two modes of neural response, excitation and inhibition, and the latter was inconsistent with the then-known physiology. Neurophysiological support for Hering ultimately arrived (DeValois, Abramov and Jacobs, 1966), but not until after Jameson and Hurvich (1955) developed psychophysical methods for measuring opponent processes and provided a firm quantitative foundation for the Hering theory that was further developed by Vos and Walraven (1972), Ingling (1977), and Guth, Massof, and Benzschawel (1980), among others.

The method of Jameson and Hurvich capitalized on the opponent nature of hue sensations. To determine the strength of redness, for example, they measured the energy of a superposed green light which was required to cancel the redness. The assumption was that the strength of redness at a particular wavelength and luminance level is proportional to the greenness required to produce an equilibrium state, that is, neither red nor green. Similarly, the strength of blue could be measured by adjusting the energy of

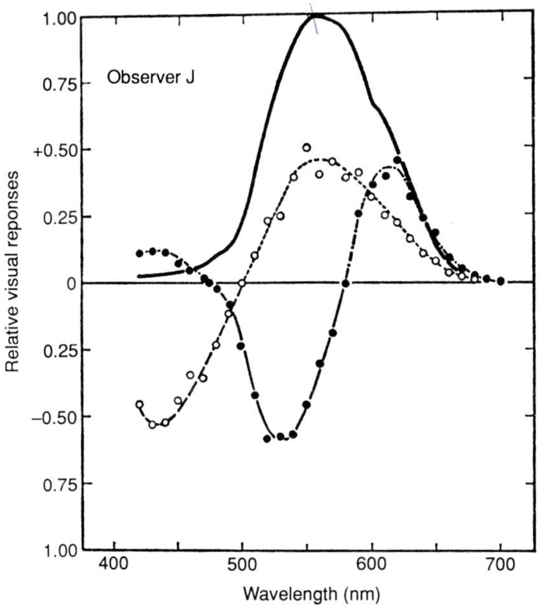

FIG. 2 Opponent-hue cancellation functions obtained for one observer are plotted as a function of wavelength (data from Jameson & Hurvich, 1955). The white function (solid line) is the observer's spectral luminosity function. From Jameson (1972).

a yellow light to produce a blue–yellow equilibrium. Figure 2 presents data obtained by Jameson and Hurvich for one subject's opponent processes, plotted as a function of wavelength. The red lobes (note that redness occurs at short and long wavelengths) of the red–green process (filled circles) are plotted with opposite signs to the green lobe, just as blue and yellow (open circles) are plotted with opposite signs. This convention in plotting is consistent with Hering's idea that red and green are opponent sensations and they are derived from opposite modes of neural response.

Notice in Fig. 2 that, in addition to the opponent-hue cancellation functions, Jameson and Hurvich show a unimodal curve (line) based on spectral sensitivity measurements in a neutral state of adaptation. They assumed that this function, or the spectral luminosity function of the CIE standard observer, represents the whiteness spectral response function and that blackness would be identical except for a sign inversion. This is because blackness, a fundamental color, exists only by virtue of contrast. To measure blackness requires, therefore, that one uses conditions of spatial (Werner, Cicerone, Kliegl & Dellarosa, 1984) or temporal (Volbrecht, Werner & Wooten, 1989) contrast. Measurements of blackness induction, representing one of the two dimensions of Hering's achromatic opponent process, are presented in Fig. 3 for one observer measured at two different luminance levels (see also Fuld, Otto & Slade, 1986). All spectral sensitivity functions are plotted in the same direction for comparison; filled circles represent blackness induction, and open circles represent spectral sensitivity measured by methods originally used in obtaining the CIE average observer. The log spec-

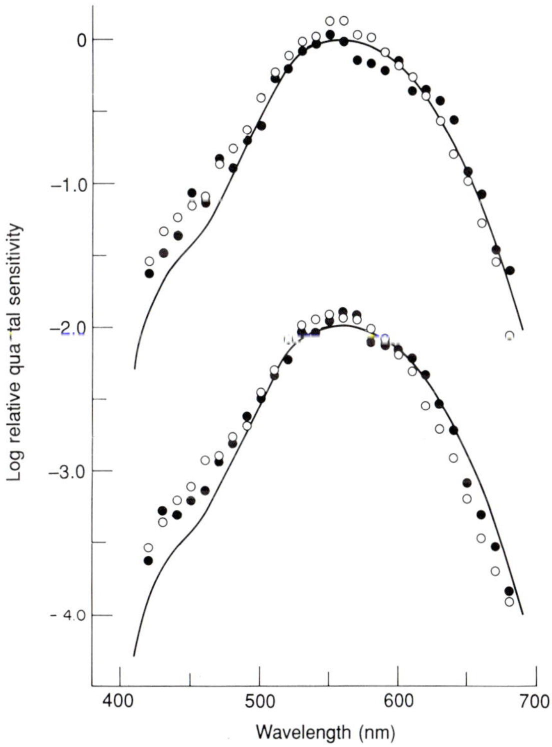

FIG. 3 Log quantal sensitivity is plotted as a function of wavelength for one observer. Filled circles represent the efficiency of blackness induction; open circles represent spectral sensitivity measured by heterochromatic flicker photometry. Smooth curves represent the spectral sensitivity of the CIE standard observer fit to each data set. Different data sets represent two different luminance levels for measurements. From Werner et al. (1984).

tral sensitivity of the latter is shown by the smooth curves in Fig. 3 and is similar to that shown on an arithmetic scale in Fig. 2. It appears that Jameson and Hurvich were correct in assuming that Hering's achromatic process has this spectral sensitivity.

If the psychophysically measured opponent-process functions represent the physiological substrates for perceived color, then it should be possible to relate opponent-cancellation functions such as those in Fig. 2 to color-naming data. Hurvich and Jameson (1955) proposed that the ratio of red–green or yellow–blue chromatic response, at each wavelength, relative to total chromatic activity (red–green plus yellow–blue) measured by a cancellation procedure, should produce a ratio that is related to hue-scaling data. A test of this prediction is provided in Fig. 1. The circles show the opponent-cancellation function predictions and the squares show hue-naming data from the same group of three observers. The close correlation between the two sets of data is consistent with the Hurvich–Jameson–Hering view that opponent processes are the basis for perceived color.

D. Coupling of Receptors to Opponent Mechanisms

To further investigate the physiological basis of color perception by psychophysical methods, one can ask how the three types of cone photoreceptor might be linked to the opponent-cancellation functions. Jameson and Hurvich (1968) proposed a model in which the opponent mechanisms receive input from a linear combination of the three classes of cone receptor. Tests of this model support the linearity of the red–green process for many conditions, but the yellow–blue system appears to receive a nonlinear input (Larimer, Krantz & Cicerone, 1975; Werner & Wooten, 1979; Elzinga & de Weert, 1984; Ejima & Takahashi, 1985; Ayama & Ikeda, 1986; Akita, Takahashi & Ejima, 1987).

A typical property of the yellow–blue hue-cancellation code is shown in Fig. 4. The energy ratio of a yellowish to a blue light (E_λ/E_{465}) at yellow–blue equilibrium (yellow and blue have cancelled each other) is plotted as a function of the retinal illuminance of the 465 nm light. The data show a systematic deviation from the linear prediction; as the intensity is increased, more than a proportional increase in the yellow light is required for cancellation. The amount of this nonlinearity depends on the wavelength of the yellowish light; as the wavelength is increased, the nonlinearity becomes more evident.

Ejima and Takahashi (1985) proposed that the results in Fig. 4 can be explained by a yellow–blue code in which signals from the long-wave cones enhance the gain of the signals from the short-wave cones, an effect called sensitization, while the signals from the middle-wave cones have the opposite effect, that is, they attenuate the gain of the short-wave cones. This type of interaction could be accomplished if the gain of the signal from the short-wave cones is controlled by the difference signal between the middle- and long-wave cones, so that the sensitivity of the blue

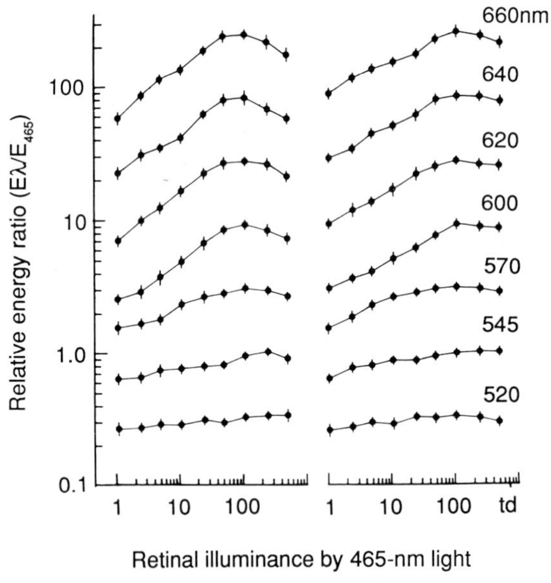

FIG. 4 Relative energy ratios of long-wave lights (wavelength indicated near each curve) to 465 nm light at yellow–blue equilibrium plotted as a function of the illuminance of the 465 nm light for two observers. If the energy ratio remained constant, as required for a linear system, all curves should be parallel to the abscissa. From Ejima and Takahashi (1985).

response is enhanced with an increase in the long-wave cone excitation and attenuated by an increase in the middle-wave cone excitation. Ejima and Takahashi have shown that this model can account for various nonlinear properties of the yellow–blue process such as the noninvariance of unique red (a red that is not tinged with either yellow or blue), nonlinearity of the cancellation function, and linear additivity of the blue chromatic response.

The nonlinearity of the yellow–blue cancellation code is also strongly influenced by the size of the stimulus. The sensitization of the blue response in yellow–blue hue cancellation occurs at a lower intensity level when the stimulus size is increased. This implies that L and M cones that control the sensitivity of the S-cone signal have a large spatial summation area. There is much physiological and psychophysical evidence that the short-wavelength cone mechanism may lack distinct spatial center–surround antagonism (Tansley & Boynton, 1978; Creutzfeldt, Lee & Elepfandt, 1979; Foster, 1981; Zrenner & Gouras, 1981; Zrenner, 1983a; Takahashi & Ejima, 1984). The finding that in the yellow–blue opponent process the S-cone contribution occurs within a larger spatial summation area than for the other two cone types, together with the lack of a distinct spatial center–surround antagonism, corresponds to the poor spatial resolution of the S-cone system mentioned above.

More recent investigations have provided evidence which might link cone antagonistic signals identified under threshold conditions to hue sensations. Pugh and Larimer (1980) concluded that the site of the blue–yellow hue interaction postulated by the opponent-colors theory is identical to the site of chromatic antagonism identified by the threshold measurements, similar to those that are explained along with Fig. 18 later in this chapter (Section IV,H) (see also Friedman, Thornton & Pugh, 1985; Takahashi & Ejima, 1987). Figure 5 is a schematic diagram that represents the hypothesized interaction between S, M, and L cones. The gain in the S-cone signals is assumed to be controlled by the L − M difference signal.

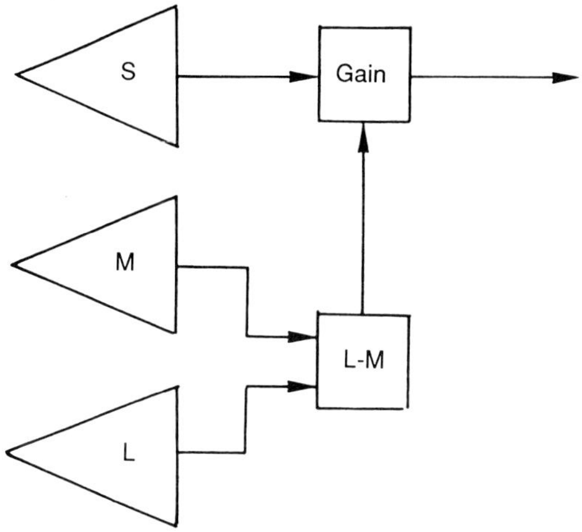

FIG. 5 Schematic diagram representing the hypothesized interaction between the short- and longer wavelength cones in the yellow–blue hue-cancellation code. The gain of the signal from the short-wavelength cones is assumed to be controlled by the difference in signals coming from the long- and middle-wavelength cones.

From recordings in S-cone-driven ganglion cells, Zrenner and Gouras (1981; Zrenner 1983a) proposed a circuit in which the L- and M-cone signals control the S-cone signals by modifying the S-cones' membrane characteristics via horizontal cells by means of a hyperpolarizing transmitter. The model can account for the effects of sensitization and desensitization found in S-cone-driven ganglion cells in response to long-wavelength adapting lights. The hypothesis derived from hue-cancellation data by Ejima and Takahashi (1985) is in good accord with this model. Details on the underlying physiological mechanisms are presented in Section IV,H.

III. PHOTOPIGMENTS, CONES, AND PRIMARY CHROMATIC MECHANISMS

A. Number of Spectrally Different Cone Mechanisms Necessary for Color Vision

The minimum requirement for discriminating color is a system having two receptor types with different spectral sensitivities and a nervous system that compares their responses (see Boynton, 1979). This becomes clear when considering the color-matching of a monochromat, an individual with only one spectral channel (i.e., all receptors have the same spectral sensitivity). Such a subject can adjust the intensity of a standard light on one side of a bipartite field to match completely any stimulus in the other half of the field. All the subject must do is adjust the intensity such that his receptors absorb the same number of quanta from each side of the field—if this were not done, he could discriminate the stimuli only on the basis of a brightness difference.

If the subject has two receptor types with different but overlapping sensitivities, then he cannot adjust a single standard wavelength to match all other wavelengths but could match any wavelength with a mixture of two others. Such an individual is known as a dichromat. Of course, the nervous system that processes the responses of these receptors must somehow preserve the differences in response; if it simply summed the responses of these receptors, this would be equivalent to having a single channel whose spectrum were the combined function—the subject would still be color-blind.

As outlined above, normal humans are "trichromatic"; they need three primaries to match any stimulus presented to the central 1° of the retina, which contains three types of cones and relatively few rods. However, normal human observers can be dichromatic under certain circumstances: (1) when stimuli are very small and limited to the central fovea, such that vision is tritanopic, lacking S cones (Willmer & Wright, 1945); (2) when the light spectrum is limited to wavelengths longer than about 540 nm (see Boynton, 1979); and (3) when the eye is dark adapted and stimuli are very dim and limited to long wavelengths, so that one cone type in conjunction with the rods can provide a form of color vision (Smith & Pokorny, 1977; Stabell & Stabell, 1982). Under other conditions, the same observers can be "tetrachromatic": when the stimulus is viewed peripherally, four primaries may be required because discriminations are dependent on all three types of cone and the rods (Trezona, 1976).

B. Spectral Characteristics of the Cones

The above psychophysical findings can be understood in terms of the photopigments contained in the outer segments of the retinal receptors. These photopigments determine the ability of the receptor to absorb incident light. In other species, the sensitivity of the photoreceptors depends not only on the photopigment in the receptor, but also on colored oil droplets located in front of the outer cone segment (see Chapter 4, this volume). In mammals, however, the photopigments set the fundamental spectral limits, and any understanding of color vision must start with these pigments.

1. Spectrophotometric Measures of Photopigments

Primate cone pigments have strenuously resisted efforts to extract sufficient quantities for *in vitro* studies. Two related spectrophotometric methods have been used to study their properties *in situ*. The first method, *reflection densitometry*, was applied to the living eye to measure light reflected from the fundus and hence not absorbed by any pigments (Campbell & Rushton, 1955; Weale, 1959, 1965).

The second method, *microspectrophotometry* (MSP), measures the light absorbed by single receptors in excised retinas (for reviews, see Bowmaker, 1984; Levine & MacNichol, 1985, Chapter 4, this volume). There are several major problems associated with MSP, including postmortem changes and light scattering (see MacNichol, 1986). In practice, where optical density (absorbance) falls to a level below 10% of peak density, the results must be attributed to "noise." Also, the different cone types are not equally prevalent, which creates great sampling problems. Unless the measurements are rigorously screened, the results will yield a distorted representation of that cone type (MacNichol, 1986; Harosi, 1987).

(a) MSP and Primate Cones. Dartnall (1953) noted that rod photopigments from a wide range of animal species have similar shapes when the proportion of absorbed quanta is plotted as a function of frequency (wave number, reciprocal of wavelength). Cone photopigments also have similar shapes if relative quantal absorption is plotted on an axis whose units are normalized with respect to each pigment's peak frequency (MacNichol, Levine, Mansfield, Lipetz & Collins, 1983; Mansfield, 1985). Thus, a particular pigment is often adequately characterized by its wavelength of maximal density (λ_{max}). Of course, when the top of the density curve is flat, the peak must be located by fitting some smooth function to the data points.

Table 1 shows three mean values of λ_{max} for macaque (*Macaca fascicularis*) and baboon (*Papio papio*) cones obtained in several different laboratories and using different types of instruments. In spite of the technical difficulties of this research, the results are reassuringly similar for the M and L cones. However, there are large discrepancies in the values for the S cones. The differences are even greater than they appear; the table gives values in terms of wavelength, but, as discussed later, frequency is the more appropriate dimension for describing light absorption by pigments. Therefore, a 10 nm difference at short wavelengths produces a much greater shift in the peak than would a 10 nm step at longer wavelengths. The reasons for the differences probably include higher light scatter at shorter wavelengths (MacNichol, 1986) and small sample sizes.

Table 1 also shows means from a large sample (108) of human cones, including five S cones (Dartnall, Bowmaker & Mollon, 1983). Note that the mean λ_{max} for all three human cones are shorter than those for macaques. This could be due to greater light scattering in these measurements, possibly because of tissue deterioration. However, it is also possible that the cones differ for the two species. Rayleigh matches (red plus green mixture that matches a standard yellow) have been obtained psychophysically from macaques and human trichromats, and consistently macaques require slightly more green in their mixtures (DeValois, Morgan, Polson, Mead & Hull, 1974; Oyama, Furusaka & Kito, 1979; Jacobs, 1983a; discussed also in Chapter 4, this volume).

2. Action Spectra

The ability of a receptor to respond to light is based on the ability of its photopigment to absorb quanta. Therefore, there should be a close agreement between

TABLE 1 Wavelengths of Maximal Density (λ_{max}) for Primate Cone Photopigments (in nm)

Method of measurement	Cone type		
	S	M	L
Microspectrophotometry			
Macaque (Bowmaker Mollon & Jacobs, 1983)	415	535	567
Macaque (MacNichol et al., 1983)	429	532	567
Baboon (Bowmaker et al., 1983)	432	535	566
Macaque (Bowmaker, 1984)	420–430	535	565
Macaque (Harosi, 1987)	431	534	566
Human (Dartnall et al., 1983)	419	531	558
Possible subpopulations			
Macaque (MacNichol et al., 1983)	—	532–543	—
Macaque (Bowmaker et al., 1984)	—	535–543	—
Human (Dartnall et al., 1983)	—	528–534	554–563
Action spectra			
Macaque (Baylor et al., 1987)	430	531	561
Human (Schnapf et al., 1987)	—	530	560

the receptor's relative spectral sensitivity (action spectrum) and the absorption spectrum of its pigment. To make this comparison, it should be kept in mind that in MSP the light usually passes transversely through a receptor and therefore the measurement is of a very dilute pigment; this limiting case is appropriate for characterizing the ability of the pigment molecule to catch quanta. In contrast, under physiological conditions, light passes through a much greater length of the receptor, and the effective concentration of the pigment is much higher. If the fraction of absorbed light (absorptance) is measured, it is found that increasing the concentration changes the shape of the pigment's spectrum: it makes it broader (Dartnall, 1957).

Thus, for comparison with a receptor's action spectrum an absorptance spectrum must be used that takes account of the length of the receptor's outer segment. The comparison should be made on the basis of the number of quanta absorbed and not on total energy absorbed. This is based on the accepted notion that when a pigment molecule absorbs a quantum of visible light, the effect is the same regardless of the individual quantum's frequency (energy). Absorption of a long wavelength (low frequency, low energy) quantum has the same effect as absorption of a short wavelength (high frequency, high energy) quantum. This is the "principle of univariance," according to which a receptor can only report the rate at which its pigment is absorbing quanta and cannot report the frequencies of the individual quanta (Naka & Rushton, 1966). More formally, a receptor's response, R, can be described as some function of light absorbed by a photopigment at a given wavelength:

$$R = f(IA_\lambda) \qquad (1)$$

where I is the number of quanta and A_λ denotes the effective fraction of incident quanta absorbed by the photopigment at each wavelength, λ. For each stimulus, the intensity is simply scaled by the value of A at that point on the spectrum; on logarithmic coordinates this self-similar functional form will generate parallel response-versus-intensity curves (see Sirovich & Abramov, 1977).

Figure 6 shows data from single neurons and receptors that illustrate the above property of univariance. In Fig. 6A are data of Graham and Hartline (1935) from a single fiber in the lateral eye of the horseshoe crab (*Limulus polyphemus*). Note that any response measure (e.g., frequency of spike firing, or latency to first spike) plotted as a function of intensity will generate parallel curves for different wavelengths; the separations between curves are dependent on the differences in log sensitivity of the pigment function A_λ. In Fig. 6B are records and the corresponding response-versus-intensity functions from a single rod of the tiger salamander (*Ambystoma tigrinum*) held in a suction electrode (Cornwall, MacNichol & Fein, 1984). This is a particularly important experiment because it affords a direct test of the notion that action and absorptance spectra are identical: in this case, the receptor's responses were recorded together with its absorption by MSP in the same apparatus, at the same time, and illuminating the same portion of the receptor. Spectral sensitivity is defined as the reciprocal of the intensity needed to elicit some constant, criterion response. Since the response-versus-log intensity curves are parallel, any criterion can be used and the relative intensities can be found by interpolation on the curves for the different wavelengths. The results are shown in Fig. 6D, and the coincidence between the two spectral measures is excellent. Finally, Fig. 6C shows similar data from a primate cone, also in a suction electrode (Baylor, Nunn & Schnapf, 1987). The lower half of Fig. 6C shows an original recording in response to a short flash. The corresponding response-versus-log intensity curves are shown in the upper half for two wavelengths.

(a) Action Spectra of Primate Cones. Spectral sensitivities have been measured from macaque cones by recording photocurrents from individual outer segments pulled into a suction electrode (Nunn, Schnapf & Baylor, 1984; Baylor et al., 1987; see Chapter 5, this volume) as shown in the example of Fig. 6C. The mean results from 5 S cones, 20 M cones, and 16 L cones are shown in Fig. 7 plotted as open circles. The λ_{max} values of the smooth curves are, respectively,

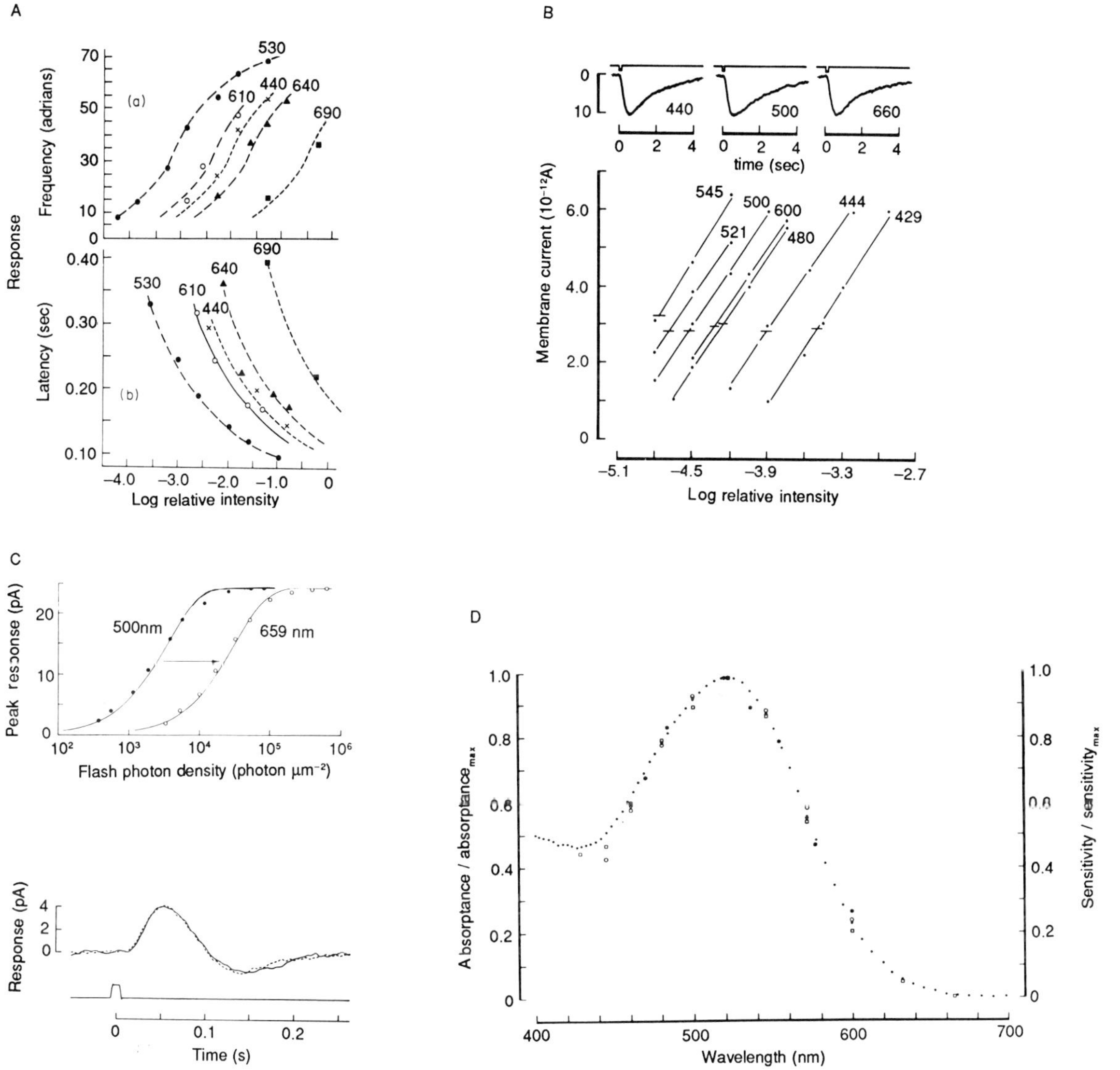

FIG. 6 Data from single neurons and photoreceptors, illustrating the property of univariance. (A) Recordings from a single fiber of the lateral eye of horseshoe crab (*Limulus*) in response to monochromatic test lights of various wavelength (unpublished data of Graham & Hartline, 1935, after Sirovich and Abramov, 1977). The plots of discharge frequency versus relative intensity reveal parallel functions indicating univariance, that is, only one spectral type of photoreceptor is involved. (B) A similar experiment as in A was carried out by Cornwall, MacNichol, and Fein (1984) in an isolated rod of tiger salamander responding with a univariant hyperpolarization to all three wavelengths shown at top; again, response-versus-intensity functions for seven wavelengths (below) are univariant. (C) Similar data were obtained by Baylor, Nunn, and Schnapf (1987) in isolated macaque cones. The electrical responses (bottom) to the two wavelengths, of which response-versus-intensity functions are shown at top, are practically identical. (D) From the data shown in B, an action spectrum is plotted, based on a fixed criterion response (symbols, right-hand ordinate). The data fit the microspectrophotometric data obtained simultaneously (dotted line) very well (Cornwall et al., 1984).

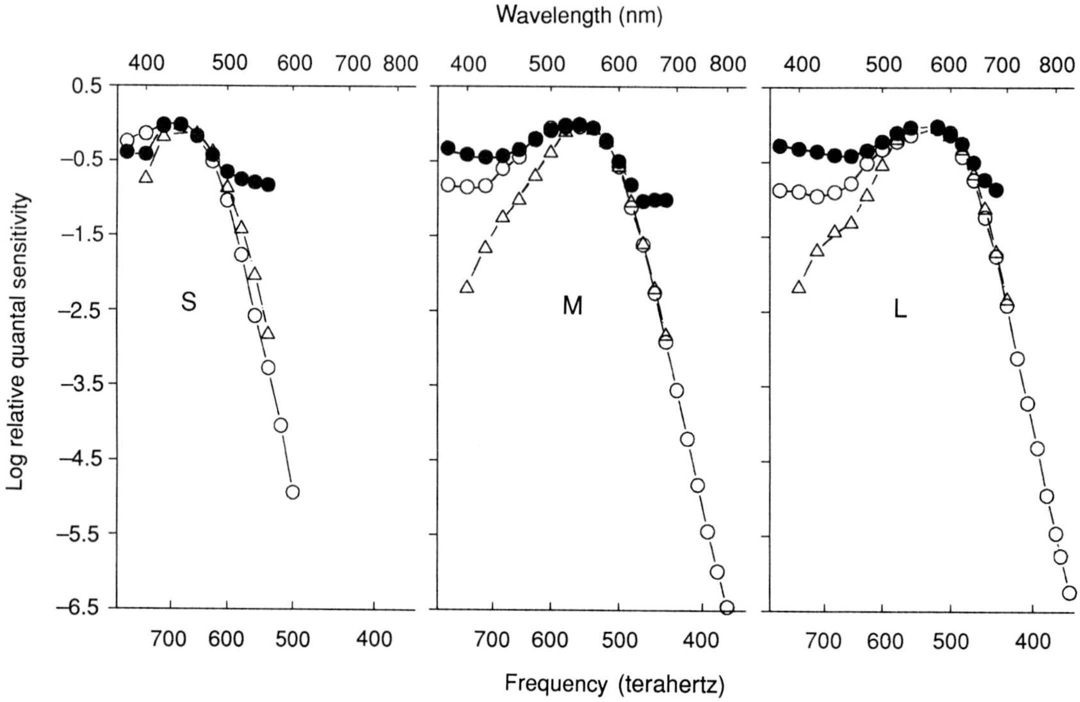

FIG. 7 Spectral sensitivities of the three types of primate cones, S, M, and L, on a linear frequency scale (bottom) and a wavelength scale (top). Three sets of data, obtained with different methods, are shown: microspectrophotometric data from macaque (solid circles, from Harosi, 1987), data from isolated macaque cones (open circles, from Baylor et al., 1987), and data from human psychophysics (triangles, from Smith & Pokorny, 1975).

430, 531, and 561 nm. For comparison, Fig. 7 also shows some representative MSP curves from macaques (Harosi, 1987). The agreement between the two sets of data in the short-wavelength region is not very good. The discrepancy in these data is most likely caused by the fact that the data in Fig. 7 were from different animals, and there is always an uncertainty about proper correction for lens absorption and density of macular pigment in an individual animal. Fig. 7 also illustrates a point made earlier: MSP has a small "dynamic range": density values less than 10% of the peak value are meaningless due to inherent noise (MacNichol, 1986). A remarkable feature of Fig. 7 is the linearity with which the long-wavelength limb of the curve descends over several decades of sensitivity. The action spectra of human cones from a single eye have also been measured in a similar fashion, and the results agree very closely with those from macaques (Schnapf, Kraft & Baylor, 1987).

For comparison, Fig. 7 also includes action spectra of human cones derived from psychophysics (Smith & Pokorny, 1975). These curves describe the spectral sensitivities of M and L cones in the two major types of dichromats whose foveas contain only one of these cone types; the S-cone curve was obtained by calculation from color matching data of trichromats, using the M and L cone results. For M and L cones, the agreement with the single-cone action spectra is good at longer wavelengths. However, there are big deviations at shorter wavelengths. This is common when comparing psychophysics with MSP or with excised receptor preparations: in the former, one is measuring light delivered to the eye and not light reaching the receptor. Ocular media, particularly the lens and macular pigment, selectively absorb the shorter wavelengths and so reduce sensitivity measured at the cornea (Ruddock, 1972; Werner, 1982; Werner, Donnelly & Kliegl, 1987). (The data of Smith and Pokorny are corrected for these factors.) Over the fovea there is an additional wavelength-selective filter, the macular pigment, that can further distort results. These factors also vary greatly among individuals.

C. Variations among Cones

1. Retinal Distribution

It has been known for some time that cones are found throughout the retina but are densely packed in the fovea (Østerberg, 1935). Detailed counts have been made of cone densities across the retinas from several human eyes (Curcio, Sloan, Packer, Hendrickson & Kalina, 1987). Some of these results are shown in Fig. 8. Two interesting features should be noted: first, there is large variation among individuals in foveal densities; second, there are marked asymmetries across the retina. Specifically, the cone density in the nasal hemiretina is greater at any given eccentricity than the temporal retina; there are no marked asymmetries in the superior-inferior meridian. This asymmetry may be the basis for several observations that color vision is usually "better" on the nasal retina; color zones extend further into it (Ferree & Rand, 1919, Uchikawa, Kaiser & Uchikawa, 1982), chromatic contrast sensitivity is higher (Noorlander, Koonderink, Den Ouden & Edens, 1983), and the spectrum locus on a chromaticity diagram is less constricted in this hemiretina (Stabell & Stabell, 1982). Figure 9 shows that S, L and M cones are rather differently distributed over the retina (Marc & Sperling, 1977). The data in Fig. 9 were obtained from a baboon retina; a similar distribution is believed to exist for the human retina, but with the M and L ratios reversed. Human psychophysical data show that there are approximately twice as many L as M cones (Vos & Walraven, 1971; Cicerone & Nerger, 1989), with densities decreasing monotonically from the fovea to the periphery, while S cones are sparse, with a maximum density at 2° eccentricity, as shown by psychophysical methods (Williams, Hayhoe & MacLeod, 1981).

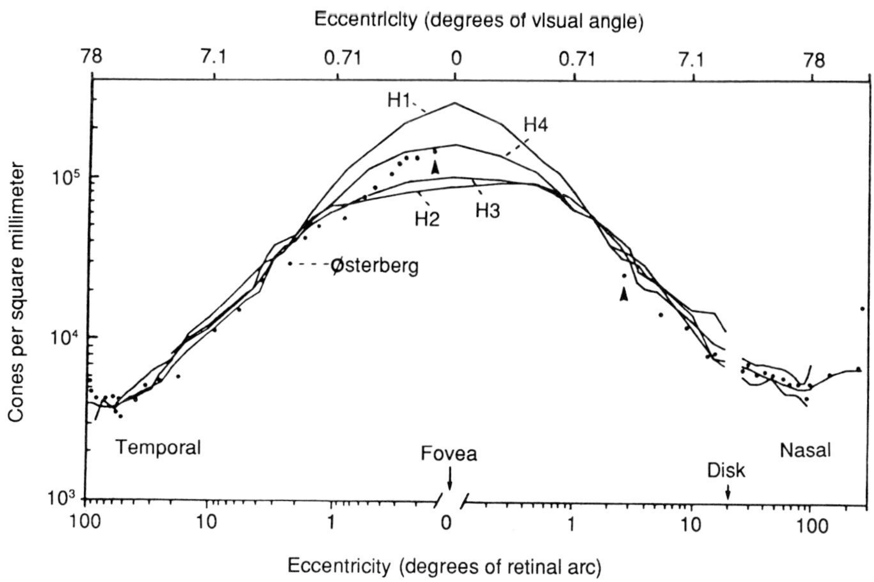

FIG. 8 Retinal distribution of human cone density across the horizontal meridian, obtained in several eyes (H1–H4); the data are compared with Østerberg's (1935) results. From Curcio, Sloan, Packer, Hendrickson, and Kalina (1987). Copyright 1987 by the AAAS.

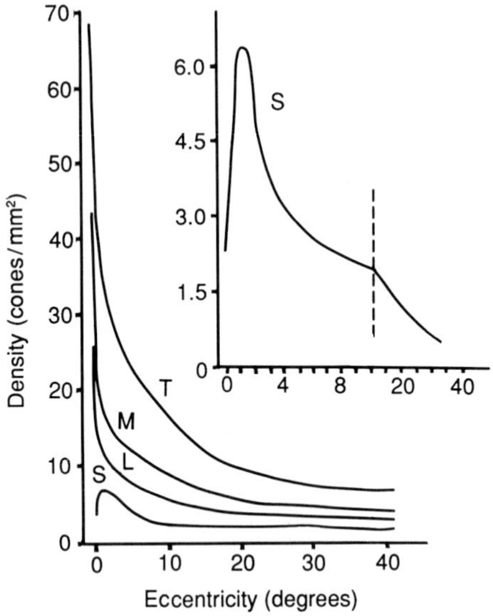

FIG. 9 Density of three classes of baboon cones (L, M, S, respectively, and T = total) isolated by tetrazolium blue, a dye that selectively stains active neurons, so that the populations can be separated by illumination with appropriate wavelengths. The inset shows the S-cone distribution on a magnified scale. From Marc and Sperling (1977). Copyright 1977 by the AAAS.

2. Population Variation

There are significant variations in the color matches made by individuals classified as normal trichromats (Alpern, 1979). These variations are often due to differences in preretinal absorption. However, large differences are still found in data from Rayleigh matches; at these longer wavelengths, the differences in ocular transmission are quite small. This raises the possibility that there may be small but real differences in the photopigments across individuals.

The New World squirrel monkey (*Saimiri sciureus*) provides a very interesting example of polymorphic color vision. From a variety of psychophysical tests (including Rayleigh matches, spectral neutral points, and wavelength discrimination) it has been concluded that male squirrel monkeys are dichromats but that the females are either dichromats or trichromats (Jacobs, 1984, 1987). MSP of squirrel monkey cones, including animals whose color vision had been studied psychophysically, showed that there were individual differences in the cone photopigments (Mollon, Bowmaker & Jacobs, 1984; Bowmaker, Jacobs, Spiegelhalter & Mollon, 1985). All individuals appear to have had the same short-wave cone pigment with λ_{max} at 433 nm. The other possible pigments peaked at 536, 550, or 564 nm; if the individual was a dichromat, the second pigment was any one from this set, whereas trichromatic individuals could have had any pair from this set in addition to S cones (Jacobs, 1987; see also Chapter 4, this volume). From psychophysics, it was possible to predict which pigments would be found by MSP. Given this polymorphism in color vision, the question arises whether a similar variation exists in Old World primates.

Neitz and Jacobs (1986a) collected Rayleigh matches from a large group of color-normal humans (200 individuals) and found that the frequency distribution of the match points of males was bimodal. The distribution from females was unimodal with its peak at the minimum of the male distribution. This sex difference suggests that the variation is linked to the X-chromosome. From calculations based on the ratios of the primaries used in color matching, they concluded that there was individual variation in the λ_{max} of the L cones but not the M cones. Since there were two subpopulations of males, each of which differed from the females, this suggests that there may be three different variants of the L cone photopigment in normal humans.

The genetic basis for these variations among human cones is beginning to be understood. Each photopigment molecule is formed from the vitamin A derivative retinal joined to an opsin. The different opsins shift the pigment spectrum. The genes on the X chromosome that specify cone opsins in humans have been identified (Nathans et al., 1986a,b; Nathans, 1987). Some males have the two genes expected from classical notions about trichromacy. However, most males have either three or four such genes that are able to produce the amino acid sequences found in human opsins. This polymorphism is related to the polymorphism already noted for color matches. Neitz, Neitz, and Jacobs (1987) obtained Rayleigh matches and DNA samples from males in both subpopulations. The samples were analyzed to identify the number of opsin genes carried by each individual. Those with only two X-linked opsin genes could show one form of Rayleigh match or the other. Those with three opsin genes needed somewhat more red in their matches than did those with four genes. It is possible not only that there are real differences among trichromats, but that some "trichromats" may have more than three photopigment types.

D. Identifying Cone Inputs

When responses are recorded from neurons beyond the receptors, it is difficult to pinpoint which cone types provide the input. At the most elementary level, one would like to determine how many cone types contribute to the response without necessarily identifying them. Even this is not simple. Consider a cell that has input from two spectrally different cones, the responses of which are of opposite polarity (opponent cell): All that is certain is that the inputs are from at least two spectral mechanisms that differ in spectral sensitivity. These two inputs need not be from only two individual cone types; each could be a combination of cone responses. If this were the case, it would not be apparent from the spectral responses which cones are involved since an opponent cell signals the difference between two *weighted* spectral inputs. The resulting wavelengths of maximal excitation and inhibition of the cell's response could take on almost any value, depending on the scaling of the inputs relative to each other. In general, however, the cell's excitatory and inhibitory maxima will lie outside the limits of the maxima of the antagonistic inputs.

A popular technique used to identify the receptor inputs is chromatic adaptation (Stiles, 1959; Wald, 1964). An adapting light is chosen such that it affects the response to one of the inputs to a cell far more than the other. That response will be selectively desensitized so that the cell is largely driven by the other input. In this way, the response properties of the cell can now be studied in relative isolation.

Even when using the technique of chromatic adaptation, it is difficult to determine whether the chromatically isolated responses are driven solely by a single cone type. The usual approach has been to show that the action spectrum of the responses remaining after chromatic adaptation either matches the absorption spectrum of one of the cone types in the particular species or conforms to the general form of a photopigment spectrum. Further evidence for a single cone type can be obtained by determining whether the isolated responses are univariant, for example, showing that the curves relating spectral responses and log intensity are parallel. Alternatively, one can show that a given test wavelength can be "silently substituted" for all other wavelengths, provided their intensities have been appropriately adjusted (Estévez & Spekreijse, 1982). Unfortunately, such tests of univariance are insufficient for asserting that responses are driven by a single cone type, as is explained in the next section.

It is not possible to apply, at the level of a single cell, the techniques usually applied to specify the number of different receptor types. As described above, the number of independent primaries that a subject needs to match the appearance of any light is the number of spectrally different receptors in that subject's eye. But for a spectrally opponent cell, two primaries are probably always enough to match its responses to any wavelength. A method that is related to color-matching is based on the assumption that the spectra of the cone types are known. In this case it is possible to calculate values for various mixtures of stimuli that should be equivalent for any cell with the postulated cone inputs. This approach has been used with some success to identify which cones contribute to a cell's response (Abramov, 1968; Derrington, Krauskopf & Lennie, 1984). Note, however, that the validity of this approach depends on accurate knowledge of the cone spectra.

E. Pigments and Pseudopigments

In many cases in which chromatic adaptation is used to isolate an input to a cell, the spectrum of the mechanism does not correspond to the absorptance of any receptor in that species (Abramov, 1972). Figure

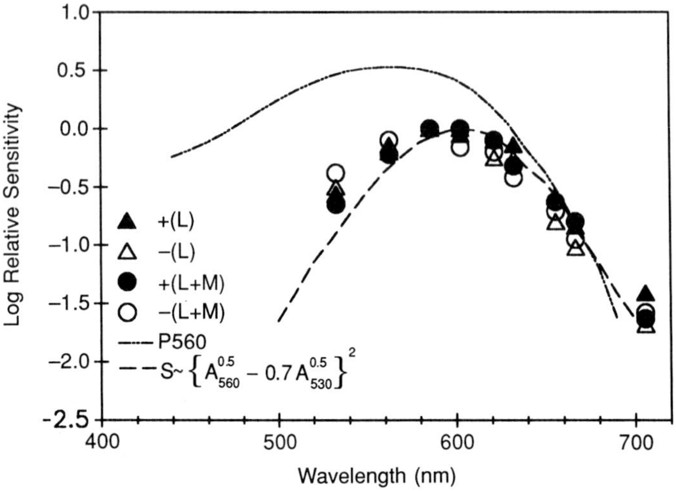

FIG. 10 Symbols represent spectral sensitivity functions from a set of L−M color opponent cells that were chromatically adapted with short-wavelength light in order to isolate L−cone sensitivity (unpublished data of R. L. DeValois; the four symbols correspond to the four types of spectrally opponent cells identified by DeValois et al., 1966). The resulting action spectra are much narrower than the L−cone pigment absorption, derived from a Dartnall nomogram (P560). The data can be described by a function (broken line) constructed from the formula shown, indicating that there is still some opponent input from the M cone (A_{530}) weighted with the factor 0.7. The formula corresponds to the definition of a pseudopigment (Sirovich and Abramov, 1977).

10 shows the spectrum of long-wavelength mechanisms from different types of opponent cell in the macaque LGN, which clearly disagree with the spectrum of the L cones; the spectrum of the isolated mechanism is too narrow and is shifted too far into the long-wavelength end of the spectrum.

As Sirovich and Abramov (1977) demonstrated, univariance is necessary if all the responses are functions of the same photopigment, but it is not sufficient to identify that condition. When responses are driven by only one receptor type, as Eq. (1) shows, the response is a function of stimulus intensity scaled by the absorption spectrum of the photopigment. But the isolated mechanism can also behave as if only one photopigment were involved, when in fact the cell's responses are a function of a combination of inputs from several different cone types.

The narrowing of the spectral response shown in Fig. 10 stems from some remaining opponent M cone input that could not completely be eliminated by chromatic adaptation. This is indicated by fitting the data points with a function that is represented by the equation given in Fig. 10. The validity of action spectra attributed to a single receptor mechanism depends very much on the wavelength composition and strength of the light used for chromatic adaptation. Since the spectral sensitivities of cone mechanisms overlap and since cones cannot be saturated easily by light (see Chapter 5, this volume), isolation of an individual cone mechanism usually is not possible through the entire range of the visible spectrum.

In summary, the mosaic of primate cone photoreceptors contains three populations which differ in their spectral sensitivity, density, and retinal distribution, so that essentially three different neuronal images of the outer physical world are created by postreceptoral neurons for further processing. At the level of ganglion cells, the information from the 6 million cone photoreceptors has to be compressed so that the central 100,000 ganglion cell axons can forward it to the LGN and visual cortex.

IV. NEUROPHYSIOLOGICAL MECHANISMS OF COLOR OPPONENCY IN RETINAL GANGLION CELLS

In primates, the retinal neurons directly connected with photoreceptors, bipolar cells and horizontal cells, show no sign of opponent interaction between spectrally different cones. Horizontal and bipolar cells are, however, instrumental in establishing the receptive fields of color-opponent neurons. Horizontal cells contribute to the spatial organization of the receptive fields of these neurons, while bipolar cells are responsible for the formation of the ON- and OFF-pathways described in Chapter 6. Color opponency in its strict sense is first observed in the ganglion cells of the primate retina (Wiesel & Hubel, 1966).

Several groups of ganglion cells can be distinguished in the primate retina. A full account is given in Chapter 6 of this volume. The two main pathways shall be mentioned here briefly: (a) a group with large cell bodies, fast conduction-velocity, large dendritic and receptive field size, and short transient (phasic) responses that project mainly to the magnocellular layers of the LGN; and (b) a group of smaller ganglion cells with slower conduction velocity, smaller dendritic and receptive field sizes, sustained (tonic) responses, in cat also called X–cells, that project to the parvocellular layer of the LGN. These latter cells form the most important retinal substrate for opponent-color processing.

These parallel pathways, called Y and X in the cat and M and P in the monkey, are further discussed in relation to cortical neurons in Section V of this chapter. The organization of color information by the retinal ganglion cells is presented here.

A. Organization of Color-Opponent Ganglion Cells

By means of glass micropipettes, electrical responses can be recorded directly from ganglion cells (for methods, see Zrenner, 1983b). Figure 11a shows a simplified circuit that links the photoreceptors to a color-opponent ganglion cell. When red light (solid bars) is projected onto the cell's receptive field, L cones (black spots) excite the cell through its center, so that it responds with a tonic, sustained discharge during the entire period of stimulation. When the red light is turned off, the cell is silent. Illumination by green light (dotted bar) produces the reverse result, that is, M cones inhibit the cell via the receptive field surround. When the green light is turned off, the cell's activity is high; an OFF-discharge is observed. Consequently, the cell's responses to red and green lights are almost 180° out of phase. In this example the L cones in the center of the receptive field cause excitation of the ganglion cell in response to *increments* of red light, and are called ON-center cells. Cells that are excited by *decrements* of red lights are called OFF-center cells. The reverse spatial organization of L and M cones occurs as well.

Light of a wavelength lying between the middle and long wave parts of the spectrum stimulates both center and surround about equally and does not produce a modulated response (e.g., yellow in the cell shown in Fig. 11a, dotted/solid bar). In this case, inhibition and excitation mutually cancel each other. The cell shows only a relatively weak, continuous discharge. The spectral region between the absorption maxima of the two cone types, in psychophysical terms, represents the neutral point of a cell. This spectral antagonism, when a cell is excited by one part of the visible spectrum and inhibited by another, is called color opponency. Color opponency implies that the mutual antagonism between two spectrally different cone mechanisms is strongest for spectral regions where the different cone types involved are both stimulated simultaneously. In the L–M opponent cell shown in Fig. 11a this would be the yellow region in the spectrum, in S–L or S–M opponent cells, the blue–green region.

Excitation and inhibition act not only through spectrally different cone mechanisms, but the receptive field of a color-opponent ganglion cell is also spatially organized as an antagonistic center–surround structure. Excitation and inhibition therefore depend on the locus of stimulation as first shown in limulus by Hartline (1949), in mammalian eye for spectrally nonopponent neurons by Kuffler (1953), and in color-opponent ganglion cells of rhesus monkey retina by DeValois (1965), Wiesel and Hubel (1966) and DeValois, Abramov and Jacobs (1966).

B. Various Types of Color-Opponent Cells

Color-opponent ganglion cells can be classified on the basis of their spectral and spatial properties. Fig-

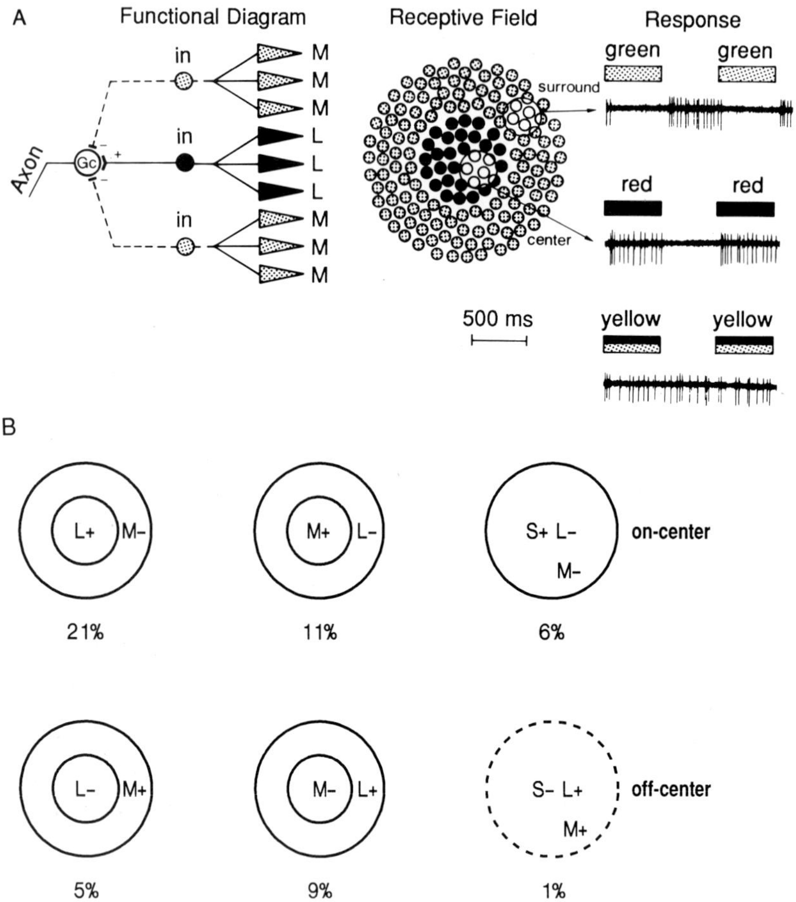

FIG. 11 (A) Simplified functional diagram showing receptive field structure and responses of a color-opponent ganglion cell. In this cell, the L cones in the center act excitatorily (+), and the M cones in the surround act inhibitorily (−). Yellow light, which stimulates both L and M cones, produces no modulated response since excitation and inhibition cancel each other. The number of receptors (dotted and filled circles) is arbitrary. (B) Spatial structure and frequency of incidence of the six most common varieties of color-opponent ganglion cells. From Zrenner (1983a).

ure 11b illustrates the most common receptive field structures in macaques, with their percentage of occurrence indicated. The remaining 48% are not color-opponent cells. There are several additional *rare* trichromatic types of ganglion cells (De Monasterio, Gouras & Tolhurst, 1975).

The most common type of ganglion cell (21% in the macaque sample shown here) has a receptive field where the L cones form an excitatory center with inhibitory M cones in the surround ($L^{+}-M^{-}$). The second most common type of cell (10%) is characterized by excitatory M cones in the center and inhibitory L cones in the surround ($M^{+}-L^{-}$). Cells with an S cone input are rare (only 6%), and those which *inhibit* a ganglion cell are especially rare (0.3–3%) according to several studies (Malpeli & Schiller, 1978; Zrenner & Gouras, 1980, 1981; Creutzfeldt et al., 1979; Valberg, Lee & Tigwell, 1986). Cells that are inhibited by M and L cones through the center of the receptive field are more frequent (9 and 5%, respectively).

It is difficult to judge whether L or M cones form the antagonistic mechanism of ganglion cells with S-cone input. The data derived from spectral sensitivity measurements suggest that both L- and M-cone mechanisms act synergistically in these cells to antagonize S-cone inputs (De Monasterio et al., 1975). Often, however, chromatic adaptation does not reveal more than one antagonistic cone mechanism in S-cone driven ganglion cells.

OFF-center neurons are generally less common than ON-center neurons: their ratio is about 2:3

(Gouras & Zrenner, 1981). All these cell types can be found side by side in the retina. In a single penetration, the electrode often makes contact with two, three, or four different types of ganglion cells in sequence. However, their distribution across the retina changes regularly with eccentricity.

C. Determination of Cone Inputs to Opponent Cells

Chromatic adaptation can be used to identify the receptors that have input to a certain ganglion cell with careful consideration to limitations described in Section III,E. Figure 12 shows spectral sensitivity functions of three populations of retinal ganglion cells; sensitivity is based on a constant threshold criterion, namely, the reciprocal of the number of quanta per second per square micrometer necessary to evoke a fixed change in impulse rate at the various wavelengths (usually 40 spikes per second). If the pigments of the L and the S cones are bleached strongly with light containing short and long wavelengths (μ, representing the wavelength composition of the background), one cell population reveals input from the M cones (circles) with a sensitivity maximum at 535 nm; if the pigments of the M and L cones are bleached by a strong orange–red adapting light, a second cell population is revealed with input from the S cones (triangles), and a sensitivity maximum is observed at 440 nm. These data agree reasonably well with the corrected microspectrophotometric data of Bowmaker, Dartnall, and Mollon (1980) over a rather large part of the visible spectrum (solid lines). If strong, steady short-wavelength adapting lights are used, the L-cone mechanism is revealed in another cell population (squares) with a maximum at 567 nm. Since the goal is not to determine the shape of a photopigment but only to distinguish L, M, and S cones from one another, this technique is sufficient to identify the cone mechanisms that have input to a color-opponent ganglion cell. The spectral identification of the cone mechanisms involved is indispensible for understanding the underlying retinal circuitry.

D. Spectral Sensitivity of Color-Opponent Cells

Figure 13 shows the spectral sensitivity functions of the various color-opponent cell types in the presence of a white adapting light, demonstrating how the cones interact in normal daylight. Sensitivity is based

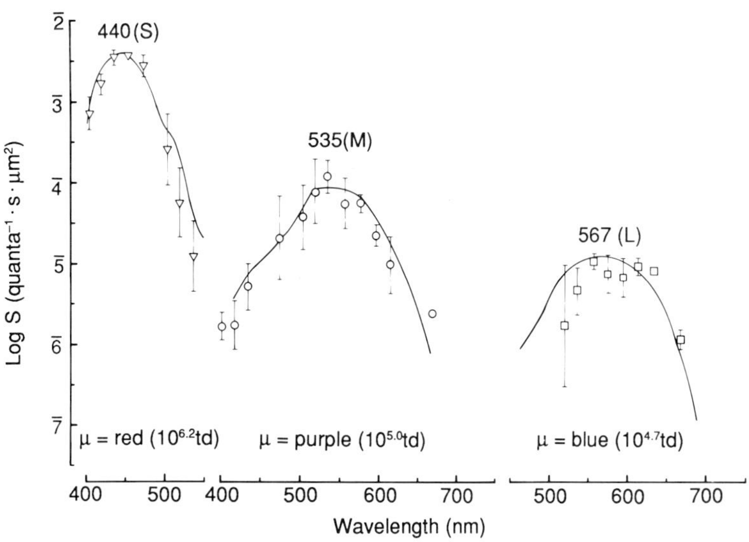

FIG. 12 Action spectra of three populations of retinal ganglion cells of rhesus monkey based on a constant response criterion for monochromatic wavelengths (stimulus size 15°, duration 200 msec). Isolated by the appropriate background illumination, indicated below each function, three spectrally different cone mechanisms are revealed (n = 3 cells, means ± standard deviations are shown). The functions are compared with the pigment absorption spectra (solid lines) of Bowmaker, Dartnall, and Mollon (1980), obtained by microspectrophotometry in macaque photoreceptors, with λ_{max} values indicated above each function. From Wienrich and Zrenner (1981).

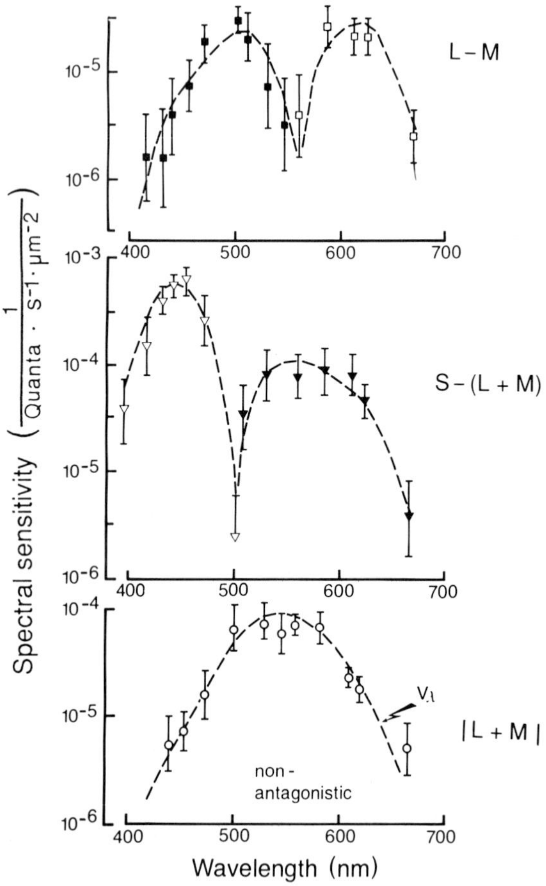

FIG. 13 Action spectra of eight L–M opponent cells (squares), three S–(L + M) opponent cells (triangles), and three nonantagonistic tonic ganglion cells (circles), recorded in the presence of a bright white Ganzfeld background (means ± one standard deviation are indicated). Open symbols indicate sensitivity based on thresholds for excitatory responses, that is, just detectable increase of spike frequency increments in response to increments of the irradiance of the test flashes (15° in diameter). Closed symbols indicate sensitivity based on threshold for inhibitory responses, that is, just detectable decrease of spike frequency in response to increments of irradiance. Dashed lines represent the results of a linear subtraction of L and M cones (top) or S and (L + M) cones (center) or the V_λ (daylight luminosity) function (bottom). From Zrenner (1983a).

on a constant threshold criterion. At each wavelength, the irradiance (quanta sec^{-1} μm^{-2}) was determined that produced either a certain impulse increment for ON-responses (open symbols, representing excitation) or an impulse decrement for OFF-responses (closed symbols, representing inhibition). The reciprocal of this value was plotted as sensitivity on the ordinate. L^+-M^- opponent cells (top) with overt opponency have a sensitivity maximum near 610 nm for excitatory responses, a second peak at 500 nm for inhibitory responses, and a neutral point at 565 nm. The bandwidth of each spectral branch is smaller than an individual cone function (cf. Fig. 12); however, it can be described quite well by a linear subtraction of the L and M functions of Fig. 12 as indicated by the dashed lines derived from the functions given by Bowmaker et al. (1980). The second type of L–M opponent cells (not shown here) is very similar in spectral sensitivity except that the M cones mediate excitation, whereas L cones provide inhibition. Such cells are often called "red–green opponent" cells.

There is another distinct cell type, usually excited maximally near 440 nm and inhibited maximally near 560 nm (or vice versa), as shown in the center of Fig. 13. Its spectral sensitivity is described by calculating the difference between the S function and the additive combination of the L and M functions as shown by dashed lines in the center of Fig. 13. Such cells are therefore often called "blue–yellow" opponent.

These color-opponent cells respond *qualitatively* differently in the several spectral regions and are therefore not well suited for signaling the brightness of two spectrally different stimuli. There is, however, a third cell type, constituting about 20% of tonic cells, which responds in a non-color-antagonistic manner, either with excitation or inhibition. Its sensitivity closely follows the photopic (daylight) luminosity function V_λ (Fig. 13, bottom). This cell type is well suited to code brightness or darkness and has a spectral sensitivity function similar to that of the phasic ganglion cells. However, the latter have the highest incidence in the retinal periphery (Zrenner, 1983b, p. 42), and respond to all luminance changes of any wavelength with a short monotonic transient discharge. Therefore, one may assume that phasic cells serve as luminance difference detectors for signaling new events in the retinal periphery. The fovea can then be directed toward these events for closer analysis. Other such correlations between neurophysiology and psychophysics are discussed in Section V.

E. L–M Opponent versus S–(L + M) Opponent Cells

As mentioned above, either L versus M cones or S versus L + M cones build up the main types of color-opponent cells. S–(L + M) opponent cells have large receptive fields (0.35 to 2.0°) with excitatory zones covering about the same area as the inhibitory zones. L–M opponent cells are concentrically structured with center diameters of 0.08° to 0.25°, that is, receptive fields are smaller and show a clear spatial antagonism. Due to the large coextensive field size, the spatial resolution of the S-cone system is rather poor, as was also demonstrated in blue cone monochromatic human observers (Zrenner, Magnussen & Lorenz, 1988). L–M and S–(L + M) antagonistic cells have clear differences also in the time course of their responses. In Fig. 14, the first impulse in a S–(L + M) driven cell is delayed longer (for about 30 msec) than that of an L–M cone driven ganglion cell. Furthermore, it should be noted that the response duration of S-cone driven cells is considerably longer than that of the 500 msec test flash. There is a delay of 100–200 msec after the offset of a stimulus before the spike frequency of the S-cone driven cell returns to the original level. This is similar to the "aftereffect" of rods (Steinberg, 1969). The return becomes slower as the strength of stimulation increases. In contrast, excita-

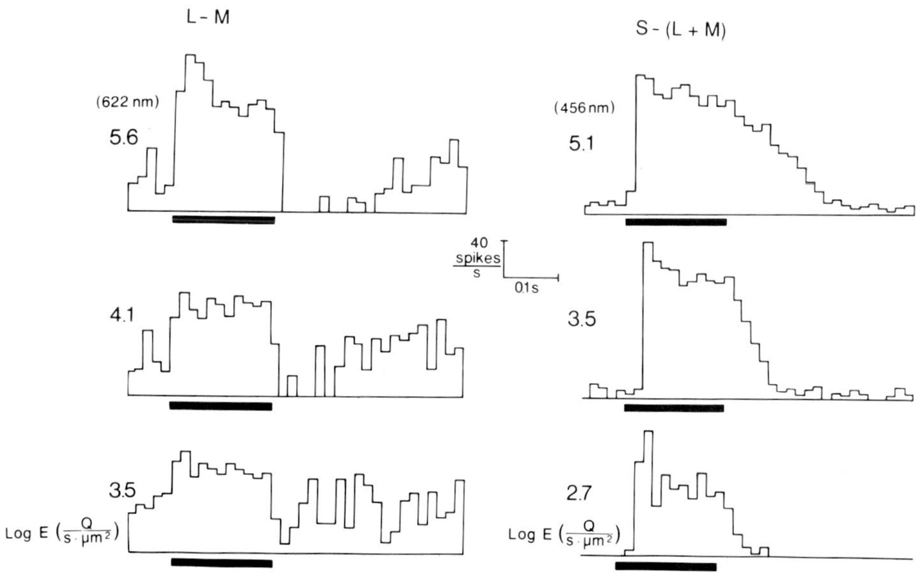

FIG. 14 Response profiles (histograms showing impulses/sec versus time) of cells with L–cone (left) and S-cone driven (right) center mechanisms. In order to isolate the center mechanism, a short-wavelength background was applied to the L–M and a yellow background was applied to the S–(L + M) cell. The irradiance *E* of the test flash (quanta sec^{-1} μ^{-2}) is indicated beside each record. Black bars symbolize the test flash duration. Note the differences in the time course of L and S driven center mechanisms. Modified from Zrenner and Gouras (1981).

tion in L–M opponent cells ends abruptly with the termination of the test flash. Moreover, in S-cone driven ganglion cells, no inhibitory (impulse-free) phase after the offset of the test light can be observed.

These two features of S-cone driven cells, the long latency at the onset and the lack of inhibition at the offset of light, apparently limit their their temporal resolution. This observation is supported by experiments (Zrenner & Gouras, 1981) revealing a low maximal flicker fusion frequency of 35 cycles per second (Hz) in S-cone driven ganglion cells, while L and M driven cells reach a much higher flicker fusion frequency of 60–70 Hz, that is, they can resolve a rapid sequence of stimuli much more easily. Thus, in many respects, the S-cone system is more similar to the rod system than to the M- and L-cone systems. This nicely parallels psychophysical findings on S-cone temporal resolution, established by Brindley, Du Croz, and Rushton (1966).

F. Variations in Color Opponency That Can Enhance Wavelength Discrimination

Interestingly, the neutral point of color-opponent cells where inhibition and excitation cancel each other can vary considerably, depending on the balance of strength of the two cone mechanisms involved. Variable spatial stimuli such as spots and slits can cause either the center or surround mechanism to dominate, thereby favoring one of the cone mechanisms (Wiesel & Hubel, 1966; Gouras, 1968; De Monasterio & Gouras, 1975). Temporal variables can cause phase shifts between the responses of cone mechanisms and thereby change their interaction from antagonistic to synergistic (Zrenner & Gouras, 1978; Gouras & Zrenner, 1979; Zrenner, 1983a,b). As explained below, there are also intrinsic variations within a certain functional category of color-opponent ganglion cells that are not dependent on the mode of stimulation.

The two cone mechanisms involved in antagonistic interactions are not equally strong in each cell; one of them usually dominates. This is demonstrated by the variation of neutral points in the action spectrum of

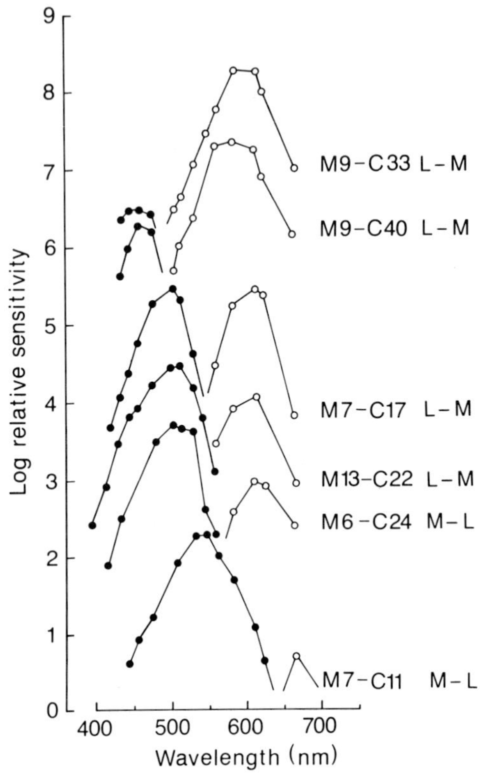

FIG. 15 Action spectra of six L–M opponent cells, recorded under identical conditions (white background, 20,000 td Ganzfeld stimuli of 200 msec duration). Note the intrinsic variation of the neutral point from 480 to 630 nm. The action of L cones is indicated by open symbols, that of M cones by filled symbols. Action spectra are shifted arbitrarily along the *Y*-axis for comparison. Adapted from Zrenner (1983a).

such cells (Fig. 15) based on threshold response criteria. The L-cone mechanism (open symbols) strongly dominates in the uppermost cell's action spectrum, while M cones (closed symbols) provide only little inhibition in the short-wavelength part of the spectrum. The strength of the L and the M mechanism is about balanced in the cell's spectrum shown in the center of Fig. 15. In contrast, the M-cone mechanism strongly dominates in the lowermost spectrum. Figure 15 demonstrates that there is an almost continuous gradation in color opponency concerning the weight of the opponent mechanisms involved so that in L–M opponent cells, under identical stimulus conditions, the neutral point can vary from 630 to 480 nm. A similar range was found for LGN cells by DeValois, Abramov and Jacobs (1966).

At low luminance levels and with sinusoidal modulation around the white point, Derrington et al. (1984) found smaller variations of the relative contribution of L and M cones to color-opponent cells. The variation of cone contributions to color-opponent cells increases considerably at higher photopic levels and when increment threshold techniques are employed, as shown in Fig. 15. In cells which receive input from S cones, the strength of color-opponency does not vary to the same extent. The spectral sensitivity functions of all ganglion cells having input from S cones are strikingly similar in shape and absolute sensitivity despite their different retinal locations.

If one considers the L–M opponent cells as a singular heterogeneous system, a graded degree of opponency emerges. Could such an arrangement improve the visual system's abilities? Since the number of spectrally different analyzers is greatly enhanced by such a graded scale of color-opponent cells, the heterogeneity of L–M color-opponent cells provides a greater range of responsiveness to different chromatic borders within each area of the retina, as outlined by Zrenner (1983b). Many chromatic borders excite the cell equally and therefore produce no response gradient when moved through the cell's receptive field. However, there is a small fraction of cells whose neutral point lies *between* the spectral loci of the two colors forming the chromatic border. These cells and only these cells can respond maximally by changing from excitation to inhibition or vice versa. For instance, two colors with close spectral loci (e.g., 630 and 640 nm) would have little effect on most cell types in Fig. 15. One cell type (lowermost in Fig. 15), however, has its neutral point between the two spectral loci and would respond with a reversal of polarity. If both wavelengths were presented successively to its receptive field, the cell would signal this small difference in wavelength strongly as a polarity reversal.

Since the neutral points of the various types of L–M cells are spread continuously throughout the visible spectrum, there is always a cell which is reversed in polarity by successive color contrast (even if differences in spectral composition are small) and thereby provides a strong neuronal signal. Therefore, the heterogeneity of the L–M opponent tonic system can greatly enhance the visual system's capacity to discriminate a large variety of chromatic borders within each part of the visual field, but particularly in the fovea, where cone dominance values are most evenly distributed (Zrenner, 1983b; Zrenner & Gouras, 1983).

G. Temporal Variables in Color-Opponent Cells

It is often suggested in the literature that opponent cells with a two-peaked spectral sensitivity function constitute a color channel, while cells with a single-peaked broadband spectrum constitute an achromatic ("brightness") channel. However, this distinction is not exclusive as under certain circumstances color-opponent cells act as brightness detectors as well. (Abramov, 1972; DeValois and DeValois, 1975).

Color-opponent cells change their action spectra with temporal frequency of stimulation (Gouras & Zrenner, 1979; Zrenner, 1983b). This is shown in Fig. 16 (lower half, triangles). At low flicker frequencies (5 Hz, triangles), L–M color-opponent cells have two sensitivity maxima, one for excitation and one for inhibition, separated by a neutral point near 560 nm. At higher flicker frequencies (33 Hz, crosses), the wavelength of the neutral zone becomes most effective, and the spectral dichotomy and color opponency are lost. The spectral sensitivity function becomes broadband and single-peaked and resembles that of a luminance detecting cell.

This spectral transition was seen by Zrenner and Gouras (1978) and Gouras and Zrenner (1979) in all 21 macaque cells they studied with low and high frequencies. This abrupt change in sensitivity, caused by a phase shift between the center and surround responses, is shown in Fig. 16, top (Gouras & Zrenner, 1979; Zrenner, 1983b, Ch. 5). At low frequencies (5 Hz), the excitation provided by the center (622 nm

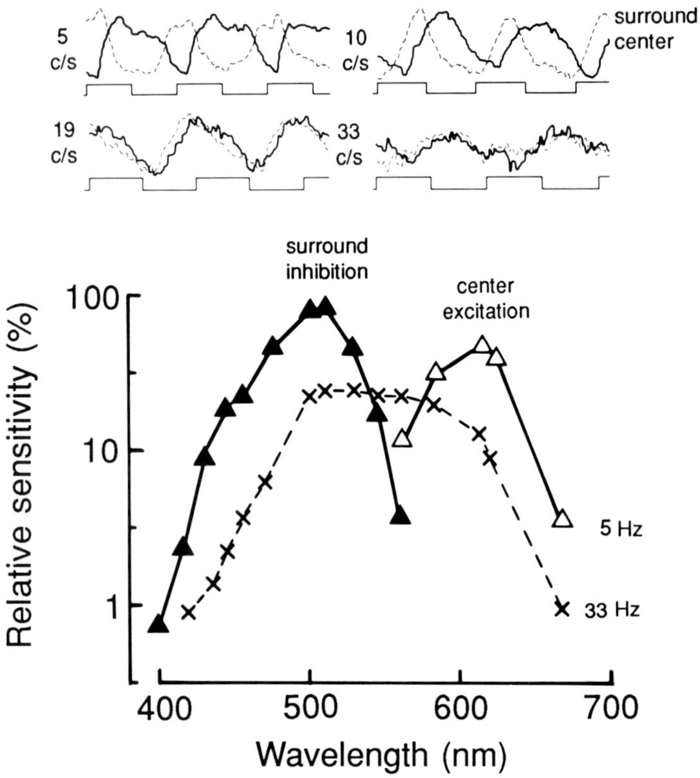

FIG. 16 Action spectrum of an L–M opponent ganglion cell, based on a flicker threshold criterion at low (5 Hz) and at high (33 Hz) frequencies of stimulation in the presence of a white adapting light of 30,000 td. The cell loses color opponency at higher flicker frequencies owing to a phase shift between center and surround (shown at top). (See Zrenner & Gouras, 1978; Gouras & Zrenner, 1979.)

stimulus, solid line) and the inhibition provided by the surround (456 nm stimulus, dashed line) are almost 180° out of phase; the sum of both responses is therefore zero at low frequencies, and the cell shows no modulated response to light. At higher frequencies a latency change occurs, which is different for the center and surround, so that the phases of inhibition and excitation slowly synchronize (10 and 19 Hz in Fig. 16). Near 29 Hz this synchronization is almost perfect, and the sum of the two responses results in a very strong flicker response, especially for wavelengths that stimulate center and surround equally. Since center and surround respond in the same manner under such conditions, both their spatial and their color opponency is lost.

At higher frequencies, spectral sensitivity functions of color-opponent cells are single-peaked and broadband. This might explain why the photopic luminosity (V_λ) function obtained by flicker photometry is such a simple, stable, and single-peaked curve. However, it also suggests that the V_λ function is a rather artificial function, not reflecting trichromatic spectral sensitivity under normal, that is, *nonflickering*, daylight conditions. If the daylight spectral sensitivity function is measured in the presence of a white background with single flashes of long duration, a three-peaked function emerges (Sperling & Harwerth, 1971; King-Smith & Carden, 1976; Zrenner, 1977; Zrenner & Krüger, 1981); an example is shown in Fig 17.

The determination of sensitivity (based on the increment threshold criterion) for 26 monochromatic wavelengths in human observers reveals a function with three peaks (Fig. 17, left) if the flicker frequency is low (1 Hz) but a single-peaked function if the repe-

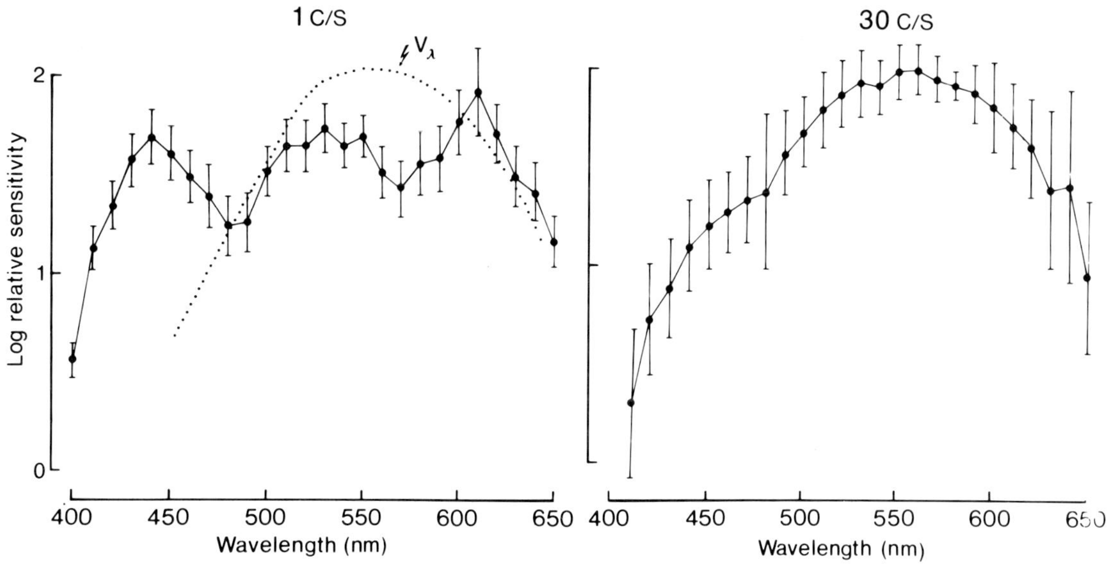

FIG. 17 Psychophysical relative sensitivity, shown on the left, in man, determined by single light flashes of long duration (1 Hz) and by flicker detection (30 Hz). Sensitivity does not follow the V_λ function. From Zrenner and Krüger (1981).

tition rate is high (Fig. 17, right). Without doubt, the function on the left is created by L−M and S−(L + M) color-opponent cells, with sensitivity dips near 560 and 490 nm, similar to those observed in monkey (Fig. 13). However, the action of opponent mechanisms can no longer be observed if the repetition rate is increased (Fig. 17, right), similar to the findings in the macaque visual system (Fig. 16). The spectral sensitivity then approaches the V_λ function, which is also based on a flicker criterion. The cell type best suited to carry information with a V_λ characteristic is the magnocellular, nonopponent (phasic) type, but under certain spatial, temporal, and spectral conditions the parvocellular (tonic) system can take over this task.

Apparently, The V_λ function requires that center and surround excitation of color-opponent cells be synchronized. This synchronization is achieved not only by fast flickering stimuli but also by flashes of short duration. If a light is switched on and immediately switched off again, the ON- and OFF-discharges occur quasi-simultaneously (Zrenner, 1983b). Consequently, it becomes much more difficult to judge the color of flashes of short duration.

H. Special Interaction of S Cones with Other Cones

There are several examples in which the sensitivity of S cones is controlled by L and M cones, as shown in Figs. 4 and 5. Another such interaction is demonstrated by the phenomenon of transient tritanopia (see Stiles, 1959; Das, 1964; Mollon & Polden, 1977; Polden & Mollon, 1980; Pugh & Mollon, 1979). Transient blindness for blue test lights ("tritanopia") is observed in the first few hundred milliseconds after the offset of strong yellow adaptation lights although the S cones are not stimulated by the yellow adapting light. Pugh and Mollon (1979) hypothesized that L (and/or M) cones that are modulated by the yellow adapting light control the sensitivity of S cones.

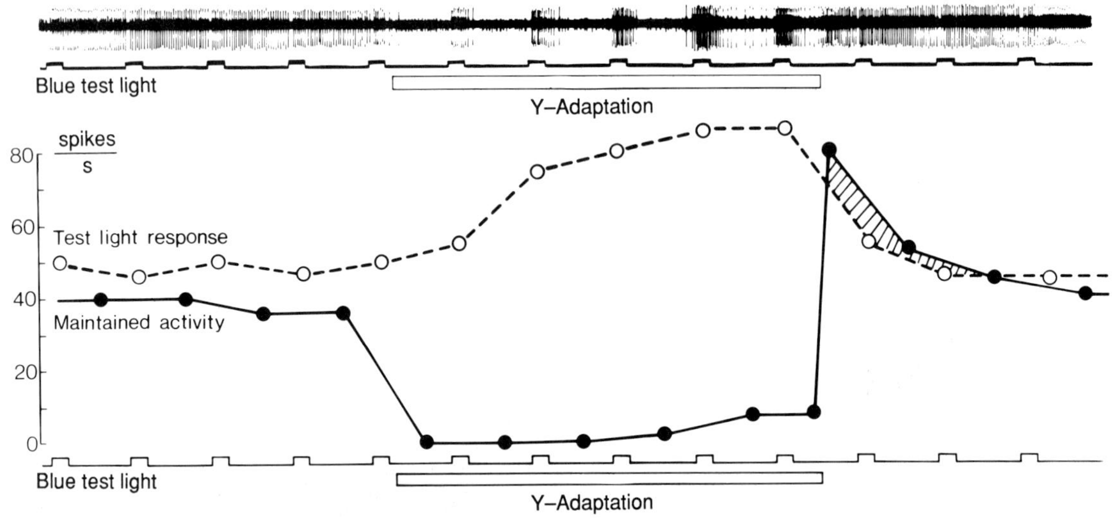

FIG. 18 The response of a blue-sensitive ganglion cell (spikes per second) during the presentation of a blue test light (open circles) is separated from the resting activity (filled symbols show activity *between* the test light presentations). Both functions show a characteristic behavior when a yellow adapting light, μ (open bar), is presented (retinal illumination of 30,000 td). The hatched area indicates the period during which the continuous activity surpasses the response to the test light. This phase indicates relative response decrements. From Zrenner and Gouras (1981).

An example of such sensitivity control is shown in Fig. 18, which is based on recordings from S-cone driven retinal cells (Zrenner & Gouras, 1981). When test pulses (456 nm) of 200 ms duration were presented at 1 sec intervals, the cell responded only with a small increase in impulse frequency, imposed on a high spontaneous discharge rate. When yellow light (30,000 td) was switched on for about 6 sec (open bars), the cell's spontaneous activity was strongly inhibited, apparently through the action of longer wavelength sensitive cones on which yellow light acts exclusively. After some seconds of yellow adaptation, the spike frequency evoked by the blue test lights increased from about 50 to 80 spikes/sec (Fig. 18, open circles). This appears paradoxical, since the sensitization of the cell is caused by *light* adaptation which usually desensitizes the cell. At the offset of the yellow light, an OFF-discharge of such strength occurs that the test stimulus can produce no further increase in spike frequency, since the continuous activity surpassed the test light response (hatched area, indicating relative response decrements). This resembles a paradoxical desensitization of the cell during the first seconds of dark adaptation, probably an electrophysiological correlate of Mollon and Polden's (1977) psychophysically determined "transient tritanopia." A neurophysiological model that can explain this psychophysical threshold phenomenon was brought forward by Zrenner (1983b). It was linked to psychophysics by Ejima and Takahashi's (1985) observations on the yellow–blue cancellation code (see Figs. 4 and 5). Interestingly, psychophysical studies show a similar interaction between L and M cones as well, albeit much less pronounced (Reeves, 1981).

The physiological observations outlined in this chapter demonstrate that chromatic processing and thereby color appearence strongly depend on temporal variables; the illusion of the Fechner–Benham top is a good perceptual example. The experiments on single ganglion cells of monkey illustrate that information on color is carried in the visual system usually at the expense of temporal as well as spatial information. A direct correlation between a color space used in psychophysical experiments and color-opponent ganglion cells is very difficult. Nevertheless in the next section a first step toward such an integration is attempted.

V. DETECTION OF LIGHT AND DISCRIMINATION OF COLOR

In relating physiological responses to psychophysical data, it is important to differentiate between various stimulus conditions. For example, the detection of light increments on a dark or a steady white background is based on cell types different from those that are responsible for the representation of light decrements. Different types of cells may thus mediate perception under different stimulus conditions.

A. Threshold Measurements on a White Background

For comparison of cell sensitivity with a psychophysical threshold task, an experiment will be described where chromatic spots of increasing luminance were presented on a steady white background. The fact that sensitivity functions to such spots peak at several wavelengths (see Fig. 17) has been used to infer the existence of chromatic channels in the human visual system (Sperling & Harwerth, 1971; King-Smith & Carden, 1976; Mullen, 1987). Responses to such a series, typical of those obtained from cone-opponent parvocellular and non-opponent magnocellular neurons of the macaque monkey, are shown in the histograms of Figs. 19 and 20. Fig 19A shows response histograms of a blue ON–center cell with S–L cone input to a 4° stimulus, of a M–L cone driven green ON–center cell and of a M–L cone driven red OFF–center cell. With increasing luminance, responses increase, approach saturation, and then decrease. Figures 20A,B display similar histograms for ON- and OFF-center magnocellular units, respectively. The transient responses of these cells contrast with the sustained cell discharge of the parvocellular unit shown in Fig. 19A.

In Figs. 19B and 20C,D, symbols represent the mean firing rates, plotted as a function of luminance contrast. For cells shown in Fig. 19B contrast threshold (indicated by horizontal dashed lines) depends on wavelength, with the highest incremental sensitivity occurring for short-wavelength stimuli. The S–L ON-center cell is almost 1 log unit more sensitive at about 460 nm than the M–L ON-center cell, which is again about 1 log unit more sensitive than the M–L OFF-center cell. Obviously, the activity of the OFF-center cells is so strongly suppressed (Zrenner, 1983a) by the white background that a much stronger stimulus is necessary to activate them.

For the magnocellular neurons in Fig. 20, contrast sensitivity depends on luminance contrast, not on wavelength. This would be expected if the cell's spectral sensitivity is similar to the human photopic luminosity function V_λ. These cells have been shown to have all the requirements for a physiological mechanism to mediate flicker photometry (Lee, Martin & Valberg, 1988).

B. Modelling Cell Responses

The solid curves in Fig. 19B were obtained with a mathematical model that simulates a cell's response, N, assuming that the cone inputs to the cell each follow a saturating function as luminance increases, and that spectral opponency is due to differences of signals from two different cone mechanisms. A cone mechanism is a spatially integrated pool of cone input over the cell's receptive field (center and surround):

$$N = A_L V_L + A_M V_M + A_S V_S + f_0 \qquad (2)$$

where

$$V_i = S_i^{0.7}/(S_i^{0.7} + \sigma_i^{0.7}),\ i = \text{L, M, S} \qquad (3)$$

S_i is the relative absorption by the receptors. The constant σ is the absorption giving a half-maximum response and is thus a measure of sensitivity, and V is the normalized response of a receptor mechanism.

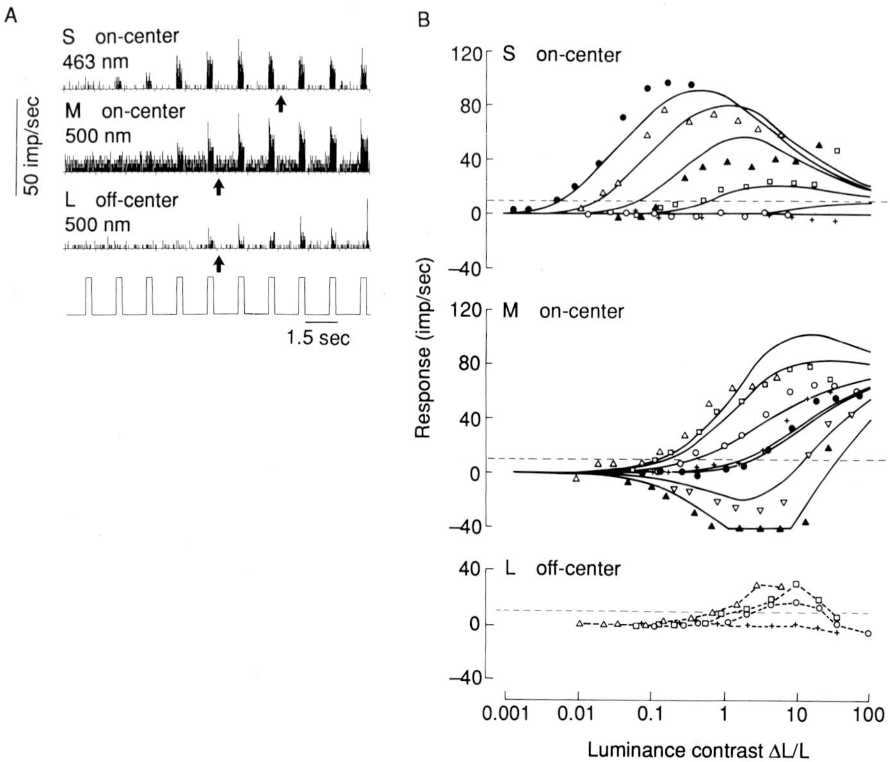

FIG. 19 (A) Histograms of luminance-increment responses of a sustained parvocellular S–L cell with S-cone driven ON-center, an M–L cell with M-cone driven ON-center and an M–L cell, with L-cone driven OFF-center to a 4° spot of 300 msec duration superimposed on a steady white, 110 cd/m² background. In each run, 10 stimuli were presented, increasing in luminance in 0.3 log unit steps. Arrows indicate identical luminance contrasts of $\Delta L/L = 1$. For the M–L OFF-center cell, ON-responses gradually change to OFF-responses as luminance contrast increases. (B) Sustained responses plotted as a function of luminance contrast for the same three types of cells as in A (maintained activity subtracted). The threshold is highly dependent on the wavelength of the stimulus. For the same wavelengths, the contrast sensitivity of the ON-response of the M–L OFF-cell is about 1 log unit less than that for the M–L ON-cell. The solid curves are predicted from a model of cone combinations and response behavior. No modeling was done for the L OFF-center cell. (From Valberg & Lee, 1989.)

The amplitude A is a measure of the strength of the input of a receptor mechanism and may enter this Eq. (2) with a positive (excitation) or a negative (suppression) sign, or be zero. f_0 is the response to removal of stimulation ("dark response"). There are two free parameters for each cone mechanism (A and σ), and since the majority of cells have input only from two opponent cone types, a total of four free parameters may describe cell responsiveness over a 5 log unit range of luminance. A more detailed account of the model has been given by Valberg, Lee, and Tryti (1987).

For the magnocellular units of Fig. 20, responsiveness is largely wavelength independent, indicating that these cells have L + M cone inputs adding up to the human luminosity function (V_λ). These responses have not been modeled, and a common smooth curve has been drawn through the data points.

In Fig. 21 the contrast sensitivities obtained with

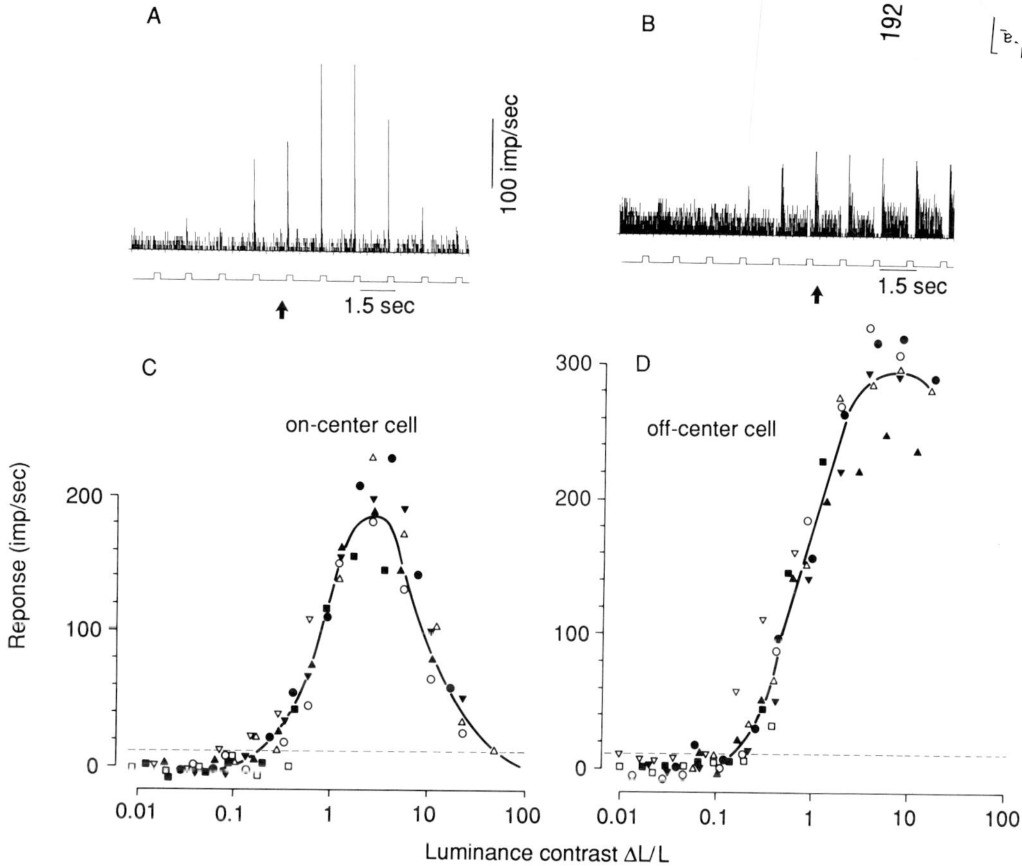

FIG. 20 (A and B) Histograms as in Fig. 19A, but for a transient magnocellular ON-center and an OFF-center cell tested with 589 nm spots. Arrows mark contrast at unity. (C and D): Transient responses (first 45 msec) plotted as a function of luminance contrast for different wavelengths of the stimulus; same cells as in A and B. Contrary to sustained cells, threshold responses of these transient cells are nearly wavelength independent. (From Valberg & Lee, 1989.)

stimuli of different wavelengths in the two ON-center cells of Fig. 19 are shown by filled circles (S–L cell) and open triangles (M–L cell). For comparison, two additional cells are presented (open circles and filled triangles), to complete the set of the four main types of ON-center color-opponent cells. The luminance units in Fig. 21A are transformed to radiance units in Fig. 21B, and only the sensitivity envelope is drawn (solid curve), that is, the most sensitive parts of the cells in Fig. 21A. The curves are derived from the model described above. Below about 480 nm, S–L ON-center cells were the most sensitive (filled circles). Between 480 and 560 nm, M–L ON-center cells were most sensitive (open triangles), whereas above 580 nm, L–M ON-center cells were most sensitive (open circles). Around 570 nm, M–S ON-center cells (filled triangles) sometimes exceeded the sensitivity of M–L cells and L–M cells.

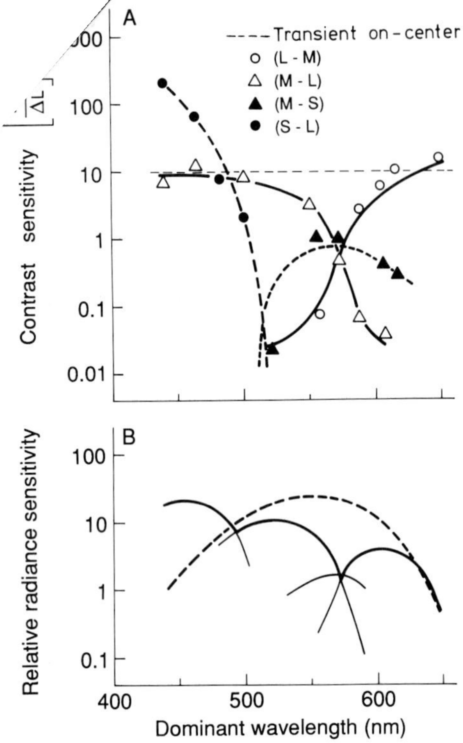

FIG. 21 (A) Spectral luminance contrast sensitivity of the ON-response of four parvocellular layer cone-opponent ON-cells and one magnocellular layer ON-cell. (B) Sensitivity of A plotted in radiance units. The S–L, blue and M–L, green ON-center cells are those of Fig. 19. The curves are those derived from the response model. The horizontal dashed line in A and dashed curve in B represent a transient magno cell for the same 4° spot size. (From Valberg & Lee, 1989.)

Figure 21A also shows data for a transient ON-center magnocellular unit (dashed horizontal line). The contrast sensitivity of this cell exceeds that of the parvocellular units by about 1 log unit for the mid-spectral stimuli. At the spectral ends, however, the S–L ON-center cells and L–M ON-center cells are the most sensitive.

C. Comparison of Psychophysical and Cell Sensitivities

The sensitivity envelope of the four ON-center opponent cells in Fig. 21, with peaks at 605, 530, and 450 nm in Fig. 21B, resembles human psychophysical chromatic sensitivity for test spots on a white background (see Fig. 17). Several studies have shown that detection and chromatic thresholds are similar at the spectral ends (Abney, 1913; Graham & Hsia, 1969; King-Smith & Carden, 1976; Crook, Lee, Tigwell & Valberg, 1987), where opponent cells are more sensitive than non-opponent cells. For mid-spectral lights, threshold differs between *detection* of a luminance increment and *identification* of the hue of a stimulus. This difference is called the photochromatic interval (Abney, 1913). A possible explanation for this interval can be derived from the results of Fig. 21: detection is mediated by the magnocellular neurons and chromatic discrimination by the parvocellular neurons. At the spectral ends, where the latter cells are the more sensitive, they alone can mediate both detection and discrimination. Consequently, the difference in luminance between detection and hue identification

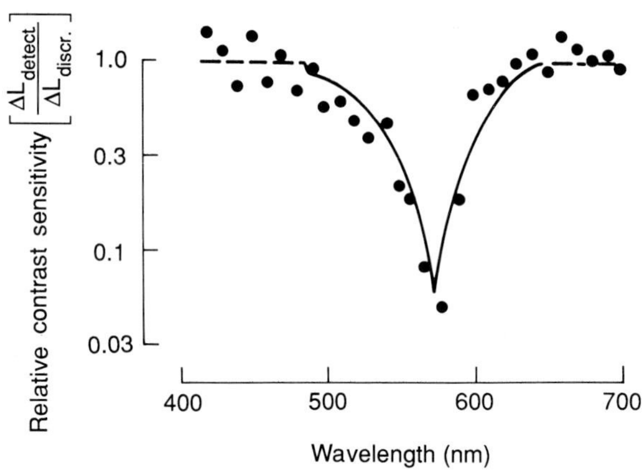

FIG. 22 The solid curve represents the difference between non-opponent magnocellular contrast sensitivity and the envelope of parvocellular color-opponent cell sensitivity (model curves of Fig. 21). In the wavelength range where transient magnocellular units detect the stimuli before the sustained parvocellular units, it would be expected that detection thresholds would be lower than chromatic discrimination thresholds. The dashed parts of the curve indicate the spectral region where opponent cells are more sensitive than nonopponent cells, and where detection and discrimination thresholds should be the same. The data points represent the human foveal photochromatic interval between detection and color identification as determined by Graham and Hsia (1969). (From Valberg & Lee, 1989.)

should correspond to the difference in sensitivity between magnocellular and parvocellular units. In Fig. 22, this sensitivity difference (of Fig. 21A) is compared to the size of the foveal photochromatic interval (dots) on a dark background (Graham & Hsia, 1969). The curve fits the data well. These results have recently been confirmed more directly by using the same stimuli in psychophysical threshold experiments and neurophysiological cell recordings in the macaque (Crook et al., 1987).

Differences in psychophysical thresholds for detection and chromatic thresholds are found to be larger on a dark than on a bright background (Spillmann & Conlon, 1972; King-Smith & Carden, 1976; Mullen, 1987). This is in accord with the finding that retinal phasic non-opponent cells become increasingly more sensitive than cone-opponent cells when background luminance decreases. A similar relation between physiology and psychophysics of the photochromatic interval holds in the spatial domain (Spillmann & Seneff, 1971).

D. Correlations between Neurophysiology and Psychophysics

The results presented above suggest that different classes of visual neurons may be involved in detection and discrimination of color stimuli depending on stimulus conditions. For example, with a steady white background, detection can be achieved either through the magnocellular, non-opponent or through the opponent ON-center cells of the parvocellular system, depending on which class is more sensitive to a given stimulus. OFF-center opponent cells are too insensitive near threshold to play a role.

The notion that the most sensitive neurons are responsible for detection and discrimination seems reasonable near threshold, but under suprathreshold conditions combinations of cell outputs are likely to be responsible for the percept. For example, in a natural viewing condition when stimuli are both brighter and darker than some mean level, parvocellular opponent OFF-center units display the highest sensitivity to dark colors, but they do not respond well to stimuli brighter than the adaptation level, when parvocellular ON-center cells are most active (Schiller, Sandell & Maunsell, 1986; Chapter 7, this volume). Thus, ON- and OFF-center systems share the task of representing the entire scale of luminance ratios, ON-cells being best suited for coding of the brighter colors of self-luminous objects, and OFF-cells for coding the colors of darker, reflecting surfaces, with some overlap between them.

It is possible to expect purely chromatic signals, with elimination of response to achromatic stimuli, by subtracting outputs of cells with opposite cone inputs (i.e. subtracting outputs of L–M and M–L ON-center cells, and of L–M and M–L OFF-center cells in the red–green dimension). The coding of the third dimension, lightness (for objects) or brightness (for light sources), may be provided by adding the activities of opponent ON-center cells (for instance L–M and M–L ON-cells) to yield a "brightness" signal, and of OFF-center cells to provide a signal for "blackness" of surface colors. Such a combination of sustained ON- and OFF-cells could form the B- and D-systems postulated by Jung (1961, 1973), Baumgartner (1961), and Spillmann (1971).

By analyzing the coding of object colors through a set of linear combinations of geniculate-opponent cell outputs, it was possible to reconstruct an equidistant color space (Valberg, Seim, Lee & Tryti, 1986). In this space, the perception of hue is related to the relative activities of the different opponent cell systems, and saturation to response magnitude. Nevertheless, in order to identify the various attributes of color and lightness of unrelated, single stimuli and of related stimuli in complex scenes (Evans, 1974), the ON- and OFF-cell afferents carrying this information must maintain their identity so that comparison between them leads to a proper location in sensory color space. Such channels may coexist with cell systems having response properties that result from combinations of outputs of the same cells. By interchanging information between divergent and convergent pathways (e.g., sums and differences of cone outputs and of opponent signals at different stages), other perceptual attributes like blackness–brightness, grayness–fluorence (Evans, 1974), or the Abney effect (Kurtenbach,

Sternheim & Spillmann, 1984) may also be accounted for. Thus, one may hypothesize that cortical mechanisms derive perceptual attributes from configurations of relative activities in several pathways. Although anatomical and physiological findings suggest that parallel streams within the cortex process spectral information (Chapter 6, this volume), the neural loci for such an analysis remain unknown.

VI. SEGREGATION OF FORM, COLOR, MOVEMENT, AND DEPTH PROCESSING IN THE VISUAL SYSTEM

Recent electrophysiological findings suggest that visual signals are not processed by a single hierarchical system (Lennie, 1984; Livingstone & Hubel, 1984). Rather, the same input is fed into at least three separate processing systems in the brain, each having different functions. One system deals with the perception of shape, another with color, and a third with movement, location, and spatial organization. Thus, the same stimulus is analyzed in several different ways to describe different aspects of the environment.

The idea that the visual system processes information along several separate pathways is far from new and probably dates back to the mid-1800s, when it was observed that the optic nerve splits into several subdivisions after leaving the eye. It may seem strange to think of vision as multipartite rather than as a single process, or that perception of the shape of an object, its color, location, and motion are processed by different parts of the brain, but anatomical, physiological, and psychological studies all strongly indicate that this is the case. The fact that an object's shape, color, position, and motion appear unified, despite being analyzed separately, can be compared to the multimodal experience of listening to someone speak. The sound of the voice is heard by the auditory system and the movement of the lips is analyzed by the visual system, without one being aware that the two are processed independently.

The first major subdivision in the visual pathway becomes apparent in the ganglion cell layer of the retina. This layer contains two intermixed cell types that differ in size and in the way they integrate the signals from the cones that form the magno- and the parvocellular system at the LGN as described above and in Chapter 6 of this volume. The leftmost part of Fig. 23 summarizes some of their most salient properties.

A. From Lateral Geniculate Nucleus to Primary Visual Cortex

From the LGN, the nerve signals proceed to the first cortical visual area (Fig. 23), the primary visual cortex or Visual Area 1 (V1) of primates. This area is a folded sheet of neurons about the size of a credit card but three times as thick, located at the back of the brain. The geniculate fibers project to the middle layer of Area V1, where the segregation of different kinds of information is maintained. Signals from the magnocellular layer of the LGN go to the top half of this layer (4Cα), and signals from the parvo-cellular layer go to the bottom half (4Cβ). Signals then go from this middle (input) layer (4) to the upper (output) layers (2 & 3) of V1.

Until the mid 1980s, it was not known how this prominent functional segregation continued. It was clear that some segregation must exist at higher stages, well beyond Area V1, because cells with different visual functions have been described in quite separate parts of the brain. For example, Zeki (1978a,b) found that, in monkeys, a higher visual cortical area located in the middle temporal lobe (MT) has a high proportion of cells selective to movement or to stereoscopic depth. Another higher area, Visual Area 4 (V4), seems to be selectively involved in color perception. However, it was not known how these higher visual areas were related to each other and to the subdivisions at lower levels. Thus, there was strong evidence for functional segregation at levels before information reaches V1 and at levels several

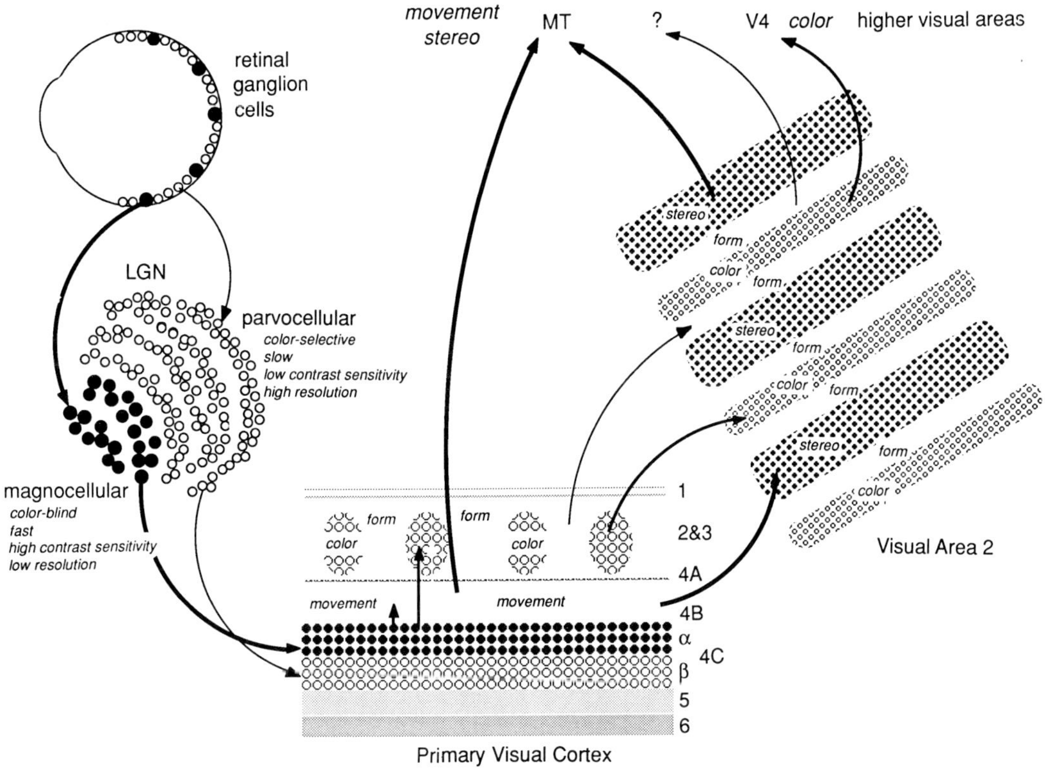

FIG. 23 Diagram of functional segregation in the primate visual system. See text for details. From Livingstone & Hubel (1988). Copyright 1988 by the AAAS.

stages beyond, but little evidence for segregation within V1 or the next stage, V2. Recent work (Livingstone & Hubel, 1984) on functional segregation at these intermediate levels has, in a sense, completed the puzzle.

One way to determine the functional segregation in Areas V1 and V2 was developed by Wong-Riley (1979), who found that staining V1 for a mitochondrial enzyme revealed a fine pattern of dark and light regions in the upper layers. The dark regions turned out to be slightly irregular ovoids, about 0.2 mm in diameter, arranged in a vaguely regular mosaic. These regions were called blobs, because of their shape (Livingstone & Hubel, 1984). This stain made it possible to identify three subdivisions in the output stage of V1: the blobs (layers 2 & 3), the surrounding interblob regions (layers 2 & 3), and layer 4B (Fig. 23). As a result, the connections and response properties of each subdivision could be identified.

The following pattern emerges. The two pathways evident at lower levels seem to be rearranged into three subdivisions at this stage: the interblobs receive input from the parvocellular system, layer 4B receives input from the magnocellular system, and the blobs receive input from both, as indicated in Fig. 23 and Table 2. When tested for selectivity to shape, position, distance, movement, chromaticity, contrast, and size, the differences in the visual response properties of cells in the three subdivisions of Area V1 were dramatic. As described by Livingstone and Hubel (1984), the blobs contain cells highly selective for chromaticity or for contrast but not for shape or movement of

TABLE 2 Subdivision of Information Processing in the Parvocellular and Magnocellular Systems of the Lateral Geniculate Nucleus

	Parvo- and magnocellular system	Parvocellular system	Magnocellular system
Area of V1 receiving input from LGN	Blobs	Interblobs	Layer 4B
Area of V2 receiving output from V1	Thin stripes	Pale stripes	Thick stripes
Information carried	Color	Form	Stereopsis and depth
Higher visual area receiving output from V1 and V2	V4	?	MT

the stimulus. In comparison, interblob cells respond selectively to the orientation of edges but neither to color nor movement. For example, an interblob cell may respond only to a vertical bar regardless of how it moves or whether the bar is black, white, or any other color; yet it will not respond to any bar at any orientation other than vertical. Cells in layer 4B are also unselective for color, but are selective for stimulus orientation and for direction of movement: a typical cell may require horizontal edges moving upward.

B. From Primary Visual Cortex to Higher Visual Areas

The information from the primary visual cortex is transmitted to the next processing stage, Area V2, a region of the cortex adjacent to V1. The mitochondrial stain of Wong-Riley (1979) revealed that V2 is also differentiated into three subdivisions, but here the subdivisions form three different kinds of stripes (which are called pale stripes, thin stripes, and thick stripes because of the way they appear when stained). How are the three subdivisions of Area V2 related to the three subdivisions of V1? Looking at their connections and their response properties, one notices that the color-selective blobs provide input to the thin stripes, which continue processing color information. As sketched on the right in Fig. 23 and in Table 2, information from the orientation-selective interblobs is transmitted to the pale stripes, which further process the information in a way that suggests that the pale stripes are involved in form analysis. A detailed account is given by Hubel and Livingstone (1987). Information from the magnocellular system is relayed to the thick stripes, which analyze the signals to extract information about stereoscopic depth (see Table 2). At still higher cortical stages, these pathways may continue to be independent. The thick stripes project to the middle temporal area, a region concerned with movement and stereopsis (Maunsell & Van Essen, 1983; Shipp & Zeki, 1984, 1985). The thin stripes project to Area V4, an area that appears specialized for processing of color. The projections of the pale stripes are not yet clear.

From studies of cortical lesions in monkeys, Mishkin, Ungerleider, and Macko (1983) have proposed that still higher visual areas fall into two major subdivisions. Parietal lobe areas seem to be important for location, and temporal lobe areas for the recognition of objects in space ("where versus what"). The object localization pathway probably represents the continuation of the magnocellular pathway, and the object recognition pathway the continuation of the parvocellular pathway. Table 3 presents a summary of the physiology and anatomy discussed so far.

In humans, the strongest evidence that color, movement, and form perception are carried by separate pathways comes from clinical neurology. Localized brain damage from strokes can produce very specific types of blindness, such as selective loss of the ability to recognize faces, loss of ability to detect movement (Zihl, von Cramon & Mai, 1983), or loss of color vision without loss of form vision (see Section VII).

TABLE 3 Correlation between Human Perception and the Physiological Properties of the Magnocellular and Parvocellular Divisions of the Lateral Geniculate Nucleus[a]

System/attribute	Color selectivity	Contrast sensitivity	Temporal resolution	Spatial resolution
Magnocellular system				
Physiology	No	High	Fast	Low
Movement perception				
Movement detection	✓	✓	✓	✓
Apparent movement	✓	✓	✓	✓
Depth cues				
Stereopsis	✓	✓	✓	✓
Interocular rivalry	✓			✓
Parallax	✓			
Depth from motion	✓	✓		
Shading	✓	✓		
Contour lines	✓			✓
Occlusion	✓			
Perspective	✓	✓	✓	
Linking properties				
Linking by movement	✓	✓		
Linking by colinearity (illusory borders)	✓	✓	✓	✓
Figure–ground discrimination	✓			
Parvocellular–interblob system				
Physiology	Yes	Low	Slow	High
Shape discrimination				
Orientation discrimination	✓	✓	✓	✓
Shape discrimination	✓	✓	✓	✓
Parvo- and magnocellular–blob system				
Physiology	Yes	High	Slow	Low
Color determination	✓		✓	✓
Flicker photometry	✓		✓	

[a]A check mark indicates that the psychophysical results are consistent with the physiology, and a blank indicates that the experiment has not been done.

C. Dividing Tasks between Specialized Cortical Systems

The parvocellular–interblob–pale stripe system carries high-resolution information about borders. Cells in the early stages of this system are color selective, but at higher levels the color information is transformed in such a way that cells respond to chromatic borders but not to uniform chromatic fields. This system uses color differences to detect borders that might be invisible to the color-blind magnocellular system. Nevertheless, it cannot specify the hues forming the border. It is assumed that in this system orientation information is used for perceiving shape, because much of the information about the shape of objects is represented by their borders. The slow time course and high resolution of the parvo–interblob–pale stripe system are probably important for our ability to see detail in the stationary elements of a scene.

The parvocellular and magnocellular–blob–thin

stripe–V4 system (Table 3) carries information about color and shades of gray, but not information about movement, shape discrimination, or stereopsis. The acuity of this system is several times lower than that of the interblob system. It may increase the efficiency of the form system's color information or carry color information itself with reduced spatial resolution.

The magnocellular–4B–thick stripe–MT pathway (listed in Table 3) is characterized by cells that are selective for movement and for stereoscopic depth. This system has very high temporal resolution—cells respond quickly, and their responses decay rapidly, even when the stimulus is maintained—so this system is especially sensitive to moving and flickering stimuli. It is well suited for detecting motion but not very good at scrutinizing stationary images. This pathway seems to be "color-blind": it is unable to see borders defined only by color contrast.

D. Possible Consequences of Parallel Processing for Perception

The fact that different aspects of vision are subserved by different subdivisions of the brain should have obvious consequences for human perception. The question is whether the functional segregation is as complete as the anatomy and the physiology suggest.

Movement perception may be "color-blind" (Gregory, 1977; Cavanagh, Tyler & Favreau, 1984). For example, Cavanagh et al. displayed red and green moving stripes on a TV screen and found that when the red and green were equiluminant, the perceived speed of movement was greatly reduced, or the stripes even appeared to stop moving completely. Other studies had shown that motion perception also exhibits the other three characteristics of the magnocellular system, high contrast sensitivity, low spatial resolution and fast temporal resolution. All these observations are consistent with the idea that motion perception is mainly a function of the magnocellular system and not the parvocellular system.

Stereopsis is the ability to judge depth using differences between the images in the two eyes (see Chapter 12, this volume). The visual system can interpret these small differences as distance. Lu and Fender (1972) found that people cannot see depth in random-dot stereograms when the dots presented to each eye are equiluminant. This suggests that stereopsis is also "color-blind," consistent with the distinguishing characteristics of the magno- and parvocellular systems. The properties of human stereopsis and motion perception lead to the conclusion that these two functions are probably carried out almost exclusively by the magnocellular system.

Shading is an important cue for the perception of depth and shape. Under most natural light sources, shading consists mainly of differences in brightness rather than hue. Therefore, depth information conveyed by shading is primarily luminance-contrast information, so the part of the visual system coding "shape from shading" need not carry any color information. (see Chapter 11, this volume). Cavanagh and Leclerc (1985) found that shape from shading is "color-blind," that is, a shadow can be any hue, it need only be darker than the rest of the surface to convey a sense of depth. This observation seems to have been known to artists. For example, in Matisse's self-portrait the shadows are a peculiar green, but they still create a normal three-dimensional effect. A black-and-white photograph shows that the shade of green used for contouring is indeed darker than the rest of his skin.

Apparently the magnocellular system subserves movement perception and the ability to use many kinds of depth cues to judge distance and spatial relationships. Why should this particular pair of functions be carried by one system? A possible answer comes from Gestalt psychology. Most natural images contain a rich assortment of visual elements such as edges of many orientations, homogeneous surfaces, colors, and textures. Perception requires principles of organization of all these elements. The Gestalt psychologists suggested that certain visual properties are used to group together parts of an image and to separate objects from each other and from the ground.

These linking features include direction and velocity of motion, colinearity (a house is not perceptually split in two by a telephone pole or a wire crossing in front of it), depth, lightness and texture (different parts of the same object usually have the same surface properties). The fact that all these functions fail at equiluminance suggests that the ability to link together related parts of the scene, to discriminate figure from ground, and to perceive the correct spatial relationships of objects might all be carried by the magnocellular system. Indeed, an image in which all colors are equiluminant appears disorganized, and figure–ground distinctions become difficult.

The parvo–magno–blob system has a severalfold lower acuity than the interblob system. This lower resolution of the color system compared to the form system can explain a phenomenon that was already discussed by Helmholtz and Hering in the nineteenth century, namely, that two colors can interact with each other depending on their spatial arrangement. Usually, when regions of different colors are juxtaposed, the colors oppose each other (simultaneous contrast), so that each tends to appear less like the other. But when the two colors are interlaced in a fine pattern, the opposite happens: they come to look more like each other, that is, they blend or "bleed" (assimiliation). Color contrast and assimilation have received much attention from color vision psychophysicists (see Hurvich, 1981), and some theoretical models are presented in Chapter 15.

The acuity difference between the parvocellular–interblob system and the parvocellular and magnocellular–blob–system implies that the shape of an image that is too small for the color system to resolve cannot be discriminated. As a consequence, colors become assimilated when the pattern exceeds the resolution of the color system (Fach & Sharpe, 1986; see also Chapter 7, this volume). The phenomenon of color assimilation can be readily observed in pointillist paintings. Individual brushstrokes or dots can be seen, although the colors still blend. Thus, there is a relatively narrow range of pattern sizes over which one can discriminate a pattern but still perceive color blending, the range between the resolution of the color system and the resolution of the form system. The television industry takes advantage of the low resolution of the color system by transmitting the color part of the image at a lower resolution than the black-and-white image, thereby reducing the amount of information transmitted.

These few examples demonstrate how knowledge about the segregation of functions in the visual system can be useful in devising ways to enhance the visibility of blurry or low contrast images and in designing video systems for robotics or automatic navigation. From what is known about the sensitivity of the magnocellular system to contrast, movement, and stereopsis, one would predict that hard-to-see objects would become more visible if either motion parallax (by moving the object or the observer) or retinal disparity (by stereo-viewing two images of the same scene taken from different positions) were introduced. Although the proposed links between visual pathways and perceptions still have to be proved, there is increasing evidence that the links do exist.

VII. COLOR VISION AND BRAIN DAMAGE

It is remarkable that so many of our ideas and discoveries about the cerebral mechanisms of primate color vision have come from studying deficient color vision in subjects where the anomaly is retinal. This contrasts strikingly with the study of pattern and object perception. Here, too, there is a long tradition of examining perceptual disorders for clues about normal mechanisms, but patients with cerebral rather than retinal abnormalities have provided the most illuminating information. This difference may reflect a simple fact, namely, that trichromacy and wavelength discrimination are determined and adequately described by retinal mechanisms, whereas the perception and recognition of shape require extensive cerebral computational analysis of the relatively simple signals from the eye.

A. Chromatic and Achromatic Disorders

During almost a century of neurological investigation of patients, only a handful have been described in which presumed geniculate or pregeniculate damage has selectively impaired either the perception of color or of lightness. For example, the patient described by Hyvärinen and Rovamo (1981) had a remarkably poor ability to discriminate black–white gratings but could discriminate isoluminant red–green gratings. The complementary disorder was reported by Bender and Bodis-Wollner (1978); who described several patients able to perceive achromatic but not chromatic contrasts. Patients such as these have not yet been examined with modern brain-imaging methods such as computer tomography, and the precise locus of their damage is unknown. However, on the basis of existing knowledge about the organization of the visual pathways one can ask which lesion would produce such disorders.

The optic tract in primates is classically described as containing a single topographic representation of the contralateral half of visual space, that is, each region on the retina is represented in one region of the tract, regardless of cell type. If true, this means that a localized pregeniculate lesion could not selectively impair a single quality of vision unless it involved only one cell type, or more exactly one axon type, in a population of fibers in which all functional classes were intermingled. However, if different functional classes were segregated in the optic tract it would not be surprising for one of them to be occasionally selectively damaged. In the optic tract of the cat the thickest axons, believed to arise from retinal α cells (that correspond to some extent to the magnocellular system of primate), lie ventrally whereas the putative axons from retinal β cells lie dorsally (Guillery, Polley & Torrealba, 1982; Torrealba, Guillery, Eysel, Polley & Mason, 1983); the latter cell type corresponds to some extent to the parvocellular system of primates. It has been shown that a similar segregation according to axon diameter is also present in the optic tract of Old World monkeys (Reese & Guillery, 1987).

In monkeys, the fine dorsal axons of the tract arising from retinal P_β cells form the parvocellular system whereas those of the ventral aspect of the tract from the retinal P_α cells form the magnocellular system (Perry, Oehler & Cowey, 1984). It should thus be possible to damage them selectively. To test this idea, Reese and Cowey (1988) implanted a small pellet of horseradish peroxidase (HRP) in either the dorsal or the ventral aspect of the optic tract in several monkeys. The dorsal implant labeled predominantly retinal P_β cells with very few α cells, whereas the ventral implant labeled chiefly P_α cells. Such a reversal is never seen after implants in the optic nerve, suggesting that the segregation into two classes of fibers is not yet present. In addition, the dorsal implants gave rise to anterograde (forward) labeling in the parvocellular layers of the dorsal lateral geniculate nucleus (dLGN), whereas the anterograde labeling following a ventral implant was concentrated in the magnocellular layers. It is known that P_β cells and the parvocellular layers of the dLGN are concerned with wavelength discrimination, and that the P_α cells and the magnocellular layers of the dLGN transmit broadband information (see Shapley & Perry, 1986). This evidence provides a possible anatomical basis for the rare reports of selectively impaired discrimination of color or achromatic contrast. There is an obvious, as yet not performed, test of this hypothesis. Sectioning of the dorsal half of the optic tract in monkeys should impair chromatic and sectioning of the ventral half should impair achromatic contrast thresholds, and sectioning of the ventral half should not produce a total lack of vision in any part of the visual field.

B. Cerebral Achromatopsia in Humans

Patients with cerebral achromatopsia perceive the world as devoid of color. Although colors are still experienced, they are faint, desaturated, and sometimes dark. Not surprisingly, hue discrimination is poor, and it is sometimes so bad that the patient is virtually color-blind. Yet, the retina retains its trichromacy, with normal spectral sensitivities for the three channels, as shown by using the Stiles two-color increment threshold method (see Mollon, Newcombe, Polden & Ratcliff, 1980). This implies that the experience of color and the discrimination of hue require extrastriate visual mechanisms. What, and where in the brain, might they be?

The localization of the cortical damage that leads to cerebral achromatopsia is far from precise, but there is good agreement about its general location on the ventral aspect of the occipital and temporal lobes within the lingual and fusiform gyri (see Meadows, 1974; Damasio, Yamada, Damasio, Corbett & McKee, 1980, for reviews). In all patients, there is probably damage of higher visual areas, including parts of Brodmann's Areas 19, 21, 36, and 37. The perceptual disorder is commonly but not universally associated with object agnosia, but in patients with the pure color disorder the cortical damage seems little different. The first notable feature of this brain damage is that it is much more ventral and medial than the position in Old World monkeys of cortical Area V4, which has often been implicated in extrastriate mechanisms of color vision on electrophysiological grounds (Zeki, 1983a,b; Van Essen, 1985).

As there is good evidence for parallel processing of chromatic and achromatic contrast in the dLGN, striate cortex, and foveal projections from the latter (Livingstone & Hubel, 1984; Shipp & Zeki, 1984, 1985; Van Essen, 1985; Shapley & Perry, 1986), it would be interesting to know whether the discrimination between shades of gray was relatively spared in patients with cerebral achromatopsia. This was examined by Heywood, Wilson, and Cowey (1987) in a patient whose achromatopsia was not accompanied by object agnosia. The patient arranged equiluminant colored stimuli in a random fashion over most of the color circle. When presented with a series of grays, in which the discriminability between adjacent stimuli is matched to that of the hues for normal observers, the achromatopsic patient performed substantially better. This is shown in Fig. 24, where the patient's perfor-

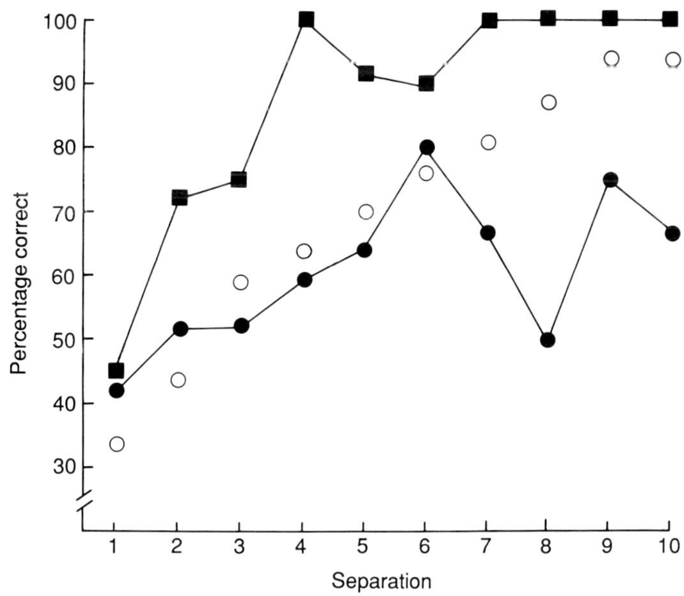

FIG. 24 Solid circles show the performance of a patient when asked to select the odd color out of three simultaneously presented colors (two of which were identical). Random selection would yield 33% correct responses. The colors presented in each trial were always from the same part of the color circle (red, yellow–green, or blue), but the difference between them varied from 1 to 10 steps on a Munsell scale of hue. Squares show the patient's performance when asked to discriminate between grays, in which case the abscissa refers to separation in arbitrary units on the Munsell reflectance scale. Open circles show the performance of monkeys in which much of Area V4 had been removed. The monkeys were presented with the same Munsell colors but in a task where random responding would yield 50% correct. Their scores have therefore been appropriately adjusted for guessing so that they are directly comparable to the scores of the patient. (For full details, see Heywood & Cowey, 1987, and Heywood, Wilson & Cowey, 1987.)

mance is plotted against perceptually equivalent steps between chromatic and achromatic stimuli. It is evident that the patient can discriminate much better between shades of gray than between hues.

C. Achromatopsia in Monkeys

According to Zeki (1973, 1978a,b, 1983a,b) cortical Area V4 is specialized for the processing of both wavelength and color. Although many neurons in V4 respond to achromatic contrast and to features like orientation and length (Desimone, Schein, Moran & Ungerleider, 1985), the primary role of V4 probably lies in the processing of hue and color. Therefore, its removal might lead to a condition resembling achromatopsia in man. Heywood and Cowey (1987) tested this hypothesis by removing Area V4 bilaterally in monkeys that had been trained to discriminate between hues and between grays. Discrimination was assessed by presenting three stimuli side by side, in a row. The central stimulus was identical to one of its neighbors; the third stimulus—the odd one out—served as the positive stimulus. The hue separation or the lightness separation was systematically varied. Figure 25a,b,c compares performance before and after removal of Area V4 on hue discrimination in the red region of the color circle. The performance of monkeys after removal of V4 was significantly impaired at the smallest hue separations. In comparison, unoperated control animals (UNOP) or monkeys in which the so-called face cell area in the superior temporal sulcus (STS) had been removed were not impaired (data not shown). Results similar to those shown in Fig. 25 were obtained with a range of yellow–green or blue hues. After removal of Area V4, the animals were impaired when, instead of varying hue, the saturation of a particular red stimulus was varied (Fig. 25d). However, when the stimuli were gray (Fig. 25e), the three groups were indistinguishable. The evidence thus far indicates that monkeys in which Area V4 has been removed show the same dissociation between hue and gray discrimination that was reported for the achromatopsic patient by Heywood et al. (1987).

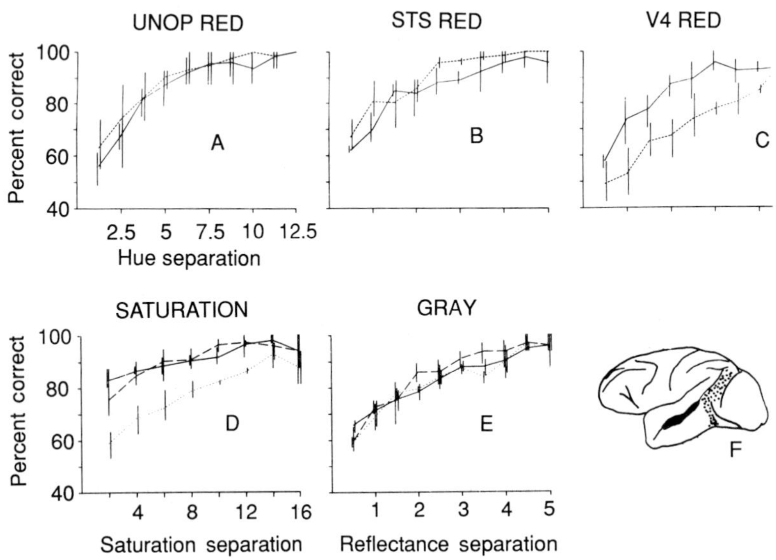

FIG. 25 Graphs A, B and C show the percent correct discrimination of three groups of monkeys, before and after surgical removal of V4, when presented with Munsell hues. The hue separation is given in Munsell units on the abscissa. The vertical bars show the full ranges of scores contributing to each mean. Postoperatively (dashed line), all animals in Group V4 were impaired. Graph D shows the postoperative performance of all three groups when discriminating the saturation of a red stimulus. Graph E shows that the three groups were indistinguishable when required to discriminate between neutral gray stimuli, despite the fact that this was a difficult task for normal monkeys. In F is shown the position of the cortical ablation of V4 (dotted) or the upper and lower banks of the rostral superior temporal sulcus, STS (black). (For full details see Heywood et al., 1987.)

D. Cerebral Achromatopsia and Color Constancy

Although cerebral achromatopsia in man can exist without any other form of visual agnosia (e.g., Case 1 of Damasio et al., 1980; Heywood et al., 1987), the nature of the color disturbance is not yet fully established. The common symptom of a world that looks drab, or completely colorless, suggests that although the retina may still be trichromatic (Mollon et al., 1980), the cortical mechanism for *comparing* the output of the three different channels is missing. If so, one might expect isoluminant chromatic gratings to produce normal evoked responses when the latter are measured over striate cortex. When this was done (Damasio et al., 1980) both achromatopsia patients showed negligible occipital responses to red–green reversing checkerboards but normal responses to black–white checkerboards. This finding suggests that the lesion may be interrupting the chromatic channel *before* it reaches the striate cortex.

Could color constancy be selectively disturbed in achromatopsia? Our ability to perceive color as largely unchanging despite wide variations in the spectral composition of incident, and therefore in reflected light, is usually taken for granted. But the brain must be comparing wavelength composition if the light is reflected from adjacent regions (Land, 1983; D'Zmura & Lennie, 1986) and using the relationship between these regions to determine the color as opposed to the wavelength of the light. As there are neurons in Area V4 that demonstrate qualities of color constancy in that they respond selectively to particular colors despite wide variations in the wavelengths falling on their receptive fields (Zeki, 1983a,b), one may ask whether impairing this mechanism could explain achromatopsia. A disturbance of color constancy was reported in two monkeys following ablation of Area V4 (Wild, Butler, Garden & Kulikowski, 1985), but there was no clear evidence that wavelength discrimination was intact. If the latter were impaired, as in the study by Heywood and Cowey (1987), color constancy can hardly be normal. Furthermore, if the sole or principal defect lies in color constancy, there is no reason why the world should look colorless or why it should be difficult to make hue discriminations when the hues are adjacent and identically illuminated. The weight of evidence therefore suggests that in achromatopsia the defect lies at an earlier stage of processing than that concerned with color constancy.

VIII. CONCLUSION

The 1960s, 1970s, and 1980s have brought remarkable insights into the mechanisms of color vision. The structure of the photopigments of the three different classes of cones has been described, the electrical responses of the three different cone mechanisms have been recorded in individual outer segments of macaque, and the differences in the individual properties of the electrical responsiveness of the three cone mechanisms have been clarified. Color-opponent mechanisms have been carefully studied in retinal ganglion cells and in the lateral geniculate nucleus, and the spatial and temporal properties of this opponent stage have been rather completely described. It has become clear that in the retina a large number of spectrally different "chromatic analyzers" are built from the three cone mechanisms. The separation of pathways for chromatic and achromatic information, starting at retinal ganglion cells, has been followed up through the lateral geniculate nucleus to the primary visual cortex and beyond. The segregation of pathways in higher visual areas has been described anatomically. Furthermore, the processing of chromatic information in certain cortical substructures such as blobs and the attribution of chromatic processing to certain visual areas such as V4 have been clearly established. In a marvelous way, the several disciplines, neurophysiology, neuroanatomy, and neuropathology, have collaborated to establish the neurobiological substrates of color perception. This knowledge has been linked in many ways to psychophysical and perceptual findings.

Nevertheless, there are still large pieces missing from this puzzle. Despite much effort, a direct correlation between classical color metrics and neurophysiological mechanisms is not yet possible. Other important questions for future research involve color constancy, the contribution of rod to cone vision, and simultaneous color contrast, to name only a few. Promising models have been developed in these areas, but experiments linking neurophysiological mechanisms to perceptions are still lacking. The fascinating field of color vision is still wide open and promising for those who take up these challenges.

ACKNOWLEDGMENTS

The authors were supported by the following grants: German Research Council grants ZR 1/1-2, ZR 1/1-3, and SFB220, TP B7 to E.Z.; research grant 60450015 from the Japanese Ministry of Education and Science, and a travel grant from the Alexander von Humboldt Foundation to M.A.; grant No. N001488K0201 of the Office of Naval Research and a Presidential Young Investigators award from the National Science Foundation to M.L.; NATO Collaborative Research Grant 650/83 and the Norwegian Research Council for Science and the Humanities to A.V. A. Valberg's experimental work was done in Göttingen, in collaboration with Dr. B. B. Lee at the Max-Planck-Institute for Biophysical Chemistry. MRC Grant G971/397/B; to A. C.

9

THE PERCEPTION OF MOTION

Robert Sekuler, Stuart Anstis, Oliver J. Braddick, Thomas Brandt, J. Anthony Movshon, and Guy Orban

I. INTRODUCTION

Of the many important contributions to the study of motion perception, three stand out as towering landmarks in a long and provocative scientific literature. Like their physical counterparts, these intellectual landmarks can serve to orient travelers who are unfamiliar with the surrounding territory. Also, these landmark contributions have influenced much of the current work on motion perception. As a result, they provide a convenient and natural entree to our discussion.

The first modern study of motion perception was done by Sigmund Exner a century ago. Although other scientists before him also made significant contributions, Exner (1888) was the first to appreciate that, as a perceptual quality, motion was special. Physically, motion can be described as a spatial change over time. But Exner demonstrated that perceptually, motion was not merely the stepchild of the perception of space and the perception of time. In one study (Exner, 1888), he placed two sources of electrical sparks so close to one another that an observer could not distinguish the two. Despite the impossibility of resolving the sources spatially, when the sparks were presented with the appropriate time interval, observers experienced compelling motion—the spark seemed to move from one location to another. In other words, observers experienced motion even though they could not *spatially* resolve the two endpoints of the motion. Exner also succeeded in demonstrating that observers could experience motion even though they could not *temporally* resolve its sources.

The second landmark in our brief history of motion perception is Max Wertheimer's 1912 monograph. For anyone who delves into it, Wertheimer's monograph is a remarkable source of stimulation. Many readers will be familiar with the monograph's main experiment: a compelling sensation of motion can be produced by a brief, sequential presentation of first one then the other of two, spatially adjacent lines. But the monograph also anticipates issues that many vision researchers are working on today. For example, Wertheimer provided a good demonstration of motion inertia, a phenomenon central to perceptual theory which is described below. He also provided a good demonstration of hysteresis, a form of "memory" that has proved to be of much theoretical importance (Williams, Phillips & Sekuler, 1986). But that is just a small, highly selective sample; Wertheimer's entire monograph is worth reading for enlightenment as well as for stimulating research ideas.

And finally, the third landmark exploration of motion perception is Werner Reichardt's studies in the late 1950s and early 1960s. These studies constitute a genuine *paradigm shift*, in Thomas Kuhn's sense (Kuhn, 1970). Reichardt's elegant mathematical model (1961) shifted the field from its prior status—an enterprise geared to the uncoordinated collection of interesting facts—to a field with a consensus about research methods and priorities. Reichardt's model, for the first time, stimulated people to think about how the visual system might extract motion information from the stimulus on the retina. His work, though now over a quarter-century old, remains very much alive today.

Most current models of motion extraction are elaborations on Reichardt's original model. Basically,

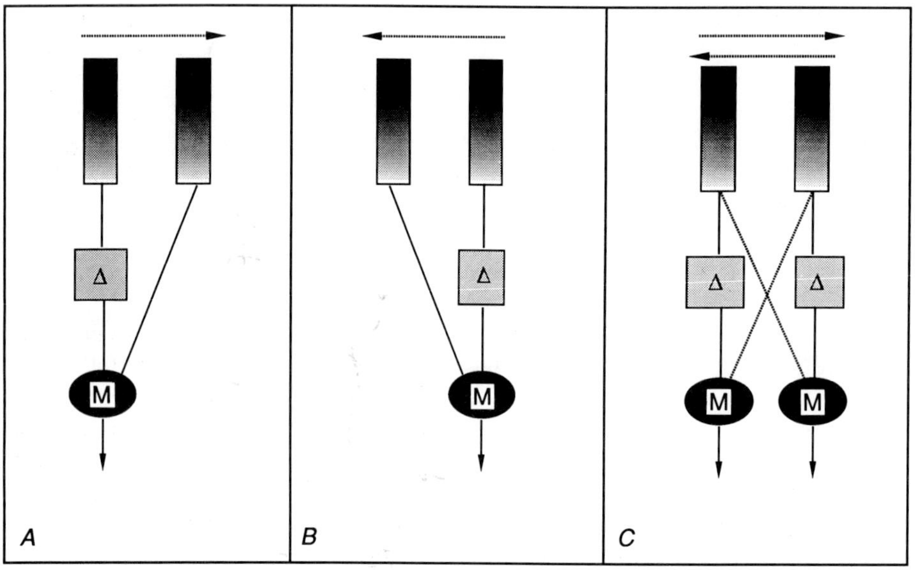

FIG. 1 Basic scheme of Reichardt's motion detector. (A) Signals from two photoreceptors (shaded rectangles) are sent to unit M where the signals arriving at various instants are multiplied. The signal from the left receptor reaches the multiplier after some delay, Δ, relative to the signal from the right receptor. As a result, the multiplier unit responds well to a pattern moving in the direction of the arrow at top. A stimulus would be particularly effective if it first stimulated the left receptor and then, with delay Δ, stimulated the right receptor. Under these conditions, the product of the two signals would be large, as would be the output of unit M. (B) A second group of photoreceptors and associated multiplier unit. The position of the delay, Δ, makes this group respond poorly or not at all to rightward motion. Its preferred direction of motion, shown by the arrow at top, is leftward. (C) A more complete Reichardt unit, with two pairs of receptors, multiplier units, and delays. The left multiplier unit would respond well to a pattern that travels across the retina from left to right (with appropriate velocity); the right multiplier would do the same for a pattern traveling from right to left (again, with appropriate velocity). A final, subtraction unit, not shown, would convert the difference between the two M units' outputs into a directional response.

the scheme assumes that the visual system compares the signals that arise, over time, from different photoreceptors. If some pattern travels across the retina, its effect on receptor R_a at time t will be strongly correlated with its effect on another receptor, R_b, at some slightly later time, $t + \Delta$. There will be a strong cross-correlation, with lag Δ, between the signals from the two receptors. Note that the spatial separation between the two receptors acts to delay one signal relative to the other. Figure 1 illustrates the kernel of Reichardt's model. Note that this simple scheme makes use of only two receptors (shaded rectangles). Poggio and Reichardt (1973), extending the basic scheme, have shown that a motion detection model with n inputs and a single output can be reduced to the sum of 2-input pairs, the case illustrated in Fig. 1. [See Sekuler, Pantle, and Levinson (1978) for more details.] Reichardt's work opened the way for the development of detailed, quantitative accounts of motion perception (Reichardt, 1987).

Although the mathematical precision, clarity, and force of Reichardt's contribution makes today's work on motion more coherent, there is still an enormous variety of approaches to motion. There is a good reason for this variety, despite what seems to be quite a broad consensus.

II. THE MANY FUNCTIONS OF MOTION

Since motion plays so many different perceptual roles, researchers can emphasize or concentrate on certain aspects only. Such choices necessarily lead researchers along different paths. Let us briefly review some of motion's many roles (see Nakayama, 1985, for a more thorough treatment).

Motion is particularly important for segregation of figure and ground. When an object moves relative to a background, producing differential speeds or different directions in the retinal image, the visual system converts those differences into perceptual separation of figure and ground (shape from motion; see Chapter 11, this volume). Motion also segregates, or sorts, objects into different depth planes (depth from motion; again, see Chapter 11, this volume). When any single region of the retina is stimulated by different velocities, the visual system is challenged (shearing; see Koenderink & van Doorn, 1978). Different velocities usually mean different objects, or parts of objects. But in the natural world, two (or more) objects cannot occupy the same place at the same time. The visual system seems to resolve the apparent contradiction of different velocities within a single region by assigning those different velocities to different depth planes. The processes responsible for such depth assignments, structure from motion, are currently being actively investigated by vision scientists, physiologists, and people interested in computer vision.

Finally, one of the main motives for studying motion perception is a desire to understand how motion helps us avoid colliding with objects, keeps us moving along the straight and narrow, and helps to maintain our posture. As shown later, motion's different functions probably require that a variety of different neural computations be carried out, most likely by different neural circuits.

A. Stimuli

Scientific research is limited—or empowered—by the tools that are available. By probing with a sufficiently complex and rich stimulus, the motion system can be forced to reveal its richness. For this purpose, stimuli belonging to the family of random dot cinematograms are especially good. All members of this family have two features in common: first, a random spatial arrangement of their elements, which is designed to minimize visible contours; second, some rule or rules that govern the way in which those elements are displaced from one frame of the display to the next. [See Chang (1986) for a discussion of these stimuli.]

1. Correspondence Problem

Random dot cinematograms present a special challenge to the visual system in the form of the *correspondence problem*. The term "correspondence prob-

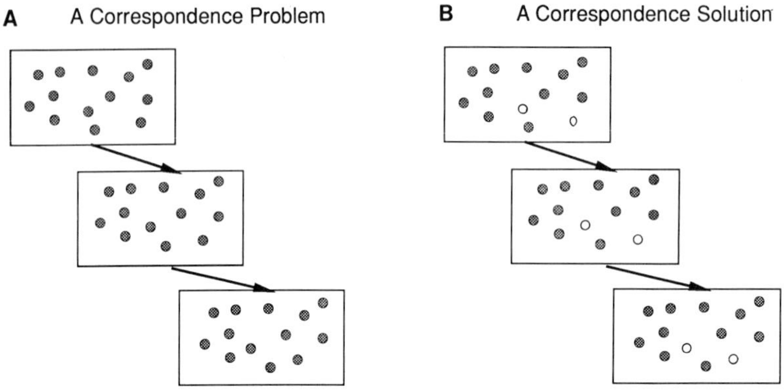

FIG. 2 Each panel shows three frames of a simple random dot cinematogram. Some dots have been shifted from the first frame (top) to the second frame (middle) and then to the third frame (bottom). If the frames were presented as a random dot cinematogram, the shifted dots would immediately manifest themselves in apparent movement. In (A), some effort is required to identify the shifted dots in still frames. In (B), the three frames of the cinematogram are shown with the shifted dots highlighted for ease of identification.

lem" denotes the challenge of matching elements in one frame with elements in a succeeding frame. From top to bottom, Fig. 2a illustrates three successive frames of a random dot cinematogram. Some subset of dots from the first frame (top) has been shifted in the second frame (middle) and shifted again in the third frame (bottom). In Fig. 2b the shifted dots are highlighted for ease of identification.

Though effort is needed to find the subset of shifted dots in Fig. 2a, when the same frames are shown as a cinematogram the visual system extracts the subset with no effort at all. More specifically, if the three frames illustrated in Fig. 2 were spatially superimposed and shown in rapid succession, the displaced set of dots would appear to move upward and to the left. The visual system has little trouble extracting coherent motion of the shifted dots. Even with enormously dense and complex displays, perceived motion can still be easily extracted.

"Matching" may not be the proper term for what the visual system is actually doing, but it is a term in common use. There are various possible strategies for solving the correspondence problem. One strategy might be a point-by-point match. This approach may actually be employed when the cinematogram contains just a few elements. But when the cinematogram contains several thousand elements and only relatively few are being shifted in a coherent fashion, a point-by-point match becomes unfeasible. An alternative employs a more global strategy, one heuristic or another from the "bag of tricks" to which Ramachandran and Anstis (1986a) have called attention.

2. Aperture Problem

The correspondence problem is not the only challenge that the visual system must overcome in its quest to extract useful information about object motion. Another significant obstacle, the *aperture problem* (Section IV,B) arises from the limited field of view, or receptive field, assigned to any visual neuron. Imagine that you see the world through the narrow local window of a single receptive field. This restricted field of view necessarily creates ambiguities. Suppose an infinitely long edge is moving through the receptive field. Any one of a large number of combinations of directions and speeds could mimic perfectly the velocity of that edge. So, to that neuron, many combinations of directions and speeds ought to be indistinguishable. Yet, except in some very special circumstances, perceivers do not make the sort of confusions that one neuron would. As seen later in this chapter (Section IV,B) Movshon, Adelson, Gizzi, and Newsome (1986) have developed an ingenious scheme to circumvent this apparent neuronal limitation.

B. Percepts and Physiological Links

The ease or difficulty with which one experiences motion in displays depends on a number of spatial and temporal variables. For example, if the elements from one frame to another are shifted by very large steps, the sensation of motion breaks down: instead of motion, one set of dots seems to disappear and then reappear at a different location. This upper limit is now called d_{max}, the largest displacement between successive presentations for which observers still obtain a coherent sense of motion. The existence of such a limit has been known for some time; Wertheimer (1912) noted it, and Korte (1915) formalized it in one of his laws of apparent motion. More recently, this spatial limit, d_{max}, has become an indispensible tool for understanding motion perception. Among other virtues, d_{max} can be quite useful for bridging the gap between psychophysics and physiology. As this chapter shows, measurements such as d_{max} can be made in several different domains: on single neurons, in human and animal observers. Such comparisons allow connections to be made across the domains. At various points in the chapter, we note particular linking propositions, statements that assert some link between physiological (Φ) and psychophysical (Ψ) domains. (See Chapter 3, this volume.)

Returning to the nature of test stimuli, it is worth pointing out that random dot cinematograms can vary in a great many different ways. Consider first, the lifetime (exposure duration) of each individual element. In some random dot cinematograms, individual elements have a short life expectancy; they exist for a short time and then disappear to be replaced by other random elements (Mather & Moulden, 1980; Siegel & Anderson, 1988; see Chapter 4, this volume). This renewal scheme minimizes the probability that individual dot paths are being tracked. For example, one could not compute a dot's direction by comparing the points at which it entered and exited the display area.

The successive displacements of the elements in a cinematogram can be governed by various sorts of rules. For example, a simple rule can be used, causing all the moving elements to be displaced in unison, all in the same direction and at the same pace. This represents the extreme of narrow-band directional content: only one direction is present. However, there are other possibilities. Random dot cinematograms can contain many different, spatially intermingled, directions of motion, all present simultaneously. For example, the elements in a given local area may be displaced over a series of frames, not by some constant step and direction, but by directional values drawn from a *distribution* with some given mean direction and covering a range of directions (Watamaniuk, Sekuler & Williams, 1989).

With this latter scheme, a perceiver may experience two contradictory percepts: (a) different directions of local motions and (b) a coherent flow in the direction of the mean of the directional distribution (Williams & Sekuler, 1984). One sees individual dots moving randomly, but at the same time one also perceives the overall flow of the dots in some dominant direction. This global percept enables one to use the concept of metamerism to study the mechanisms of motion perception (Richards, 1979). Two stimuli are said to be metameric if, despite physical differences, they are perceptually indistinguishable. Under appropriate circumstances, metamers reveal what information the visual system retains and what information it discards. Although best known and exploited in color vision, metamers also exist in the domain of motion: radically different distributions of directions are able to produce perceptually indistinguishable motions.

In using psychophysical "confusions" to study the number or type of underlying mechanisms, one postulates a particular type of linking proposition, the Converse Identity proposition (Chapter 3, this volume). One formulation of the proposition states that "statistically indiscriminable sensations imply statistically identical states of the nervous system." Symbolically, this proposition can be stated as

$$\text{Identical } \Phi \rightarrow \text{Identical } \Psi$$

III. SPATIAL LIMITS TO MOTION

A. d_{max}

In analyzing human motion perception and its possible neurophysiological basis, we have learned much

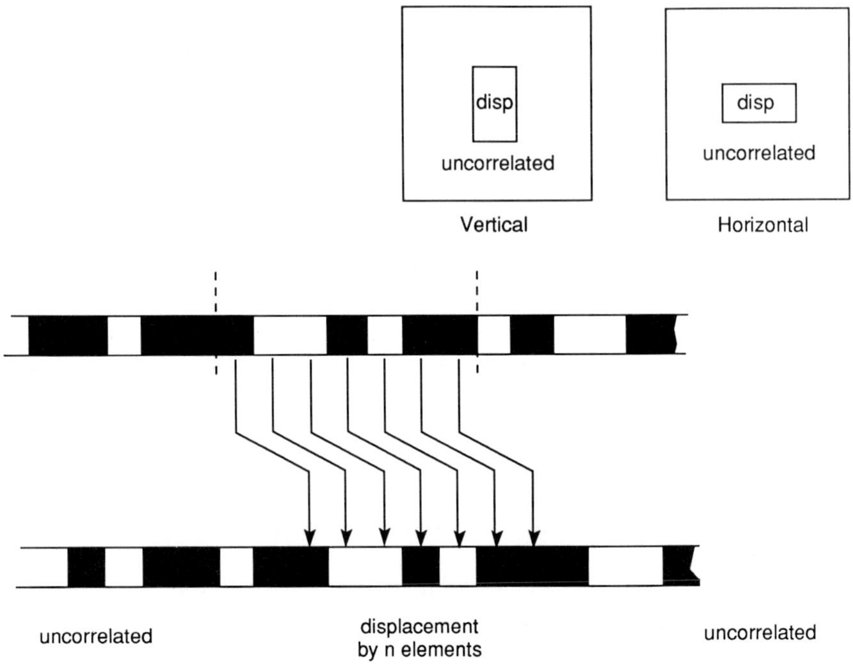

FIG. 3 Construction of a random dot cinematogram. Two patterns of random dots are presented in rapid succession: a typical row from the first and second pattern is shown. In a random dot cinematogram of this kind, only the dots within a central region undergo a coherent displacement, and the subject is asked to report the shape (vertical or horizontal) of this region. An alternative method is to displace all the dots in the pattern, requiring the subject to report the direction of motion. From Braddick (1974).

from experiments on apparent motion using random dot cinematograms such as the one illustrated in Fig. 3. As indicated earlier, a key parameter from these experiments is d_{max}, a spatial limit on apparent motion. This parameter has particular significance when one tries to relate the psychophysics of motion to the physiology of direction-selective neurons; it presumably represents the spatial range of the interactions that underlie directional selectivity within the receptive fields.

Earlier studies (Braddick, 1974) suggested that d_{max} was a quite closely defined parameter. It seemed to fall between 15 and 20 min of arc, regardless of variations in the size and spacing of the elements of the random dot patterns. This measure is striking because it represents a distance much smaller than the range for apparent motion in the classic work of Wertheimer (1912). Recall that in those studies, Wertheimer, and others after him (e.g., Neuhaus, 1930), quantified the range for which one could see motion when spatially offset lines or spots were alternated, and he typically found this range to be at least several degrees of arc (see also Jung & Spillmann, 1970). The term "short-range process" was coined by Braddick (1974) to indicate a motion process that would be particularly responsive to cinematogram displays. It was meant to contrast with the longer range process that yields perceived motion in patterns which contain a small number of clearly defined elements. Although more recent work (see below) shows that the spatial limit cannot be thought of as an invariant 15–20 min arc, the idea of a distinct short-range process seems still to be valid.

In fact, two demonstrations show that, under the right conditions, d_{max} can be extended a good deal beyond 15–20 min arc. In one study, Baker and Braddick (1985) constructed random dot cinematograms in which dot displacements occurred within a pair of strips on either side of the fixation point. By varying the separation of the strips, d_{max} could be measured at several different eccentricities of viewing. The results in Fig. 4 show that d_{max} increases with retinal eccentricity in an orderly fashion, and, at 10 degrees from the fixation point, displacements as large as 90 min

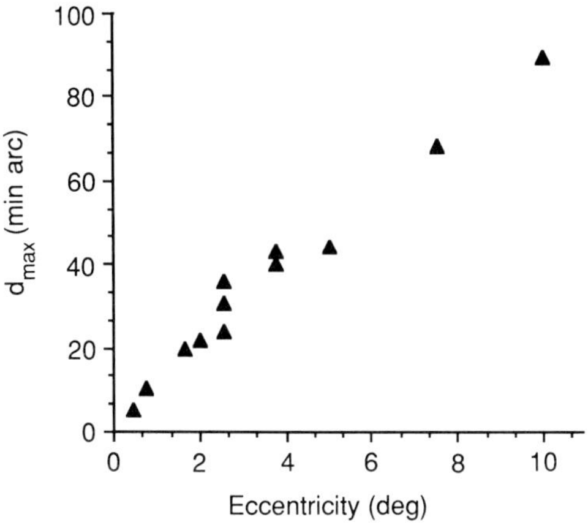

FIG. 4 Variation of d_{max} with eccentricity, e. The display consisted of dots displaced upward or downward within two vertical strips. The width and length of the strips are scaled as e changes so that the width is always equal to $e/3$ and length always equals $2e$. Moreover, the outer edges of the vertical strips are maintained at distance e on either side of the fixation point. After Baker and Braddick (1985).

can be perceived as coherent motion. This increase is not entirely unexpected, since most spatial parameters of vision increase with eccentricity (see Chapter 10, this volume). Therefore the maximum range of motion detection is no exception to the rule. However, two features of this result are worth noting. First, the increase in d_{max} with eccentricity implies that direction of large displacements (or high velocities) can be perceived more accurately in peripheral than in foveal vision. This is one of the few ways in which the performance of peripheral vision is actually superior to that of the fovea. Second, the function relating d_{max} to eccentricity does not have the same form as that found for parameters such as minimum angle resolvable (acuity) (see Chapter 10, this volume). Most likely, task-dependent variations in scaling with eccentricity suggest that different visual functions depend on different subpopulations of visual neurons.

B. Determinants of d_{max}

So, d_{max} should not be thought of as a constant; its value depends on the location tested in the visual field. Eccentricity is not the only variable that alters d_{max}; an equally potent variable is the pattern's spatial frequency content. The elements in the random dot cinematogram illustrated in Fig. 3 had quite sharp edges, and this is important in determining the measured d_{max}. For example, if one takes such a cinematogram and adjusts the displacement so that it just exceeds d_{max}, the sensation of motion will cease, as one would expect. However, with the displacement still set at the same value, one can immediately restore the sensation of motion by simply squinting and thereby blurring the image. Thus, blurring, which removes the high spatial frequencies in the pattern, has effectively increased d_{max}. This may also explain why d_{max} is larger in the periphery of the visual field.

Cleary and Braddick (1985) tested the effects of spatial frequency on d_{max} in a more systematic way. They filtered random dot patterns so that they contained only certain narrow bands of spatial frequencies. In three different cinematograms, the center frequencies of these narrow bands were 1.3, 2.7, and 5.3 cycles/degree. Results with these three filtered cinematograms are shown in Fig. 5. The y-axis shows the percentage of errors in observers' directional reports. The values on the x-axis are not expressed in terms of minutes of arc, as the values in some preceding figures had been. Instead, x-axis units are the number of cycles of the center frequency of the band, for each cinematogram. Plotted in this way, the three functions are virtually identical, and in particular d_{max} (taken as the lowest displacement for which the error rate rises to 20%) falls at about the same value for all three cinematograms. However, this constant number of cycles will occupy very different spatial extents (e.g., one cycle of the 5.3 cycle/degree cinematogram covers only about one-fourth the distance covered by one cycle of the 1.3 cycle/degree cinematogram). That is, the similar d_{max} values in Fig. 5 imply a factor of four variation in d_{max} expressed in the usual, angular distance units. Chang and Julesz (1983) have reported rather similar results.

Thus, within a given region of the visual field d_{max} is a function of the spatial frequencies present in the image. Roughly speaking, if a random dot cinematogram consists of big blurry patches, one can see them move over large displacements. There is a great deal

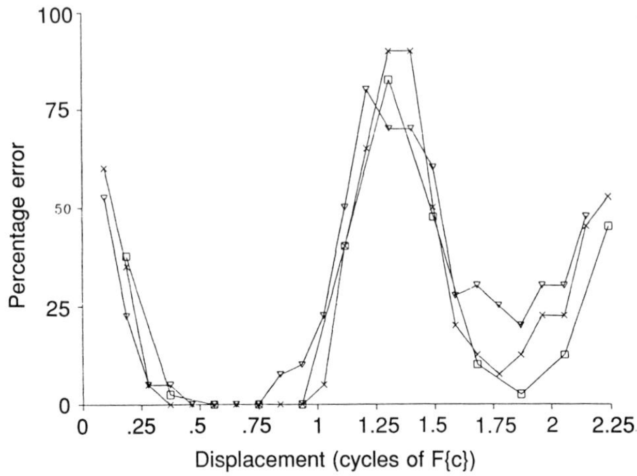

FIG. 5 Directional judgments for displacements in narrow-band (0.5 octave) spatially filtered random dot cinematograms. The three curves are data from patterns whose center spatial frequencies are in the ratio 1:2:4. Displacements are plotted on the *x*-axis as multiples of the period of the center frequency for each pattern. d_{max} is taken as the displacement for which the error rate (*y*-axis) reaches 20% on the first rising part of the curve. The error rate exceeds 50% when the displacement size is between 25 and 50% of the period of the pattern. From Cleary (1988).

of evidence that the visual system contains receptive fields, or channels, with different spatial frequency properties. These results suggest that at any particular location in the visual field, the overall scale of those receptive fields differ, not only in the scale of patterns to which they are sensitive, but also, proportionally, in the scale of displacements that they can detect (cf. Chapter 10, this volume).

There are some other significant features in these data. Figure 5 shows that in terms of the characteristic spatial frequency of a narrow-band cinematogram, d_{max} turns out to be just about one cycle of that frequency. (There are also some interesting oscillations in performance for displacements above one cycle, but we are not concerned with those here.) Several current theoretical models of motion processing imply that the limiting displacement ought to be somewhere between a quarter and half a cycle (e.g., Adelson & Bergen, 1985; Van Santen & Sperling, 1985). The form of the data casts some doubt on such "quadrature phase" models. It implies that correlation mechanisms that underlie motion perception are not necessarily confused by the similarity between one cycle and the next. Therefore, they must be using additional information than simply matching the locations of individual zero-crossings or peaks in the one-dimensional signal. This additional information might be contained in the detailed shape of the waveform, combined information from a range of orientations, or an extended area of the pattern.

A second important implication comes from considering the original, unfiltered, cinematogram. This contains a broad band of spatial frequencies, including the low frequencies which are known to yield a large d_{max}. However, d_{max} for this broadband pattern can still be increased by blurring, which does not add to these low frequencies but simply attenuates the high spatial frequencies. Thus, we conclude that the presence of high frequencies (fine detail) can interfere with the use of motion information potentially available in the low frequencies. That is, although each spatial frequency channel has its own d_{max}, in this situation they do not act independently. This inaccessibility of information carried in the low spatial frequencies when high frequencies are present is reminiscent of the way a static picture can be made unrecognizable by segmenting it into sharp-edged blocks (with high spatial frequencies), as in the well-known "Abraham Lincoln" demonstration (Harmon, 1971). When optically blurred, Lincoln's photo becomes immediately visible. Clearly, independent frequency channels are by no means the whole story, neither with respect to suprathreshold pattern recognition nor with respect to motion perception.

What do these results imply for defining a distinctive short-range process in motion perception? As we have seen, d_{max} varies as a function of the spatial frequencies in the retinal image, and as a function of retinal eccentricity. If this limit is so variable, does the division between "short-range" and "long-range" processes have any meaning at all? Perhaps the perceived motion ascribed to a distinct long-range process occurred in conditions when low spatial frequency information could be used, and consequently

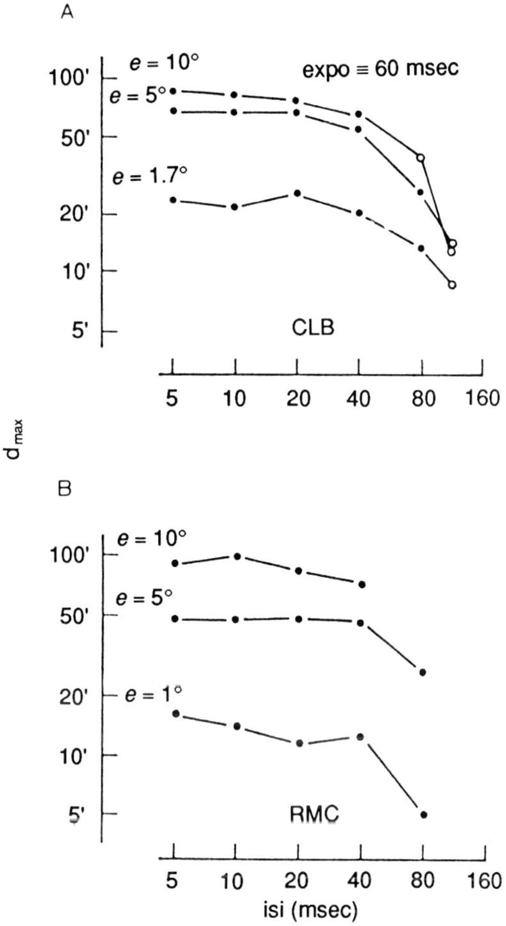

FIG. 6 d_{max} as a function of the interval (isi) between dot pattern exposures, for three different eccentricities with each of two subjects (A and B). For isi values higher than the rightmost point of each curve, the direction of motion could not be reported for any size displacement, so d_{max} can be taken as zero. Each pattern was exposed for 60 msec. From Baker and Braddick (1985).

d_{max} was large. However, the short-range process was not defined solely in terms of its spatial limit. Even though various manipulations can affect the value of d_{max}, certain temporal properties seem to be characteristic of the short-range process.

Take for instance the eccentricity variation mentioned before. Figure 6 shows the results of measuring d_{max} at different eccentricities while also varying the interval between the first and second exposure. As the interval approaches 100 msec all the curves fall off in a similar manner. This temporal variation does not seem to change with eccentricity. And indeed, there is a similar effect with variation in spatial frequency: similar limiting intervals seem to hold regardless of the cinematogram's spatial frequency content. Again, with respect to the more classical kind of apparent motion displays (e.g., Wertheimer, 1912) these are relatively short intervals. Therefore the distinctive temporal aspect of the short-range process holds up across spatial variations, and a different, "long-range" process must be invoked to account for the apparent motion with single elements that can be seen with considerably longer delays.

C. Physiological Correlates of d_{max}

At the beginning of this section, it was suggested that d_{max}, a psychophysical variable, should be related to physiological measures of the range of direction-specific interactions within receptive fields. Figure 7 illustrates some data which may allow us to make this connection. The basic strategy is to measure a neuron's response to a stimulus that is displaced laterally from one brief presentation to the next. As the displacement gradually increases, one notes the displacement at which the responses cease to be directionally selective (e.g., the response to a displacement to the left becomes as strong, or as weak, as that to a displacement to the right). This procedure is analogous to the psychophysical assessment of d_{max}. The data shown in Fig. 7 were gathered by Mikami, Newsome, and Wurtz (1986) from single neurons in macaque monkeys. The stimuli were not random dot patterns as used in the psychophysical d_{max} experiments, but thin bars that appeared to step across the visual field in a series of flash exposures. Triangles represent measurements on directional cells in Area V1, known as the primary visual cortex. As the regression line (dashed) indicates, the physiological analog for d_{max}

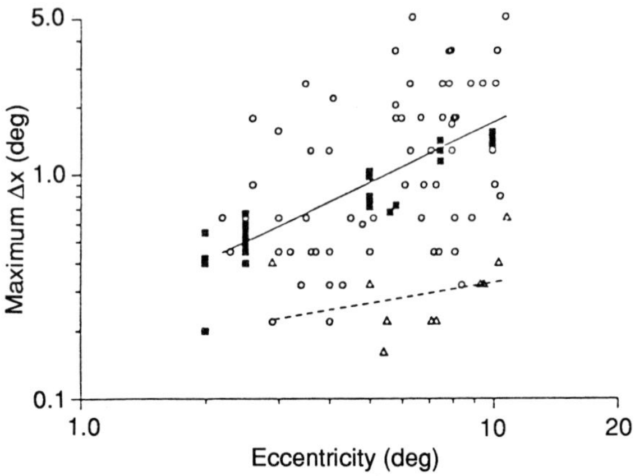

FIG. 7 Maximum displacement for directional response in macaque cortical neurons. Triangles and dashed regression line: cells in Area V1. Circles and solid regression line: cells in Area MT. The squares show human psychophysical data for comparison, taken from the results illustrated in Fig. 4. From Mikami et al. (1986).

varies somewhat with retinal eccentricity. Mikami et al. also studied neurons in cortical area MT, which is believed to be specialized for motion processing. In Area MT, the analog for d_{max} not only grows more rapidly with eccentricity, but also reaches higher values than for V1 cells at comparable eccentricities. Mikami et al. (1986) have plotted some of Baker and Braddick's (1985) data on these same axes (squares). The human psychophysical data seem to correspond much more closely to the maximum displacement for cells in Area MT than in Area V1.

Obviously there are problems in relating the performance of single cells to an observer's performance on some psychophysical task. For one thing, the observer presumably uses the signals coming from a very large number of cells. There are usually differences between stimuli. For instance, the stimulus used by Mikami and associates made many steps as it traversed the receptive field. As we see below, the psychophysical d_{max} is higher when the stimulus takes more than two steps. Nonetheless, it is striking that psychophysically we can detect the direction of displacements that are greater than those that elicit directional responses from any cell in Area V1. It is equally striking that psychophysical performance falls within the range of displacements processed by Area MT cells. Apparently, a major portion of the "machinery" for extracting motion information from successive exposures lies beyond Area V1, that is, beyond the first major direction-selective stage in the magnocellular stream (see Chapter 6, this volume).

When directionally selective units are probed, their directional selectivity does not depend on the stimulus passing right across the receptive field. Rather, any small region of the field shows directional responses (see Barlow & Levick, 1965). In fact, studies such as those by Mikami et al. in macaque cortex (1986) show that the largest displacement which produces a directional response is normally considerably smaller than the cell's receptive field. This has led to the idea that a receptive field is made up of many local subunits each of which is directionally selective (Emerson, Citron, Vaughn & Klein, 1987). Each subunit can generate a signal that contributes to the cell's overall directional response. Yuille and Grzywacz (1988) offered an explicit computational account of how motion information might be integrated over space. Their model gives an excellent account of various psychophysical demonstrations that neighboring regions in the visual field interact cooperatively to produce an overall sensation of motion (Chang & Julesz, 1984; Williams et al., 1986).

IV. INTEGRATION OF INFORMATION

A. Integration of Directional Information

Under certain conditions, stochastic displays can give rise to a percept of global motion, an effect that can shed considerable light on the visual system's strategy for integrating motion over space. To examine this phenomenon, Williams and Sekuler (1984) developed special random dot cinematograms in which all dots drew their successive displacements from a rectangular distribution characterized by some particular directional range. On any frame of the display, the direction in which any single dot moved was (i) independent of its own history of movements and (ii) independent of the movements of other dots. When the distribution of directions covered a broad range of directions, for example, 270–360°, the observer saw only the local, random motions of individual dots. When the distribution of directions covered a narrower range, for example, 90–180°, the observer continued to see those local random motions, but now also saw a global, coherent flow in the general direction of the mean of the distribution.

Williams and Sekuler (1984) measured the probability with which global motion was seen, as a function of the directional distribution's range. They found that as the distribution changed, so did the percept, from random, incoherent motions to global flow, or vice versa. Moreover, the perceptual change tended to be quite abrupt, making for frequency-of-seeing curves that were quite steep.

B. Integration over Time

After exploring a number of the parameters that determined when stochastic motions would yield a global percept of flow, the obvious challenge was to characterize the system that might produce such behavior. Williams et al. (1986) suspected that cooperativity might be involved. Since hysteresis, a form of memory, is regarded as a reliable marker for cooperativity, they set out to determine whether the percept of global flow exhibited hysteresis. In the typical experiment, a trial began with a random dot cinematogram that contained either a narrow or a broad distribution of directions. Then, after some random interval, the distribution changed slowly over successive frames. This change in the direction distribution caused the percept to change, either from global flow to random noise (when the starting distribution was narrow) or from random noise to global flow (when the starting distribution was broad). The dependent measure was the direction distribution at which the percept changed from one state to the other.

The basic finding is simple: the dependent measure varied strongly with the starting state of the stimulus (and, correlatively, the starting state of the percept). If the initial conditions had promoted a percept of global flow, the percept switched states at a relatively broad distribution; if the initial conditions had not promoted a percept of global flow, the percept switched state at a far narrower distribution. Quantitative estimates of the effect of starting state were obtained under several different stimulus conditions. After studying several control conditions, Williams et al. (1986) concluded that the percept, once established, did indeed exhibit a resistance to change, that is, the percept exhibited hysteresis. The results of these experiments were well fit by a model that involved cooperative and competitive interactions among direction-selective units. A network comprising such interactions decides among alternative percepts on a "winner-take-all basis" (Feldman & Ballard, 1982).

C. Integration and d_{max}

One should expect that the visual system would combine motion information not just over space but over time as well. In integration over space, there is one range, within the subunit of the receptive field, that is related to d_{max}, but there is also a larger range over which there are interactions among separate subunits. Analogously, there might be two time constants in the motion system. One time constant might relate to the maximum interval for a single displacement. However, if the subject is presented with a sequence of more than two exposures, information may be integrated over a period much longer than the interval between a single pair of display frames. Figure 8 illustrates this idea with some data from Snowden and Braddick (1987). Using random dot cinematograms, d_{max} was measured as a function of the number of successive exposures per trial. Note that as this number increases, d_{max} increases as well. As Fig. 8 shows, d_{max} increases up to between four and six displacements (see also Nakayama & Silverman, 1984). Clearly, the motion system is gaining extra informa-

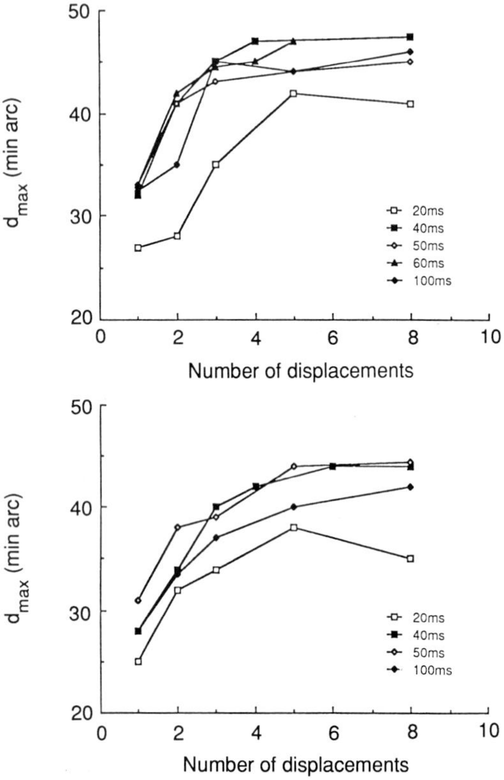

FIG. 8 Increase of d_{max} with increasing number of displacements in a sequence: d_{max} as plotted refers to the size of each individual displacement in the sequence. The different symbols refer to different rates of presentation: the value given in the key is the stimulus onset asynchrony, that is, the time between the onset of successive pattern exposures. Upper and lower panels show data for two different observers. From Snowden and Braddick (1987).

tion from temporal integration over successive displacements. The detector's basic directional response requires two exposures within less than 100 msec, but Fig. 8 shows that this response is enhanced by temporal integration over at least 300 msec.

The results of Fig. 8 show integration over time, but one should not conclude prematurely that the asymptotic performance is determined by the temporal limits of integration. At least over the range shown in Fig. 8, when the entire train of displacements is speeded up or slowed down, the asymptotic number of steps of d_{max} remains constant. The time to reach asymptote varies between about 100 and 400 msec, depending on the rate of presentations. Of course, motion does inevitably involve both time and space: in taking n steps, each of a given d_{max}, the stimulus traverses a particular distance.

Figure 9 is taken from Mikami et al.'s (1986) experiment on the relation between receptive field width and d_{max} for macaque Area MT neurons. As mentioned before, the receptive field widths tend to be much larger than d_{max}, implying some form of subunit structure. The graph plots the ratio between field width and d_{max}. Note that this ratio shows a shallow gradient with eccentricity; between four and seven steps of d_{max} would fit within one receptive field. This finding resembles the kind of asymptotic value found by Snowden and Braddick (1987), suggesting that the limit might be set by the width of the receptive field.

However, further experiments by Snowden and Braddick (1989) suggest that the limiting factor may be neither spatial nor temporal, but simply a constant number of steps. Such a limit might reflect the effec-

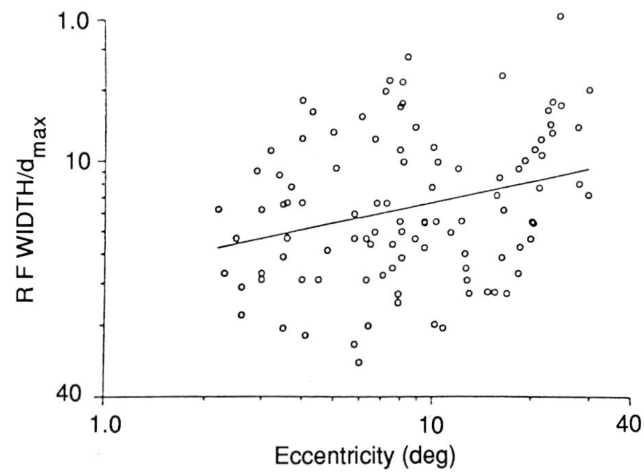

FIG. 9 Ratio of receptive field (RF) width to maximum displacement for directional response, for neurons in macaque Area MT. The plotted regression line indicates the shallow increase of this ratio with receptive field eccentricity. From Mikami et al. (1986).

tiveness with which signals can be propagated from one detector to the next, across a cooperative network. The idea that linked detectors combine information by means of mutual facilitatory and/or inhibitory interactions can be contrasted with the simpler idea of subunits, each having an independent directional response, whose outputs are summated in the motion detector. (Of course, such combinations must have limits on its temporal and spatial range, even if they are not the major factor in these experiments.)

These results imply that in order to understand how neural structures determine psychophysical performance in motion perception tasks, it will not be sufficient to examine the performance of an isolated motion detector. Our perception of motion depends on integrating a number of local neural responses. Clearly, further psychophysical experiments need to be done to characterize this integration. For instance, how far can successive steps at different effective velocities, or in different directions, be integrated? It is hoped that there will also be advances in physiological knowledge that will clarify the neural basis of this integration and of other factors that affect d_{max}.

V. HEURISTICS FOR MOTION PERCEPTION

A. Correspondence Challenges and Correspondence Solutions

In order to extract apparent motion from complex displays, the visual system somehow solves a very difficult problem. Among the thousands of possible element-to-element matches, only one is correct. How does the visual system determine which parts of successive images reflect a single object in motion?

Ramachandran and Anstis (1986a) have suggested that early stages of visual processing of motion uses various heuristics, or rules of thumb, that the human visual system has acquired through millions of years of evolution. These heuristics have been adopted not for mathematical elegance or aesthetic appeal, but merely because they worked. One can learn much about these rules of thumb by watching the visual system as it struggles to solve the correspondence problem.

These rules reflect the fact that in the real world objects move in characteristic, predictable ways. For example, if one's arm moves, neighboring parts of the arm tend to move together. Or, as a football spirals through the air, its parts tend to travel en masse (no piece of the pigskin or the laces are likely to peel off on its own independent course).

The visual system seems to make the correct assumption. At a macroscopic level the physical world is not a chaotic, amorphous mess. The visual system capitalizes on the world's predictable physical properties and limits the matches it must consider by dealing only with matches that would yield perceptions of motion that are plausible in the real, three-dimensional world. Later on, we return to speculate how this scheme might be implemented. To examine the notion that the visual system assumes the world has order, Anstis and colleagues fashioned motion displays that could be interpreted in more than one way and then observed how this ambiguity was resolved (Anstis & Ramachandran, 1986a; Ramachandran & Anstis, 1986b). The resulting percepts, or interpretations, suggested that the visual system was making three different but quite sensible assumptions about the real world: (1) inertia, namely, that moving objects tend to continue moving in the same direction, showing minimal changes in velocity over time; (2) rigidity, that extended surfaces tend to move all in one piece, showing minimal changes in velocity over space; and (3) that moving objects tend to cover and uncover predictable regions of the background.

1. Assumption One: Inertia

The visual system makes one assumption that may remind you of Newton's first law of motion: objects in motion tend to continue their motion along the same path. [Note the resemblance between this statement and the Gestalt law of good continuation (Bruce & Green, 1985).]

Perceptually, once motion is experienced there is a tendency to continue to experience it, even after the motion has actually stopped. Wertheimer's monograph (1912) offered an intriguing demonstration of this fact. He produced apparent motion by a series of alternating presentations of two vertical lines. During the alternations, without warning to the observer, Wertheimer occluded one, leaving the remaining line to appear at its normal time in the sequence. Observers continued to see motion for several "cycles" after the line had been occluded.

Anstis and Ramachandran (1986b) gave an elegant demonstration of this phenomenon in the case of rotary inertia. Figure 10 illustrates one arrangement that shows inertia in rotary motion. First, consider control measurements, which evaluate motion perception with no inertia. The display alternates between a pair of crosses that are rotated 45° relative to one another. These crosses can be thought of as a plus sign and a letter x. When these two spatially overlapping figures are alternated, the apparent motion they set up is ambiguous. Rotation is seen, but it can be either clockwise or counterclockwise (anti-clockwise, if the demonstration is performed in Great Britain). The bottom part of the figure illustrates what happens when an inertia-inducing constraint is added. This constraint is another, tilted, cross, oriented toward eleven o'clock on the watch face. This constraining cross, in frame 1, precedes the sequence of the other two crosses. Now the first two presentations, a tilted cross followed by a plus sign, produce strong motion in a clockwise direction. Interestingly, this strong apparent motion continues when the third element, the letter x, is presented. The first, unambiguous jump, imparts a perceptual rotary inertia that converts the previously ambiguous motion into one that inevitably is seen as clockwise. This may be termed a form of motion bias (priming).

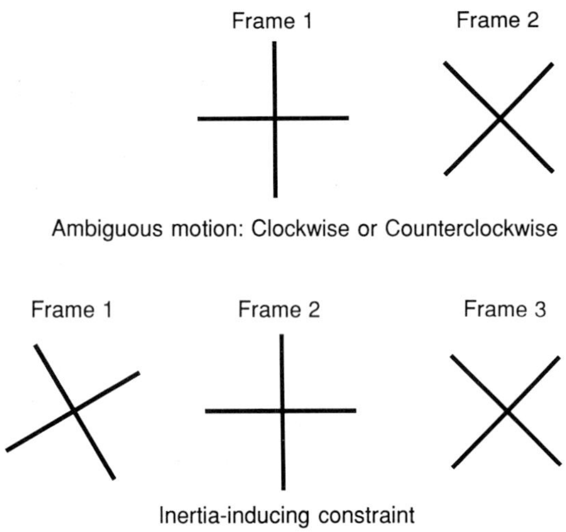

FIG. 10 An arrangement for demonstrating rotary inertia. The top row illustrates the two-frame sequence in a control condition. The display alternates between two, spatially overlapping crosses that are rotated 45° relative to one another. The resulting apparent motion is ambiguous; rotation is perceived either clockwise or counterclockwise. The bottom row illustrates a three-frame sequence designed to show inertia. Note that a new, third cross has been added before the original sequence. The relative orientations of the first and second targets produce strong clockwise motion. This strong motion persists when the third element is presented and the sequence repeated.

2. Assumption Two: Rigidity

Another assumption that could limit possible correspondences is the assumption that objects are rigid; that is, all points on a moving object are assumed to move in synchrony. Though many interesting objects are not rigid in the strict sense, most exhibit at least some local rigidity, a tight coupling between the movements of closely neighboring parts. The tendency for neighboring components to move in similar ways lends considerable redundancy to the motions of neighboring elements within image space. This redundancy would make it economical for the visual system to extract salient features, such as clusters of elements, rather than individual elements, from a complex display and then search for corresponding features in successive images.

This strategy, if it could be implemented, would certainly reduce the number of potential matches without increasing perceptual errors. Take a leopard leaping from a branch of one tree to a branch of another. [Note the resemblance between this statement and the Gestalt law of common fate (Bruce & Green, 1985).] According to the rigidity assumption, a viewer who picks out any salient feature of the leopard, such as its basic shape, and finds the same feature in a second frame need not compare every black spot on the animal at moment t_0 with every single black spot at moment t_1. A highly efficient system might take advantage of the spatial redundancy by attempting to match features on a coarse scale. Consistent with this idea, Ramachandran, Ginsburg, and Anstis (1983) found that the visual system often detects correspondence between regions of similar low spatial frequencies before it detects more detailed outlines or sharp edges. The same heuristic might also account for the way in which a cinematogram's spatial frequency content influences d_{max} (see above).

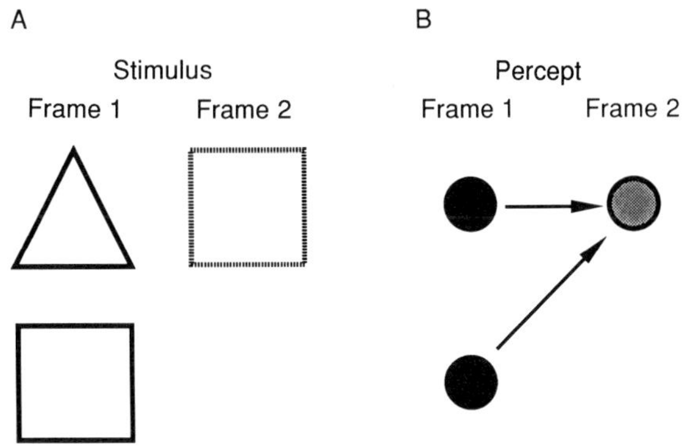

FIG. 11 (A) Display whose first frame comprises a triangle and a square, and whose second frame comprises just a single square located adjacent to the position previously occupied by the triangle. (B) Diagram of the percept produced by the display. The square appears to move obliquely upward and to the right; the triangle appears to move horizontally, ultimately being occluded by the square.

3. Assumption Three: Covering and Uncovering

The visual system appears to make a third assumption, which is a corollary of the other two: a moving object will progressively cover and uncover portions of a background. J. J. Gibson (1968), among others, has called attention to the importance of this fact. When an object, which is normally opaque, temporarily occludes a background, the background still exists; it does not disappear. To see how the third assumption affects perception, consider Fig. 11. Figure 11A illustrates a display in which a triangle and a square below it are presented and then are replaced by another square adjacent to the triangle and directly to its right. As Fig. 11B suggests, one sees the triangle appear to move horizontally, and to hide behind the obliquely moving square, which now appears to occlude a triangle that is not, in fact, being displayed. The visual system seems to assume that an object continues to exist, even if the system has to fabricate the supporting evidence (Anstis & Ramachandran, 1985).

But consider even more complex stimuli. What strategy could the system adopt when presented with many objects simultaneously in apparent motion? The visual system behaves economically, perceiving all objects in a field as moving in the same direction, unless there are unambiguous cues to the contrary.

Figure 12 provides an example of another spatial constraint, one that operates on a more global scale (Ramachandran & Anstis, 1985). Figure 12 shows nine ambiguous quartets of dots, with two dots (either black or shaded) from each quartet appearing in each frame. Under proper conditions, observers report that the dots in each pair sometimes move vertically and sometimes horizontally, though in opposite directions. The percept fluctuates more or less randomly. The interesting point is that all the quartets move in the same direction at any given time. If the dots in any one quartet appear to move vertically, the dots in all the quartets do likewise. Then suddenly they all change step together and move horizontally; the dot quartets entrain each other. There is a strong tendency toward seeing spatial coherence, or, if you like, uniformity across the field (see also Chapter 11, this volume).

The visual system behaves as though it took advantage of certain rules of thumb about the properties of objects in the real world. Naturally, if this viewpoint is more than an interesting metaphor, we need some idea of how such behavior is possible. How might such "assumptions" be implemented, either in neural hardware or in software? Figure 8 gives some hint of

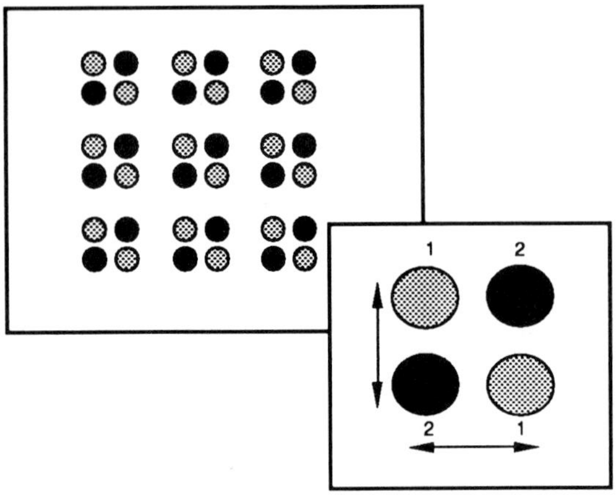

FIG. 12 (Bottom) Quartet of disks that produces a randomly fluctuating percept. When the pair of lighter disks (labeled "1") is presented in alternation with the pair of darker disks (labeled "2") the percept varies randomly. The disks will seem to move either up and down or left and right (as indicated by the arrows). (Top) When many quartets are presented in an array, the random fluctuations of individual quartets seem to be synchronized: at one time all seem to move up and down, and at another time all seem to move left and right.

a reductionistic explanation of this phenomenon. As was noted earlier, Braddick has shown that when the total excursion of some stimulus occurs in a series of small, successive displacements, d_{max} increases. The result is that one is more likely, than otherwise, to see motion in a straight line. Among the interesting questions that remain, though, none is more intriguing than the question of the genesis of these assumptions. Are they represented in neurons that are "hard-wired" from birth to implement those assumptions or strategies? Or do those assumptions become wired into the system as the result of some kind of natural selection at the neural level, a kind of neural Darwinism (Edelman, 1987; see Chapter 13, this volume)?

Because this process depends on the viewer's own experiences with his or her environment, the resultant neural connections would be likely to reflect the properties of objects and motions in that environment. Alternatively, does the perception of motion require some higher level of cognition? Time—and further research—will tell.

VI. CORTICAL MECHANISMS

A. Initial Stages

While various psychophysical phenomena of motion perception are still fresh in mind, let us consider some of the neuronal mechanisms that might contribute to the psychophysical effects that have been discussed so far. Basically, in the visual cortex of cat and monkey three types of cells seem most likely to play major roles in motion perception. Two of these cell types, direction-selective and velocity-tuned cells, seem well suited to provide estimates of local motion as opposed to global motion. The third, more recently discovered type is a motion-segregation or parallax cell. This type of cell may be especially relevant to several of the psychophysical effects described earlier.

When one asks what sort of cells contribute to perceived motion, the first answer that comes to mind is the direction-selective cell (Pasternak, 1986, 1987; Pasternak & Leinen, 1986). In fact, a preponderance of direction-selective cells in one region, such as Area MT, suggests that the region is involved in processing motion information (Albright, 1984; Newsome, Wurtz, Dursteler & Mikami, 1985; Newsome & Pare, 1988). But directional selectivity is not easily defined. It is not only a matter of having a preferred direction of motion, a direction to which the cell responds more vigorously than to any other. Nor is it only a matter of directional asymmetry, in which the cell responds strongly to one direction and little or not at all to the opposite direction. Rather, directional asymmetry may be characterized by some ratio of responses to the motion in the optimal direction over responses to motion in the opposite direction. One commonly used formula is

$$\text{Direction Index} = (R_{pd} - R_{npd})/R_{pd} \times 100,$$

where R_{pd} is the net response to stimulation in the preferred direction, R_{npd} is the net response to stimulation in the direction opposite the preferred direction, and "net response" signifies the difference between the response elicited by the stimulus and the mean spontaneous activity of the cell.

By such an index, cells vary widely in directional asymmetry. Various researchers have advocated using a high value of this ratio, typically an index of 50, as a cutoff between direction-selective and nonselective cells. However, cells' indices of direction asymmetry form a continuous distribution, not a bimodal one.

To make matters even more complex, for many cells, direction selectivity depends on the speed of the moving test target (Orban, Kennedy & Maes 1981). One can then argue that statements about any cell's directional selectivity must be contingent statements, specifying the velocity for which selectivity has been assessed. For this reason, Orban et al. (1981) introduced the mean direction index (MDI) which is a weighted average of direction indices measured at different velocities, using the response strength at different speeds as weighting factors. Finally, the direction selectivity of some cells changes with the sign of the target's luminance contrast (Albus, 1980; Yamane, Maske & Bishop, 1985; Orban, Gulyas, Spileers & Maes, 1987). For such cells, a bright bar on a dark background may yield a different index of selectivity than will a dark bar on a bright background. Perhaps the mean of the mean direction indices for light and dark bars might be a good index of the overall direction selectivity of a cortical cell.

The properties of direction-selective cells might help account for some of the phenomena of apparent motion. A cortical cell's direction selectivity depends on interactions between distinct regions within the receptive field. Indeed, in Area 17 of the cat, if one masks the entire receptive field except for a central strip some 0.3° wide, the mean direction index of cortical cells is reduced to that of lateral geniculate nucleus (LGN) cells. If a moving target is illuminated stroboscopically, direction selectivity to that target is abolished if the gaps between successive flashes are separated too much, either in space or in time (Duysens, Maes & Orban, 1987). This may explain why the short-range motion process in apparent motion operates over short spatial and temporal intervals.

It is important to appreciate that not all direction-selective cells are actually involved in encoding motion of an outside object. Indeed most physiological studies have used a single, isolated stimulus to measure direction selectivity, an artificial condition quite different from those occurring outside the laboratory. Recent results (Orban, Gulyas, & Vogels, 1987; Orban, Gulyas, & Spileers, 1988) demonstrate that in about half the cells in Areas 17 and 18 of the cat, direction selectivity for a foreground stimulus is modified dramatically by the motion of a textured background stimulus (see the solid curve in Fig. 13A and the dashed curve in Fig. 13B). These cells have been implicated either in motion segregation (see below) or in the extraction of depth from motion (Orban, Gulyas & Vogels, 1987). [Related observations have been made by Von Grünau and Frost (1983) in cat lateral suprasylvian gyrus and by Allman et al. (1985) in Area MT of the owl monkey.] Other cells, for which the direction selectivity does not depend on background motion, are most likely to encode motion of an object in the world. Presumably, they could signal the direction of object motion per se, without being strongly affected by the particular moving background against which the object happened to appear.

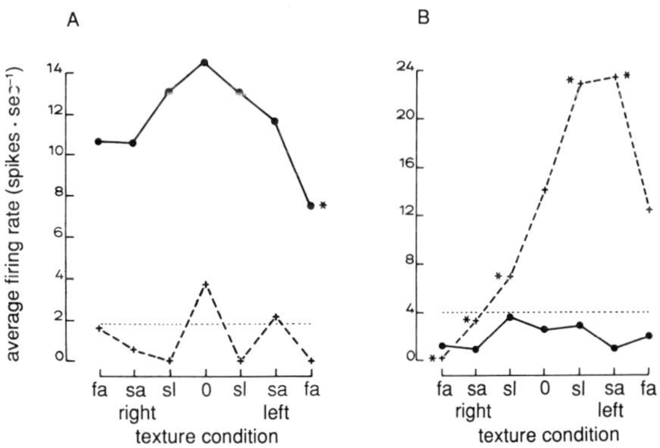

FIG. 13 Responses of cortical cells (cat Area 17) to opposite directions of bar motion as a function of texture motion. The texture was either stationary (0), or moved in the left or right direction, at the same speed as the bar (sa), four times slower (sl), or four times faster (fa). The dotted horizontal lines indicate the significance level; an asterisk indicates a response in the preferred direction that is significantly different from the responses to that direction in the control condition (texture stationary). The neuron in A remains direction selective for all texture motion conditions; the neuron in B loses direction selectivity when the texture moves in phase with the bar. From Orban, Gulyas, and Vogels (1987).

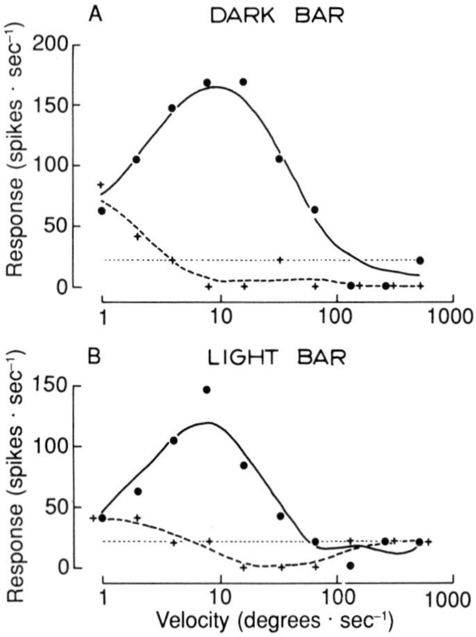

FIG. 14 Responses of a velocity-tuned cell (cat Area 18) to light (B) and dark (A) bars moving in a preferred direction (to the right) or in a nonpreferred direction (to the left). The cell is tuned to the same speed (9.5°/sec) for light and dark bars. For both bars, the cell is not direction selective at 1°/sec, at slow and high speeds, but it becomes completely direction selective at medium speed. From B. Gulyas, L. Lagae, and G. Orban (unpublished).

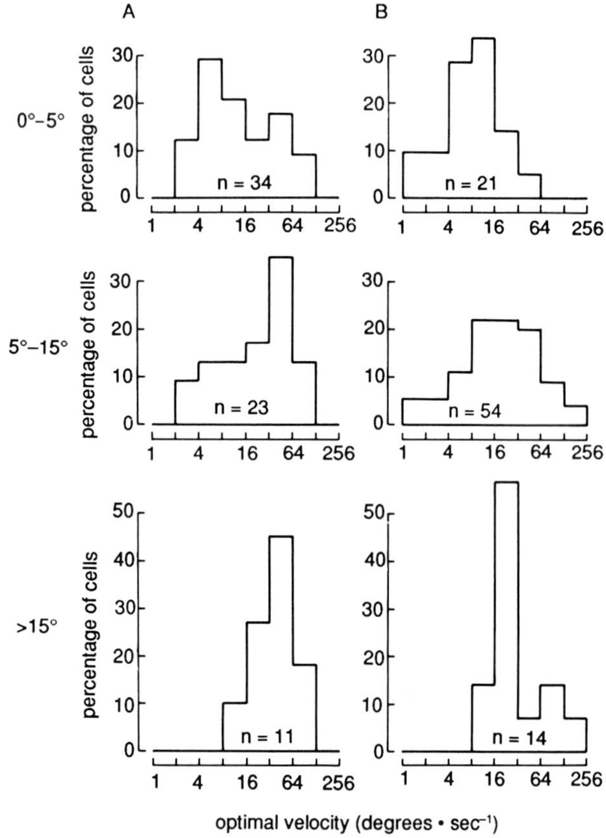

FIG. 15 Percentage of cells plotted as a function of optimal velocity for cells in Areas 17, 18, and 19 of the cat (A) and of Area MT cells with strong velocity tuning in the macaque (B). Distributions are plotted for three ranges of eccentricities (as indicated to the left of the histograms). The third range of eccentricity shown at the bottom extended up to 35° in the cat and up to 25° in the monkey. The data in B are plotted from Maunsell and Van Essen (1983b). From Orban (1985). Copyright © 1985, Martins Nijhoff Publishers, Dordrect, Holland. Reproduced by permission of Kluwer Academic Publishers.

Another type of cell that may be important in motion perception is the velocity-tuned cell (Fig. 14). Note that here the cell's response is a distinctly nonmonotonic function of velocity, for both light and dark moving bars. Velocity-tuned cells typically respond optimally to some intermediate, moderate level of stimulus velocity. Orban and colleagues (Orban et al., 1981; Duysens, Orban, van der Glas & deZegher, 1982) showed that at very high or very low velocities, velocity tuning was absent in Areas 17, 18, or 19 (Fig. 15). The same holds for Area MT of the monkey where many cells are velocity tuned (Maunsell & Van Essen, 1983a,b,c).

This observation leads one to expect that velocity discrimination, measured psychophysically, might also be best at corresponding, moderate stimulus velocities. Velocity discrimination measurements in humans, cats, and monkeys confirm that this is so (Orban, DeWolf & Maes, 1984; Vandenbussche, Orban & Maues, 1986a,b).

In each species, the just noticeable difference in velocity is a U-shaped function of reference velocity. Also note that whereas humans and monkeys give very similar results (minimal just noticeable differences of about 5–7%), cats do more poorly overall (minimal just noticeable differences of about 50%), although under optimal spatiotemporal conditions they may discriminate differences in velocity of about 15% (Pasternak, 1987). It is worth noting that these U-shaped functions remain invariant when measured with random dot patterns rather than moving bars (DeBruyn & Orban, 1986).

Striking though the analogy is, could the resemblance between psychophysical data and physiological data be merely coincidental? Of course one can never rule out such a possibility. However, one can strengthen the argument by exploring other dimensions of analogy. In particular, one can exploit the fact that velocity-tuned cells do not constitute an entirely homogeneous class. Orban (1985), working in both monkey and cat, has shown that the optimal stimulus velocity for velocity-tuned cells varies with receptive field eccentricity. Figure 15 groups cells into three different ranges of eccentricity, 0–5°, 5–15°, and greater than 15°. Note that the optimal velocity increases with retinal eccentricity. One would expect velocity discrimination to show a similar dependence on eccentricity. Orban, Van Calenbergh DeBruyn, and Maes (1985) found, with human observers, that indeed this is the case.

To push the analogy even further, note that velocity-tuned cells lose their tuning when they are tested with slow (2–15 Hz) stroboscopic motion (Fig. 16). Human observers show a comparable disruption of velocity discrimination when they, too, are tested with stroboscopic motion (Fig. 17). A striking example of this is provided by MacKay's (1958) displacement illusion.

In addition to direction- and velocity-tuned cells there is a third group of cells that ordinarily show no selectivity for direction, but do show selectivity under special conditions. Recognizing their potential perceptual role, Orban and Gulyas (1988) have called such cells "motion-segregation" cells. Although mo-

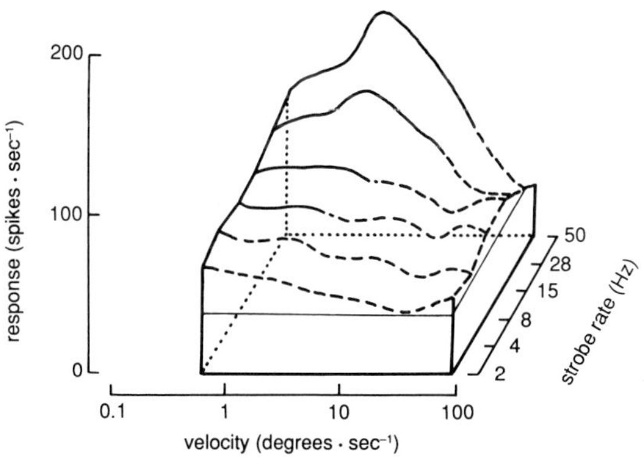

FIG. 16 Three-dimensional plots of response rate in the preferred direction as a function of apparent velocity and strobe rate of a cat Area 17 velocity-tuned cell. The dashed parts of the velocity–response curves indicate responses below the significance level. Horizontal thin lines indicate mean spontaneous activity. From Crumieux, Orban, and Duysens (1984).

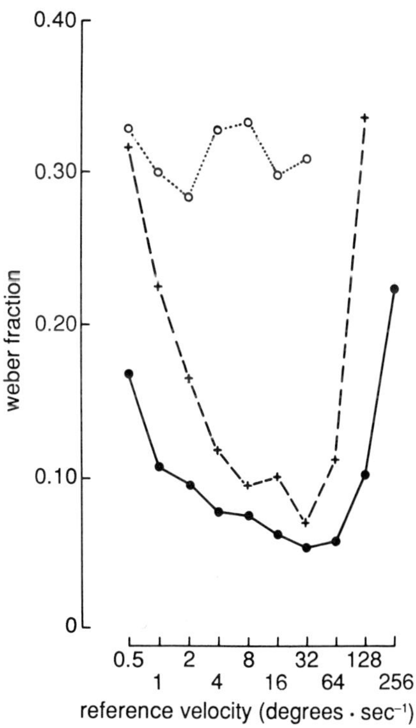

FIG. 17 Just noticeable differences in perceived velocity expressed as Weber fractions ($\Delta\omega/\omega$) and plotted against stimulus velocity (ω). Data are averages from two human subjects. The loss in velocity discrimination at 10 Hz is not due to a reduction in total energy. From B. DeBruyn and G. Orban (unpublished).

tion-segregation cells fall into several distinct classes (Orban, Gulyas & Vogels, 1987), only one is presented here, the so-called anti-phase cell.

When anti-phase cells are tested with a moving bar in the conventional manner (a single moving stimulus with no background movement) they show no direction selectivity. At first glance, then, one might falsely think that these cells play no role in motion perception. However, the cell's response does change markedly when a moving background is introduced. In fact, in the presence of a background of moving, random noise, these cells become strongly directionally selective, and this selectivity is quite complex (Hammond & Smith, 1982, 1984; Hammond, Ahmed & Smith, 1986).

Whatever the direction of the moving background, and whatever the direction of a moving bar superimposed on that background, the cells respond most strongly when the bar moves in a direction opposite to the background motion (Fig. 18). Because they are selective for target motion in a direction opposite to background motion, these cells can be labeled "anti-phase cells" (Orban, Gulyas & Vogels, 1987).

Anti-phase cells fall into two classes. In Area 17 of the cat (Fig. 18) and in Area V1 of the monkey, anti-phase cells exhibit selectivity only along one particular axis of movement. The other class of anti-phase cell, found in Area V2 of the monkey, exhibits selectivity regardless of the axis of motion. So long as foreground and background motions occur in opposite directions, it does not matter much what either direction is. This second class of anti-phase cells re-

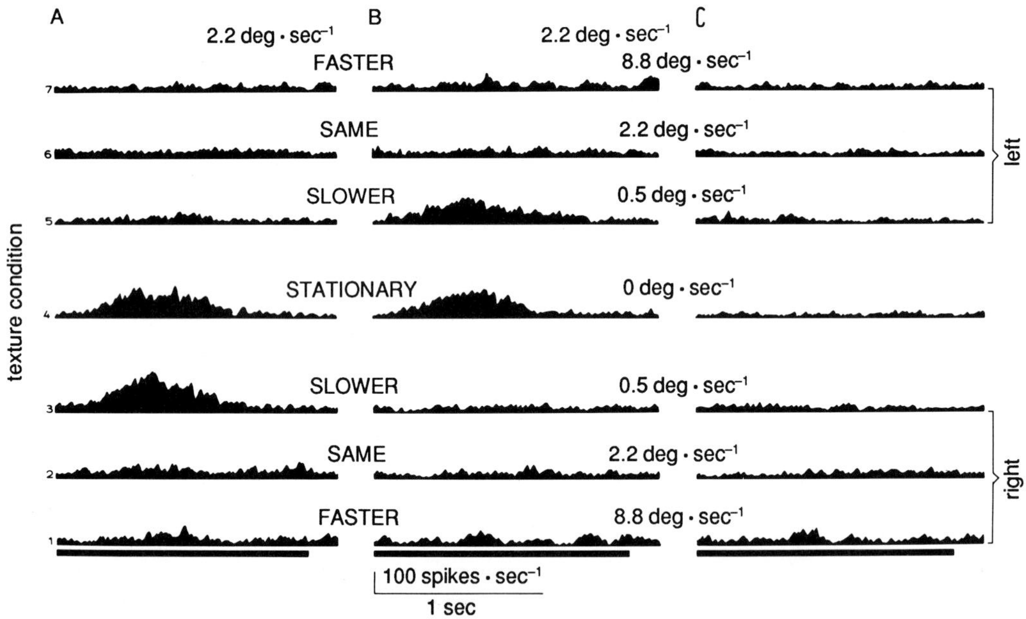

FIG. 18 Poststimulus time histograms (PSTHs) representing the average response ($n = 20$) to a light bar moving horizontally over the texture (A), to the same bar moving in an opposite direction over the texture (B), and to the texture moving on its own (C). This cell was recorded from layer 6 in Area 17 of the cat, and its receptive field was centered 3.4° from fixation. Each row of PSTHs corresponds to a background condition indicated by a number between 1 and 7. Conditions 1 to 3 correspond to texture motion to the left, condition 4 corresponds to a stationary texture, and conditions 5 to 7 to the texture moving to the right. In conditions 2 and 6, the texture moves at the same speed as the bar (2.2°/sec); in conditions 3 and 5, slower than the bar (0.5°/sec); and in conditions 1 and 7, faster than the bar (8.8°/sec). From Orban, Gulyas & Vogels (1987).

sembles the opposed-motion cells found by Frost and Nakayama (1983) in the pigeon tectum.

What perceptual role might be played by motion-segregation cells, including anti-phase cells? They all share a potential for signaling the presence of a difference, in speed or direction, between target and background motion. Commonly, such differences arise when target and background lie in different depth planes. Moving objects occupying different apparent depth planes and traveling in different directions set up shearing patterns of optical flow (Nakayama, 1985). Under some conditions, such shearing gives rise to strong kinetic contours, separating motion in one depth plane from motion in another. The perceptual conditions needed to see the kinetic contours have been studied by Koenderink and van Doorn (1978), among others. These studies add support to the idea that direction-segregation cells, rather than direction-selective or velocity-tuned cells, are involved in the creation of kinetic contours (Orban & Gulyas, 1988). For instance, if one measures the difference in direction of travel for two adjacent random dot cinematograms necessary for producing a kinetic contour, one finds that the direction difference has to approach 30°, a value some 20 times higher than the difference threshold for direction. Interestingly, such large critical differences in direction are precisely what one would expect if motion-segregation cells, not direction-selective cells, played a key role in kinetic contours. Thirty degrees is about the smallest difference between foreground and background motions that elicits a strong response from motion-segregation cells.

The lesson, then, is that motion involves a great many different features, and that the nervous system makes use of several different cell classes to produce those features. Direction selectivity, though surely important, is not the alpha and omega of motion perception.

B. Area MT and the Aperture Problem

One of the major problems of motion analysis is the way in which local motion signals are integrated to provide information about the motion of complex objects and patterns. This class of problem was termed the "aperture problem" because it is readily made explicit when considering measurements of motion made through finite apertures (Movshon et al., 1986). Figure 19A illustrates the problem by considering the motion of two diamond figures, one moving down and one moving to the right.

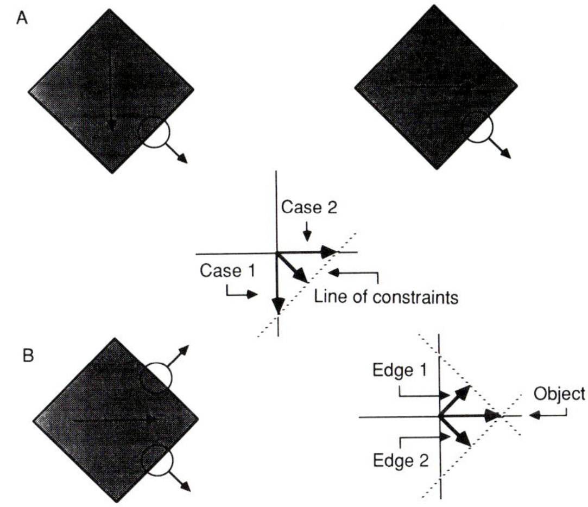

FIG. 19 The aperture problem. (A). Two diamonds, one moving downward and one moving to the right, showing that locally measured motions (circles) do not unambiguously reflect the overall motions of objects. (B) One formal solution to the aperture problem based on using the intersection of the constraints set up by local measurements to resolve their ambiguity.

Although the global motion of these two figures is quite different, a local measurement of motion made in the circles drawn on the lower right-hand border of each diamond would yield the *same* value in each case. The local motion of a border is usually seen as being orthogonal to the border, as shown by the arrows linked to the circular apertures of measurement. This situation is formalized in the lower diagram of Fig. 19, a graph in which the angle of a vector represents direction of motion and its length represents speed. The local measurement of motion made in each of the apertures is not sufficient to define the motion of the whole object: there is an *ambiguity* concerning the motion measured locally. The true motion of the border consists of the measurable component *orthogonal* to the border and some unmeasurable (and therefore locally unknown) component *parallel* to the border (dashed line in Fig. 19). The measurable component is represented by the oblique vector directed down and to the right, and the unmeasurable component is represented by the dashed line orthogonal to it. The motion of the local border thus does not specify object motion completely, but imposes the *constraint* that the motion of the object containing the border must fall somewhere along the dashed line. The true motions in the two cases illustrated (the vertical and horizontal vectors) both correspond to different points along this "line of constraints."

The existence of these constraints makes possible a simple formal solution to this class of aperture problems, if measurements made over two or more contours are combined (Adelson & Movshon, 1982). The form of this solution is shown in Fig. 19B. Measurements made along the upper right border of the figure ("edge 1") provide one line of constraints; measurements made along the lower right border ("edge 2") provide a second line of constraints; the intersection of these two lines ("object") is the only motion consistent with the two constraints, and must therefore yield the motion of the object.

The neural implementation of this model requires that some set of directionally selective neurons integrates signals from several local measurements of motion. Because of the larger spatial scale of Area MT receptive fields and the fact that Area MT receives directionally selective inputs from Areas V1 and V2, it is natural to suppose that MT might be the site of this integration. It turns out that this is indeed the case. Area MT also contains two distinct kinds of directionally selective neurons. *Component* direction-selective neurons, like neurons in Area V1, provide signals about the local motions of individual contours or orientations. *Pattern* direction-selective neurons, found only in Area MT, carry more fully integrated information about motion that emerges from the combination of signals about motion from several different contours or orientations (Movshon et al., 1986). These neurons provide motion signals that are invariant with the orientation of moving contours and represent a degree of abstraction of motion information not seen at lower levels of the visual pathway.

Our knowledge of the functional characteristics of neurons in the portions of the motion pathway beyond Area MT is relatively sketchy. Even the anatomy is not yet fully understood, and it is likely that areas such as Areas MST (medial superior temporal), 7a, and VIP (ventral intraparietal) will ultimately prove to have complex functions related to several different aspects of motion processing. For example, some neurons in Areas MST and 7a respond to complex patterns of motion but not to the simple rigid motion of objects across the visual field. Motter and Mountcastle (1981) have shown a pattern of directional responsiveness in parietal neurons that lends itself to an analysis of optic flow produced by locomotion through the environment. More recently, Saito, Yukie, Tanaka, Hikosaka, Fukada, and Iwai (1986) reported several complex patterns of response in MST neurons, including preferences for rotations, both in the frontoparallel plane and in depth, as well as for optic flow patterns of the kind suggested by Motter and Mountcastle. Still other data suggest a role for the higher areas of the motion pathway in the control of smooth pursuit eye movements (see, e.g., Lisberger, Morris & Tychsen, 1987). Moreover, signals related to motion must also be involved in such basic perceptual tasks as segmentation of complex images (see Nakayama, 1985; DeYoe & Van Essen, 1988). Further analyses of this complex and important neural system will surely yield new insights into the brain's processing of visual images.

VII. MOTION PERCEPTION BY A MOVING OBSERVER

Up to this point, this chapter has emphasized the dependence of motion perception on *afferent* signals. Although such an emphasis is justified, it neglects *efferent* influences on the perception of object motion. Such influences are clearly important. For example, motion perception is strongly influenced by factors such as concurrent self-motion, eye movements, or oculomotor disorders (Brandt & Dieterich, 1988). Although the physiological underpinnings of these effects are not yet understood (Galletti, Bataglini & Aicardi, 1988), they do represent important boundary conditions for the entire field of study.

Under normal everyday conditions, an observer moves freely about within his or her environment. As a result, motion signals arising from the retina subserve two quite different tasks: the observer must control his or her own motion and, at the same time, must also perceive the motion of objects. These two tasks can sometimes be in conflict. For example, while one drives down the road it is difficult simultaneously to perceive movement of roadside tree tops. This fortuitous discovery prompted a series of experiments on object motion perception in the presence of self-motion perception or eye movements. Concern for highway safety lends added importance to the possibility that self-motion and object motion interact. To take but one example, accurate perception of changes in headway, the distance between cars, is essential to safe driving. If a driver's ability to perceive object motion were impaired by movement of his or her own car, the driver would be much disadvantaged when the situation demanded rapid response to changes in headway.

Mean response times to change in headway, the intercar separation, have been taken under actual road conditions and compared with measurements made in the laboratory by nonmoving observers. Laboratory tests simulated a car's rear end, using an ellipse whose size was varied electronically. Measurements were made with two different reference headways, 20 and 40 m. As Fig. 20 shows, detection of headway change is much more difficult under actual road conditions (a) than under static laboratory conditions (b and c). Figure 20 also shows that it makes no difference whether the simulation involves an ellipse (b) or a horizontal bar (c) that changes in size. In either case, detection of change is much better than on the road. These results suggest that extrapolations from static, laboratory conditions to predictions of detection on the roadway may underestimate roadway reaction times by as much as several hundred milliseconds (Probst, Krafczyk, Brandt, & Wist 1984; Probst, Krafczyk & Brandt, 1987).

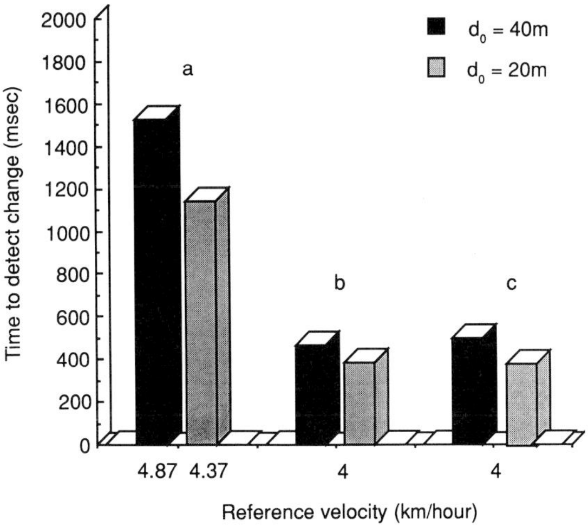

FIG. 20 Object motion perception under actual road and simulated conditions. Mean response times were determined for the perception of changes in headway at distances of 20 and 40 m under actual conditions (a) and simulated conditions without concurrent self-motion (b and c). In measurements for actual road conditions, the subject was in a moving car. In the laboratory, an approximation of the perceptually effective area of the rear of the leading car was simulated by an electronically generated ellipse of equivalent retinal size. Headway changes were simulated by adjusting the retinal ellipse area. The times to detect changes in headway were significantly higher for the actual road condition. Under static conditions in the laboratory there was no difference between the detection of a gradual change in area of the ellipse (b) and a horizontal bar with the same but one-dimensional movement (c). After Probst et al. (1984). Copyright 1984 by the AAAS.

The next experiment deals with the perception of frontoparallel, object motion while the observer's eyes, head, or trunk are also in motion. Figure 21 shows that the threshold for detection of object motion increases during concurrent head motion and fixation of the moving target. Data are shown for several different rates of oscillation about the vertical axis, ranging from 0 to 1.5 Hz. The oscillations had an amplitude of plus and minus 20°. Notice also that similar results can be obtained without eye or head movement; neck stimulation produced by rotating the

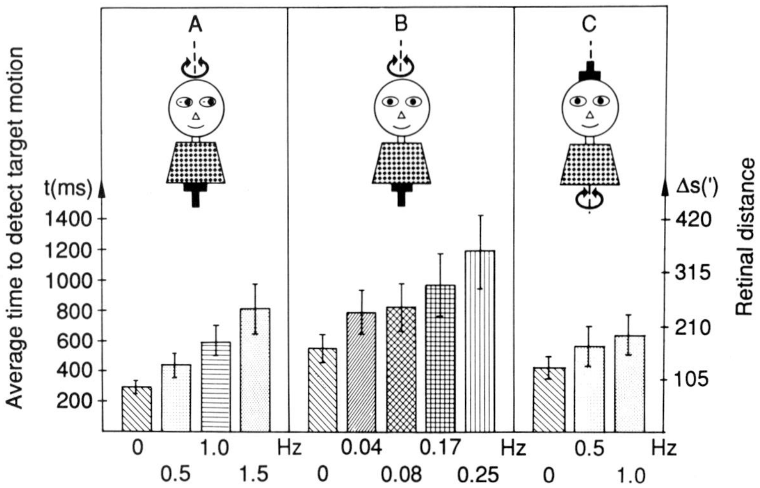

FIG. 21 Object motion perception with head or trunk oscillations. Mean response times (in milliseconds) are plotted as a function of oscillation. Target speed was 5°/sec. There were three modes of simultaneous body motion. The target was fixated during horizontal head oscillation with vestibular–ocular reflex (VOR) (A), with fixation suppressed (B), or with the head fixed by the helmet and pure cervical stimulation provided by trunk oscillations (C). The abscissa shows different frequencies of oscillation. Response time to detect object motion increases with increasing frequency of either head or trunk oscillations.

trunk relative to the head can also elevate the threshold for object motion (Brandt, 1982; Probst, Brandt & Degner, 1986).

Finally, consider the perceptual consequences of certain oculomotor disorders. The patients whose perceptions are described had an acquired palsy of the oculomotor, trochlear, or abducens nerve (i.e., the third, fourth, or sixth cranial nerves). All these patients had difficulties in object motion perception (Brandt & Dieterich, 1986; Dieterich & Brandt, 1987). For example, Fig. 22 shows motion perception in a patient's affected and unaffected eyes. The figure also shows the performance of age-matched control observers. The dependent variable is the time required to detect a moving object. Generally, paresis seems to be associated with a suppression of motion perception.

Though suppression of perception of object motion is decidedly abnormal in patients with eye muscle paresis, such suppression confers certain benefits. The perceptual suppression reduces or eliminates the oscillopsia (illusory perceptual jitter) that would otherwise accompany head movements. This is partly confirmed by the fact that the perceived amplitude of oscillopsia in these patients is always smaller than the net retinal slip. Figure 23 shows that the same holds

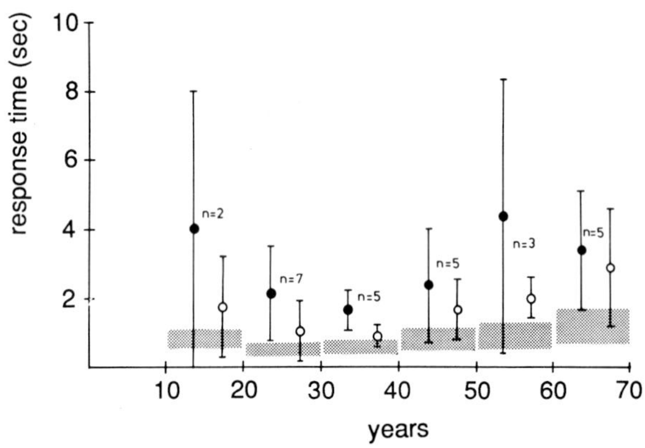

FIG. 22 Response times (means and standard deviations) required to detect horizontal object motion as a function of subject age. The stimulus moved at a constant angular velocity of 24 min/sec. The shaded areas represent results from a control group, 60 neurological patients without ocular motor disturbances ($n = 10$ for each decade from 10 to 70 years). Response times are shortest at about 20 years of age, with increasing mean values and standard deviations in the elderly. For comparison, the data from 27 patients with acquired extraocular eye muscle pareses are shown. These patients exhibit longer response times for monocular vision with the affected eye (filled circles) as well as the normal eye (open circles). Impairment of motion perception is more pronounced for the affected eye.

FIG. 23 Object motion perception as a function of the eccentricity of horizontal gaze in patients with congenital nystagmus and acquired downbeat nystagmus. Thresholds for detection of object motion (24 min/sec; means and standard deviations) as a function of the eccentricity of horizontal gaze in patients suffering from congenital nystagmus and acquired downbeat nystagmus are compared to normals. Thresholds are indicated, on the left ordinate, as Δt (exposure time in seconds) or, on the right ordinate, as Δs (displacement of stimulus in minutes of arc). Normals first show only a slight increase in thresholds with eccentric gaze and then show a more pronounced increase on lateral gaze of 40°. However, whether the ocular oscillation is congenital or acquired, the patients' thresholds are significantly raised. There is a large increase in threshold for directions of gaze beyond 20°. As a result the amplitude of the nystagmus is increased.

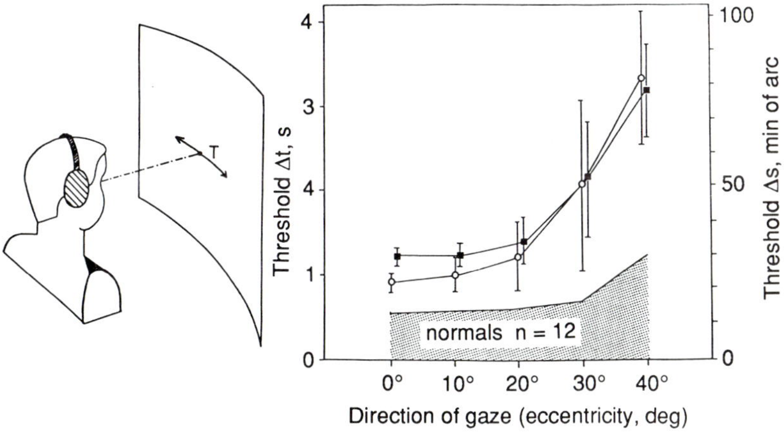

for patients with an acquired downbeat nystagmus (quick involuntary vertical oscillations of the eye; usually a sign of central nervous system dysfunction) or congenital nystagmus (Dieterich & Brandt, 1987).

VIII. CONCLUSIONS AND SPECULATIONS

This chapter has tried to reinforce the notion that the field of motion perception is not completely unified. The diversity of motion becomes particularly clear when one considers the physiological processing of motion information. Different aspects of motion may be processed, or made explicit, at different stages of the magnocellular stream. As DeYoe and van Essen (1988) emphasize, "motion cues can be used in a diverse range of computational tasks, only some of which are directly related to the perception of object motions *per se*." Thus, although the magnocellular stream has often been linked to motion perception, that link, or those links, may turn out to be quite complex and varied (Van Essen & Maunsell, 1983).

For example, suppose we assert that some particular psychophysical aspect of motion processing emerges at one stage of the magnocellular stream. This assertion assumes what Teller (1984) terms "transparency," the assumption that subsequent stages of the system do nothing to undo this emergent achievement. In other words, those subsequent stages must be transparent. The heterogeneity of neural properties at any one stage of the magnocellular stream presents quite a different challenge. Many people have recorded from cortical regions that may be involved in motion processing. Nearly every one of those researchers (e.g., Orban, 1986) has commented on the extraordinary cell-to-cell variability in directional selectivity. Because some of the cells at one stage in the magnocellular stream have properties that parallel human psychophysics in some interesting way, one might be tempted to link psychophysics to the behavior of such cells. However, this fails to account for what the remaining cells in the area are doing, or are not doing. Can we explain how the system filters out those responses? Or do those responses act as kind of noise?

Researchers interested in motion perception have recently begun to explore these questions. For example, Newsome and Wurtz (1988) used a neurotoxin, ibotenic acid, to create a localized, chemical lesion in Area MT of the monkey. Such lesions produced large, temporary losses in the ability to initiate smooth pursuit eye movements. There is an even more dramatic, hypothetical experiment in which one might ask what everyday vision would be like if one did not have Area MT. This question is interesting, because of a clinical report of a patient who purportedly had lost the tissue of Area MT and neighboring areas (Zihl, von Cramon & Mai, 1983). This patient was extraordinarily impaired on many different tests of movement perception, particularly tests that involved moderate and faster motions (as opposed to very slow motion). One might assume, then, that loss of Area MT would impair motion perception in a similar manner as the brain lesion impaired performance in this patient. Yet, if a macaque monkey's Area MT is removed bilaterally and *in toto*, the monkey has no trouble moving around or even responding to objects such as people who move toward the monkey or near it (A. Cowey, unpublished observations).

One possibility is that those signals on which we base motion perception come through Area MT, when Area MT is available. However, various studies show that if Area MT is destroyed, a relatively short period in which motion perception is severely impaired is followed by a rapid recovery of function. Unfortunately, the patient described by Zihl et al. (1983) never experienced anything like the recovery that the monkeys do, perhaps because the patient's damage was more extensive.

To return to the first example given at the beginning of this chapter: Exner's demonstration that motion is not merely a derivative from separate analyses of time and space. This demonstration notwithstanding, it is entirely possible that some everyday problems of motion perception could be solved by analyzing *where* things are and *when* they are there, without actually making the motion signal explicit. In other words, target motion does not in and of itself guarantee that the target is processed by a specialized motion-processing system. For example, when a target moves extremely slowly, does perception of that target necessarily depend on the special "machinery" normally involved with motion perception? A major challenge for future research is learning to define the conditions under which Exner was right.

ACKNOWLEDGMENTS

Preparation of this chapter was supported by grants to the authors from U.S. Air Force Office of Scientific Research, Natural Sciences and Engineering Research Council of Canada, British Medical Research Council, National Institutes of Health, and National Research Council of Belgium.

10

THE PERCEPTION OF FORM
Retina to Striate Cortex

Hugh R. Wilson, Dennis Levi, Lamberto Maffei,
Jyrki Rovamo, and Russell DeValois

I. INTRODUCTION

The successive transformations of spatial and temporal information in the retina, lateral geniculate nucleus (LGN), and striate cortex provide the basis for form vision and pattern discrimination in cats, primates, and humans. The resultant cortical representation facilitates the extraction of salient features, such as the location and orientation of lines and edges, but it also imposes restrictions on pattern discrimination. Following the pioneering neurophysiological research by Enroth-Cugell and Robson (1966) and the psychophysical studies of Campbell and Robson (1968), recent vision research has utilized the concepts of systems theory (both linear and nonlinear) to elucidate the nature of the cortical representation of spatial information (see DeValois & DeValois, 1988). As a result, the responses of single units or cells are now described in terms of their spatial filtering characteristics, which may be equivalently described either as a spatial receptive field or in the Fourier domain as a sensitivity to sine and cosine gratings as a function of spatial frequency, orientation, and phase. In addition to single-unit filtering characteristics, it is also crucial to determine the spatial sampling capabilities of two-dimensional arrays of neural elements in order to estimate their ability to represent accurately spatial information in accordance with the sampling or Nyquist theorem (see Eq. 2, p. 234). Finally, evidence that different stimulus attributes, such as motion, depth, and color, are processed in parallel and partially independently in striate and extrastriate cortex (see Chapters 6, 7, 8, and 11, this volume) is discussed. The plan of this chapter, then, is to review the spatial sampling and filtering characteristics of the visual system beginning with the photoreceptor array and proceeding to the ganglion cells, LGN, and striate cortex. In each instance, anatomical, physiological, and psychophysical data are integrated to emphasize the substantial agreement arising from these diverse approaches. Following this, pattern discrimination is discussed as a manifestation of the spatial information processing capabilities of the system. Finally, important issues raised by the current state of our understanding are discussed.

II. OPTICAL FILTERING AND PHOTORECEPTOR SAMPLING

Grating acuity provides a fundamental measurement of the spatial capabilities of the visual system. It is usually measured by requiring a subject to determine whether a small patch of a square wave grating 5–10 cycles in width has vertically or horizontally oriented bars. Typical grating acuities for young adults with normal vision range from about 30 cycles per degree (cpd), which corresponds to 20/20 vision, to just below 60 cpd (20/10 vision), with the average being about 42 cpd or 20/14. For reference, the width of one's thumb at arm's length is approximately 2°, so that the grating resolution limit corresponds to 60–120 cycles across the thumb at this distance. A more complete description of visual function is provided by the contrast sensitivity function (CSF), which measures the visibility of sine or cosine gratings as a function of their spatial frequency.[1] Designating the mean luminance of the display by L_{mean} and the spatial frequency by ω, a vertically oriented cosine grating of contrast C is described by the intensity distribution $I(x)$:

$$I(x) = L_{\text{mean}}\,[1.0 + C\cos(2\pi\omega x)] \qquad (1)$$

To measure the CSF, the value of C is adjusted until the pattern is at the visibility threshold (typically 75% correct discrimination in a two-interval forced choice paradigm), and this procedure is repeated for a range of spacial frequencies ω.[2] The sensitivity at each spatial frequency is defined as the reciprocal of C at threshold, and the CSF is then a plot of sensitivity versus spatial frequency.

Measurement of the CSF in the fovea results in a curve with a peak sensitivity of 100–300 occurring at 3–5 cpd and a decline in sensitivity at both lower and higher spatial frequencies, as shown by the open circles in Fig. 1. This curve shape is typical for measurements taken at low temporal frequencies (e.g., below 2 Hz) and at photopic luminances (see Kelly, 1972a, for data on the effects of light adaptation). When the CSF is measured at different retinal eccentricities, results such as those shown in Fig. 1a are obtained (Rovamo, Virsu & Näsänen, 1978; Rovamo & Virsu, 1979; Virsu & Rovamo, 1979). It is clear that for a fixed size of grating the maximal sensitivity, peak frequency, and highest resolvable spatial frequency all decrease with increasing eccentricity. Thus, the first question that must be answered in studying form vision is, why does the CSF vary in these characteristic ways as a function of eccentricity?

From the early work by Østerberg (1935) and more recent data of Curcio, Sloan, Packer, Hendrickson, and Kalina (1987, see open squares in Fig. 2) it is well known that the density of human cones declines dramatically as one moves outward from the fovea into the peripheral retina. However, the ratio of cones to ganglion cells is roughly constant from 0° to 10° (Perry & Cowey, 1985). Therefore, Virsu and Rovamo (1979; Rovamo & Virsu, 1979) reasoned that if the area of a cosine grating patch was adjusted at each eccentricity so as to stimulate the same number of ganglion cells, then one might expect the peak sensitivity to be the same at all eccentricities. Second, they reasoned that if spatial frequency were measured relative to the reciprocal of ganglion cell receptive field spacing at each eccentricity, then the peak frequencies and the high frequency cutoffs should be the same at all eccentricities. As shown in Fig. 1b, these predictions were confirmed experimentally by Rovamo and Virsu (1979), and this result has been extended to suprathreshold contrast matching by Swanson and Wilson (1985). It should be said here that Rovamo and Virsu (1979) believed that the reciprocal of ganglion cell receptive field spacing was directly related

[1] In this chapter the terms cosine grating and sine grating will be used interchangeably. The only difference is the phase relative to the fixation point, and contrast thresholds for the two are identical.

[2] In addition to the two-interval forced choice procedure, several others are frequently used to measure the CSF. These include a single interval seen/not seen procedure and the method of adjustment.

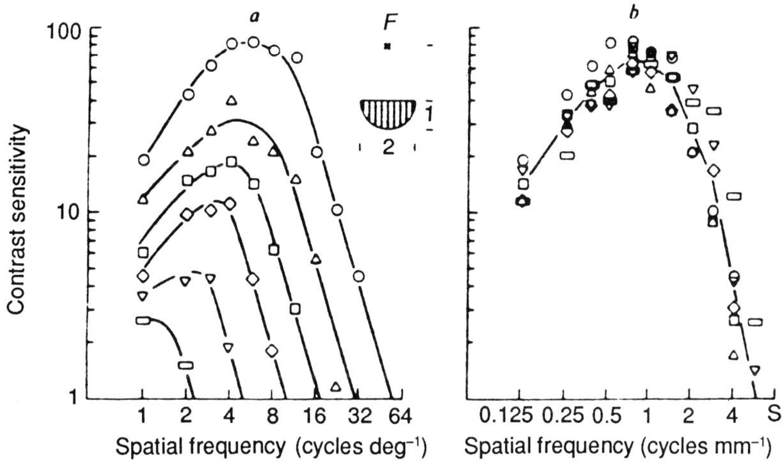

FIG. 1 Contrast sensitivity as a function of spatial frequency and retinal eccentricity. (a) Sinusoidal test gratings of 1° × 2° were used at different eccentricities as shown in the inset. Different curves refer to different eccentricities. From the highest curve downward these were 0°, 1.5°, 4°, 7.5°, 14°, and 30°. (b) Contrast sensitivity data gathered with a grating patch that was scaled in size by the inverse of the local ganglion cell spacing. When spatial frequencies are plotted in units proportional to local ganglion cell spacing, the CSF at all eccentricities assumes a common shape. From Rovamo et al. (1978). Copyright © 1978 Macmillan Journals Limited.

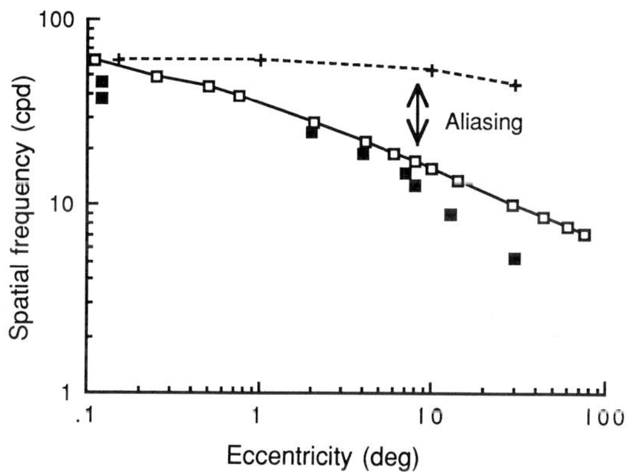

FIG. 2 Relationship between the optical line spread functions of the human eye, the Nyquist limit of the foveal cone mosaic, and psychophysically measured grating acuity. The quality of the ocular media is constant out to eccentricities of about 10° and is sufficient to transmit spatial frequencies up to about 60 cpd (dashed line). Open squares and the solid line represent the Nyquist limit imposed by the spacing of the foveal cones, and solid squares show typical grating acuity data. Note that grating acuity falls slightly below but parallel to the cone Nyquist limit at all eccentricities less than 20°. As the optical quality is significantly higher than the Nyquist limit beyond about 1°, aliasing should occur in the near periphery (arrow).

to distances in visual cortex, but subsequent research has indicated that this is not quite correct (see Section III).

Let us examine the basis for grating acuity and its variation with eccentricity in greater detail. As light intensity can never fall below zero, the maximum possible contrast for the cosine stimulus in Eq. (1) is unity. Thus, acuity may be defined as the highest spatial frequency resolvable with a grating of unity contrast. Typical grating acuities at a range of eccentricities are shown by the solid squares in Fig. 2. What limitations are placed on grating acuity by the optics of the eye and the density of photoreceptors? Campbell and Gubisch (1966) have measured the line spread function for the optics of the human eye and have reported that under ideal conditions it is about 1.2 min arc wide at half-height. From their measurements it is possible to calculate that the optics of the eye will reduce the contrast of the image of a 60 cpd grating by a factor of about 100, rendering the grating lines unresolvable. As optical quality does not change very much within the central 20° (Jennings & Charman, 1981), it follows that 60 cpd may be taken as a reasonable estimate of the central acuity limit imposed by the optics. This is shown by the dashed line in Fig. 2. As the acuity data (solid squares) fall far below this except at the center of the fovea, it is clear that the optics do not limit grating acuity other than in the fovea.

The role of cone density in limiting grating acuity can be determined from the sampling or Nyquist theorem. In the present context this theorem is most conveniently stated as follows:

Nyquist Frequency: Consider a system that encodes spatial patterns by values at a series of uniformly spaced sample points. If the spacing between samples is Δx, then the system can exactly represent sine or cosine gratings of all spatial frequencies up to the Nyquist frequency, ω_N, where

$$\omega_N = \frac{1}{2\Delta x} \tag{2}$$

In other words, such a system can exactly represent any cosine grating for which there are at least two spatial samples per cycle. From Fourier analysis, which demonstrates that any spatial pattern may be described as a sum of sine and cosine gratings of various orientations and contrasts (e.g., Bracewell, 1965; Gaskill, 1978), it follows that a system with discrete spatial samples can exactly encode any pattern that contains only frequencies below the Nyquist frequency ω_N. The foveal cones comprise an almost perfect hexagonal mosaic (Hirsch & Hylton, 1984), and therefore visual acuity should be limited by the Nyquist frequency for the cones. From the data of Curcio et al. (1987) it is easy to estimate cone spacing at various eccentricities by taking the square root of cone density. [For a hexagonal array the spacing of neighboring rows of cones along the principal axes is $\sqrt{3}/2$ closer than the individual cones themselves.]

The resulting estimates of the Nyquist frequency for the cones are plotted by the open squares and solid line in Fig. 2. It is clear that typical grating acuities (solid symbols) are parallel to but slightly below the cone Nyquist limit, thus indicating that grating acuity is largely determined by the variation of cone spacing with eccentricity from 0° to 10°, as had been suggested by Rovamo and Virsu (1979).

In comparing acuity as determined by the Nyquist frequency for the cones in Fig. 2 with the acuity limit imposed by the optics an interesting point arises. The optics of the eye will only transmit spatial frequencies up to the cone Nyquist limit in the fovea, and thus foveal optics and cone spacing are tailored to one another. In the periphery, however, the cone Nyquist frequency falls rapidly, while the optical transfer function remains almost constant out to 10°. As a consequence, grating frequencies higher than the Nyquist limit for the cones are imaged on the peripheral retina. This should lead to spatial aliasing, whereby frequencies above the Nyquist limit appear as distorted gratings of lower frequency. Recent psychophysical evidence has indeed indicated the presence of spatial aliasing in perifoveal vision (Coletta & Williams, 1987; Smith & Cass, 1987; Thibos, Cheney & Walsh, 1987). However, the deleterious effects of peripheral aliasing are reduced somewhat by the irregularity of the peripheral cone mosaic, which is apparently perturbed by the presence of rods (Yellot, 1982, 1984). It may be noted that aliasing can also occur in the fovea if blurring by the optics is eliminated through the use of laser interference fringes (Williams, 1985a,b, 1986). Indeed, the lowest spatial frequency at which aliasing is first perceived has been used to estimate the foveal Nyquist frequency and hence the foveal cone spacing psychophysically (Williams, 1985a). The result, about 35 sec arc, is in excellent agreement with anatomical data (Curcio et al., 1987).

III. SPATIAL SAMPLING, CORTICAL MAGNIFICATION, AND HYPERACUITY

Signals from the cones are transferred via bipolar cells to retinal ganglion cells, whose axons project to the LGN. There they synapse onto relay cells that in turn project to layer IV of striate cortex. Two distinct classes of ganglion cells have been identified in the monkey: the Pα, which project to the LGN magnocellular layers; and the Pβ, which project to the parvocellular layers. To carry the spatial sampling analysis of the visual system further, it is necessary to know the numbers of ganglion, LGN, and cortical neurons per cone. Comparison of ganglion cell and cone densities in the monkey suggests that the ratio is approximately 1 : 1 in the fovea, but beyond about 10° eccentricity this ratio decreases so that there is only about one ganglion cell for every two cones (Perry & Cowey, 1985). Thus, the foveal ganglion cells appear to have the same Nyquist limit as the cones, thereby accurately representing spatial information, while the peripheral ganglion cells actually undersample the cone mosaic. In the LGN this difference between central and peripheral representations is further accentuated, as there are two to three LGN relay cells per ganglion cell axon for the foveal representation, but only about one per two ganglion cell axons for the periphery (Connolly & Van Essen, 1984).

Although there is general agreement on the basic features of the mapping from the photoreceptors to striate cortex, Schein and De Monasterio (1987) have argued that the variation with eccentricity is significantly different for the magno- and parvocellular pathways. They conclude from a careful examination of the available data that the density of parvocellular (P-cell) afferents to striate cortex is almost constant at all eccentricities. In contrast, the density of magnocellular (M-cell) afferents increases about tenfold from fovea to far periphery. P-cells have small receptive fields, slow axonal conduction velocities, and color-opponent responses, whereas the M-cells have higher contrast sensitivity, larger receptive fields, faster conduction velocities, and broadband luminance responses. Therefore, different visual functions might be expected to show very different eccentricity variations. It is the P-cell afferents that appear to be directly related to cortical magnification (see below). As our discussion of the eccentricity variation of psychophysical properties focuses mainly on acuity tasks requiring small receptive fields, most of the following discussion is related to P-cell properties.

Given these data on spatial sampling at subcortical levels, it is convenient to focus on the overall mapping from retina to striate cortex, where the accentuation of central vision is even greater (Dow, Snyder, Vautin & Bauer, 1981; Van Essen, Newsome & Maunsell, 1984). On average there are about 1,000 striate cells per incoming LGN axon for the fovea, but only about 100 for the far periphery (Connolly & Van Essen, 1984). Combining this with the estimates of ganglion cell to LGN convergence above, it follows that there should be about 100 times more striate cells per cone in the foveal representation than in the far periphery. This is close to independent estimates by Dow et al. (1981). Reasons for this profusion of cortical cells will become clear subsequently.

Figure 3 summarizes the mapping from visual space (A) to LGN (B) and onward to striate cortex (C) in the macaque, where it is apparent that over 40% of the striate area is devoted to processing information from the central 5° of the visual field. To describe the mapping from retinal coordinates to striate cortex Daniel and Whitteridge (1961) introduced the notion of the cortical magnification factor, which is defined as millimeters of cortex per degree of visual angle. The cortical magnification factor, M_C, has been shown to be accurately described by the following relationship:

$$M_C = \frac{M_F}{1 + \frac{E}{E_2}} \quad (3)$$

where E is the retinal eccentricity in degrees, and E_2 is the eccentricity at which magnification has changed by a factor of 2. The foveal magnification, M_F, has generally been reported to fall in the range from 6 to 13 mm/degree (Daniel & Whitteridge, 1961; Van Essen et al., 1984).

Before discussing estimates of E_2, it may be noted that if one views M_C as an approximation to the derivative of radial cortical distance, D, with respect to visual angle, simple integration yields an expression for the mapping from retina to cortex:

$$D = \int_0^E \frac{M_F}{1 + \frac{E'}{E_2}}\, dE' = M_F E_2 \ln\left(1 + \frac{E}{E_2}\right) \quad (4)$$

Here D gives the distance from the mapping of the foveal center to the mapping of a point at eccentricity E. Although E_2 does vary somewhat with polar angle (Van Essen et al., 1984), Eq. (4) nevertheless provides a reasonable first approximation. This deri-

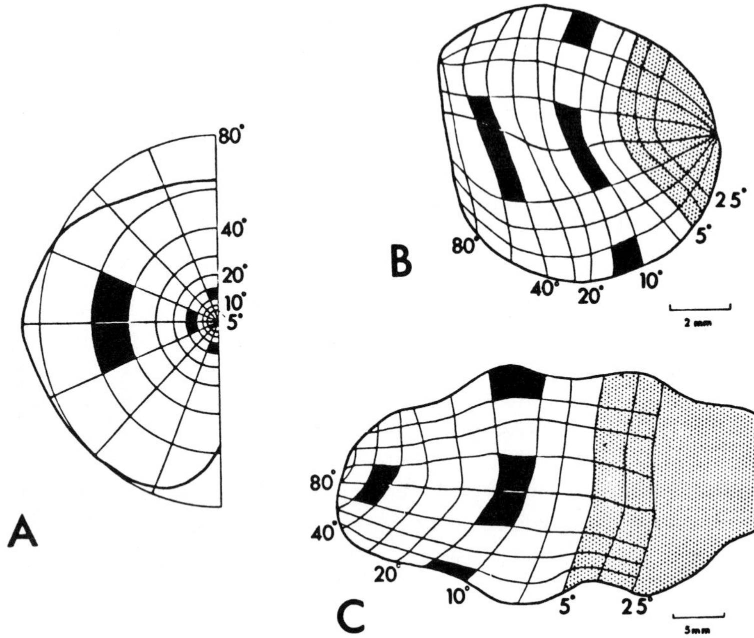

FIG. 3 Representation of the visual field (A) in the lateral geniculate nucleus (B) and striate cortex (C) of the macaque. The spherical visual field has been divided into small, approximately square regions by a grid of isoeccentric and isopolar circles. The bold line represents the outer perimeter of the visual field. The transformations of the grid are shown in the LGN and striate cortex, where several visual field compartments have been darkened to facilitate comparison. The representation of the central 5° field (stippled) occupies about 40% of the cortex. From Connolly and Van Essen (1984).

vation and its perceptual consequences were first pointed out by Fischer (1973) and subsequently exploited by Schwartz (1980, 1984). An elegant anatomical confirmation of this analysis was subsequently provided by Tootell, Silverman, Switkes, and DeValois (1982). Using 2-deoxyglucose to map metabolic activity in the cortex, they stimulated a monkey with a pattern of concentric circles equally spaced on a logarithmic scale (Fig. 4A) and obtained the pattern of cortical activity shown in Fig. 4B, in accordance with the prediction from Eq. (4).

The variation of cortical magnification with eccentricity given by Eq. (3) suggests that many visual functions might be equated in central and peripheral vision by applying a scale factor F of the form

$$F = 1 + \frac{E}{E_2} \tag{5}$$

to each linear dimension of the peripheral stimulus at eccentricity E. As mentioned previously, this notion was first suggested by Rovamo and Virsu (1979), who showed that this transformation could account for the variation of the CSF with eccentricity. However, they estimated their value of E_2 from cone and ganglion cell spacing data and assumed that it also reflected cortical magnification values of E_2. As the foregoing resume of spatial sampling from retina to striate cortex has shown, the variation of cortical properties with eccentricity is much more rapid than the retinal variation. Are there psychophysical tasks reflecting these differences in mapping at different levels of the visual system? A review of the literature suggests that there are two critical values of E_2 that are significant for spatial vision in primates and humans: a value between 1.5° and 4° and a second one between 0.3° and 0.9°. It will be argued that these two critical values of E_2, which will be referred to by average values of 2.5° and 0.6°, represent limitations imposed by cone sampling and cortical magnification, respectively.

Figure 5 summarizes the falloff of vernier acuity for abutting line segments (filled squares and circles) and of grating acuity (open squares and circles) with eccentricity. The dashed line indicates the ratio of peripheral to foveal cone spacing derived from the data of Rolls and Cowey (1970), while the solid line shows

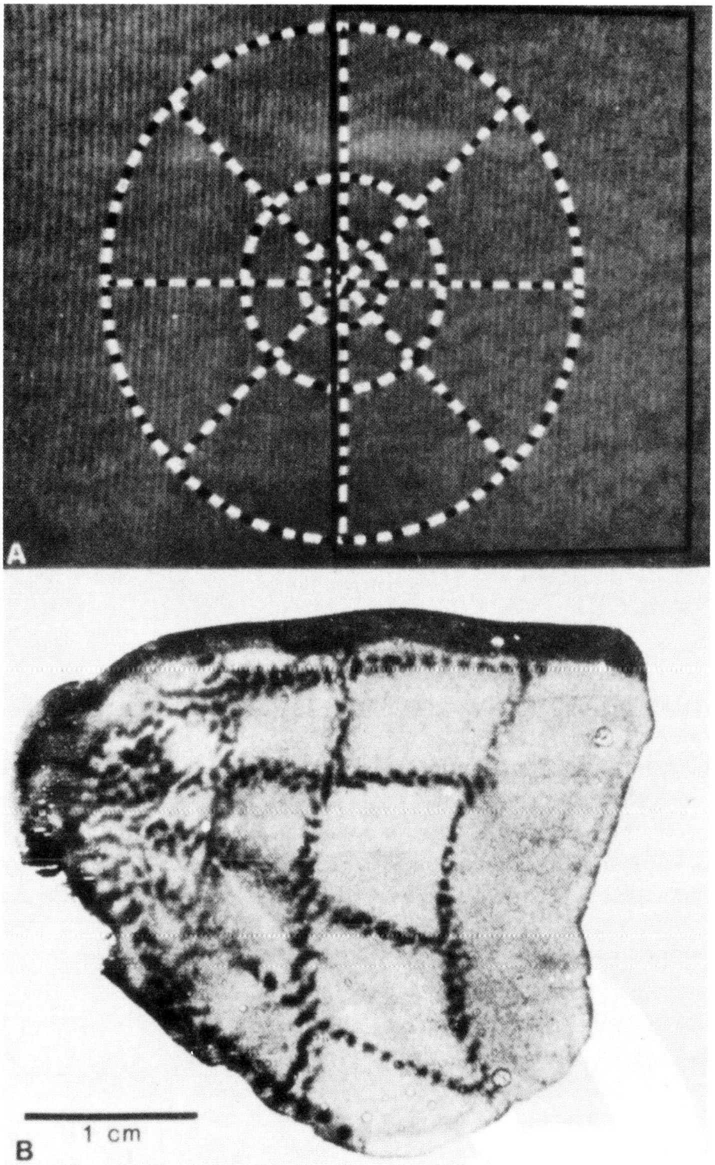

FIG. 4 Neural activation pattern in macaque striate cortex produced by the visual stimulus in A. B shows the pattern of 2-deoxyglucose activity produced in the cortex. Note that the concentric circles in A have exponentially increasing spacing from the center outward, while the retinocortical logarithmic mapping has transformed this into the relatively even spacing in B. From Tootell et al. (1982). Copyright 1982 by the AAAS.

the reciprocal of cortical magnification relative to the foveal value as estimated from data by Dow et al. (1981) in the rhesus monkey. Clearly, grating acuity is proportional to cone spacing, as shown previously in Fig. 2, while vernier acuity follows cortical magnification. Also included in Fig. 5 are estimates of the reciprocal of human cortical magnification, and it is striking that they scale with eccentricity at the same rate as the monkey magnification data. The human magnification estimates were obtained by Cowey and

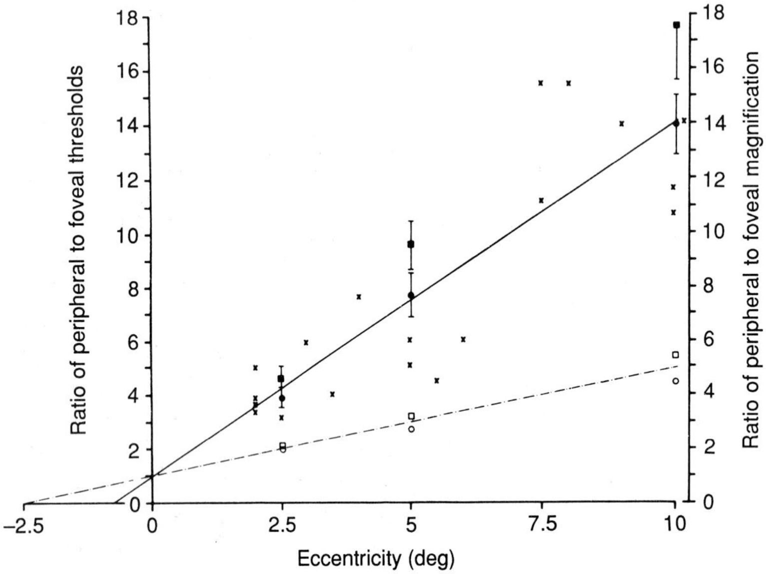

FIG. 5 The dashed line illustrates the increase in cone spacing with retinal eccentricity, using data from Rolls and Cowey (1970). Note that the data have been normalized to a foveal value of unity. The dashed line has a value of $E_2 = 2.5°$, as can be seen graphically by its intersection with the x axis at $-2.5°$. The solid line shows the variation in macaque inverse cortical magnification with eccentricity, based on the data of Dow et al. (1981) as reanalyzed by Levi et al. (1985). The solid line has a value of $E_2 = 0.77°$. Also shown are estimates of the variation in inverse human cortical magnification with eccentricity (x) from Cowey and Rolls (1974). The open circles and squares show the variation in grating acuity with eccentricity for two observers, while the respective filled symbols show the change in vernier acuity of the same observers. Note that vernier acuity falls off 3–4 times faster with eccentricity than does grating acuity. From Levi et al. (1985).

Rolls (1974) based on data provided by Brindley and Lewin (1968), who plotted the distribution of phosphenes evoked by direct stimulation of the visual cortex in a patient with electrodes implanted at fixed distances. Analysis of the human data suggests that E_2 is about 0.8°, albeit with a large standard deviation (Levi, Klein & Aitsebaomo, 1985). To summarize, there is a close correspondence between the change of human and monkey cortical magnification with retinal eccentricity and the change for vernier and other hyperacuities. This suggests that spatial sampling at the cortical level plays a crucial role in limiting the accuracy of spatial localization, a topic to which we return later.

Table 1 summarizes anatomical data and psychophysical tasks which fall into the two broad categories defined by these different rates of eccentricity variation. Let us examine these two classes in more detail. For tasks exemplified by grating acuity and contrast sensitivity (Rovamo & Virsu, 1979), E_2 falls in the range from 1.5° to 4°, with much of this variation due to measurements made along different meridia. For example, E_2 is about 4° along the temporal horizontal meridian in visual space, but it decreases to about 2° on the inferior vertical meridian. These figures are consistent with the variation in angular separation between adjacent P_β ganglion cells and cones near the fovea. Also listed in Table 1 with approximately the same value of E_2 is the variation of cortical receptive field size (Dow et al., 1981). It is of interest that the variation of ganglion cell spacing and the diameter of cortical receptive fields scale together, as it suggests that cortical receptive fields on average receive their retinal input from a fixed number of neighboring ganglion cells at each eccentricity. In agreement with this, psychophysical estimates of the variation of human spatial filter size (analogous to receptive field size, see below) with eccentricity also fall into this class (Swanson & Wilson, 1985).

A number of psychophysical tasks involving judgments of relative position are clearly characterized by a different value of E_2. These tasks are generally referred to by the term hyperacuity (Westheimer & McKee, 1977), because under optimal conditions judgments of relative position are about ten times finer than the separation of bars at the grating acuity limit. The hyperacuity data of Bourdon (1902), as replotted by Weymouth (1958), suggested that posi-

TABLE 1 E_2 for Structures and Functions[a]

Structure/function	Source
E_2 between 1.5° and 4°	
Cones	Østerberg (1935), Curcio et al. (1987)
Pβ ganglion cells	Perry & Cowey (1985), Schein & De Monasterio (1987)
Cortical receptive field size	Dow et al. (1981)
Resolution	Wertheim (1894), Weymouth (1958), Westheimer (1979*a*), Levi et al. (1985), Coletta & Williams (1987)
Contrast sensitivity	Rovamo et al. (1978), Koenderink et al. (1978), Swanson & Wilson (1985), Watson (1987)
Slow velocity discrimination	McKee & Nakayama (1984), Wright (1987)
E_2 between 0.3° and 0.9°	
Inverse cortical magnification (M^{-1})	Dow et al. (1981), Tootell et al. (1982), Van Essen et al. (1984)
Optimal 2-dot vernier acuity	Westheimer (1982)
Abutting vernier acuity	Bourdon (1902), Levi et al. (1985)
Interference zone for vernier acuity (crowding)	Levi et al. (1985)
Optimal 3-dot bisection	Yap et al. (1987), Klein & Levi (1987)
Stereoacuity	Fendick & Westheimer (1983)
Phase discrimination	Klein & Tyler (1981)

[a]Summary of visual structures and functions and their variation with retinal eccentricity. E_2 is the eccentricity at which the foveal value has increased by a factor of 2. Values of E_2 fall into two groups, one related to cortical receptive field size and one related to inverse cortical magnification.

tion acuity declined more rapidly with eccentricity than did spatial resolution. A careful study by Westheimer (1982) provided definitive evidence that vernier acuity (the ability to judge whether two line segments are collinear) declined more rapidly than grating acuity. Table 1 lists a variety of position acuity tasks, including vernier acuity, stereoscopic acuity, discrimination of spatial phase, and bisection of spatial intervals, for which the E_2 value falls into the range between 0.3° and 0.9°.

Several caveats are necessary in this discussion of the eccentricity variation of anatomical properties. First, there are obvious difficulties in estimating the variation of ganglion cell density in central vision, as the central ganglion cells are all located at the circumference of the foveal pit. However, estimates have been made based on reasonable assumptions, and those are reported here. Second, individual variations are known to exist in both cone spacing and area of striate cortex in both humans and monkeys. For example, the four human retinas examined by Curcio et al. (1987) showed a fourfold variation in foveal cone density, which translates into a twofold variation in spacing, although there was little variation in peripheral cone density. However, this variation agrees well with the range of foveal grating acuities of healthy young adults. In addition, the area of human striate cortex has been reported to range from about 1500 to 3700 mm^2 (Filimonoff, 1932; Stensaas, Eddington & Dobelle, 1974), and a similar range has been found in the macaque (Van Essen et al., 1984). Although this range is somewhat less than the variation of human foveal cone density, it may reflect the decreased variability of cone density in the periphery. It would be of great interest to find out whether the variations in human foveal cone density are correlated with variations in both grating acuity and area of foveal striate cortex on an individual basis.

IV. SPATIAL FILTERING FROM RETINA TO STRIATE CORTEX

So far we have examined the variations in spatial sampling at successive stages in the visual system and have related them to acuity and hyperacuity. An understanding of form vision also requires a characterization of the spatial filter or receptive field properties of the cells at each level of the system. The receptive field of a single cell may be described as that area of the retina within which changes in light intensity cause either excitation or inhibition of the cell. Although the earliest measurements were made using spots of light and lines as stimuli (e.g., Kuffler, 1953;

Hubel & Wiesel, 1962, 1968), the discussion here focuses on the more recent use of cosine gratings as a measurement tool. The major reason for the use of cosine gratings is that they stimulate the entire receptive field at once, thus improving the signal-to-noise ratio of the measurements.

Enroth-Cugell and Robson (1966) were the first to use cosine gratings to measure the receptive field properties of single cells in the visual system. Their measurements, made on ganglion cells in the cat, distinguished two distinct categories: X-cells, which are relatively linear in their responses, and Y-cells, which exhibit strong nonlinear distortions in their responses to cosine gratings (see Chapter 6, this volume). Subsequently Maffei and Fiorentini (1973) compared the responses of retinal, LGN, and cortical neurons in the cat to drifting cosine gratings. Typical results are shown in Fig. 6, where each curve represents the spatial frequency response of a single cell. All results shown in Fig. 6 were taken from cells with receptive fields in the same part of the visual field, and thus the data have been controlled for the eccentricity variation of visual properties. For all cells shown the response consisted of a modulation of firing at the same temporal frequency as the grating drift rate, which is a characteristic of linear systems (see below and Fig. 9), and the ordinate indicates the relative amplitude of this response as a function of spatial frequency. Two major points may be noted. First, at each stage of the visual pathway cells with receptive fields in the same part of the visual field can respond to different ranges of spatial frequencies. Second, spatial frequency selectivity becomes progressively narrower moving up the system from retinal ganglion cells to LGN cells to simple cortical cells (Fig. 6c). This is particularly evident as a progressively steeper decline in sensitivity on the low spatial frequency side of each tuning curve. As this low spatial frequency decline is due to the presence of lateral inhibition, this implies that additional inhibitory interactions in the LGN and cortex must be responsible for sharpening the spatial frequency tuning.

Results very similar to those in the cat have been obtained in macaque monkeys by DeValois, Albrecht, and Thorell (1982). They adjusted the contrast of

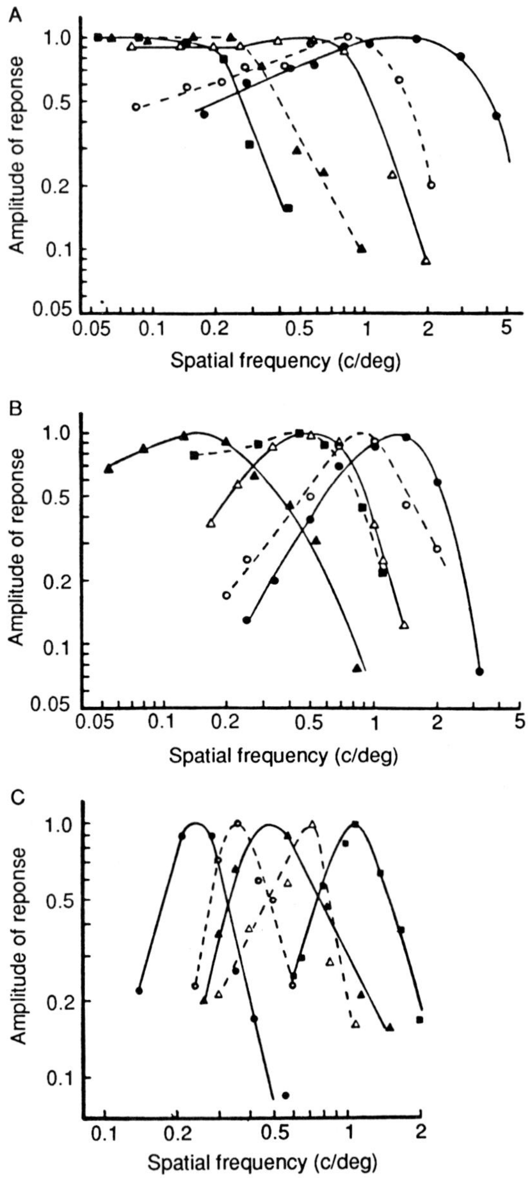

FIG. 6 Responses of retinal, LGN, and simple cortical cells in the cat to a sinusoidal grating as a function of spatial frequency. Each curve shows the response of a single neuron. The receptive fields were all located in approximately the same part of the visual field. The ordinates represent the average response amplitude to the passage of the grating over the receptive field. Experimental conditions at the three levels of the visual system were comparable. Note that spatial frequency tuning bandwidths decrease progressively at more central levels of the visual system. From Maffei and Fiorentini (1973).

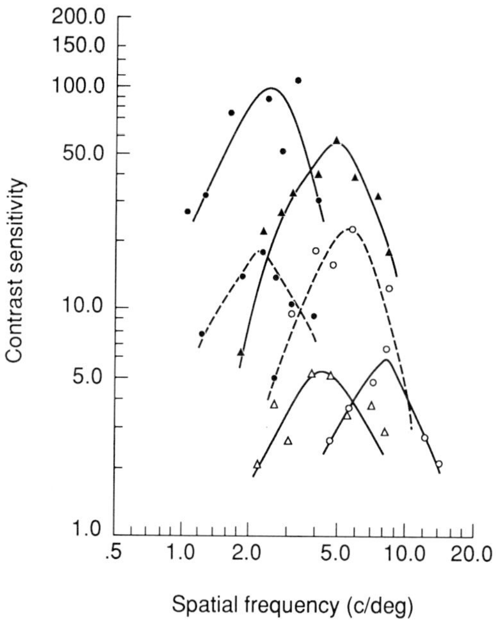

FIG. 7 Spatial frequency tuning curves for six striate cortical cells in the macaque recorded during the same electrode penetration. The symbols indicate the contrast sensitivities of the cells (reciprocals of contrasts needed to reach a specified criterion response). Note the similarity to cortical data from cats (Fig. 6) and to psychophysical results in humans (Fig. 12). From DeValois et al. (1982).

drifting gratings until the cell response just reached a criterion level. Contrast sensitivities, defined as reciprocals of these threshold contrasts, are plotted as a function of spatial frequency for six macaque striate cells in Fig. 7. As all six were recorded during a single electrode penetration, the receptive fields of all six fell at approximately the same retinal position. As with the cat cortical cells of Fig. 6, these cells exhibit relatively narrow spatial frequency tuning and display a range of optimal spatial frequencies. In both cat and monkey, therefore, spatial frequency tuning progressively narrows at successive levels of the visual system, with bandwidths (defined as the full width at half-amplitude) averaging about 1.4 octaves for cells in striate cortex.

Spatial frequency selectivity represents but one dimension of visual spatial filters. Traditionally the second dimension has been chosen to be tuning for the orientation of spatial patterns (Hubel & Wiesel, 1962). Using cosine gratings as stimuli, orientation selectivity is easily determined by measuring the cell's response to gratings as a function of orientation at the optimal spatial frequency. For retinal and LGN cells, receptive fields are approximately circularly symmetric [although small but systematic deviations from circular symmetry have been reported physiologically (Levick & Thibos, 1980) and psychophysically (Rovamo, Virsu, Laurinen & Hyvärinen, 1982; Fahle, 1986)], and they therefore respond about equally well to gratings at all orientations. In the cortex, however, Hubel and Wiesel (1962, 1968) showed that receptive fields were not circularly symmetric, but elongated, and therefore were selective for stimulus orientation. Measurements with cosine gratings reveal that average orientation bandwidths of cortical cells in the monkey vary from about $\pm 15°$ to $\pm 30°$ at half amplitude (see Fig. 13). When both orientation and spatial frequency bandwidth are measured for the same cell, it is convenient to plot them in polar coordinates. This is shown for a selection of cells from macaque striate cortex in Fig. 8, where the radial spatial frequency coordinate has been plotted on a logarithmic scale to emphasize the similarity of shapes for different spatial frequency tunings. Each cell is represented by a patch constructed by connecting its half-amplitude, half-bandwidth points in both orientation and spatial frequency. Note that even this small sample obtained at an eccentricity of 1° contains cells tuned to all orientations and to a range of spatial frequencies from about 1 to 16 cpd. On the likely assumption that a larger sample would completely fill this polar coordinate plot with overlapping patches, it follows that the population of cortical cells, at least near the fovea, provides a complete representation of the spatial frequencies and orientations in the retinal image.

The discussion thus far has dealt only with spatial frequency and orientation tuning and has ignored questions of response linearity and differences between simple and complex cells. The question of linearity becomes crucial if one wishes to derive the spatial sensitivity profiles of cortical receptive fields from their spatial frequency and orientation tuning via

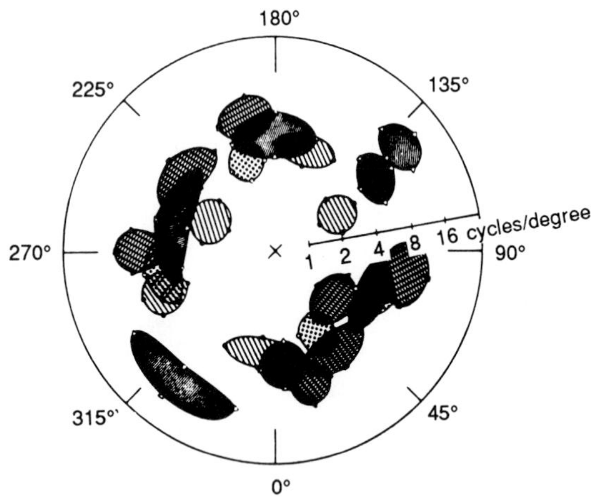

FIG. 8 Two-dimensional polar coordinate plots of the orientation and spatial frequency tuning for a sample of cortical cells recorded in one monkey at 1° eccentricity. The spatial frequency axis (radial) is logarithmic, as spatial frequency tuning shows the greatest regularity on a logarithmic scale. From DeValois et al. (1982).

inverse Fourier transformation. Two simple tests for response linearity involve the use of drifting or counterphase flickering cosine gratings. In a linear system, the average response to either of these stimuli will be a cosine at the same temporal frequency as the stimulus. The responses of a typical simple cell to each of these stimuli are shown in Fig. 9A,B. Owing to the existence of a threshold, responses to the negative half-cycles of both the drifting and flickering gratings are suppressed. However, the responses to the positive half-cycle of the drifting grating are very nearly sinusoidal (Fig. 9A), thus indicating a high degree of linearity for the suprathreshold response of this simple cell. As a consequence, it has proved possible to describe the responses of a simple cell as a linear filtering operation followed by a threshold nonlinearity, as diagrammed in Fig. 10 (Movshon, Thompson & Tolhurst, 1978a).

When these same two tests for linearity are applied to complex cells, a very different pattern emerges. As shown in Fig. 9C, a typical complex cell responds to a drifting cosine grating with a uniform increase in response that shows no evidence of sinusoidal modulation. In response to a counterphase flickering grating, complex cells respond at double the temporal frequency of the stimulus (Fig. 9D). Both results indicate that complex cells are extremely nonlinear in their responses to spatial patterns. However, detailed measurements have shown that complex cells can be described as a nonlinear pooling of responses from a spatially distributed group of subunits within the cell's receptive field (Movshon, Thompson & Tolhurst,

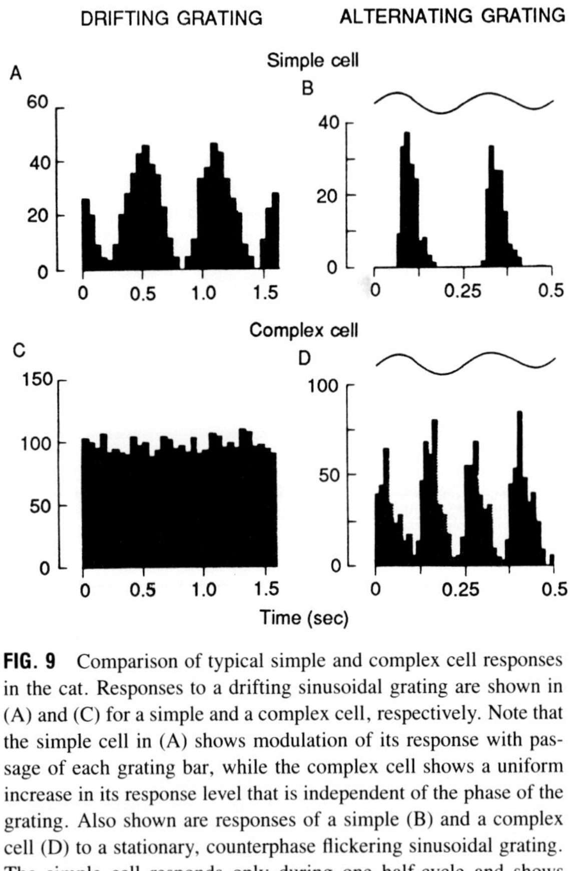

FIG. 9 Comparison of typical simple and complex cell responses in the cat. Responses to a drifting sinusoidal grating are shown in (A) and (C) for a simple and a complex cell, respectively. Note that the simple cell in (A) shows modulation of its response with passage of each grating bar, while the complex cell shows a uniform increase in its response level that is independent of the phase of the grating. Also shown are responses of a simple (B) and a complex cell (D) to a stationary, counterphase flickering sinusoidal grating. The simple cell responds only during one half-cycle and shows evidence of half-wave rectification. The complex cell, on the other hand, responds at twice the flicker frequency, thus providing evidence for full-wave rectification. These results indicate that simple cells are relatively linear except at threshold, while complex cells are highly nonlinear. From Maffei (1985). Copyright © 1985 John Wiley & Sons, Inc.

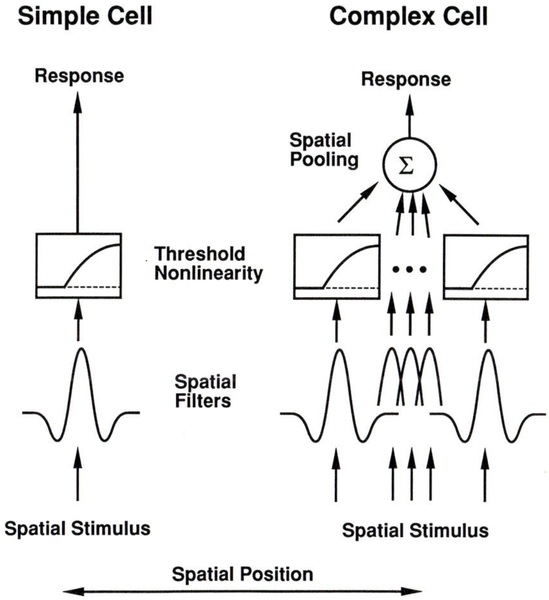

FIG. 10 Schematic diagram of the circuitry thought to produce simple and complex cell response properties. Simple cell responses (left) can be described by a linear, orientation selective spatial filter followed by a threshold nonlinearity. This nonlinearity also exhibits some response compression or saturation at high contrasts. Complex cell receptive fields (right) comprise a number of subunits, each consisting of a linear spatial filter followed by a threshold nonlinearity. Responses of a group of subunits positioned throughout the receptive field are pooled or summed to produce the complex cell response. Complex cells are tuned for spatial frequency by virtue of the filters associated with the subunits. However, they are insensitive to spatial phase as a result of the nonlinearity and spatial pooling. Many complex cells are also selective for the direction of stimulus motion. This can be incorporated into the complex cell model through appropriate inhibitory connections among the subunits prior to spatial pooling.

1978b; Heggelund, 1985). As shown in Fig. 10, the subunits of a complex cell may each be described by a linear spatial filter followed by a threshold nonlinearity. A group of these subunits with spatial filters covering a small patch of the visual field is then summed to produce the complex cell response. Thus, complex cells are tuned for spatial frequency as a result of the tuning of their subunits, but they are not selective for spatial position or phase as a result of the nonlinear subunit pooling operation. The orientation tuning of complex cells may be due either to the spatial arrangement of nonoriented subunits or, in some cases, to orientation selectivity of the subunits themselves.

A critical test of the idea that the initial spatial filtering in both simple and complex cells is linear was provided by DeValois, DeValois, and Yund (1979), who compared responses to cosine gratings with those to checkerboard patterns. The rationale was provided by Kelly (1976), who pointed out that the fundamental spatial frequency components in a checkerboard are oriented at ±45° relative to the vertical and horizontal edges defining the checks. For appropriate check sizes Kelly (1976) showed that psychophysical thresholds were determined by these fundamental components rather than by the checkerboard edges. DeValois et al. (1979) made similar measurements on individual striate cells and obtained the results plotted in Fig. 11. The simple cell shown responded optimally to a cosine grating of optimal spatial frequency oriented at 315° (−45°) relative to the vertical (squares), and the orientation tuning was such that the response fell to zero within a narrow angular range on this polar coordinate plot. When stimulated with a checkerboard, this same cell responded only when the edges were oriented horizontally and vertically (triangles), that is, at ±45° relative to the preferred cosine grating orientation. This is exactly the response expected if the orientation selective spatial filtering stage of the cell operated linearly. As similar results were obtained with complex cells, it may be concluded that the spatial filtering stage of the complex cell's subunits is also linear.

Thus, current evidence supports the notion that both simple and complex cells may be characterized functionally by a linear filtering operation followed by either a threshold nonlinearity (simple cells) or a nonlinear subunit pooling operation (complex cells, see Fig. 10). In consequence, the spatial frequency sensitivity of these filters from Fig. 6 and 7 may be inverse Fourier transformed (given appropriate phase information) to provide a description of the spatial sensitivity profile of simple cell receptive fields (see Fig. 14). It may be noted that this contemporary quantitative description of cortical cells is in rough

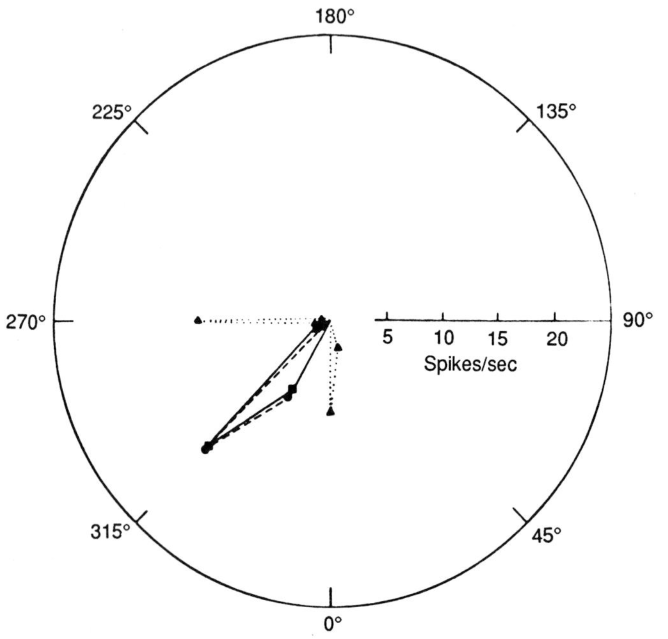

FIG. 11 Responses of a cat simple cell to a cosine grating (squares), a checkerboard (triangles), and a plaid pattern (circles). Note that the grating and plaid patterns yield the same orientation tuning, while the response lobes for the checkerboard are shifted 45° to either side. This means that the cell was responding to the fundamental frequencies of the checkerboard, which is the result expected from linear filtering, rather than to the edges of the check, as would be expected from an edge detector. From DeValois et al. (1979).

agreement with the qualitative categorizations first proposed by Hubel and Wiesel (1962, 1978).

Hubel and Wiesel (1962, 1968) originally identified hypercomplex cells as a third category of striate unit, but more recently these have been classified as subsets of simple and complex cells (Dreher, 1972). The defining hypercomplex property is the presence of powerful inhibitory zones at one or both ends of the excitatory region of the receptive field, with the consequence that these cells will respond to bars of the preferred orientation only if they are not too long. As a result, the hypercomplex property is frequently referred to as "end-inhibition" or "end-stopping." The models for simple and complex cells in Fig. 10 could be extended to include the hypercomplex property simply by introducing an additional inhibitory zone at one or both ends of the receptive field.

As discussed above, the major spatial filtering characteristics introduced at the cortical level and missing at the retina and LGN are orientation selectivity, narrower spatial frequency tuning, nonlinear spatial pooling (complex cells), and end-stopping (subsets of both simple and complex cells). In addition, one finds direction selectivity for moving patterns and tuning for disparity (Chapter 12, this volume). Thus, it is natural to ask how these new forms of spatial filtering are implemented by the cortical machinery. Hubel and Wiesel (1962, 1968) suggested a hierarchical model in which simple cell receptive fields were formed by convergent input from two to three LGN cells with aligned receptive fields. Complex cells were viewed as the next stage of processing produced by pooling of responses from a group of simple cells with overlapping receptive fields. Finally, hypercomplex cells were supposed to derive their properties from a combination of excitatory and inhibitory complex cell inputs.

Although this hierarchical scheme provided a concise description of the early data, subsequent research has shown it to be faulty in three major respects. First, as already noted, there are both simple and complex cells with end-inhibition (Dreher, 1972), so hypercomplex cells are neither a single class of cells nor the final stage in a processing hierarchy. Recent evidence suggests that end-stopping may be generated via inhibition of cells with short receptive fields by those with longer receptive fields but with the same preferred orientation (Boltz & Gilbert, 1986). Second, Sillito (1975, 1979, 1985) has provided evidence that orientation selectivity does not arise from a convergence of LGN inputs by demonstrating that when GABA (γ-aminobutyric acid, an inhibitory neurotransmitter) is chemically blocked in the cortex, both simple and complex cells lose their orientation tuning. This implies that orientation selectivity is a property of inhibitory circuits at the cortical level, a conclusion arrived at independently by Cruetzfeldt and Ito (1968).

Finally, there is evidence that complex cells (or at least a large subset of them) do not receive excitatory input from simple cells and thus must represent a parallel rather than hierarchical stage of information processing. The first evidence for this was the observation that many complex cells respond to a visual stimulus *before* simple cells (Hoffmann & Stone, 1971). Subsequently Hammond and MacKay (1977, 1978) demonstrated that complex cells in Area 17 respond to two-dimensional visual noise, while simple cells are unresponsive. Burr, Morrone, and Maffei (1981, see also Maffei, 1985) extended this result by showing that the response of a simple cell to a one-dimensional pattern at its preferred orientation could be suppressed by the presence of a grating drifting at right angles. Further experiments suggested that this suppression was due to inhibition from complex cells, which therefore appear to modulate or control the responses of simple cells. Thus, it now appears that simple, complex, and their end-stopped subclasses mainly represent parallel rather than hierarchical information processing stages. The possible functional significance of this is explored subsequently (Section X).

V. PSYCHOPHYSICAL MEASUREMENT OF SPATIAL FILTERS

Shortly after the introduction of cosine gratings as stimuli for single-unit physiology by Enroth-Cugell and Robson (1966), their value as psychophysical stimuli for the study of vision was exploited by Campbell and Robson (1968). This study demonstrated that the CSF could not be regarded as the description of a single linear system even for the purposes of predicting sensitivities to simple patterns like square-wave gratings. Instead, the CSF appeared to represent the envelope of a number of underlying sensitivity curves with narrower spatial frequency tuning than the system as a whole, a result corroborated by the work of Graham and Nachmias (1971). As a result of these pioneering studies, subsequent research focused on measurement of the spatial frequency and orientation tuning of these underlying mechanisms. These studies generally employed one of three techniques: subthreshold summation, spatial frequency adaptation, or masking.

The typical stimulus in a subthreshold summation experiment comprises two components: a test pattern and a summation pattern. In the case of cosine gratings, therefore, a frequently used stimulus was

$$P(x) = L_{\text{mean}}[1 + C_{\text{test}} \cos(2\pi\omega_{\text{test}}x) + C_{\text{sum}} \cos(2\pi\omega_{\text{sum}}x)] \quad (6)$$

where L_{mean} is the mean luminance, C_{test} and ω_{test} are the contrast and spatial frequency of the test grating, and C_{sum} and ω_{sum} are contrast and spatial frequency of the subthreshold grating. Following pilot experiments in which thresholds for both gratings were independently measured, C_{sum} would usually be set to about one-half its threshold value (hence, subthreshold summation), and the threshold value of C_{test} would then be measured. In this manner it was possible to measure the extent to which gratings of different spatial frequencies summed to generate a threshold response. The original experiments of Campbell and Robson (1968) and Graham and Nachmias (1971) may be viewed as special cases of this paradigm in which ω_{test} and ω_{sum} were in the ratio of 3:1, and both showed that frequencies in this ratio do not sum at threshold.

Attempts were then made to use subthreshold summation to measure the spatial frequency tuning of individual spatial mechanisms by reducing the ratio of ω_{test} to ω_{sum} until summation was obtained (Sachs, Nachmias & Robson, 1971; Kulikowski & King-

Smith, 1973). These studies produced exceptionally narrow bandwidth estimates on the order of 0.25 octave at half-amplitude—far narrower than measurements on cortical cells. It was later shown, however, that these narrow estimates were an artifact of the spatial beat pattern produced by the sum of two cosine gratings with only slightly different frequencies (King-Smith & Kulikowski, 1975; Stromeyer & Klein, 1975; Wilson & Bergen, 1979). Whereas a single cosine grating has the same contrast at all points across the retina, the sum of two similar frequencies produces regions of zero contrast where the two are out of phase. In consequence, fewer ganglion cells are stimulated by the grating sum, and statistical considerations (i.e., spatial probability summation) show that this will artificially raise the threshold.[3] In fact, recent experiments by Graham and Robson (1987) have shown that subthreshold summation between closely spaced frequencies is primarily dependent on the degree of spatial probability summation and is a very poor indicator of mechanism bandwidths. Subthreshold summation experiments using cosine gratings are thus not thought to provide adequate descriptions of the spatial frequency tuning of visual mechanisms.

Pantle and Sekuler (1968) and Blakemore and Campbell (1969) first demonstrated that prolonged observation of a high contrast cosine grating greatly reduces the visibility of a low contrast grating of similar spatial frequency and orientation, thus producing a notch in the CSF. On the assumption that grating adaptation reflects desensitization or fatigue of a homogeneous group of orientation selective neural units, Blakemore and Campbell (1969) estimated spatial frequency bandwidths to be of the order of 1.3 octaves at half-amplitude. This was refined and corrected for nonlinearities in the adaptation process by Georgeson and Harris (1984), who obtained an average bandwidth estimate of 1.4 octaves, in excellent agreement with the median for cortical cells in the macaque (DeValois et al., 1982).

Cosine grating adaptation has been shown to be closely correlated with the responses of single cortical neurons in the cat by Maffei, Fiorentini, and Bisti (1973). First, a low contrast cosine grating of optimal spatial frequency was drifted over the receptive field of a cortical neuron and the average rate of discharge was recorded for 1 min. Next, the contrast was set at the highest available value, and the cell was exposed to this stimulus for 1 min. Following this, contrast was lowered to its initial value, and recordings were again made. In retinal and LGN cells this adaptation procedure had no effect, but all simple cells studied showed a pronounced reduction in firing rate following adaptation and required about 30 sec to recover fully. Thus, it is likely that spatial frequency adaptation reflects a reduction in sensitivity of units in human visual cortex as well.

The third paradigm used to estimate bandwidths of orientation selective units in the human visual system is masking, which measures the threshold elevation produced by superposition of a high contrast masking pattern on a test stimulus. Thus, masking measures the degree to which a high contrast mask interferes with the visibility of a test pattern. In the experiments of interest here a high contrast cosine grating mask was superimposed on a test pattern, whose contrast was then set to threshold. By comparing test thresholds in the presence and absence of the mask, the threshold elevation could be defined as the factor by which the mask raised the test threshold.

Several studies utilized cosine gratings as both test stimuli and masks in an attempt to measure the orientation and spatial frequency tuning of human cortical mechanisms (e.g., Campbell & Kulikowski, 1966; Legge & Foley, 1980). However, when both test and mask are cosine gratings of the same orientation and spatial frequency, masking reduces to a task of grating contrast discrimination as opposed to pattern discrimination (i.e., discrimination of test plus mask contrast from mask contrast alone). Wilson, McFarlane, and

[3] If a grating stimulates an array of neural units that have mutually uncorrelated noise, then the probability that at least one unit will accurately detect the grating will be greater than the probability that any individual unit will detect the grating. When the neural units are distributed in space, this is referred to as a spatial probability summation.

Phillips (1983) provided a solution to this problem by using patterns that were localized in space and band pass in spatial frequency as test stimuli instead of cosine gratings. These patterns, mathematically defined by the sixth spatial derivative of a Gaussian function with a 1-octave spatial frequency bandwidth, appeared as a blurred bright vertical bar flanked on either side by blurred dark bars. The rationale was that these patterns should have a luminance profile closely matched to the sensitivity of cortical receptive fields of appropriate size (see Fig. 14). When these test stimuli were added to masks of a slightly different orientation, the appearance at threshold was always of a spatial deformation running down the center of the mask, so that the subject's task was always one of pattern discrimination. In addition, the use of a slightly different orientation for test and mask was shown to control for spatial phase effects and spatial probability summation.

Masking data were obtained foveally on each subject using this paradigm for a range of test and mask spatial frequencies spanning the range from 0.25 to 22 cpd in 0.5-octave steps (Wilson et al., 1983). The resulting data were corrected for a compressive, power law contrast nonlinearity associated with masking (Nachmias & Sansbury, 1974; Legge & Foley, 1980; Legge, 1981), and they were then analyzed to compensate for the overlap between neighboring tuning curves. The results showed that a set of six spatial frequency tuned mechanisms could account for all 14 sets of masking data for each subject, with the data fit being adequate to account for 96% of the variance.[4] The normalized spatial frequency tuning curves for these six mechanisms are plotted in Fig. 12, where

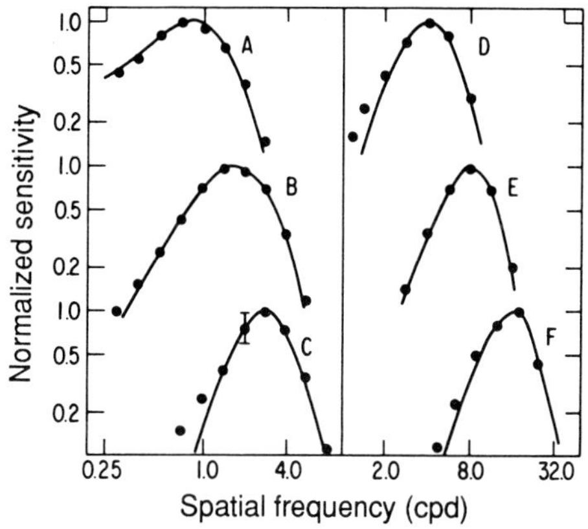

FIG. 12 Spatial frequency tuning of six visual mechanisms measured with a psychophysical masking technique. The data, obtained with foveal fixation, are averages for three subjects. Peak frequencies increase progressively from 0.8 cpd in A to 16 cpd in F. The curves show the fits of the Fourier transform of Eq. (7) to the data. Note that the bandwidth of these curves decreases from A to F. The left and right sides of the graph have different abscissas. From Wilson and Gelb (1984).

the data represent averages for three subjects. Note that these curves are remarkably similar in both shape and bandwidth to the curves for single cells in monkey cortex plotted in Fig. 7 (DeValois et al., 1982) and cat cortex in Fig. 6 (Maffei & Fiorentini, 1973). In fact, the comparison with monkey single-unit data is very close quantitatively.

It may be noted that the full bandwidth at half-amplitude of the tuning curves in Fig. 12 decreases from A to F as peak spatial frequency increases from 0.8 to 16 cpd. These bandwidths in octaves are shown as a function of peak spatial frequency by the filled squares in Fig. 13A. For comparison, average bandwidths of macaque striate units from the DeValois et al. (1982) study have been plotted with dotted squares. Both human masking and monkey physiological data agree in showing a progressive decrease in bandwidth from about 2.5 to 1.25 octaves with increasing spatial frequency. A similar trend has also been found in cat visual cortex (Tolhurst & Thompson, 1981). Using band-pass noise masks, similar results were obtained by Stromeyer and Julesz (1972) in humans.

[4] Although six filters provide an excellent fit to the oblique masking data, it is difficult to rule out a larger number. Indeed, given the increase in filter size with eccentricity, there must be a much larger number of filter sizes within 2°–4° of the fovea. This may be one reason why physiologists have tended to find a wide range of different receptive field sizes at the cortical level. However, receptive field sizes for X- and Y-cells in the cat retina do form two distinct classes at each eccentricity (Cleland, Harding & Tulunay-Keesey, 1979), and it is likely that the same is true of primate M- and P-cells.

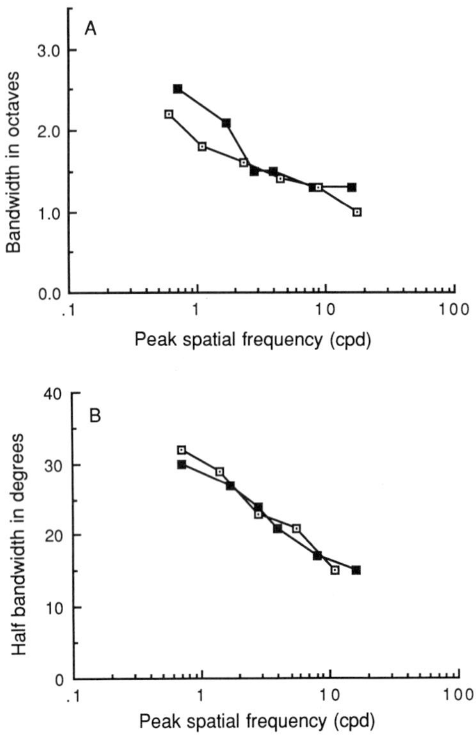

FIG. 13 Spatial frequency (A) and orientation (B) bandwidths of human foveal mechanisms compared with average data for single units in macaque visual cortex. Data are plotted as a function of the peak spatial frequency of the mechanism or cell. The human data were obtained using a psychophysical masking technique, and the data in A reflect variations in curve widths from Fig. 12. Spatial frequency and orientation tuning in both humans and macaques become narrower as peak spatial frequency increases.

Phillips and Wilson (1984) used a variant of this masking paradigm to measure the orientation tuning of human visual mechanisms. Rather than masking a test stimulus with cosine gratings covering a range of spatial frequencies at a fixed orientation, each test stimulus was masked by a cosine grating of the same spatial frequency over a range of orientations. The data were again corrected for contrast nonlinearities in masking and for overlap of neighboring orientation channels. The resulting bandwidth estimates (half-bandwidth in degrees at half-amplitude) are shown as a function of test spatial frequency in Fig. 13B (filled squares). Again, there is very close quantitative agreement with average bandwidth data for single units in macaque striate cortex (dotted squares) reported by DeValois et al. (1982): both sets of data show bandwidths decreasing from $\pm 30°$ at low spatial frequencies to $\pm 15°$ at high. Thus, both monkey striate cells and human spatial mechanisms are more narrowly tuned for orientation and spatial frequency at high spatial frequencies.

These masking studies have made it possible to provide a quantitative description of two-dimensional human spatial filters. Experiments showed that these could be described by a product of one-dimensional functions in Cartesian coordinates but not in polar coordinates (Daugman, 1984; Phillips & Wilson, 1984), and the following function was shown to provide an accurate fit to the data:

$$RF(x,y) = A\left\{\exp\left(\frac{-x^2}{\sigma_1^2}\right) - B\exp\left(\frac{-x^2}{\sigma_2^2}\right) + C\exp\left(\frac{-x^2}{\sigma_3^2}\right)\right\}\exp\left(\frac{-y^2}{\sigma_y^2}\right) \tag{7}$$

This function describes a vertically oriented filter with even symmetry; filters of other orientations can be generated by a simple rotation of coordinates. The smaller filters have both central and secondary excitatory regions by virtue of their narrow spatial frequency tuning, while the larger ones have only one excitatory region [corresponding to $C = 0$ in Eq. (7)]. Multiple sidebands of decreasing amplitude have been reported for receptive fields of cortical cells (Bishop, Coombs & Henry, 1971; Maffei & Fiorentini, 1976; Andrews & Pollen, 1979). The curves in Fig. 12 show the fit of the Fourier transform of Eq. 7 to the spatial frequency tuning data, while the two-dimensional spatial sensitivity of several filters is pictured in Fig. 14. Owing to the close quantitative agreement between human and monkey data in Fig. 13, the filters depicted in Fig. 14 may also be regarded as pictures of typical cortical simple cell receptive fields. It should be noted that Eq. (7) describes a filter with even symmetry, although the psychophysical masking results only provide amplitude

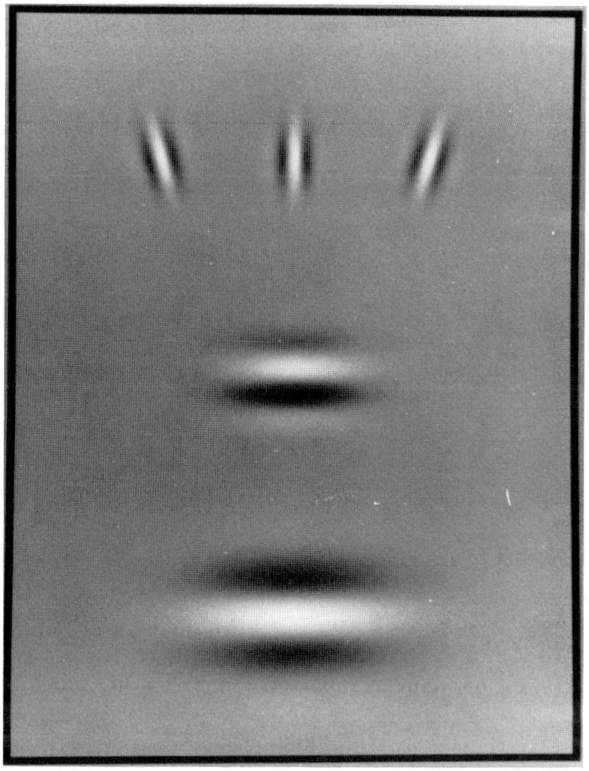

FIG. 14 Gray scale representations of two-dimensional, orientation selective filters in the human visual system. Excitatory regions are plotted in light shades from middle gray to white, while inhibitory zones range from dark gray to black. Orientations of the smallest filters at the top are separated by 15°, which is approximately the difference between neighboring orientation columns in the monkey cortex. At a distance where the width of the black frame subtends 1.14° the peak spatial frequencies of the filters are, respectively, 16, 8, and 5 cpd (top to bottom). Note that the center filter is odd symmetric, while the remaining ones have even symmetry. Owing to the good quantitative agreement (see Fig. 13), these pictures represent both human spatial filters and the receptive fields of typical simple cells in macaque striate cortex.

information and not phase. Therefore, Fig. 14 also depicts a receptive field with odd symmetry, as odd symmetric units have also been reported physiologically (Pollen & Ronner, 1981, 1983).

No theoretical significance need be attached to Eq. (7) aside from the fact that it provides an accurate quantitative fit to masking data. Indeed, a variety of other mathematical functions have been fit to both psychophysical and physiological spatial frequency sensitivity data. The most common of these other functions is the Gabor function, $G(x,y)$, which is defined as

$$G(x,y) = A \sin(2\pi\omega x + \phi)\, e^{-x^2/\sigma_x^2 - y^2/\sigma_y^2} \quad (8)$$

for a vertical filter. This is just a sine wave of variable phase multiplied by two-dimensional Gaussian function that may have different space constants in the x and y directions. Depending on the phase ϕ a Gabor function may have odd or even symmetry, or it may be asymmetric. Gabor functions have been shown to provide reasonable fits to tuning curves for cortical neurons and have also been espoused for theoretical reasons (Marcelja, 1980; Daugman, 1985). In particular, it has been stated that Gabor functions simultaneously minimize uncertainty in spatial position and spatial frequency. However, this theoretical property does not apply to the real valued function in Eq. (8) (Stork & Wilson, 1988; Wilson, 1989b).[5] In addition, there is some evidence that the function in Eq. (7) fits both physiological and psychophysical tuning data somewhat better than Gabor functions do (Hawken & Parker, 1987; Stork & Wilson, 1988; Wilson, 1989b). Thus, a number of mathematical functions have been shown to provide reasonable fits to available data, and there are no compelling reasons at present for preferring one to another beyond empirical accuracy.

In summary, subthreshold summation studies first showed that the human CSF is actually the envelope of a number of more narrowly tuned spatial frequency selective mechanisms (Campbell & Robson, 1968;

[5] The joint minimization of spatial and spatial frequency uncertainty for Gabor functions applies only to a complex valued function that is an extension of Eq. (8), and the representation of a complex valued function in the visual system would require two functions of the form described by Eq. (8) but separated in phase by 90°. Thus, a real valued Gabor function that can be fit to a single receptive field does not minimize the joint uncertainties. In addition, the minimization depends on the precise mathematical form of the metric to be minimized, and it is only for one of an infinite number of metrics that the Gabor function provides a minimum. Thus, it is not clear whether the metric minimized by complex valued Gabor functions is functionally significant for vision.

Graham & Nachmias, 1971). However, beats produced when gratings of similar frequency are added made it difficult to estimate the bandwidths of these mechanisms. The spatial frequency adaptation paradigm (Pantle & Sekuler, 1968; Blakemore & Campbell, 1969) agreed with electrophysiology in providing average bandwidth estimates of about 1.4 octaves, and it was later shown that spatial frequency adaptation was a property of cortical cells (Maffei et al., 1973). The masking paradigm has produced both spatial frequency and orientation tuning curves that are in excellent quantitative agreement with data from single neurons in macaque striate cortex over the entire visible spatial frequency range. These data thus lend credence to the following psychophysical linking hypothesis: the spatial frequency adaptation and masking paradigms reflect the tuning properties of various classes of orientation selective neurons in human visual cortex.

VI. ANATOMY AND PSYCHOPHYSICS OF CORTICAL MODULES

Having discussed the spatial sampling and filtering characteristics of the retina, LGN, and visual cortex, let us now examine the modular representation of information in the cortex. A striate cortical module may be defined as a small chunk of cortical tissue (typically 1 mm^2 at the cortical surface) extending perpendicularly through the gray matter and containing a collection of neurons sufficient to analyze all visual information originating from a small patch of retina. Such modules are replicated throughout the cortex, thus providing for processing of the entire retinal image. The first evidence for cortical modules was reported by Hubel and Wiesel (1962, 1968, 1977), who discovered that all of the cells encountered in an electrode penetration perpendicular to the cortical surface had the same preferred orientation (with the exception of some layer IV concentric units). Tangential electrode penetrations, however, produced a progressive change in preferred orientation interspersed with occasional orientation jumps. Accordingly, it was concluded that neurons with similar preferred orientations were arranged in columns extending vertically through the cortex. This was subsequently confirmed anatomically using both 2-deoxyglucose (Hubel, Wiesel & Stryker, 1977) and voltage sensitive dyes (Blasdel & Salama, 1986).

The next reports of cortical modularity concerned ocular dominance columns. As is well known, alternate layers in the LGN receive input from the ipsilateral and contralateral retina, respectively. Lesions confined to a single LGN layer produced a pattern of degeneration in layer IV of striate cortex, the principal layer of LGN axon termination, comprised of alternate stripes or bands (Hubel & Wiesel, 1969). Injection of one eye with radioactive amino acids in later experiments resulted in labeling in both hemispheres of the entire set of ocular dominance columns receiving input from that eye (Hubel & Wiesel, 1977). The columns were found to be long narrow slabs with a width on the cortical surface of about 0.5 mm. Thus, a parallel pair of left and right eye dominance columns was about 1 mm wide in the monkey. Physiological recordings confirmed that layer IV neurons were monocular and alternated between groups driven by the left and right eyes. Binocular cells, crucial for stereopsis (see Chapter 12, this volume), were found above and below layer IV. Orientation columns, which are much narrower, were found to intersect ocular dominance columns at an angle, so that about 12 distinct orientations spanning the entire 180° range were represented within each 0.5 mm wide ocular dominance column.

It has also been reported that cells with similar preferred spatial frequencies are arranged in a columnar fashion. Evidence for this in the monkey was provided by Tootell, Silverman, and DeValois (1981) using the 2-deoxyglucose technique. A monkey was stimulated by a cosine grating of fixed spatial frequency that was rotated during the course of the experiment so as to stimulate all orientations. The resulting pattern of 2-deoxyglucose uptake showed the characteristic slablike columnar architecture in striate cortex. However, a different pattern of results has been reported in the cat (Maffei & Fiorentini, 1977), where it was claimed that spatial frequency is organized in tangential layers rather than in vertical columns. It would therefore be valuable to have further results from other laboratories investigating the columnar organization of spatial frequency. It may also be added that the presence of a range of different spatial frequency tunings among striate cells has been firmly established independent of the question whether they are arranged in a columnar fashion, as described in Section V.

The latest aspect of striate functional architecture to be discovered was the presence of a discrete chromatic system located in a periodic series of patches or blobs (Livingstone & Hubel, 1984). As first reported by Horton and Hubel (1981) and Humphrey and Hendrickson (1983), cortical staining for cytochrome oxidase revealed the presence of a periodic series of spots or blobs spaced about 0.5 mm apart and extending through layers II and III. Physiological recordings showed these blobs to contain cells with double opponent (usually red–green) receptive fields. Although it was initially reported that blob cells had no orientation tuning, it is now thought that they are tuned for orientation but with relatively broad bandwidths. In addition, it has been shown that these cells are tuned to very low spatial frequencies, which is consistent with the lowered acuity for chromatic gratings (see Chapter 8, this volume). Finally, it has been shown that the cytochrome oxidase blobs are centered on the ocular dominance columns.

Evidence for a modular columnar organization in human visual cortex has also been reported. Hitchcock and Hickey (1980) obtained evidence for the presence of ocular dominance columns using a reduced silver stain technique. The results, when corrected for tissue shrinkage, showed human ocular dominance columns to be about 1 mm wide, twice as wide as in the monkey. Horton and Hendly-White (1984) have successfully stained human cortex to reveal the presence of cytochrome oxidase blobs spaced about 1 mm apart. Thus, 2×2 mm^2 of cortical surface in human would be adequate to cover regions from both eyes and incorporate several cytochrome oxidase blobs.

From these data the following picture of cortical modules or hypercolumns in monkeys and humans emerges. Below each 1×1 mm^2 of cortical surface in monkeys, or 2×2 mm^2 in humans, are to be found one left and one right eye ocular dominance column along with two to four cytochrome oxidase blobs. Within each ocular dominance column are found orientation columns representing the full range of orientations around the clock face plus a set of spatial frequency columns with a range of peak frequencies. Each cortical module, therefore, contains a complete set of machinery to encode the orientation, size or spatial frequency, spatial position, depth, color, and motion of the stimulus falling within a small spatial region of the retina.[6] As cortical modules are roughly constant in size (1×1 mm^2 or 2×2 mm^2) throughout the cortex, the size of the spatial region analyzed by each module is dependent on the mapping from retina to cortex described by the cortical magnification factor in Eq. (3). Thus, a foveal module would process a patch about 0.10° across, while at 45° eccentricity patch size would increase to about 6°. Receptive fields of neurons within the module are displaced to provide spatial sampling of the patch. Neighboring modules process neighboring areas of visual space, and, based on estimates of the surface area of human visual cortex, the total number of modules in each hemisphere in humans would be in the range 375–925.

Psychophysical data suggest that certain spatial interference effects in hyperacuity reflect the modular structure of human visual cortex. Westheimer and Hauske (1975) first demonstrated that the presence of flanking contours within several minutes of arc of a hyperacuity target sharply degraded positional acuity. As these effects occur when the target is presented to one eye and the interfering contours to the other, they must reflect cortical rather than subcortical processes (Levi et al., 1985). Fig. 15A shows vernier acuity measured at 0°, 2.5°, 5°, and 10° using repetitive pat-

[6] The original notion was that all modules across the cortex were structurally and functionally the same and differed only in the location and spacing of their subcortical inputs. As discussed earlier, however, there are about 10 times as many striate cells per LGN input in the foveal representation as in the far periphery. Thus, the nature of cortical modules must vary to some extent across the visual field.

tern. Note that at each eccentricity, threshold varies with interline separation (abscissa). In the fovea, thresholds are more or less invariant for large separations but increase sharply at small separations. In the periphery, the results are quite similar; however, the thresholds are much higher than in the fovea, and the sharp increase in thresholds occurs at much larger interline separations. Figure 15B shows these data replotted in cortical coordinates (millimeters across the cortical surface). The specific values for the cortical axes were based on the assumption that foveal cortical magnification is 15 mm/degree, and that the value of E_2 [eccentricity at which magnification is halved, see Eq. (3)] is 0.77°. In these coordinates, the widely disparate functions seen in Fig. 15A collapse to a more or less unitary function, suggesting that, in units of cortical distance, vernier thresholds correspond to about 0.05 mm of cortical distance at all eccentricities, and position acuity is degraded when the interline spacing is less than 1 mm. A distance of 0.05 mm is approximately the distance between neighboring orientation columns as measured in monkeys, while 1 mm agrees with the spacing between human ocular dominance columns (Hitchcock & Hickey, 1980; Horton & Hedley-White, 1984). Thus, it appears that interference with vernier acuity occurs when the interfering stimuli fall within the same cortical module as the target.

There are, of course, a number of assumptions and uncertainties associated with the specification of cortical coordinates. However, the data may be simply plotted as a fraction of the effective eccentricity (i.e., eccentricity plus E_2), and the same superposition as shown in Fig. 15B will be obtained. In these psychophysical coordinates optimal vernier thresholds are approximately 1/400 of the effective eccentricity, and interference begins at an interline spacing of about 0.1 times effective eccentricity. Thus, at all eccentricities it is possible to define a functional psychophysical spatial processing module. This psycho-

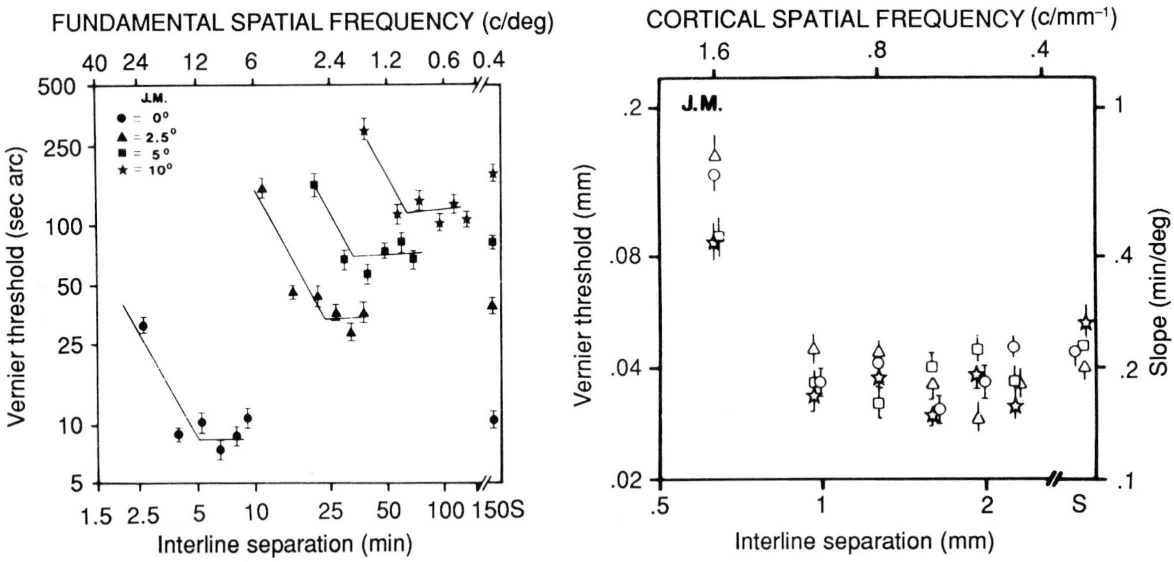

FIG. 15 Thresholds for repetitive vernier gratings (A) are plotted as a function of the interline separation (lower abscissa) or fundamental spatial frequency (upper abscissa) at 0°, 2.5°, 5°, and 10° in the lower visual field. The S shows vernier thresholds for a classical vernier target (i.e., single lines). In B the data from A are replotted with the interline separation (lower abscissa) specified in units of cortical distance. Similarly, the threshold vernier offset at each eccentricity is expressed in units of cortical distance (left-hand ordinate). The upper and right-hand axes show the data expressed as a fraction of "effective eccentricity" (i.e., eccentricity + 0.77°). From Levi et al. (1985).

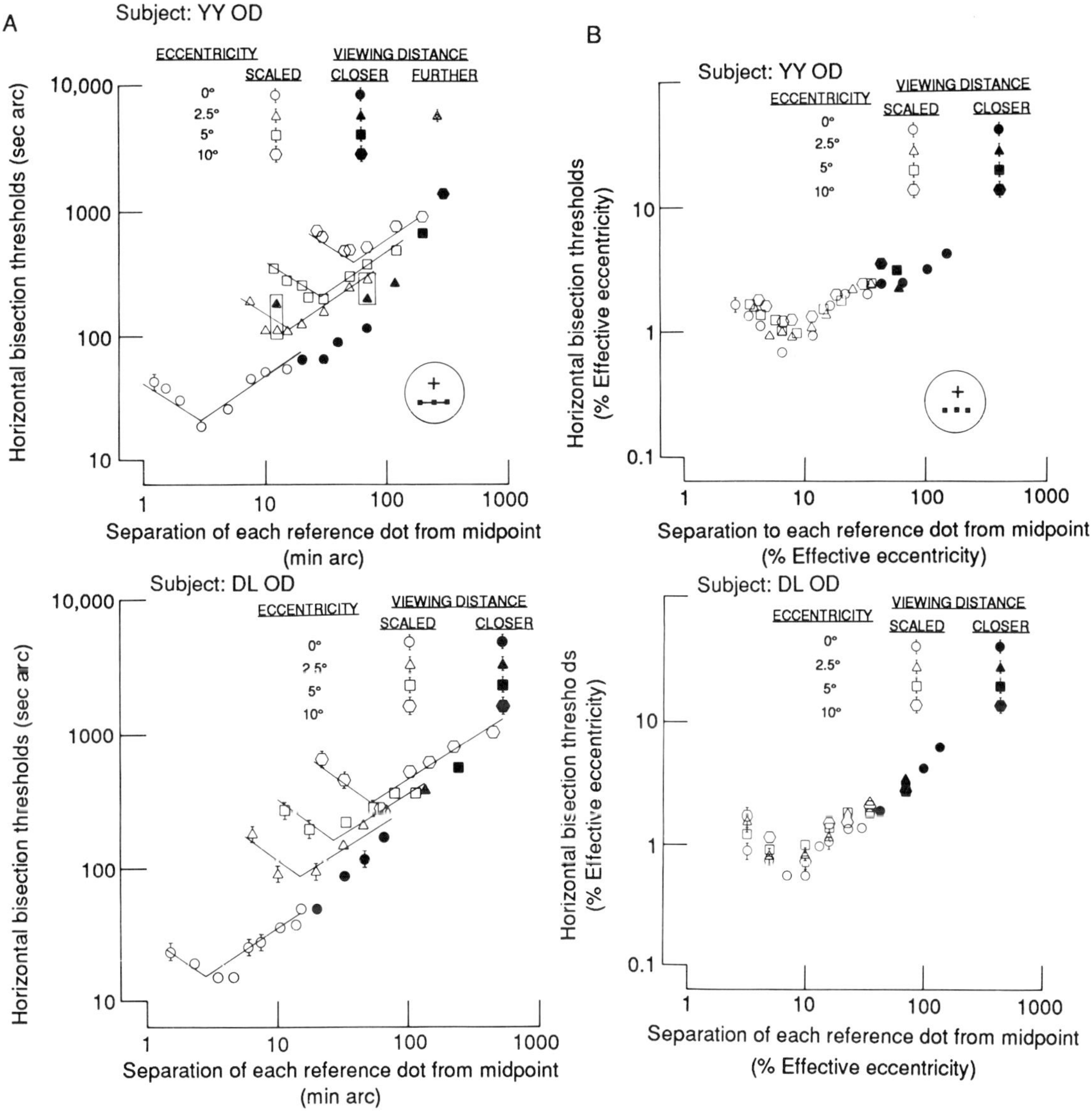

FIG. 16 In (A) three-dot bisection thresholds are plotted as a function of half the separation of the pair of reference dots at 0°, 2.5°, 5°, and 10° in the lower visual field. In (B) the data from (A) are replotted with the dot separation and bisection thresholds expressed as a percentage of "effective eccentricity" (i.e., eccentricity + 0.77°). From Yap et al. (1987).

physical module has a width of about 0.1 times the effective eccentricity and varies with eccentricity as do anatomically defined cortical modules.

Three-dot bisection acuity is a second hyperacuity task that scales with eccentricity in the manner just described. Figure 16A shows bisection thresholds at four eccentricities obtained with a three-dot stimulus, while Fig. 16B shows the data replotted in units of effective eccentricity (Yap, Levi & Klein, 1987). Here again thresholds at all eccentricities collapse to a single function, and the thresholds rise steeply for separations which are less than 0.1 times the effective eccentricity. This lends further support to the association between psychophysically and anatomically defined cortical processing modules.

VII. PSYCHOPHYSICS AND PHYSIOLOGY OF PATTERN DISCRIMINATION

In the foregoing we have analyzed the visual system in terms of its spatial filtering and sampling characteristics from photoreceptors to striate cortex and have documented a striking convergence between psychophysical, electrophysiological, and anatomical results. On the basis of these results it should be possible to develop an understanding of visual pattern discrimination capabilities. Chief among these are the visual hyperacuities, where discrimination thresholds are typically 5–10 times smaller than the closest spacing of foveal cones (Westheimer, 1979a). Indeed, a number of quantitative models for pattern discrimination have recently been developed and applied to a range of hyperacuity tasks (Wilson & Gelb, 1984; Klein & Levi, 1985; Watt & Morgan 1985). A common characteristic of these approaches is that all are based on the calculated responses of spatially localized filters or receptive fields tuned to a range of spatial frequencies. As the Wilson and Gelb (1984) model has been applied to a greater range of pattern discrimination tasks, it is discussed first and the other models then contrasted with it.

The Wilson and Gelb (1984) model for spatial pattern discrimination employs visual filters whose spatial frequency and orientation tuning were measured in the masking studies described above (Wilson et al., 1983; Phillips & Wilson, 1984). The spatial frequency tuning of the six filters measured in the fovea is shown in Fig. 12 and their two-dimensional spatial sensitivity in Fig. 14, while the quantitative similarity of their spatial frequency and orientation bandwidths to those of monkey striate cells is indicated in Fig. 13. The complete foveal model was based on responses of these six spatial frequency tuned mechanisms, each including a range of orientations spanning 180° in 15° (high frequencies) to 30° (low frequencies) increments (Wilson, 1986). As shown in Fig. 17, a spatial stimulus is filtered in parallel by the six mechanisms and then passed through a contrast nonlinearity of the type found in cortical simple cells: a threshold at low contrasts followed by a compressive power law at suprathreshold contrasts. The shape of this function has been measured psychophysically by masking in several laboratories (Nachmias & Sansbury, 1974; Legge & Foley, 1980; Legge, 1981; Wilson et al., 1983). Following this, Gaussian noise is added to the mechanism responses, and the resultant noisy signals then serve to provide a representation of the stimulus in a multidimensional mechanism response space. To represent a spatially localized attribute of a stimulus, such as a vernier offset, the model incorporates the responses of the six classes of spatial frequency and orientation tuned mechanisms along with their spatially nearest neighbors. Comparison of neighboring spatial responses serves to provide information about spatial localization and phase within the model.

Given any two spatial patterns, the model schematized in Fig. 17 will produce two different spatial representations in the multidimensional mechanism response space, and, given the presence of physiological noise, each of these will be represented by a Gaussian distribution about its mean. Thus, discrimination between any pair of patterns should be a monotonic function of the distance between the means of their respective mechanism response distributions. The response $R_{\omega\theta}(x,y)$ of a mechanism tuned to spatial frequency ω and orientation θ will be a nonlinear function F of the integral of its spatial filter $RF_{\omega\theta}(x,y)$ multiplied by the intensity distribution of the pattern, $P(x,y)$:

$$R_{\omega\theta}(x,y) = \int_{-\infty}^{\infty}\int_{-\infty}^{\infty} RF(x - x', y - y') P(x', y')\, dx'\, dy' \quad (9)$$

The mathematical form for $RF_{\omega\theta}(x,y)$ is given by a suitably rotated version of the filter described by Eq. (7). As all of the constants associated with the filters and nonlinearities were measured in masking experiments (Wilson et al., 1983; Phillips & Wilson,

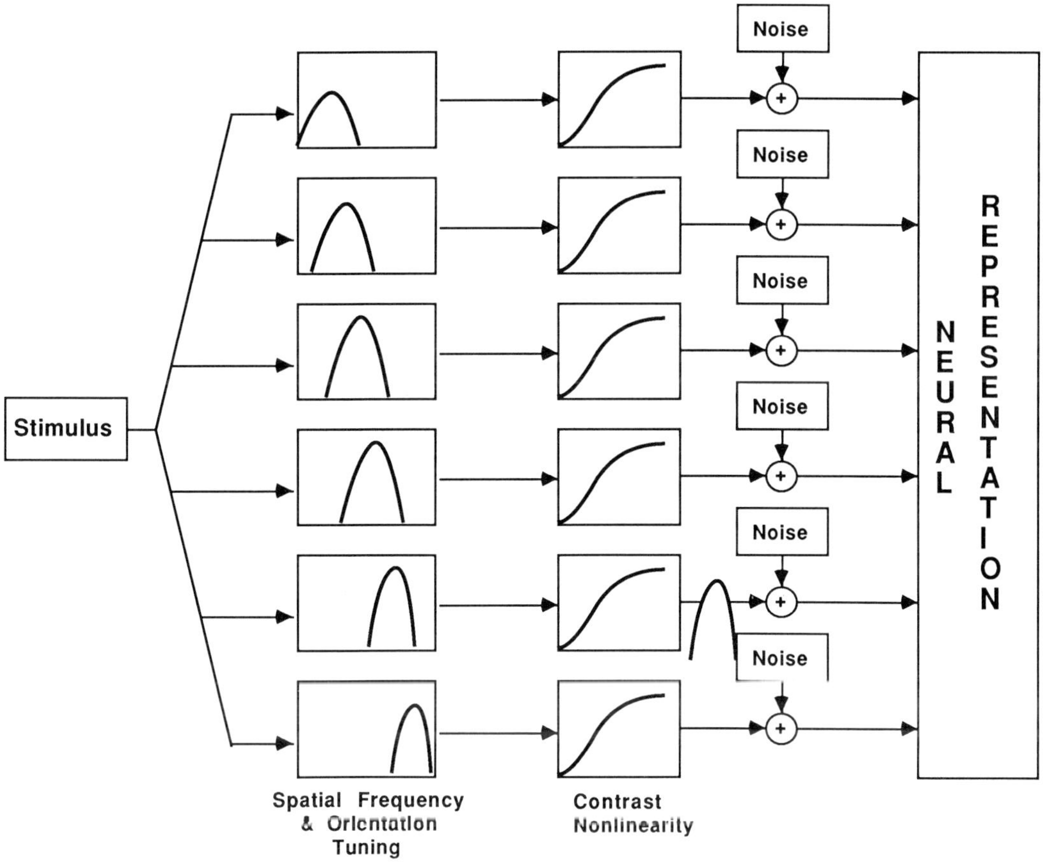

FIG. 17 Schematic diagram of a model for spatial pattern discrimination. The stimulus is first processed in parallel by an array of mechanisms tuned for both orientation and size or spatial frequency. The results of these linear filtering operations are then passed through contrast nonlinearities that are accelerated at low and compressive at high contrasts. Finally, physiological noise is added to these signals. The result of these operations is a representation of the stimulus in a multidimensional mechanism response space. The discriminability of two patterns is determined by the distance between their representations in this space.

1984), it follows that the responses of all mechanisms can be calculated directly given a knowledge of the pattern luminance distribution $P(x,y)$. Given any two patterns P_1 and P_2, the accuracy with which they may be discriminated will therefore be a monotonic function of the distance between their representations in mechanism response space:

$$\Delta R = \sqrt{\sum_{\omega=1}^{6} \sum_{\theta=0^\circ}^{180^\circ} \sum_{-\Delta x}^{\Delta x} |R_{\omega\theta}(P_1) - R_{\omega\theta}(P_2)|^2} \quad (10)$$

In Eq. (10) the summations are over the six spatial frequency tunings, the range of orientations, and the locations of neighboring spatial filters displaced by $\pm\Delta x$ (see Fig. 18). The separation between neighboring filters was set to the cone spacing for the highest frequency foveal filters and was increased in proportion to filter size for the lower frequency filters (Wilson & Gelb, 1984). Two observations may be made concerning Eq. (10). First, it is formally analogous to line element models for wavelength discrimination (Bouman & Walraven, 1972; Wyszecki & Stiles,

1982; Wilson, 1989b), except that the summation over three photopigment responses is replaced by the multiple summation over spatial frequency, orientation, and position. Thus, one may term this a line element model for spatial pattern discrimination. Second, when the two patterns generate mechanism responses that differ only slightly, the difference in responses may be approximated by a derivative of the response with respect to the appropriate stimulus variable. Accordingly, a given mechanism is most effective at pattern discrimination where the slope or derivative of its response is at a maximum.

It is natural to ask how the brain performs the differencing of mechanism responses in Eq. (10), as different sets of underlying units may be stimulated from trial to trial in any experiment due to eye movements. The answer is that responses to the first stimulus must be stored in short-term memory and then compared with responses to the second stimulus from units with comparable tuning properties. Although we are largely ignorant of the details of this short-term memory, the subtraction in Eq. (10) provides an accurate description of its role in pattern discrimination.

This line element model has been successfully applied to spatial frequency discrimination (Wilson & Gelb, 1984), a wide range of hyperacuity tasks (Wilson, 1986), and to the effects of spatial frequency adaptation on pattern discrimination (Wilson & Regan, 1984). In the case of spatial frequency discrimination, for example, the model correctly predicts increment thresholds of 2–4% for frequencies in the range 1–12 cpd, which agrees well with human psychophysical data (e.g., Hirsch & Hylton, 1982; Mayer & Kim, 1986). In virtue of the presence of just six foveal filter sizes, the model predicts that there should be alternate peaks and troughs of spatial frequency discrimination performance, as there are in wavelength discrimination. Such peaks and troughs have been reported by Hirsch and Hylton (1982), although Mayer and Kim (1986) failed to replicate this result. Failure to find evidence for peaks and troughs in spatial frequency discrimination would indicate that more than six mechanisms are involved in spatial frequency discrimination. Simulations indicate that 12 mechanisms would be adequate to produce a smooth discrimination curve. Determining whether the additional mechanisms are located in the fovea or in the near periphery would require additional experimental work.

As an example of hyperacuity predictions derived from the line element model, let us consider vernier acuity. In this task human subjects can detect an offset from colinearity in a pair of abutting lines when the offset is as little as 5 sec arc (Westheimer, 1979a, see Fig. 18A). In the pattern discrimination model developed above, the smallest filters are tuned to 16 cpd and thus have a central excitatory zone about 1.9 min arc wide, and they are spaced 38 sec arc apart, comparable to human foveal cone spacing (Williams, 1985a; Curcio et al., 1987). As shown in Fig. 18A, such a filter centered under a vernier stimulus would be expected to produce almost identical responses to aligned and offset targets. However, the vernier target will fall near the boundary between excitatory and inhibitory zones of neighboring spatial filters, and as a consequence a small offset will result in a large change in filter response. The same is true for filters oriented at about $\pm 15°$ to the vernier target axis.

This qualitative picture of filter responses in Fig. 18A leads to the expectation that these filters will support vernier thresholds significantly smaller than the width of their excitatory zones. Quantitative calculations with the model show that this is indeed true, as is shown in Fig. 18B. Here experimental (Westheimer & McKee, 1977) and theoretical (Wilson, 1986) thresholds are compared as a function of the separation between the two bars of the vernier target. For small separations both data and theory give thresholds in the 4–6 sec range, and these thresholds increase smoothly at separations above about 4 min of arc. The success of the model in generating thresholds as low as 6 sec bears out the qualitative picture in Fig. 18A. The gentle degradation of model thresholds for larger separations, which is in agreement with the data, occurs as the distance between vernier bars becomes greater than the length of the smallest filters, so that only larger filters contribute to the calculation. This model has been shown to accurately predict thresholds for a variety of other hyperacuity tasks (Wilson, 1986), including periodic vernier acuity and orien-

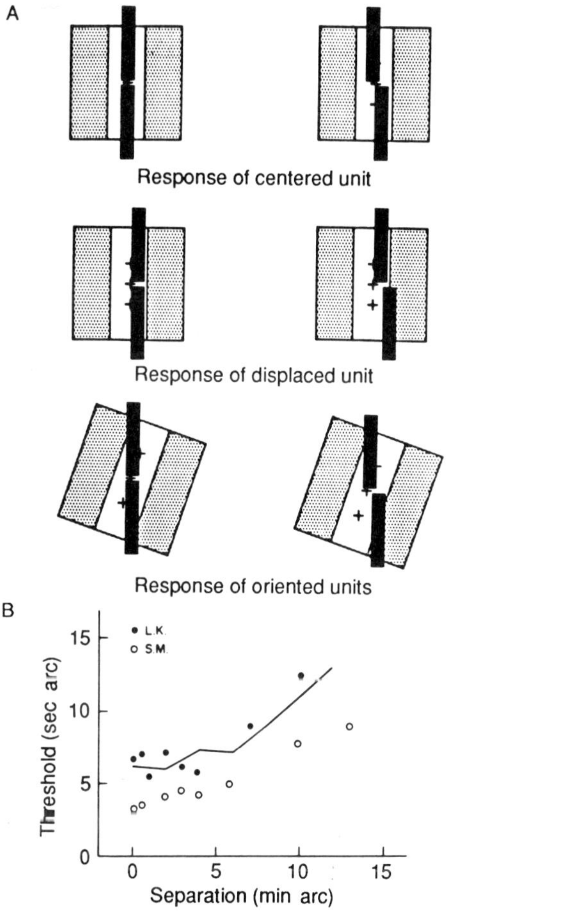

FIG. 18 In A model filters or receptive fields (excitatory region in white and + + +, inhibitory zones in gray) are shown with vernier stimuli superimposed. In the top line the filters are centered relative to the vernier target. These will produce little change in the responses to the aligned and offset targets, as both remain entirely within the excitatory region. As shown in the second line, however, a neighboring filter that is displaced slightly to the left will produce a large change in response to the vernier offset, as this displaces one bar partially into one inhibitory zone. The bottom line shows that filters at an orientation of about 15° will also produce a significant change in response to a vernier offset. Thus, the differential response to a vernier offset as small as 5 sec arc can be quite large despite the fact that the excitatory zone of these filters is about 2 min arc wide. In B model predictions (solid line) are compared with vernier threshold data for two subjects. Data and theory are plotted as a function of the separation between the near ends of the two target lines, each of which was 8 min arc long and 1 min arc wide. Data are from Westheimer and McKee (1977). The theoretical curve gradually rises from a value of about 6 sec arc as the separation between the vernier lines becomes greater than the length of the smallest receptive fields. From Wilson and Gelb (1984).

tation discrimination (Tyler, 1973), chevron acuity (Westheimer & McKee, 1977), bisection acuity (Klein & Levi, 1985), curvature discrimination (Wilson, 1985), and spatial interference with hyperacuity (Levi et al., 1985).

A critical test of the adequacy of the line element approach to spatial pattern discrimination was provided by two experiments measuring the effects of spatial frequency adaptation on spatial frequency and orientation discrimination (Regan & Beverley, 1983a, 1985). In the first experiment spatial frequency discrimination thresholds were measured before and after adaptation to a cosine grating of fixed spatial frequency, and the resulting elevations of discrimination thresholds were noted. Measured and predicted values for an adapting frequency of 5 cpd are plotted in Fig. 19. Although the maximum threshold elevation for detecting a grating occurred at the adapting spatial frequency (open circles) in agreement with Blakemore and Campbell (1969), the maximum threshold elevation for spatial frequency discrimination occurred about 1 octave above this (solid circles). In addition, the data showed a slight facilitation in discrimination near the adapting frequency and a slight discrimination threshold elevation at low frequencies.

To obtain theoretical predictions, spatial frequency adaptation was modeled as a reduction in gain or sensitivity of the mechanism most sensitive to the stimulus, an approach in agreement with the physiological evidence cited above (Maffei et al., 1973). The resultant theoretical threshold elevations for grating detection (dashed line) and spatial frequency discrimination (solid line) are shown in the top graph of Fig. 19 (Wilson & Regan, 1984). Qualitatively, the theoretical results agree with the data in showing a major elevation in discrimination thresholds approximately 1 octave above the adaptation frequency, a minor elevation at low frequencies, and a slight facilitation at the adapting frequency.

Although there are some quantitative discrepancies between theory and data, it should be stressed that the theoretical predictions were made "blind," that is, with only knowledge of the experimental conditions and adapting spatial frequency but without knowledge of the results. The explanation behind the pattern of

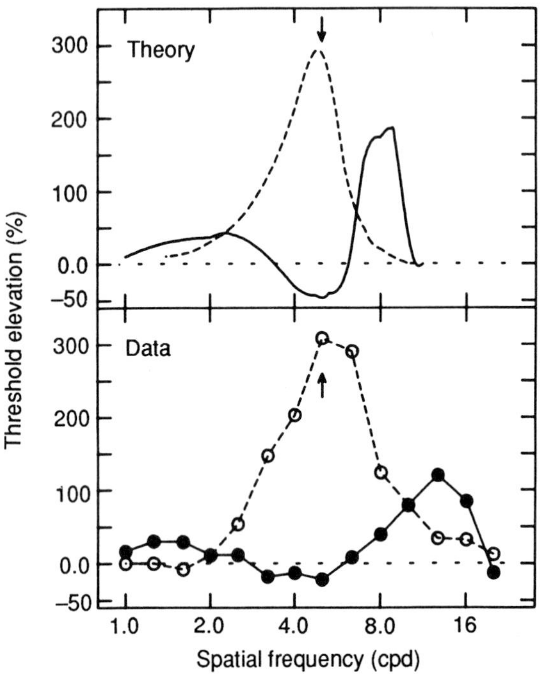

FIG. 19 Comparison of theoretical predictions and experimental threshold elevations following adaptation to a 5 cpd cosine grating (arrow). The threshold elevation for detecting a grating is plotted with open circles and dashed lines as a function of spatial frequency. As shown by Blakemore and Campbell (1969), these curves peak at the adapting frequency. Solid lines and circles show the threshold elevation for spatial frequency discrimination as a function of the base frequency. For spatial frequency discrimination, which was measured at 4 times the detection threshold, the largest threshold elevation occurs at about twice the adapting frequency, while a much smaller elevation occurs at lower frequencies. This pattern of results is a consequence of the fact that discrimination is based on the differential mechanism response (derivative of mechanism sensitivity), and Fig. 12 shows that this is greatest at about twice the peak frequency and significantly less at low frequencies. From Wilson and Regan (1984).

theoretical results becomes clear when it is recalled that discrimination is based on the differential change or slope of mechanism response to the stimuli in question. Reference to Fig. 12 shows that the tuning curves for spatially tuned mechanisms have a steeper slope at spatial frequencies above the peak and a shallower slope at frequencies below. It follows that a mechanism should be most effective at spatial frequency discrimination above its peak but much less effective below. This is the pattern of both data and theory in Fig. 19 in response to reducing the sensitivity of a mechanism by adaptation. Comparable agreement was obtained between data and theory for grating orientation discrimination following adaptation (Wilson & Regan, 1984).

The spatial frequency and adaptation experiments just discussed lend psychophysical support to the notion that pattern discrimination is based on the differential rather than the maximum response of visual mechanisms (Wilson & Regan, 1984). The differential response concept has been tested physiologically on single cells in cat visual cortex (Bradley, Skottun, Ohzawa, Sclar & Freeman, 1985, 1987), and results for spatial frequency and orientation discrimination by representative cells are shown in Fig. 20. First, the spatial frequency and orientation tuning curves of each cell were measured, and the regions of steepest change in sensitivity were estimated. For spatial frequency this was consistently found to fall at frequencies above the peak, which agrees with the psychophysical masking data (Fig. 12; Wilson et al., 1983) and threshold elevations following adaptation (Fig. 19; Regan & Beverly, 1983a; Wilson & Regan, 1984). Orientation tuning was found to be approximately bilaterally symmetric, again in agreement with psychophysics (Wilson & Regan, 1984; Regan & Beverly, 1985). Next, responses to a series of closely spaced spatial frequencies or orientations were repeatedly measured and the means and standard deviations calculated (Fig. 20A,B). These data were then used to estimate the probability of correct discrimination as a function of spatial frequency or orientation difference (Fig. 20C,D). This analysis showed that the most selective cells attained 5.25% spatial frequency and 1.85° orientation thresholds, which are only slightly higher than human psychophysical values. This was expected, as psychophysical data and models incorporate probability summation among a number of responding units [Eq. (10)], and this produces thresholds slightly lower than would be obtained from any single unit. Parker and Hawken (1985) adopted a similar analysis to show that orientation selective cells in monkey striate cortex could

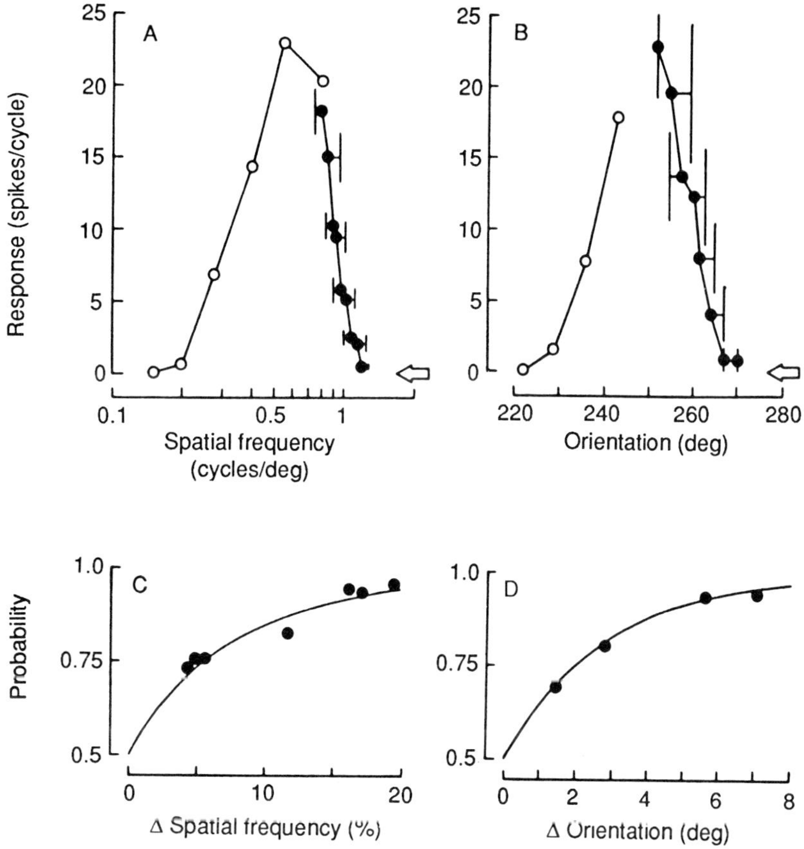

FIG. 20 Physiological measurement of spatial frequency discrimination (A and C) and orientation capabilities (B and D) of single cells in cat visual cortex. The spatial frequency tuning of the cell is shown in A by open circles at spatial frequencies at and below the peak and by solid circles at frequencies above the peak. In agreement with the psychophysical data in Fig. 12, the sensitivity curve was found to be steeper at high spatial frequencies than at low. Accordingly, sensitivities were repeatedly measured at frequencies above the peak in order to obtain means and standard errors (vertical bars indicate ±2 standard errors) as a function of spatial frequency. Based on this, it was possible to calculate the probability that two spatial frequencies differing by a given percentage could be reliably discriminated by the cell, and this is plotted in C. For this cell the 75% correct point was reached at a spatial frequency difference of 5.25%. Similar results for discrimination of grating orientation are shown in B and D. The only qualitative difference here was that the orientation tuning curve (A) was found to be approximately bilaterally symmetric. From Bradley et al. (1985).

discriminate spatial offsets on the order of 10 sec arc. Thus, single unit cortical electrophysiology provides strong corroboration for the line element or differential response approach to spatial pattern discrimination originally developed psychophysically.

Other models for hyperacuity share many features with the line element model. Klein and Levi (1985) developed a "viewprint" model, so named because it utilizes both spatial position and spatial frequency information in a manner analogous to the voiceprint of audition. Note that both spatial position and spatial frequency information are also incorporated into the line element summation in Eq. (10). The spatial filters used by Levi and Klein (1985) had spatial frequency bandwidths in the range of 1.5–2 octaves, and each was followed by a contrast nonlinearity displaying a threshold at low contrasts followed by a logarithmic nonlinear compression at high contrasts. The filters were spaced 0.2 min arc apart and covered a range of peak frequencies from 2 to 16 cpd in 0.125-octave steps. A unique feature of the viewprint model is that it utilizes mechanisms with both even (E) and odd (O) symmetry at each spatial location and then bases discrimination on differential changes in the quantity ($E^2 + O^2$). At present there is no physiological evidence for units that combine even and odd responses in this manner. Calculations using this model are otherwise similar to those of the line element model and have been shown to account successfully for bisection and two line separation hyperacuities (Klein & Levi, 1985).

Nielsen, Watson, and Ahumada (1985) have also

developed a discrimination model based on the responses of spatial frequency and orientation selective filters. Peak spatial frequencies of the filters spanned the range from 0.25 to 32 cpd in 1-octave steps, which is similar to the distribution of filters in the line element model except for the addition of the lowest and highest frequency filters. Thus, this model also represents a stimulus as a point in a multidimensional filter response space. There are three major differences between this and the line element model. First, the spatial frequency bandwidth of all filters in the Nielsen et al. (1985) model is 1 octave, which falls below most of the physiological and psychophysical bandwidth data in Fig. 13 and below the values used by Klein and Levi (1985). Second, the model does not incorporate a suprathreshold compressive nonlinearity and thus is limited to pattern contrasts near threshold. Finally, the outputs of these filters are analyzed by an ideal observer routine (Watson, 1983).[7] In applications of this model to spatial phase discrimination predictions were frequently a factor of 10 better than human psychophysical performance, which suggests that human subjects are far from ideal observers in utilizing the information conveyed by the mechanism responses.

Watt and Morgan (1985) have produced a somewhat different model for pattern discrimination dubbed MIRAGE. In its one-dimensional implementation MIRAGE contains four 1.7-octave bandwidth filters spaced at 1-octave intervals from 3.4 to 27.2 cpd. However, the responses of these filters are not used directly to produce a pattern representation. Rather, the convolution of each filter with the stimulus is first separated into its positive and negative parts (half-wave rectification), and these are separately averaged over all filters. Next, zero crossings, where the net response switches from positive to negative, are located; then three statistics of the activity between each pair of adjacent zero crossings are calculated. These are the centroid, which provides spatial localization; the area, which reflects pattern contrast; and the standard deviation, which is related to the width of the activity distribution. The major difference between MIRAGE and other models for pattern representation and discrimination lies in the nonlinear operations of half-wave rectification and averaging across filters followed by centroid, area, and standard deviation calculations. As a result, the independent responses of the different filters are lost in MIRAGE. Although MIRAGE accurately fits a range of psychophysical data (see also Chapter 7, this volume), there is as yet no physiological evidence for the existence of cortical units that might perform either the averaging across filters or calculation of the activity moments.

The focus to this point has been on quantitative approaches to pattern discrimination inspired by psychophysical and physiological data. A complementary approach has been to correlate psychophysics and electrophysiology in animals before and after selective brain lesions. This approach has elucidated the information transfer characteristics of the corpus callosum, the bundle of axons originating in Areas 17 and 18 along the representation of the vertical midline of the visual field (which also forms the border between Areas 17 and 18) and projecting contralaterally. The corpus callosum is generally assumed to be associated with the task of coordinating the representations of the two halves of the visual field in the two hemispheres so as to preserve perceptual continuity. Berardi, Bisti, and Maffei (1987) have recently shown by means of visual evoked potentials (VEPs) and single-unit recordings at the level of the border between Areas 17 and 18 of the cat that the gain of the callosal pathway is about 0.10 times that of the direct geniculocortical system. In addition, high spatial and temporal frequencies are strongly attenuated in the process of callosal transfer. An example of this obtained with VEP responses to cosine gratings in the monkey is shown in Fig. 21. The response to direct

[7] A typical ideal observer model is that of Geisler (1984), which incorporates known properties of the optics and photoreceptors and then calculates how effective the visual system would be in pattern discrimination if it optimally utilized all of the information available in the photoreceptor responses. This generally results in the generation of a matched filter for each stimulus used, and the computed thresholds are typically more than 10 times better than actual human performance. Watson (1983) applied the ideal detector approach to responses of model simple cells rather than to the photoreceptor responses.

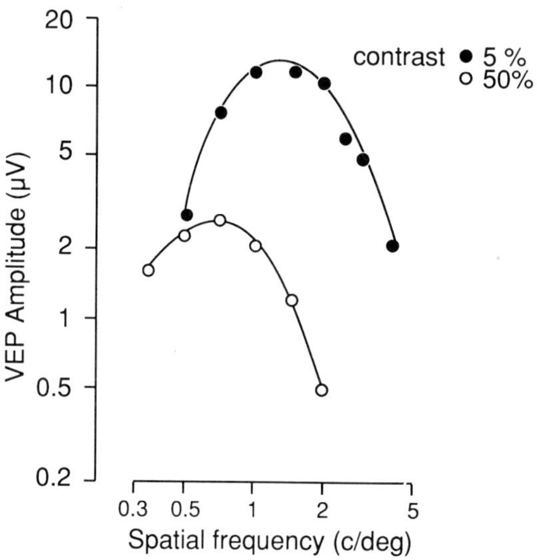

FIG. 21 Evoked potentials recorded at the V1/V2 border of a split chaism monkey in response to sinusoidal gratings of different spatial frequency, alternating in phase at 5 Hz. The data obtained for the ipsilateral eye (filled circles) represent the transfer function of the direct, geniculocortical input; the data obtained for the contralateral eye (open circles) represent the transfer function of the callosal input. The contrast of the gratings is indicated. From N. Berardi, S. Bisti, A. Fiorentini, and L. Maffei (unpublished).

ipsilateral input (filled circles) is much greater and extends to higher spatial frequencies than does the response elicited by stimulation of the contralateral, callosal pathway.

On the basis of these experiments one might expect that any interocular transfer of learning mediated by the corpus callosum could only occur when the animal was trained with high contrast patterns of low spatial and temporal frequency. This was tested by Berardi et al. (1987) using cats with a severed optic chiasm, which guarantees that only the ipsilateral retinocortical projections are preserved. These animals were trained to discriminate the orientation of a cosine grating using only one eye. Subsequent testing using the other eye revealed complete interocular transfer of learning for low spatial frequency gratings of moderate contrast. At higher spatial frequencies, however, there was no interocular transfer even at high contrasts. Berardi and Fiorentini (1987) have also provided psychophysical evidence that interocular pattern discrimination learning in humans only transfers to the contralateral field when patterns of low spatial frequency and high contrast are used. Thus, the psychophysical results agree with the expectations obtained from electrophysiology concerning information transfer cross the corpus callosum.

As a final example of the correlation between psychophysics and electrophysiology in pattern discrimination, the work of Orban, Vandenbussche, and Vogels (1984) on orientation discrimination may be cited. They gathered extensive data demonstrating that orientation discrimination is best for horizontal or vertical bars (thresholds of about 0.75°) and poorest at the 45° obliques (thresholds near 2°). Physiological measurements showed that this oblique effect was directly related to the numbers of baboon simple cells preferring horizontal and vertical as opposed to oblique orientations (Kennedy, Martin, Orban & Whitteridge, 1985).

VIII. PERIPHERAL PATTERN DISCRIMINATION

With the exception of MIRAGE, psychophysical pattern discrimination models have the general form shown schematically in Fig. 17. To extend these models to the visual periphery, it is necessary to alter both the spatial filtering and spatial sampling characteristics of the model. Swanson and Wilson (1985) performed masking experiments at an eccentricity of 8° to estimate the spatial frequency tuning of filters at that locus. The resulting tuning curves were the same as the foveal ones in Fig. 12, except that they were uniformly larger by a factor proportional to the change in grating acuity.

In the periphery, physiologically measured cortical receptive field sizes change less with eccentricity than does cortical magnification, and thus there must be less overlap of peripheral receptive fields and consequent spatial undersampling of the image. As discussed above (see Fig. 5), the rate of increase of filter size is correlated with grating acuity, while the more rapid increase in the interval between spatial samples is related to the peripheral change in hyperacuity. Levi and Klein (1987) have examined the role of spatial sampling in central and peripheral vision by asking observers to judge whether a briefly flashed test line bisects two reference lines. Each line was made up of discrete samples (dots), and the number of samples was systematically varied. If this visual task is limited by the spatial sampling grain, thresholds would be expected to be highest with a single sample and to fall in proportion to the square root of the number of discrete samples. In foveal vision, even with a single dot, thresholds were smaller than the intercone spacing, and adding discrete samples had only a small effect on thresholds (Fig. 22A). However, at 2.5° in the periphery the results were markedly different (Fig. 22B). First, the threshold for a single sample was elevated by a factor of 10, which makes it larger than the intercone spacing at 2.5°. This indicates that it is the cortical sampling grain rather than the cone mosaic which limits position discrimination in the periphery. Second, in the periphery adding samples had a pronounced effect on bisection thresholds. The slope of the descending line is -0.5, suggesting that in the periphery position thresholds decline in proportion to the square root of the number of samples (up to about 10), which would be expected of an ideal detector with uncorrelated noise at an early stage of visual processing.

In a theoretical study, Wilson (1989a) has shown that peripheral vernier acuity can be explained by altering three aspects of the foveal line element model previously described. First, the size of the visual filters must be increased in proportion to the ratio of foveal to peripheral grating acuity (Swanson & Wilson, 1985). Second, the spacing of neighboring filters must be increased by an even greater factor to reflect spatial undersampling. Finally, spatial uncertainty concerning the exact location of the filters must be introduced. This means that at cortical levels the exact location of peripheral receptive fields in visual field coordinates must be imprecisely known due to the irregularities in sample spacing that are known to be present even at the level of the photoreceptors. Although the foveal cones are hexagonally packed in a regular mosaic (Hirsch & Hylton, 1984), peripheral cones show significant disorder (Hirsch & Miller, 1987). French, Snyder, and Stavenga (1977) demonstrated that such spatial position uncertainty has the effect of reducing the spatial signal-to-noise ratio of the neural representation, and this has been shown to have a large quantitative effect in degrading peripheral vernier acuity (Wilson, 1989a,b). In an experimental study, Nyman, Greenlee, and Laurinen (1988) showed that irregularity in sample spacing had no effect on pattern detection but caused a large impairment of pattern discrimination capabilities. However, this position uncertainty may also serve to minimize some of the deleterious effects of spatial aliasing by spreading aliased frequencies into broadband noise (Yellot, 1982, 1984).

It is a striking feature of two-bar separation discrimination that once the separation is greater than a few minutes of arc, thresholds are approximately proportional to the separation. Thus, there is a Weber's law for position acuity, and this holds for separations up to at least 10° (Burbeck, 1987). There are two general classes of explanations for this Weber's law behavior, one based on the differential responses of spatially localized filters (Klein & Levi, 1985; Wilson, 1986) and one based on spatial sampling at the cortical level. As the separation between the lines increases, larger filters would be the only ones responding to both lines, and this would produce larger thresholds. However, for very large separations this explanation is implausible, as evidence for sufficiently large filters has never been found (Burbeck, 1987). For very large separations, therefore, Weber's law for position must be based on the spatial sampling grain in the peripheral visual field. The notion here is that the spatial grain of the visual cortex (reciprocal of cortical magnification) increases linearly with eccentricity; thus, the position of the reference lines becomes increasingly uncertain as their eccentricity increases. Levi, Klein, and Yap (1988) directly tested the hypothesis that Weber's law at large separations is

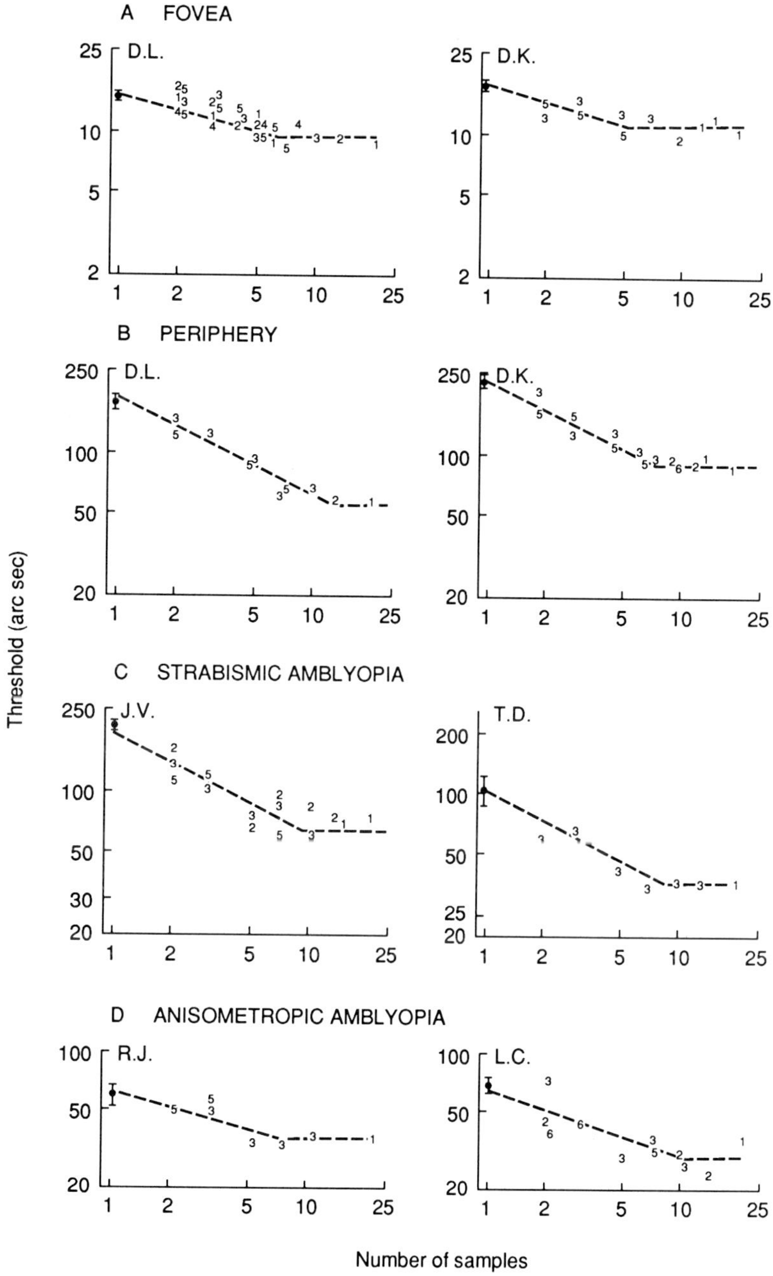

FIG. 22 Bisection thresholds are plotted as a function of the number of discrete samples of the stimulus. The numbers in each graph represent the size of the interspaces in minutes of arc. (A) Data for two normal observers with foveal fixation. (B) Data obtained at 2.5° in the lower visual field. (C) Data for the amblyopic eyes of two observers with strabismic amblyopia. (D) Data for the amblyopic eyes of two observers with anisometropic amblyopia. Note that the anisometropic data have the same dependence on sample number as normal foveal data, whereas the strabismic data resemble those from the normal periphery. From Levi and Klein (1987). Copyright © 1987 Macmillan Magazines Ltd.

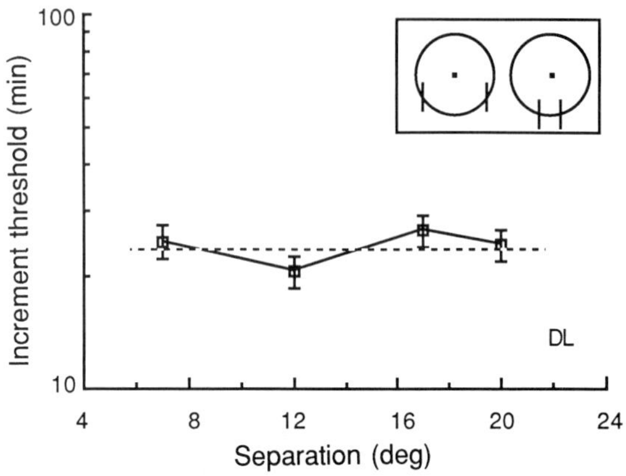

FIG. 23 Two-line separation discrimination under isoeccentric discrimination conditions. As shown in the inset, the target lines were always located on a circle (not visible) of constant 10° eccentricity. Under these stimulus conditions, increment thresholds are constant (dashed line) for a wide range of line separations. As Weber's law is not obtained for these isoeccentric conditions, it appears that Weber's law behavior for large separations is dependent on conditions in which the eccentricity of stimulation increases with stimulus separation. From Levi et al. (1988).

due to reduced cortical magnification in the periphery. In their experiments subjects were required to discriminate the separation between two lines that always fell at the same eccentricity. This was accomplished by placing the lines on a circle (not visible) of constant 10° eccentricity (see inset in Fig. 23). Under these conditions, discrimination thresholds were constant over a wide range of separations, as shown by the data in Fig. 23.

Clearly, there is no Weber's law for position when stimuli are presented at a fixed eccentricity. Rather, for eccentricities greater than about 0.5°, the human observer can localize a line with an accuracy that corresponds to about 1/10 of a cortical module. Thus, for small separations, pattern discrimination is dependent on the differential responses of spatial frequency tuned filters and their spacing, whereas for large separations, which inevitably involve peripheral stimulation, discrimination is limited by the accuracy of the spatial representation in the peripheral visual field. This accuracy is a fixed fraction of eccentricity, which leads to Weber's law when eccentricity is varied [see Eq. (3)]; however, it also appears to be a constant distance across the cortex, so that Weber's law does not hold with respect to cortical distance.

IX. PATTERN DISCRIMINATION IN ABNORMAL VISION

In the foregoing it has been shown that pattern discrimination in foveal and peripheral vision can be understood in terms of the filtering and spatial sampling characteristics of the visual system. In the fovea the filters are smaller (tuned to higher spatial frequencies), and the spatial sampling is regular and approximately at the Nyquist spacing for the high frequency cutoff of each filter. In the periphery the filters are larger (tuned to lower frequencies), and spatial sampling is both irregular and below the Nyquist limit. In this section amblyopia and albinism are briefly examined as instances of spatial sampling changes that result in reduced vision.

Amblyopia (Greek: amblyos, dull; opia, sight) is a developmental anomaly of spatial vision which is usually associated with the presence of strabismus (inability of both eyes to fixate on a common point, e.g., cross-eyed individuals) or anisometropia (unequal refractive errors in the two eyes) early in life (see Chapter 14, this volume). As a result, the deviated or defocused eye exhibits significantly reduced acuity. Amblyopia is of particular interest because the retina appears to be normal, and thus the abnormalities apparently reflect cortical processing. Moreover, several lines of evidence suggest that strabismic and anisometropic amblyopia are fundamentally different (Hess, Campbell & Zimmern, 1980; Levi & Klein, 1982, 1985; Hess & Pointer, 1985; Levi, Klein & Yap, 1987). Figure 24 compares the vernier and grating acuities for a group of amblyopes. For anisometropes (A's) the data fall along a straight line with a slope of unity, which implies that the two acuities are affected in the same way by the amblyopic process. In contrast, the data for strabismic amblyopes (S's and

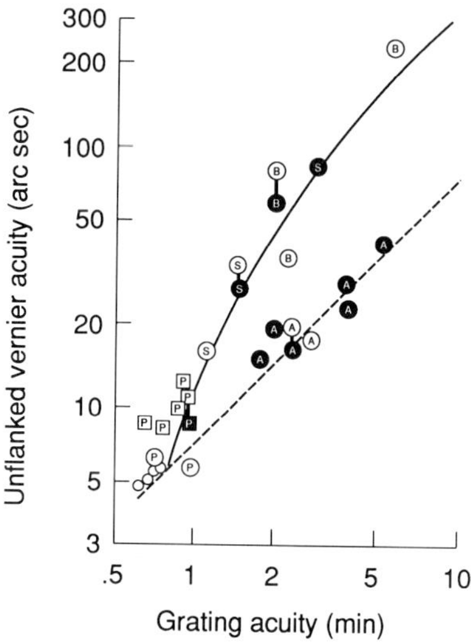

FIG. 24 Vernier acuity (ordinate) plotted against grating acuity (abscissa). Data are shown for normal observers (open circles), preferred eyes of anisometropic amblyopes (P's in circles), preferred eyes of strabismic amblyopes (P's in squares), and amblyoic eyes of strabismics (S's), anisometropes (A's), and subjects with both forms of amblyopia (B's). The black letters represent data obtained with a two-line vernier target, while white letters were obtained with repetitive vernier gratings. The dashed line has a slope of 1 and indicates the prediction if vernier and grating acuities were degraded to the same degree. The solid line shows the relationship between vernier and grating acuities in the normal periphery. Note that strabismic data follow the curve for the normal periphery, while anisometropes show comparable degradation of both acuities. From Levi and Klein (1985).

B's) deviate from this line in a direction indicating that vernier acuity is degraded to a greater degree than grating acuity. The solid line in Fig. 24 shows the relationship between vernier and grating acuities in the normal periphery, and it also provides a reasonable fit to the strabismic data.

Based on these results, Levi and Klein (1985) suggested that the performance of anisometropes could be accounted for on the basis of a reduced signal-to-noise ratio of their small (high spatial frequency) filters caused by the effects of early visual experience with one defocused retinal image. On the other hand, the reduced positional acuity of strabismic amblyopes is qualitatively and quantitatively similar to that in the periphery of normal subjects. Since the retina of strabismic amblyopes appears to be normal, Levi and Klein (1985) suggested that the central visual field of strabismic amblyopes is *cortically undersampled.* Figure 22C, which shows the influence of the number of samples on the position thresholds of a strabismic amblyope, demonstrates the strong similarity between the central visual field of strabismics and normal peripheral vision. In contrast, anisometropes show a dependence on the number of samples identical to the pattern for the normal fovea (Fig. 22D). Like the normal periphery, the strabismic fovea shows marked positional uncertainty with a single sample, while thresholds improve in proportion to the square root of the number of samples. Indeed, spatial uncertainty owing to cortical undersampling in strabismic foveal vision has been shown to give rise to characteristic spatial distortions (Hess, 1979; Bedell and Flom, 1981). Wilson (1989a) has shown that the vernier acuity of anisometropes can be quantitatively predicted on the basis of the reduced signal to noise ratio of small spatial filters, whereas the data of strabismic amblyopes require the assumption of spatial undersampling and uncertainty.

The central vision of human albinos presents a very different example of reduced spatial acuity. Albinism comprises a number of genetic disorders, all of which are characterized by disruption of melanin synthesis, low acuity, nystagmus, and abnormal retinocortical projections (for reviews, see Witkop, Jay, Creel & Guillery, 1982; Cucchiaro, 1985; Kinnear, Jay & Witkop, 1985). In addition, albino retinas in both human (Fulton, Albert & Craft, 1978) and green monkey (Guillery, Hickey, Kaas, Felleman, Debruyn & Sparks, 1984) have much lower foveal photoreceptor densities than do normals. To determine the consequences of this reduced density, Wilson, Mets, Nagy, and Kressel (1988) measured both grating and vernier acuities on two young albino adults using horizontally oriented patterns so as to minimize image degradation due to nystagmus. Both grating acuity (9.1 cpd) and vernier acuity (48 sec) were much worse than in the normal fovea. However, the ratio of grating to vernier acuity fell within the range measured for the fovea of normals and was significantly above the ratio for the normal periphery. In this respect, albino central vision is like that of anisometropic amblyopes and differs from that of strabismics.

To further explore spatial information processing in albinos, they were tested on a spatial frequency discrimination task using horizontal stimuli with a 1-octave bandwidth and frequencies in the range from 0.25 to 4 cpd (Yo, Wilson, Mets & Ritacco, 1989). As shown in Fig. 25, average discrimination for two albinos (dotted squares) was at least as good as the average of three normal observers (solid squares) at all spatial frequencies tested. As these normal data were obtained in the fovea, where grating acuity was about 42 cpd, the normal observers were tested again at a peripheral locus at which their grating acuity was found to be 9.1 cpd, the same as for albino central vision. The peripheral discrimination thresholds for normals (Fig. 25, diamonds) were 2–3 times higher than thresholds for albino central vision. Unlike the case of the strabismic amblyope, therefore, the central visual system of the albino does *not* resemble the periphery of normals.

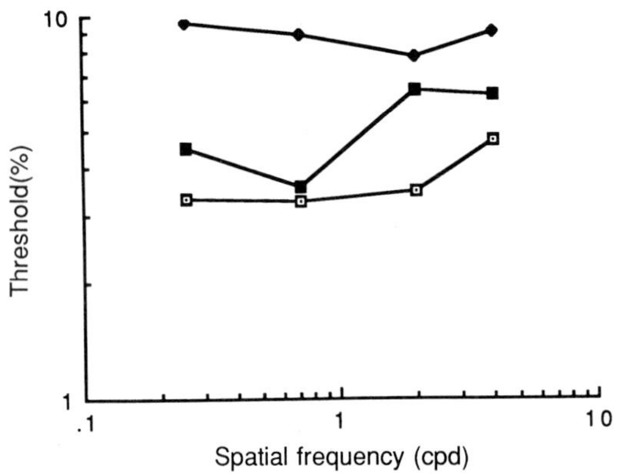

FIG. 25 Comparison of spatial frequency discrimination by albinos and visually normal young adults. Albino thresholds (dotted squares) over the range 0.25–4 cpd were slightly better than averages for foveal viewing by normals (solid squares), although the differences were not statistically significant. However, when normal subjects repeated these experiments at an eccentricity at which their grating acuities were equal to the average central grating acuity for albinos (9.1 cpd), their thresholds (diamonds) were significantly higher. Thus, albino central vision is not comparable to normal peripheral vision. Rather, it resembles a magnified or low spatial frequency version of normal foveal vision. From Yo et al. (1989).

Given that the central cones of albinos have been reported to be spaced about 3.5 times farther apart than normal adult foveal cones (Fulton et al., 1978), one would expect orientation and spatial frequency selective mechanisms to be tuned to frequencies 3.5 times lower than in normals. Calculations using the line element approach demonstrated that introduction of this factor provided a quantitative explanation of albino grating acuity, vernier acuity, and spatial frequency discrimination (Wilson et al., 1988; Yo et al., 1989). Thus, it appears that albino central vision is a spatially "stretched" or magnified version of normal adult foveal vision. As foveal cones in the normal human infant are also known to be more widely spaced than in the adult (Yuodelis & Hendrickson, 1986; see Chapter 13, this volume), it may be speculated that albinism involves an arrest of retinal development. A similar hypothesis has been advanced in regard to the poor spatial vision of a complete rod monochromat (Greenlee, Magnussen & Nordby, 1988). There are indeed anatomical and psychophysical similarities between infant and albino vision (Wilson et al., 1988). The line element approach has also been successfully applied to infant spatial vision by increasing spatial filter dimensions in proportion to the increased foveal cone spacing of infants (Wilson, 1988).

X. IDEAS AND ISSUES

The foregoing has documented current anatomical, physiological, and psychophysical understanding of the roles of spatial sampling and filtering as they relate to form vision in the retinostriate pathway. From the perspective of pattern representation in the visual cortex, foveal information is known to be processed in parallel by a number of different filters tuned for both spatial frequency and orientation. Furthermore, these filters appear to provide Nyquist sampling at their high spatial frequency cutoff so as to accurately encode all of the information present in the optically limited image falling on the foveal cones. The cortical representation of peripheral information is somewhat different. As it has long been known that peripheral grating acuity declines progressively from its foveal value, it was first thought that the peripheral representation was a larger scale or lower spatial frequency version of the foveal representation. However, this has been found to be only part of the story, and current evidence indicates that the peripheral representation is degraded both by spatial undersampling relative to the optical quality of the retinal image and by spatial uncertainty concerning the exact positioning of individual filters. As a manifestation of this, receptive field sizes follow the change in grating acuity with eccentricity, doubling in their linear dimensions in 2°–4°; while hyperacuity, which doubles in 0.3°–0.9°,correlates with cortical magnification. It was then shown that many aspects of spatial pattern discrimination, including spatial frequency discrimination and hyperacuity, could be accurately predicted based on the differential responses of spatial arrays of visual filters.

In this section, the focus is on issues raised by the current state of our understanding of cortical information processing. These issues may be grouped into four categories: (1) significance of image representation on multiple spatial scales; (2) role of distinct cell types in pattern representation; (3) significance of eccentricity variation in visual processing; and (4) implicit versus explicit representation of spatial information.

A. Image Representation on Multiple Spatial Scales

Evidence from both electrophysiology and psychophysics clearly indicates that the retinal image is processed in parallel by mechanisms having a range of filter sizes or peak spatial frequencies, and this holds true even if one restricts consideration to processing at a single eccentricity. As the ensemble of cells in a cortical module appears to cover a polar coordinate representation of orientation and spatial frequency (see Fig. 8), it has been suggested that the function of these filters is to perform a two-dimensional Fourier transform on the retinal image (Robson, 1975, 1983), although the obvious eccentricity variation of visual properties would necessarily require that this transformation be done independently on many small patches of the image. Two problems confront this notion, however. First, for an array of spatial frequency tuned mechanisms to perform a true Fourier transform on a local patch of the image, it would be necessary for their spatial frequency bandwidths to remain constant on a linear scale. This means that bandwidths would have to decrease proportionally to peak frequency on an octave scale, for example, varying from 2 octaves at 1 cpd to 1 octave at 2 cpd, to 0.25 octave at 8 cpd, and this is clearly contradicted by both the psychophysical and physiological data in Fig. 13. The second problem is more philosophical: as a Fourier transformation is an exact and invertible linear transformation of the spatial information, it is difficult to see what advantages it would afford the visual system. Pattern recognition would then be transformed into the problem of recognizing two-dimensional Fourier spectra, and this is identical to the problem of recognizing two-dimensional spatial patterns. To put it metaphorically, spatial Fourier transformation has no greater advantage for visual pattern recognition than does translation from Finnish to Italian for language recognition.

As spatial frequency bandwidths of cortical cells and psychophysical mechanisms do not decrease fast enough with peak spatial frequency to perform a Fourier transform, it follows that cortical image representation must utilize both spatial position and spatial frequency information. Accordingly, it has been proposed that the visual cortex provides a Gabor function representation of visual images (Marcelja, 1980; Daugman, 1985). As a Gabor function is defined by a sine wave modulated by a Gaussian envelope [see Eq. (8)], it accordingly encodes both spatial and spatial frequency information. It has been established that Gabor functions provide a reasonable fit to many cortical receptive fields (Marcelja, 1980; Daugman, 1985), although recent evidence suggests that the difference of two or three Gaussians in Eq. (7) may provide an even better fit (Hawken & Parker, 1987). Regardless of which functional form is found to provide the best description of filter shapes, there is a common misconception about Gabor functions that needs to be cleared up. A Gabor function representation is generally not equivalent to a Fourier representation of the image within the Gaussian envelope. For the two to be equivalent, it is necessary that the bandwidth in octaves of the Gabor functions decrease proportional to peak frequency, and the results in Fig. 13 show this to be violated in the visual system.

These considerations lead to the conclusion that the cortical representation of spatial information comprises a series of spatial images on different scales of resolution or, equivalently, filtered through bandpass filters with differing peak frequencies. Thomas (1970) was the first to recognize that the retinal image was processed in parallel by a range of different receptive field sizes, implying the representation of information on several spatial resolution scales. An elegant example of such a representation is provided by the Laplacian Pyramid scheme introduced by Burt and Adelson (1983). But what utility do these multiple spatial scales provide for visual information processing? Several intriguing suggestions here come from the realm of computational vision, where interactions between representations on different spatial scales have been found useful in edge extraction and in stereopsis. For example, Marr and Hildreth (1980) have suggested that the visual system could determine whether an edge is present in a noisy retinal image by comparing estimates of edge location obtained on different spatial scales: when these independent estimates coincide, the presence of an edge in the image may be inferred reliably. A more sophisticated approach has been developed by Canny (1986), who suggested a scheme whereby edge estimates on the finest resolution scale (high spatial frequencies) could be used to predict the pattern of activity on coarser spatial scales. Where these predictions agree with the stimulus generated activity on the coarser scales it is inferred that an edge is present. In steropsis, several schemes have been suggested whereby initial disparity estimates obtained with large, low spatial frequency mechanisms could be used to optimize disparity processing at finer spatial scales (e.g., Nishihara, 1987; Quam, 1987). Although these examples are merely suggestive, they do indicate the utility of a variety of interactions between mechanisms tuned to different spatial frequencies. Certainly, the independent, parallel channel model in Fig. 17 cannot be the complete story, and the exploration of interchannel interactions is likely to be a major focus of future research.

B. Role of Distinct Cell Types in Pattern Representation

Cortical neurophysiology has revealed the presence of at least three distinct cell types: simple, complex, and end-stopped. However, psychophysics and visual modeling studies have universally utilized units with characteristics of simple cells (c.f. filter profiles in Fig. 14); complex and end-stopped units have been ignored. For example, the line element and other pattern discrimination models diagramed in Fig. 17 use only models of simple cells. What, then, are the functional roles of these latter two cell types? They are certainly not necessary to provide a complete representation of all the information in the retinal image, as simple cells tile the spatial frequency domain (see Fig. 8) and provide Nyquist spatial sampling (at least in the foveal representation). Hubel and Wiesel (1962, 1968) suggested a hierarchical processing scenario in which complex cells receive input from arrays of simple cells and in turn provide inputs to "hypercomplex" or end-stopped cells. This, however, cannot be correct, as complex cells discard all information about spatial position within their receptive fields as a result of nonlinear pooling (see Fig. 10). Thus, hyperacuity would be impossible in a visual system in which simple cells contacted only complex cells. Despite the absence of answers to these questions, speculative hypotheses may be advanced concerning the roles of these three cell types.

As most psychophysical and modeling work has centered on the role of mechanisms with the characteristics of simple cells, it is easiest to discuss their functional role. It seems most likely that they serve to extract and accurately localize luminance lines, edges, countours, and gratings. Thus, it is no surprise that pattern discrimination models based on the differential responses of model simple cells have been successful at predicting spatial frequency and orientation discrimination and hyperacuity. However, as discussed above, there is evidence that simple cells do not respond to lines and edges embedded in complex two-dimensional textures (Maffei, 1985), so it might be inferred that simple cells mainly process isolated, locally one-dimensional luminance edges and contours.

A plausible role for complex cells may be inferred from the fact that they respond vigorously to two-dimensional textures, while simple cells do not (Hammond & MacKay, 1977, 1978). If simple cell response to two-dimensional textures are inhibited by the activity of complex cells, then the following picture emerges. Relatively simple luminance edges and contours are encoded by patterns of activity in simple cells. As the complexity of detail in a small region increases, however, a point will be reached when complex cell activity becomes sufficiently strong to suppress simple cell responses in that region. As a result of nonlinear subunit pooling (see Fig. 10), a complex cell cannot encode the spatial location or relative phase of details within its receptive field. Thus, it may be hypothesized that complex cells may function to encode a few of the statistical properties of complex two-dimensional textures, such as the dominant spatial frequency, orientation, and contrast. This would result in a very efficient nonlinear information compression in the encoding of complex textured scenes. Psychophysical evidence lends support to the hypothesis that only a few statistics of complex textures are encoded (Julesz & Bergen, 1983). Also consistent with this notion is the fact that only complex cells seem capable of processing disparity in random dot stereograms (Poggio, Motter, Squatrito & Trotter 1985).

Finally, simple and complex cells with the end-stopped property may function to provide accurate localization of the ends of thin lines and the boundaries of textures, respectively. Indeed, Wilson and Richards (1988) have obtained psychophysical evidence that visual localization of texture boundaries may be due to responses of end-stopped cells. As these ideas are certainly speculative, it remains a major challenge to develop psychophysical paradigms to explore possible consequences of parallel processing by simple, complex, and end-stopped cells.

C. Significance of Eccentricity Variation in Visual Processing

Visual acuity decreases progressively from the fovea to the periphery, and the spatial sampling grain of the cortex appears to coarsen even more rapidly so as to cause spatial undersampling. The apparent disadvantages of this arrangement lead naturally to the question: Are there any functional advantages that accrue to a visual system arranged in this manner? At first glance, one might wonder why a foveal level of acuity and sampling did not evolve throughout the visual periphery, but there is a simple reason why this was impossible. For the foveal level of acuity and spatial sampling to obtain out to an eccentricity of 45° approximately 10 times as many ganglion cells would be required in the retina. Not only would this lead to an optic nerve more than 3 times greater in diameter, but it would require 10 times the surface area of visual cortex for processing. As visual areas already comprise over 50% of cortex in monkeys and a similar amount or slightly less in humans, such an expansion of the visual areas would be impossible without a very swollen head!

Granted that a foveal level of resolution could not have been attained, it is still reasonable to ask why the particular variation of visual properties observed in primates evolved. Although no definitive answer is possible, the following scenario suggests that there may indeed have been some evolutionary advantage to this arrangement. Consider a primitive hunter running across a field. As the hunter moves forward, the images of obstacles such as rocks and trees lying to either side of his path will flow outward from the center of the retina. As they flow outward, three associated changes will occur: the images will increase in size; they will move at an increased velocity on the retina; and they will generate a greater binocular disparity. These changes are mirrored by the variation of visual properties with eccentricity: receptive field size increases in the periphery; the velocity processing range shifts toward higher velocities; higher temporal frequencies can be detected (Johnson & Massof, 1984; Tyler, 1985); and Panum's fusional area for disparity processing expands (Ogle, 1950). Given the limitations imposed by the amount of cortical tissue available for visual processing, therefore, it is a plausible hypothesis that the eccentricity variation of visual properties evolved to permit efficient processing of optic flow information.

This does not fully answer the question of why the periphery should be spatially undersampled, although Yellot (1982, 1984) has pointed out that the uncertainty of receptor spacing in the periphery serves to minimize the deleterious effects of aliasing. Perhaps related to spatial uncertainty and undersampling in the periphery is the interesting observation by Bennett and Banks (1987) that perception of relative phase between gratings is seriously degraded in the periphery. Finally, there are striking temporal processing anomalies in the periphery, such as fast flicker adaptation (Schieting & Spillmann, 1987) and the fact that all temporal frequencies above about 8 Hz appear to be flickering at 8 Hz (Johnson & Massof, 1984; Yo & Wilson, 1987). If there is a functional significance to these anomalies, it is probably related to velocity processing.

D. Implicit versus Explicit Representation of Spatial Information

In striate cortex the response of single cells varies with a number of stimulus attributes including orientation, spatial frequency, contrast, velocity, and binocular disparity. In consequence, no single attribute is represented explicitly by the activity of a single cell. Rather, stimulus attributes are represented implicitly within the pattern of activity of relatively localized neural populations, perhaps at the level of the cortical module. (For an illuminating discussion of implicit as opposed to explicit representation of information in the visual system, see Ballard, 1986.) However, the stimulus requirements to drive a striate cell are clearly more specific than those for retinal and LGN neurons, and this explains the vast increase in number of cortical neurons over LGN afferents. If, for example, the cortex contained cells tuned to 15 orientations, three disparities per orientation (near, zero, far, cf. Poggio & Fischer, 1977), and three directions of motion (e.g., left, right, and stationary) with a spatial resolution equivalent to that provided by the LGN, it would require 135 neurons per afferent. As the cortex also requires three cell types (simple, complex, and end-stopped), a range of receptive field sizes to represent spatial frequency information, and cells to encode color, the number of combinations should rapidly reach or exceed 1,000, the anatomical estimate of the factor by which cells in the striate foveal representation exceed LGN afferents.

Doubtless not all of these possible combinations are explicitly represented in the cortex, but the point is that even this modest degree of complexity in single-unit stimulus requirements requires an enormous multiplicity of cells. Clearly this proliferation cannot continue at higher levels of the system. For example, given 1,000 cortical cells per LGN afferent, an explicit representation of all possible combinations of properties at four neighboring spatial loci would require 10^{12} times as many neurons as LGN inputs, more than in the entire brain! This alone shows that the "grandmother cell" concept cannot be implemented by the brain: it would require far too many neurons.[8]

As a consequence of the fact that striate cortical neurons only represent individual stimulus attributes implicitly, it follows that psychophysical experiments must require some form of comparison of responses across a population of active neural units. For example, orientation discrimination between cosine gratings of very different spatial frequencies is as accurate as it is between gratings of the same spatial frequency, and the same is true for spatial frequency discrimination between gratings differing in orientation (Burbeck & Regan, 1983). As these results could not be obtained from the response of any single neuron in the striate cortex, these tasks must require a comparison of responses from neurons tuned to a range of both orientations and spatial frequencies. For example, to extract an estimate of stimulus spatial frequency independent of orientation from the responses $R(\omega_i, \theta_i)$ of a population of cells tuned to orientation θ_i and spatial frequency ω_i, the weighted average response (Klein, Stromeyer & Ganz, 1974, Georgeson, 1980) might be used:

$$\text{Estimated frequency} = \frac{\sum_{\omega}\sum_{\theta} \omega_i R(\omega_i, \theta_i)}{\sum_{\omega}\sum_{\theta} R(\omega_i, \theta_i)} \qquad (11)$$

This expression simply weights the response of each unit by its peak spatial frequency and then divides by the sum of the responses to minimize the effects of overall response level due to stimulus contrast. A similar expression could obviously be used to obtain an estimate of orientation independent of spatial frequency. As the computation in Eq. (11) could easily be implemented by a simple neural circuit, it is evident that information implicit in the responses of neural populations in striate cortex could be plicit at higher cortical levels.

Finally, it is worth mentioning that the implicit representation of information by populations of neurons is analogous to coding in color vision, where all information is initially represented in the responses of the three cone populations. Subsequently this information is reencoded to obtain an explicit estimate of the luminance, red–green, and yellow–blue attributes of the stimulus. In addition, a continuum of stimulus wavelengths can be represented implicitly due to the spectral overlap of the cone photopigments. This analogy to color vision was in fact a major impetus for the development of the line element approach to spatial pattern discrimination (Wilson & Gelb, 1984). The Wilson and Gelb model and others like it represent local stimulus attributes as a point in a multidimensional mechanism response space, and thus all of these attributes are represented only implicitly. Obtaining explicit estimates of stimulus attributes from these models would require a further computation such as that in Eq. (11).

[8] A "grandmother cell" is a single cell that would respond only to a visual image of one's grandmother. The point is that there are not enough cells in the brain to permit single cells to have such a high degree of stimulus specificity. Rather, the image of one's grandmother is apparently represented by an abstract pattern of activity in neural networks in one or more higher cortical regions.

XI. CONCLUSION

We have attained a significant understanding of the representation of form in the striate cortex through application of the concepts of spatial sampling and filtering in physiological, psychophysical, and anatomical research. Furthermore, we know that this representation, at least in the foveal projection, is complete in the sense that it preserves all of the spatial information present in the optical image formed on the retina. Based on this it is now possible to predict the pattern discrimination capabilities of the human visual system based on the calculated responses of mechanisms with properties comparable to those of single striate units. A major focus of future research must thus be understanding how interactions among different mechanisms perform useful visual computations and the conditions under which implicitly represented information is made explicit.

ACKNOWLEDGMENTS

Preparation of this chapter was supported by research grants from the National Institutes of Health to Hugh Wilson (Grant EY02158), Russell DeValois (Grant EY00014), and Dennis Levi (Grant EY01728). Lamberto Maffei was supported by the Consilio Nazionale della Ricerche and Jyrki Rovamo by the Finnish Academy of Sciences.

11

FORM PERCEPTION AND ATTENTION
Striate Cortex and Beyond

Anne Treisman, Patrick Cavanagh, Burkhart Fischer, V. S. Ramachandran, and Rüdiger von der Heydt

I. INTRODUCTION

Consider a "snowman" seen against a blanket of snow. How does the visual system demarcate its boundaries, and how do we recognize it as a "man" even though its surface is made of snow and the nose is a carrot? We do this almost effortlessly, even though snowmen may be perceived from different angles, at different distances, and with varied shapes, sizes, and features. The visual system has a remarkable capacity to determine the spatial relationships between the features of an object before categorizing it in the appropriate semantic category.

What kind of neural circuitry could perform this deceptively simple task? The answer is far from known. The great difficulties encountered in developing computer vision systems, even on the most advanced computers, have helped us appreciate the power and sophistication of our own visual processes (Feldman, 1986; see Chapter 15, this volume). The brain solves the problem of vision by dedicating massive amounts of cortex to it: Areas involved in vision account for over 30% of the neocortex in macaque monkeys, a species whose visual system closely resembles our own. Trying to understand the workings of such a complex system is a formidable task, but it may be made easier if parts of the system can be studied in isolation.

A widely held view of object perception divides the visual process into a number of distinct functional stages. This may be misleading for a highly interactive system like the brain, but as a first approximation it can be used to guide research and to provide a framework for results. An early stage within this hierarchy is said to extract different elementary image features and to group them on the basis of similarity and spatial proximity. The areas defined by these grouping processes become the candidates for further visual processing, culminating in identification. The next stage delineates the boundaries and surfaces present, forming a three-dimensional, viewer-centered representation of objects and their backgrounds. Finally, the representations are matched to a thesaurus of stored descriptions and identified, if possible, as familiar individuals or as instances of familiar categories.

Many questions arise within this framework: What defines the inventory of elementary features? How are they detected and grouped? How are object boundaries located? At what stage or stages are two-dimensional retinal image features mapped into the properties of real objects from which they originate? What kind of object representation is formed, and what constitutes a match to objects previously experienced? How are objects recognized independently of their locations, distances, and sometimes of their orientations, while at the same time information about these spatial properties is preserved and used? For all these stages, what neural mechanisms might implement the functions we hypothesize? In dealing with processes as complex as object perception, we are unlikely to find answers by looking only at the anatomy and physiology of the visual system. Although single cells show considerable specialization in the stimuli to which they respond best (whether oriented gratings, illusory edges, or faces), it seems highly unlikely that signals from any one cell can convey meaning in isolation. We must specify the functions underlying subject performance in a given task and then see at what levels they can be linked to the pathways identified by neuroanatomical studies. Visual phenomena are used to infer the existence of separate visual mechanisms, and these in turn are checked both by converging evidence from other behavioral tasks and by possible links to physiological processes.

It is impossible in a single chapter to review all the relevant evidence. We select examples of research which seem to us to probe central issues at the different stages of object identification and to throw light on the mechanisms which may be involved. Our understanding of these complex issues is still rudimentary; the hypotheses proposed to link behavior to physiology are tentative at best.

II. EXTRACTION OF ELEMENTARY IMAGE FEATURES

The visual system encodes a number of different classes of information: It must extract features that specify textures, surfaces, and their spatial layout, features that specify events (movement, change), and finally features that define the shapes and structures of objects. These properties of the world may each be inferred from a variety of physical parameters of the retinal image. There is no simple one-to-one mapping between the two. Thus, motion across the retina may specify object shape (structure from motion) and distance (motion parallax) as well as motion of objects or of the observer. If the goal of perception is to specify the external environment, we need not expect to find anatomical specialization reflecting simple physical parameters of the retinal stimulus; stimulus cues may be functionally grouped in terms of the real properties that they help to specify. (For more detailed reviews of psychological research on feature extraction, see Anstis, 1975; Cowey, 1979; Graham, 1985; Treisman, 1986a,b).

The first class of information, specifying the spatial layout of the scene is likely to be encoded at an early stage, in order to group the parts of potential objects and to segregate them by their surface properties from their backgrounds. The second class of properties specifies "events" such as onsets, offsets, or changes of illumination (see Chapter 7, this volume) or codes properties of motion such as direction, velocity, acceleration, and looming (Regan, 1986). Finally, there may be an inventory of parts or properties used to characterize and to identify objects. Examples might be the volumetric units or "geons" proposed by Biederman (1987). These various kinds of visual information have often been treated together in accounts of early feature analysis, but this may lead to confusion. They serve different perceptual functions and are likely to reveal their effects in different behavioral tests (see Julesz, 1984; Treisman & Gormican, 1988). As a result, disagreements have arisen about the candidate members for an inventory of basic visual features (so-called primitives) from which more complex percepts are constructed, and discrepancies between inferences from physiology and psychophysics may occur. In this section, we discuss evidence relating to the early texture and surface-segregating features. In addition, we outline behavioral criteria and neurophysiological evidence that might be relevant to this "initial parsing of the visual field."

A. Visual Grouping and Texture Segregation

A prerequisite for features involved in the initial segregation of objects and background surfaces is that they should be detected in parallel across space. That is, they should allow easy, "preattentive" grouping of areas that contain them, and set up salient boundaries with areas that do not. Figure 1A shows examples where such segregation spontaneously takes place. The Gestalt psychologists (e.g., Wertheimer, 1923, 1938; Metzger, 1953, 1975) were the first to demonstrate good phenomenal grouping based on spatial proximity of local elements, on common direction of motion, and on "similarity." An historical account of this research is found in Pastore (1971). Other attempts to specify the effective forms of "similarity" found easy detection of groups and boundaries based on the simple features of color, brightness, and line orientation (Beck, 1966, 1967, 1982; Olson & Attneave, 1970; Attneave, 1971; Julesz, 1975, 1984; Treisman & Gelade, 1980). Examples are given in Fig. 1A. Julesz (1964) added binocular disparity, line ends (terminators), and intersections, and Treisman and Paterson (1984) reported evidence that closure (a wholly or partly enclosed area) also functions as a feature whose presence can segregate one area from another. The cues which support this operation of grouping and boundary formation are likely to be detected and processed early within the visual pathways.

Spatial arrangements of parts and conjunctions of features do not define bounded areas with the same salience and clarity (Beck, 1966; Treisman & Gelade, 1980). Figure 1B shows examples where the separate areas can be found only with focused attention, and with much longer reaction time. Perceptual grouping seems, then, to be determined by separate features and not by the integrated wholes that they characterize.

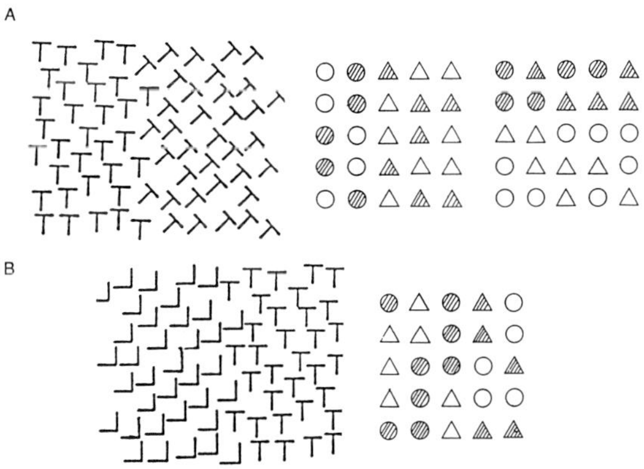

FIG. 1 (A) Examples of groups of elements that generate good perceptual segregation based on one feature (orientation, curved circles versus straight-edged triangles, shape, and color; in the experiment open shapes were red and filled shapes blue). (B) Examples of groups of elements differing only in the spatial arrangement or conjunctions of their features. No clear division is apparent between the left and right sides of the figures. From Beck (1966) and Treisman (1985).

B. Parallel Processing in Visual Search

Another visual performance test for early parallel detection of features uses visual search tasks to discover targets that "pop out" against a background of distractors (nontarget items). Such targets are detected equally quickly regardless of the number of distractors that are present. Fast and spatially parallel detection is taken as evidence that the features in question are coded early in the visual process. Targets that pop out when displays are searched usually differ from the distractors in one or more of the same set of elementary features that mediate grouping and segregation. They may possess a unique color or brightness, a unique orientation, disparity, or direction of movement, or they may be the only elements with terminators or closure (see, e.g., Neisser, 1963; Egeth, Jonides & Wall, 1972; Treisman & Gelade, 1980; Bergen & Julesz, 1983; Treisman & Gormican, 1988). Results of visual search studies suggest two further inferences: First, they are consistent with the idea that different features are processed in separate subsystems or channels, and, second, they reveal striking asymmetries in feature coding between target and distractor. These inferences are now described in greater detail.

C. Modularity of Feature Analysis in Early Vision

A module (Marr, 1982; Fodor, 1983; see also Chapter 10, this volume) is a specialized subsystem coding a particular class of properties independently of other properties. For example, stereoscopic depth might be coded independently of motion or of color. Search tasks provide evidence that early visual analysis may be modular. If a target-defining feature is coded independently of others, variation on irrelevant dimensions should have no effect on the speed of search. If, on the other hand, search depends on a more global process, heterogeneity of background elements should seriously disrupt detection of a target item, whether the variation is on the target-defining dimension or on other, irrelevant dimensions. Treisman (1988) found no interference with detection of a target (e.g., a blue bar among green bars, or a horizontal bar among vertical bars), when the distractors varied on other dimensions, although search was slower when the distractors varied on the relevant di-

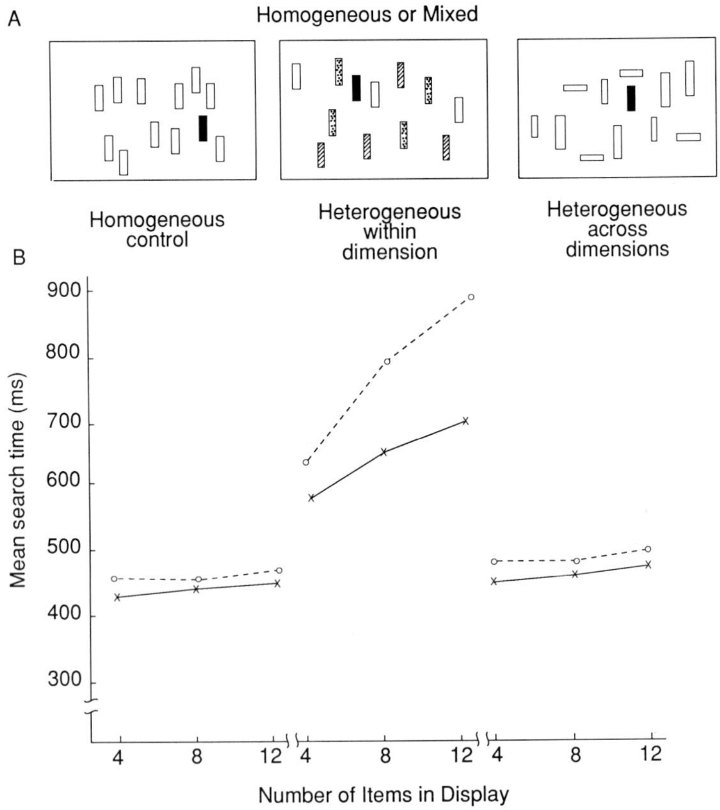

FIG. 2 (A) Examples of displays testing the effects of distractor heterogeneity, within and between dimensions. In the displays illustrated, the target is a blue bar in each case. In conditions not illustrated here, targets defined by orientation (horizontal) were presented among distractors that were either all vertical (homogeneous condition) or vertical, left diagonal, and right diagonal (heterogeneous within dimension), or vertical in three sizes and three colors (heterogeneous on irrelevant dimensions). (B) Mean search times with such displays. The results are the means for targets defined by color (blue) and by orientation (horizontal). Display size indicates the number of elements in each display, whether homogeneous or heterogeneous. Crosses indicate that a target was present in the display; circles indicate that it was not. From Treisman (1988).

mension (see Fig. 2). This finding is consistent with the idea that separate feature maps are formed in early vision, with salience defined only *within* dimensions. It conflicts with the alternative account that the locations of feature differences are detected before their nature is determined (Sagi & Julesz, 1987). On the other hand, when the target is unknown, "the odd one out" is detected more slowly than when the target is specified in advance, suggesting that it takes longer to check for its presence in several different modules than to check a single known module (Treisman, 1988).

D. Asymmetries in the Coding of Features

The failure of distractors to impair performance when variation occurs on irrelevant stimulus dimensions suggests independence of coding *across* different stimulus dimensions. Visual search results can also suggest which values *within* a dimension are coded as separable features. A surprising asymmetry between different values within dimensions has been discovered, using the visual search task (Treisman & Souther, 1985; Treisman & Gormican, 1988). Given the same physical discrimination, for example, between a curved and a straight line, search latencies may be drastically different depending on which of the two features defines the target and which the distractors. A curved line can be found quickly in a display of straight lines, whereas a straight line appears to require much slower, serial search when presented in a display of curved lines. Similar asymmetries are found with many other dimensions: a tilted line pops out of a display of vertical lines, whereas a vertical (or frame-aligned) line is harder to find among tilted lines. A pair of converging lines is easier to find among pairs of parallel lines than the reverse. A circle with a gap pops out of complete circles but not the reverse. An ellipse is found more quickly among circles than a circle among ellipses. Figure 3 gives examples of the displays and of the search functions obtained in these different tasks.

The following paradigm cases may help us to interpret the others: (1) A circle with an added intersecting line pops out of circles without lines, but a circle without a line is found only by serial search through a display of circles with intersecting lines (see Fig. 4). Thus the *presence* of an added feature seems to be detected immediately and with no effect of the number of distractors, but its *absence* does not. (2) On quantitative dimensions (such as line length, number, or contrast) search for a high value among distractors with low values is also faster than search for a low value among distractors with high values. It seems that adding a new feature or increasing the value on a quantitative dimension makes a target item more easily detectable. On the other hand, removing or decreasing the feature which distinguishes the target from the distractors makes it preattentively "invisible." By analogy, certain qualitative dimensions may also be asymmetrically coded, with one direction of change on the dimension coded as "adding a feature," or giving an increase in neural activity. This change would make a target easy to find, whereas a change in the opposite direction would make it hard. A curved line, by this analogy, appears to have an added property (curvature) that a straight line lacks; a tilted line has an added property (tilt) that a vertical line lacks.

The general rule, extracted from a number of experiments showing search asymmetries, seems to be that a stimulus that departs from a standard or reference value is coded as having an added or positive feature that the standard value lacks. An ellipse has an additional feature (elongation) relative to a circle; magenta has some additional blue relative to a standard red; converging lines have an extra property (convergence) relative to parallel lines; curved lines add curvature to the reference value of straightness. All appear to signal the *presence* of an additional unique feature besides the standard or reference value for the dimension in question. If this interpretation is correct, the direction of search asymmetry can be used to discover which stimulus in any new pair is treated as the reference value in early visual coding. For example, it appears that a dot outside a closed shape is treated as the deviation and a dot inside

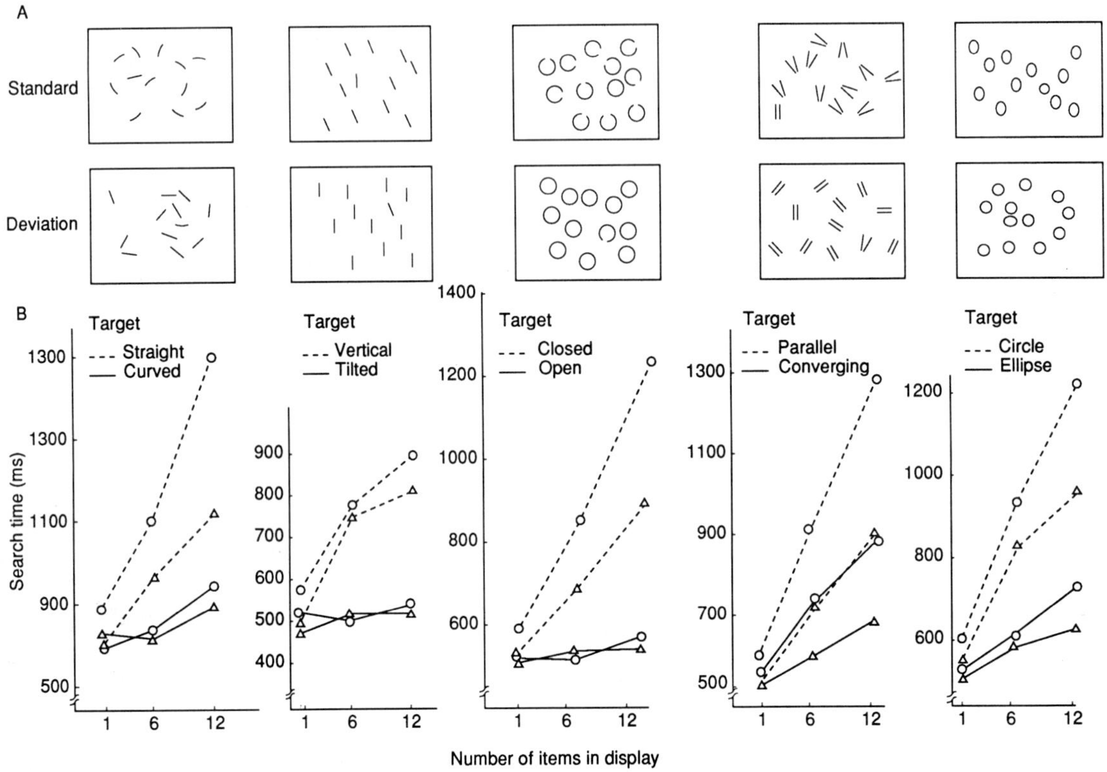

FIG. 3 (A) Examples of five pairs of displays that generate search asymmetries between target and distractor. (B) Mean search times through such displays. In each case, the dotted lines show the times for the "standard" target and the solid lines for the "deviation" target. Triangles indicate that the target was present in the display, and circles signify that it was not. Adapted from Treisman & Gormican (1988).

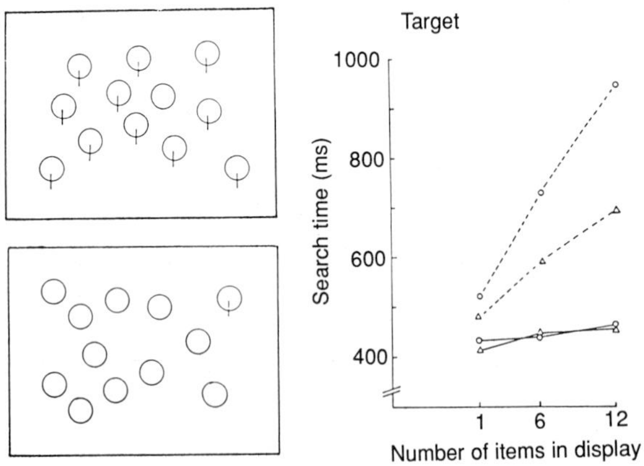

FIG. 4 Displays with a target defined by either the presence or the absence of a feature (added line), and search times for such displays. From Treisman and Souther (1985). Copyright (1985) by the American Psychological Association.

the shape as the standard. So far, no physiological correlate has been found for any of these coding asymmetries.

E. Parallel Coding versus Parallel Access to Previously Coded Features

One of the criteria to identify which features are coded as the basic elements in early visual processing is that they should be detectable preattentively. They are characterized by flat functions (near zero slope) relating search times to the number of distractor items. In addition, the mean reaction times in both search and boundary detection are typically quite short; response times to detect a target or a texture boundary average 400 to 600 msec. Some perceptual grouping phenomena, however, appear to reveal spatially parallel access after a much longer initial delay. For example, the emergence of stereoscopic depth in random dot stereograms may take several seconds (Julesz, 1971), yet the perceived depth is clearly apparent across the field as a whole, once the three-dimensional organization has emerged. (On repeated presentations, shape from depth is discerned more quickly.)

There may be other forms of perceptual grouping that share this character of slow emergence, with parallel (global) awareness of all the elements prevailing, once the organization of the field has become apparent. They contrast with other displays whose texture boundaries are found equally slowly (e.g., displays in which different areas are defined only by conjunctions of features) but which do not afford the same continued awareness of the boundaries after they have been located. For example, Ramachandran (1988a,b) has found that three-dimensional shape from shading can provide cues for perceptual grouping of this slow emerging, but global type. Thus, in Fig. 5A there is a strong tendency to perceive one set of objects (the ones that are white on top) as convex and all the others as concave. In this display, it is possible to group perceptually all the convex objects together, so that they form a separate depth plane standing out clearly from the background of concave objects. This is a surprising result, since it is generally assumed that only elementary image features like brightness and contrast, color, stereodepth, orientation, or motion can serve as a basis for perceptual grouping. The results imply that even three-dimensional shapes defined exclusively by shading can provide perceptual features that allow phenomenal grouping and segregation.

To ensure that this phenomenal grouping was not simply due to a more primitive image feature (such as luminance polarity), Ramachandran produced a control display (Fig. 5B) that was similar to Fig. 5A in terms of luminance polarity but did not convey any depth. Grouping was very difficult to achieve in this display, suggesting that the effects observed in Fig. 5A must have been based on three-dimensional shape from shading. It may take as long as 30–60 sec for depth to emerge; however, there is again a tendency for this time to decrease with repeated trials.

A

B

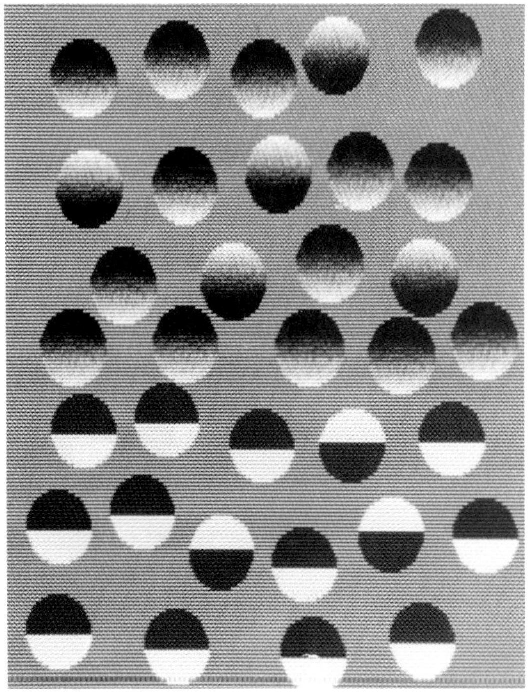

FIG. 5 Random mixture of shaded objects that have opposite luminance polarities. The objects which are light on top are usually perceived as spheres, and they can be visually grouped together and segregated from the background of concave objects. Hence, one may conclude that three-dimensional shapes defined by shading can provide tokens for perceptual grouping and segregation. (B) In the "control" no three-dimensional shapes are seen, and it is also impossible to perceptually segregate the objects on the basis of luminance polarity. From Ramachandran (1988a,b). Copyright © 1988 Macmillan Magazines Ltd.

These findings are particularly revealing because shape from shading relies on a fairly complex "interpretation" of the display in terms of an assumed source of illumination. The derivation incorporates the constraint that there is only *one* light source in the entire image (or a large portion of it), perhaps because our brains evolved in a solar system that has only one sun.

The strong sense of depth observed in Fig. 6 depends exclusively on shading. The sign of perceived depth, however, is ambiguous, for the brain has no

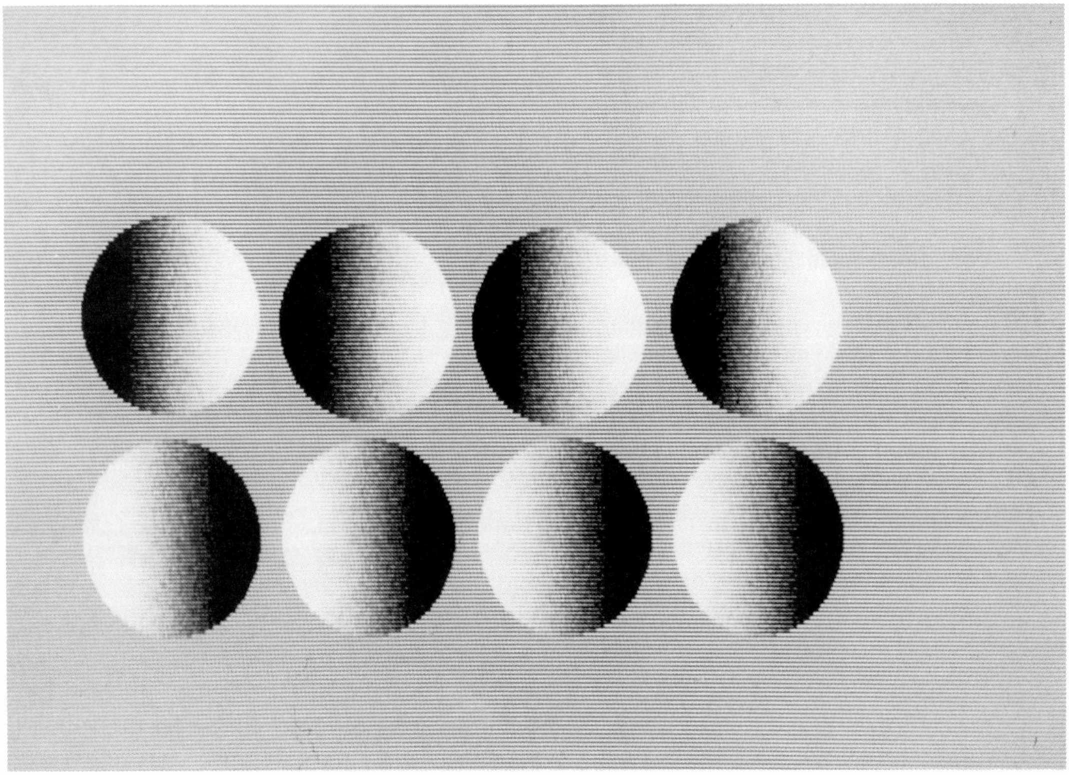

FIG. 6 Bistable display in which shapes can be perceived either as convex or concave by mentally shifting the assumed light source from left to right. When the top row is seen as convex, the bottom row usually appears concave (or flat), whereas when the bottom row is seen as convex, the top row appears concave. The effect may take some time to emerge and stabilize. The display illustrates the point that the visual system has a built-in "assumption" that there is only one light source illuminating the entire image. From Ramachandran (1987a,b). Copyright © 1987 Macmillan Magazines Ltd.

way of knowing where the light source is. It seems that when one row of objects is convex, then the mirror images are always concave (and vice versa). In fact, it is impossible to see all the objects as being simultaneously convex or concave. This observation suggests that the brain prefers a "common-light-source" assumption to a "common-depth" assumption. On the other hand, the shapes that are white on top are almost always seen as convex, and it is very difficult to generate voluntary perceptual reversals. This suggests that in addition to the single-light-source constraint, there is also a tendency to assume that the light source is at the top; an effect that is well known to artists.

While viewing these displays, one has the impression that the visual system goes through several operations before the final percept emerges. In the earliest stage the computation required for defining the three-dimensional shapes (i.e., depth) is performed. This can take several seconds. Next, the objects that differ from the others pop out (i.e., segregate) as in Treisman's displays. Once the targets have emerged, however, one has the distinct impression of being able to "hold on" to them indefinitely (hysteresis) in order to group them with other similar items in the display (grouping). Finally, after grouping has occurred, the objects are clearly segregated from irrelevant items cluttering the background (figure–ground separation). Thus, what is usually described as a one-step operation—the extraction and grouping of elementary features—may, in fact, involve several distinct perceptual capacities which contribute toward the ultimate goal of delineating figure and ground.

There is, unfortunately, no simple way to disentangle and measure these effects. One promising approach involves the use of apparent motion to determine the extent of perceptual segregation (Ramachandran, Rao & Vidyasagar, 1973a). Apparent motion of a group of items as a whole may provide converging evidence for parallel access, since all the elements must be matched to the corresponding elements in the preceding display in order to determine the extent and direction of motion. If the global motion of the group is immediately apparent, one can infer that all the items are capable of being matched in parallel. This is shown by the following experiment. Consider two frames (similar to Fig. 5A) of an apparent motion sequence. The first frame has a cluster of three convex objects on the left, whereas in the second frame the cluster as a whole is shifted to the right. The positions of the remaining elements themselves are random and uncorrelated in successive frames. The results are quite striking. As long as no depth is perceived, the elements in the display simply appear to flicker. Once depth emerges, however, the triangular cluster of convex objects jumps vividly between the two locations as the frames are alternated. (Optimum apparent motion is seen when the stimulus onset asynchrony is about 200 msec.) These results suggest that shapes defined exclusively by shading can provide cues for grouping and long-range apparent motion correspondence (see Chapter 9, this volume).

A different case of apparent motion is illustrated in Fig. 7. In this case, there is no correlation at all between the elements of the two textures in the successive displays; only the shape of the boundaries between the different areas in the two frames is correlated. Yet, when the frames are alternated, one observes vivid apparent motion between the two inner "squares." This result suggests that the long-range apparent motion system can accept previously abstracted texture borders as an input, although the individual elements constituting the apparent shape are not matched. Both the boundaries and the shape from shading, once computed by the brain, can remain perceptually available as a basis for further visual computations. Given the very long latency with which the shape from shading becomes apparent, it is possible that serial processing is required to set up the initial representation of the individual elements. Once computed, however, the results can be "held on to" and used as cues for apparent motion, global shape perception, and other visual analyses.

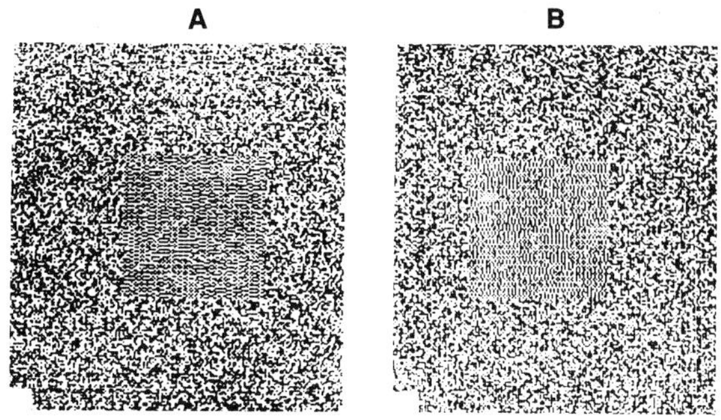

FIG. 7 Two frames of a movie (A and B), presented side by side for clarity. The square in Frame B is shifted horizontally in relation to Frame A, but the elements constituting the squares are completely uncorrelated in successive frames. When A and B are optically superimposed and alternated, the square is seen to move back and forth horizontally, suggesting that the motion system accepts texture borders as an input even in the absence of point-to-point luminance correlation. From Ramachandran, Rao, and Vidyasagar (1973a,b). Copyright © 1973 Macmillan Magazines Ltd.

In contrast, not only do stimuli defined only by arbitrary combinations of properties (e.g., red and vertical) require serial processing in most cases, but they also fail the apparent motion test. A. Treisman (unpublished) repeated Ramachandran et al.'s (1973a) experiment using conjunctions of color with orientation, color with size, and orientation with size to define sets of coherently moved elements. For example, a set of six pink bars tilted 45° to the left appeared in two different locations in alternating displays, either preserving their relative positions within the set (coherent motion) or with changes in their relative positions (incoherent motion). These six elements were embedded in a larger display of pink bars tilted 45° to the right and green bars tilted 45° to the left. Each of these background elements was slightly displaced in a random direction between the two displays, so that the targets could not be distinguished simply by contrast with a continuous background. The task was to discriminate coherent global motion of the target group from incoherent motion of its separate elements. Subjects were, in general, quite unable to do this when the target group was defined only by conjunctions of features, and, in fact, no global motion was seen. The target group did not become phenomenally salient as a whole, even once its elements had been located, and it failed to emerge in apparent motion across successive displays, even when subjects were given unlimited time to observe the alternation. The only case in which performance was above chance was when one of the features defining the target conjunction group was the larger size. In contrast, if the target group differed in a single feature rather than a conjunction, apparent motion was usually seen. For example, grey vertical bars embedded in the same background of pink and green bars tilted right and left gave significantly better performance. Thus, a difference in color, size, or orientation presumably gave access to the target group as a whole, allowing a match to be made between the displays.

F. Conclusions

These tests of perceptual grouping and segregation, search, and apparent motion suggest the existence of three classes of perceptual units: (1) simple features, which mediate rapid segregation, which pop out in search, and which create texture boundaries that can be abstracted from different successive displays to mediate apparent motion of the areas they contain; (2) more complex features of surfaces in depth, such as stereoscopic planes and shape from shading, which may be processed slowly, in some cases serially, by visual routines (Ullman, 1984) but which remain accessible in parallel once the scene has been perceptually organized; and (3) conjunctions of features that do not create new emergent properties. These are visible without difficulty when presented or attended singly. However, they appear neither to be processed in parallel nor to remain available as parallel inputs to further visual processing once they have been identified. Phenomenologically, it is difficult to maintain more than two or three of them as a salient group against the background elements. They are unlikely to play any role in segregating objects from their background. They may, however, be critical in identifying objects once they have been located.

Treisman's paradigm provides a useful method for deciding whether a given feature is "elementary" or not. For example, it is well known that orientation in two-dimensional space is an elementary feature. What about orientation in three-dimensional space? In experiments to address this issue (Ramachandran & Rogers-Ramachandran, 1988), subjects were presented with a stereogram consisting of a random array of needles tilted in three-dimensional space. For all the needles, except one, the upper ends were tilted toward the observer. (The centers of all the needles were at zero disparity.) Subjects could preattentively detect the single anomalous needle whose upper end was tilted away from them, that is, the reaction time for detecting this anomalous needle did not vary with the number of distractors.

At what stage in visual processing does popping out of elementary features occur? For example, we know that depth can be conveyed by a variety of parallel cues such as stereo disparity, shading, occlusion, and motion parallax. At least two of these (shading and disparity) constitute elementary features in the sense described by Treisman (1986a). But where does this segregation occur? Does it occur at a very early stage where there are (presumably) separate feature maps for different depth cues or at a later stage where different sources of information are combined into a common "depth map"? To answer this question Ramachandran and Rogers-Ramachandran (1988) used targets that convey conflicting depth cues. They designed a stereogram composed of small squares whose corners partially overlapped. Disparities were introduced between the two images so that for all but one square, the two cues (occlusion and disparity) were *consistent* with each other, that is, they conveyed the same depth. For the single anomalous target, on the other hand, the occlusion and disparity were of opposite sign so that they tended to cancel each other. The magnitude of depth seen in this target was considerably less than in the distractors, yet it did not seem to pop out preattentively. This result suggests that grouping must occur before the conflicting cues are combined.

III. NEUROPHYSIOLOGICAL AND ANATOMICAL EVIDENCE ON EARLY STAGES OF VISUAL CODING

A. Single Cell Recordings and Separate Neural Channels

It seems likely that the grouping and parsing phenomena attributed to early vision depend on processing in the various areas of the visual cortex in which cells respond to simple visual stimuli; these include Areas V1, V2, V3, V4, and MT. In this section, the main findings from neurophysiological recordings in these areas are outlined. As yet, there has been little attempt to relate the single-cell data directly to those from behavioral studies. One important reason is that there need not be a direct correlation between the responses of single units and the response of the system as a whole. If such a correlation is found, as it is in some specific cases, it may be very informative. In other cases, however, the correlation could be with patterns of activity across populations of individual cells; it will then be much more difficult to detect and interpret.

Most of the neurophysiological data about the striate cortex and the extrastriate visual areas come from experiments with isolated spots, edges, bars, or gratings. The main variables that have been studied are stimulus position, orientation, temporal modulation, direction and velocity of movement, side of monocular stimulation, binocular disparity, wavelength, width and length of bars, spatial frequency, and contrast. The proportion of cells that are sensitive to each of these parameters as well as their degree of sensitivity in different areas and subdivisions of the visual cortex offer important clues to their function (see Van Essen, 1985).

Any visual system must make a compromise between temporal resolution and spatial resolution. The mammalian visual system appears to resolve this problem early in the retina, where α- and β-type ganglion cells have evolved specialized functions for sharpness in time and space, respectively. Thus, when information reaches the cortex, via the separate magnocellular (originating in α cells) and parvocellular (originating in β cells) layers of the lateral geniculate nucleus (LGN), a division has occurred between the processing of pattern–color, on the one hand, and motion, depth, and spatial orientation, on the other. This division of information flow through the brain continues from visual cortex through temporal and parietal cortex. How, then, do the earliest areas (V1, V2, V3, MT) sort out the cues just mentioned for further elaboration by higher cortical modules?

A functional differentiation appears even at the beginning of cortical processing, between three parallel subsystems that are anatomically interlaced in Areas V1 and V2 as revealed by cytochrome oxidase staining (see Hendrickson, 1985, for a review) and by tracing the connections within and between these areas (Livingstone & Hubel, 1984; 1987a,b). Figure 8 provides a summary of these pathways (see also Chapters 7 and 8, this volume). The first subdivision is formed by layer 4B of Area V1 and the "thick stripes" of V2, the second by the "blobs" of V1 and the "thin stripes" of V2, and the third by the "interblobs" of V1 and the "interstripes" or "pale" stripes of V2. The first has been related to the perception of depth and motion since, in the macaque, cells in the thick stripes are often sensitive to binocular disparity and direction of movement but not to color; the second has been related to color, since most cells in the blobs and the thin stripes are unselective for orientation and direction of movement but many are wavelength selective or show color opponency; the third has been related to form perception since cells in the interblobs and the interstripes were often found to be

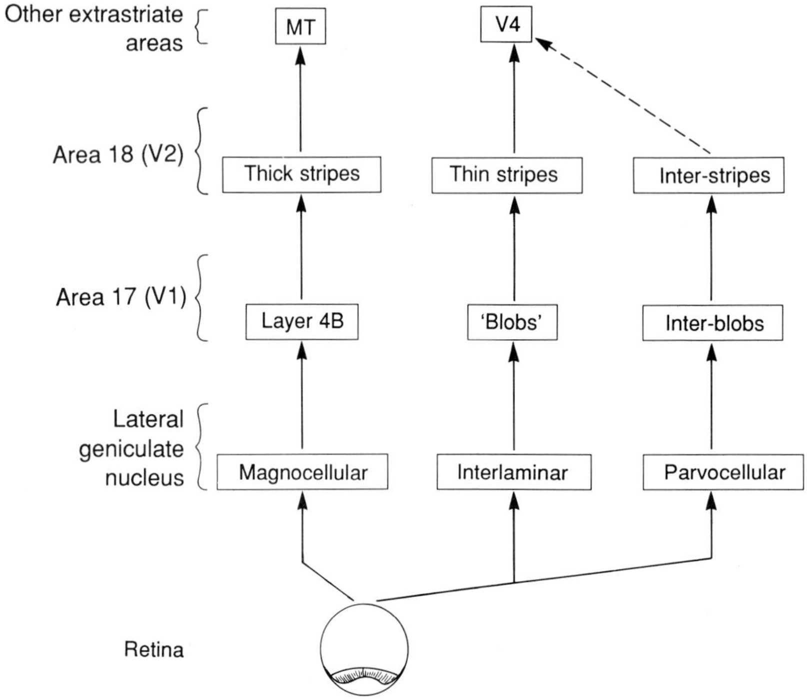

FIG. 8 Three parallel channels in the primate geniculocortical pathway. The diagram summarizes information from several sources including Hubel and Livingstone (1985) and Van Essen (1985). For clarity, the relay through layer 4C has been left out. Also, the interlaminar projection to the blobs is still somewhat controversial. After Ramachandran (1987a).

orientation selective, but not color selective (Hubel & Livingstone, 1985, 1987; Shipp & Zeki, 1985; Livingstone & Hubel, 1984b).

Further evidence comes from the projections from V2 to other areas. The thick stripes were found to project mainly to the middle temporal area (MT), the thin stripes and interstripes to Area V4 (DeYoe & Van Essen, 1985; Shipp & Zeki, 1985), which themselves are specialized, as described below. By means of a double labeling technique it was shown that individual V2 cells project either to V4 or to MT but not to both (DeYoe & Van Essen, 1985). Estimates of the numbers of specific cells in the subsystems of Area V2 do not all agree across these studies. For example, according to Hubel and Livingstone (1985, 1987) and Shipp and Zeki (1985), the thin stripes and interstripes differ markedly in the frequency of orientation-selective cells, whereas DeYoe and Van Essen (1985) find only subtle differences, if any, between these stripes.

The early anatomical segregation within Area V1 is maintained in the later stages of visual processing. There is some evidence that motion and color are analyzed by specialized cortical areas. The dichotomy into a "motion system" and a "color and form system" (Maunsell & Newsome, 1987) appears embedded in the more general distinction between two cortical streams (see Fig. 8): the occipitotemporal pathway including V4, devoted to object perception and recognition, and the occipitoparietal pathway including Area MT, concerned with perceptual localization (Mishkin, 1972; Pohl, 1973; Ungerleider & Mishkin, 1982; Desimone, Schein, Moran & Ungerleider, 1985). Thus, direction of motion is emphasized in Area MT (Dubner & Zeki, 1971; Zeki, 1974; Maunsell & Van Essen, 1983a,b), whereas processing of color is emphasized in V4 (Zeki, 1973, 1983c). Cells in Area V4 are also selective for orientation, the shape of bars, and spatial frequency, suggesting that form processing occurs here (Desimone & Schein,

1987). It is worth noting, however, that the orientation of texture elements can also be important in the segregation of surfaces by their texture. It is not always clear whether cells that are tuned to orientation are specialized to code texture elements or the orientation of global boundaries between surfaces, or both. Hammond (1978) and Nothdurft & Li (1985), for example, found different directional tuning of the same complex cells for texture motion and for motion of oriented bars. This suggests that oriented and textured stimuli may be coded by functionally different cortical pathways, which nevertheless share some of the same complex cells (Hammond, 1985).

B. Evidence from Neuropsychology and Psychophysics

Visual deficits following brain lesions in human patients have shown independent losses of at least three different attributes. Zihl, von Cramon, and Mai (1983) described a patient having difficulty perceiving moving stimuli. The patient reported that objects seemed to change position but gave no impression of motion. Botez (1975) has reported the converse, a patient who can identify objects only when they move. Cortical color blindness is an occasional consequence of brain trauma (Damasio, Yamada, Damasio, Corbett & McKee, 1980), while the reverse (luminance blindness) has also been reported (Rovamo, Hyvärinen & Hari, 1982). In the latter case, the patient complained of not being able to see anything on black and white television, even though she could see the pictures on color television without any problem. These clinical cases argue for some physical separation in the cortical representations or projections of color, luminance, and motion in the visual system.

The anatomical segregation can also be linked to psychophysical correlates. Since the magnocellular stream is "color-blind" (see Chapters 6 and 8, this volume), one might expect human motion perception, mediated by this stream, to be color-blind as well. This prediction was tested by Ramachandran and Gregory (1978) using a random dot kinematogram. A central square area in a random black and white field of dots was shifted in one display relative to another. When the two displays were alternated at the correct intervals, the square emerged from its random dot background and was seen to oscillate in apparent motion. However, when the black and white dots in the kinematogram were replaced with red and green dots at equiluminance, the appearance of the oscillating central square was lost completely. This suggested that the human motion system cannot accept purely chromatic borders as an input.

The separation does not, however, appear to be complete. Information from the LGN arrives in Area V1 through opponent-color and nonopponent or weakly opponent (luminance) pathways (DeValois, Abramov & Jacobs, 1966; Derrington, Krauskopf & Lennie, 1984). Since there is a higher area, V4, specialized for the analysis of color (Zeki, 1978a,b), it is often assumed that color information contributes only to the pathway leading to this area and not at all to the pathways involved in the analysis of motion and binocular disparity. However, several psychophysical studies have shown that color can in some conditions contribute to the perception of motion (Cavanagh, 1988) and to stereopsis (DeWeert & Sadza, 1983; Grinberg & Williams, 1985). Indeed, Ramachandran and Gregory (1978) found that although motion was lost at equiluminance in random dot kinematograms, motion could still be seen if simple line targets were used. Based on this observation, they concluded that the early motion system was color blind but that the long-range motion system can use any type of contour, including chromatic contours or even equiluminous texture borders. Other studies (Cavanagh, 1988) suggest that the contribution of color to motion passes through the opponent-color (parvocellular) pathway from the retina to the striate cortex rather than "leaking" into the magnocellular, nonopponent pathway that carries the luminance contribution to motion (see Maunsell & Newsome, 1987). These separate routes for color and luminance then converge to form a common motion pathway and a common site for motion aftereffects (Cavanagh, 1988).

Although the physiological evidence for separate

streams leading to Areas V4 (form/color) and MT (motion) is strong, the route for analysis of other perceptual dimensions such as texture and stereopsis is less clear. Texture, for example, may require a secondary analysis performed by a subset of cells in the luminance pathway. Similarly, the analysis of binocular disparity may occur in the same region, MT, as the analysis of motion (Maunsell & Newsome, 1987). This could explain the close coupling between stereopsis and motion observed by Ramachandran and Anstis (1986a,b). They presented two vertically aligned spots in Frame 1 of an apparent motion sequence followed by two spots shifted horizontally (Fig. 9A). The spots were always seen to "jump" horizontally and never crossed paths (see also Kolers, 1972; Ullman, 1979a,b), even if diagonally opposite pairs (in Frame 2) were made similar in color or "form." However, if two diagonally opposite corner spots were presented in a separate stereoscopic plane from the other two (Fig. 9B), the spots did cross paths. This was especially true if several such displays were viewed simultaneously. Thus, stereoscopic depth can change the rules of (apparent) motion processing. Motion and stereo disparity processing are closely linked in the brain. The different channels coding object shape are discussed in more detail in Section IV, together with other psychological findings concerning their interrelations.

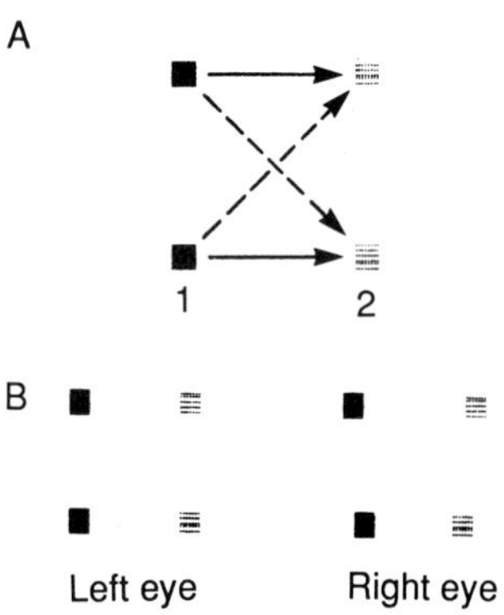

FIG. 9 (A) Two vertically aligned spots are flashed in Frame 1 (black squares) and are followed by two spots shifted horizontally in Frame 2 (gray squares). The spots never appear to cross each other's paths (dashed lines), but always seem to move horizontally (solid lines). Even if diagonally opposite pairs are made similar in color or "form," crossing is never perceived. (B) When diagonally opposite pairs occupy slightly different depth planes as in a stereogram, however, the spots cross each other's trajectories. Thus, there is a close perceptual coupling between motion and stereoscopic depth.

C. Specificity of Cortical Areas

The use of quantitative methods for assessing physiological and anatomical specificity (e.g., Schiller, Finlay & Volman, 1976a,b; Baker, Petersen, Newsome & Ullman, 1981) is obviously important in determining how strictly the different visual areas are segregated in the brain (see Felleman & Van Essen, 1987, for a synopsis of the specificity estimates of various studies of six cortical areas of the macaque). Often the differences between areas or subdivisions of areas seem to be only relative. A number of examples show this. (1) Orientation selectivity and binocular interaction are found in the thin stripes of Area V2, which are part of the "color system," as well as more frequently in the thick stripes (DeYoe & Van Essen, 1985). (2) Cells in the "color area" V4 can also be selective for orientation, spatial frequency, and even direction of motion (Schein, Marrocco & De Monasterio, 1982; Desimone & Schein, 1987). (3) Many cells in the "motion area" MT are sensitive to bincular disparity (Maunsell & Van Essen, 1983a,b). (4) Substantial numbers of wavelength-selective cells have been found in Area V3 (Felleman & Van Essen, 1987), which was previously thought to lack such cells (Zeki, 1978a,b, 1983c). Thus, even though the existence of multiple representations in extrastriate cortex is widely accepted, the routing of the pathways through these areas and the stimulus and/or response attributes processed by each are not yet clearly established.

It is sometimes assumed that successive stages of cortical processing serve to improve selectivity or "sharpen the tuning." However, there is little evidence that dimensional selectivity always increases in higher areas. For example, the width of orientation tuning is not narrower in Area V2 than in V1 (compare Burkhalter & Van Essen, 1986, versus Schiller et al., 1976a, and De Valois, Albrecht & Thorell, 1982). Cells in Area V4 are no more selective for wavelength than are retinal ganglion cells (DeMonasterio & Schein, 1982; but see Zeki, 1980). Tuning to spatial frequency appears to be broader in Area V2 (Foster, Gaska, Nagler & Pollen, 1985) and V4 (Desimone & Schein, 1987) than in V1 (Schiller et al., 1976b; DeValois, Yund & Hepler, 1982). Disparity selectivity does not differ much between Areas V1 and V2 (Poggio & Fischer, 1977; Poggio, 1984). A notable exception is velocity of movement, where cells in Area MT are more selective than cells in V1 (Maunsell & Van Essen, 1983a,b). Thus, looking at the proportions of cells devoted to one or the other parameter and their degree of selectivity, there does not appear to be any regular increase in specificity from level to level in visual cortical processing.

Perhaps a better way of studying visual cortical specificity is to try to relate physiology to behavioral function, and to ask what computational problems might be solved at a given stage (Marr, 1982). As noted earlier, the perceptual qualities of color, contour, motion, and depth depend on stimulation in a much more complicated way than the stimulus properties to which they seem to correspond, such as wavelength composition, luminance gradient, velocity, and binocular disparity. Although perception depends on these properties, the relationship is not simply one-to-one, nor is it many-to-one. For example, many different wavelength compositions can produce the same perceived hue, while a fixed wavelength can appear in many different colors while reflecting the same composition of light into the eyes. Thus, in order to see how visual information is processed in the cortex, we should analyze the stimuli in terms of the properties of the world that they reflect and that the visual system has presumably evolved to detect. If there are modules coding different properties, their function is probably to transpose image features into properties of the three-dimensional world.

Relatively few studies have explicitly used this approach (von der Heydt, 1987). Among the exceptions are studies by Maffei, Morrone, Pirchio, and Sandini (1979) and by Albrecht and DeValois (1981) using square-wave gratings with and without the fundamental component. These gratings appear similar perceptually in that the same periodicity is perceived; however, neurons in striate cortex (cat, monkey) fail to signal the periodicity of the missing fundamental grating. Zeki (1983a,b) has demonstrated that neuronal responses in Area V4 of the monkey may correlate with the phenomenology of color perception when multicolored displays ("Mondrians"; Land 1983) are used, whereas responses of single units in Area V1 are generally determined just by the spectral composition of the light falling on one small patch of retina. Movshon, Adelson, Gizzi, and Newsome (1985) have used two crossed moving gratings to show that responses in Area MT may signal the global direction of movement that is perceived in such a stimulus, whereas those in V1 signal only the directions of the grating components.

Consideration of the functional goal of retrieving real-world properties from the retinal image may help to explain many visual phenomena showing interaction between stimulus parameters that are inexplicable assuming strict anatomical segregation. Examples of such phenomena are the effect of stereo disparity on the perception of illusory contours (Harris & Gregory, 1973; Ramachandran, 1986a), the perception of shape from motion (Wertheimer, 1923, 1938; Wallach & O'Connell, 1953), and the brightness and color effects associated with illusory contours (Ehrenstein, 1941; Van Tuijl, 1975; Ramachandran, 1987a). Indeed, studies of neuronal signals in Area MT with focal and large-field motion stimuli indicate a role for this area in figure–ground discrimination (Allman, Miezin & McGuinness, 1985; Tanaka, Hikosaka, Saito, Yukie, Fukuda & Iwai, 1986). Monkeys with lesions of Area MT were impaired in the perception of motion (Newsome & Pare, 1988) as well as the perception of three-dimensional shape in motion displays (Siegel & Andersen, 1988). On the other hand, several researchers have found cells in the temporal cortex that were highly selective for stimulus form, having receptive fields that were selective for head and body parts (faces) and body movements (Gross, Rocha-Miranda & Bender, 1972; Perrett, Rolls & Caan, 1982; Schwartz, 1984; Perrett, Harries, Mistlin & Chitty, 1989).

IV. CODING OF BOUNDARIES AND CONTOURS

The visual features described so far define the groups of elements that provide the input for later identification of objects. An essential prerequisite is to locate and delineate the boundaries between the groups, since these are likely to correspond to the contours of three-dimensional objects.

If one tries to extract the contours from an image by computer, one realizes that contour is a sophisticated abstraction that involves far more than just intensity gradient detection. Mathematically, contours (specifically "occluding contours") are defined in images of three-dimensional scenes as the lines of discontinuity of the third dimension (Marr, 1977; Koenderink, 1984). At first glance, the perception of contours appears as simple as this definition; we can generally distinguish the various objects in a scene with ease, even if the objects are unfamiliar and we are not able to recognize them. This leads to the impression that the objects are delineated in the image by luminance edges or lines. Therefore, the determination of contours has often been equated with edge and line detection. Since in most cases, neither an object nor its background is homogeneous in luminance and chromaticity, the gradient across contours is variable; it may even vanish at some points and be hard to detect at others. Contours defined by intensity gradients frequently merge with background structures, or with structures on the surface of the object. Moreover, the conditions change continuously when the projection of an object moves relative to the background, as in the case of motion parallax.

A. Perception of Contour

Perception of contour is not confined to intensity or color edges. Contours can be defined by discontinuities in several other attributes, including texture, binocular disparity, and relative motion. For all the extrastriate areas up to the level of Areas MT and V4, the representation of space is fairly retinotopic (see Maunsell & Newsome, 1987). Therefore, the two-dimensional shape of a stimulus is coded on a global level by the spatial arrangement of image information for each of these attributes within one or more of these extrastriate areas. On the other hand, the nature of the local sampling of each cell, within its receptive field, varies from pathway to pathway (see Chapter 10, this volume). The structure of the receptive field for cells in a given area reveals the shape dimensions that can be assumed to be important for further processing in the visual system. In the retina and LGN, for example, information is coded by receptive fields having an antagonistic center–surround organization, and these contribute, in the striate cortex, Area V1, to the formation of receptive fields that are orientation and size selective (Hubel & Wiesel, 1968) as well as possibly curvature selective (Dobbins, Zucker & Cynader, 1987).

Information on stimulus orientation and size therefore appears to be available in Area V1 for stimuli defined by luminance. However, the explicit coding of boundaries between regions defined by other attributes may not be available until the information reaches the extrastriate visual areas. For stimuli defined by wavelength, Gouras (1974), Michael (1978), and Thorell, DeValois, and Albrecht (1984) reported size- and orientation-tuned cells selective for color in Area V1. Color-selective cells in Area V4 appear to have both oriented and nonoriented receptive fields (Zeki, 1978a,b). Many cells in Area MT (Movshon, Adelson, Gizzi & Newsome, 1986), although directionally selective, do not appear to be orientation selective, at least not for the orientation of a moving bar. Whether they are selective for the orientation of bars defined by relative motion has not been determined. Cells that respond to random dot stereograms in Area V1 do not appear to be selective for the orientation of bars presented as random dot stereograms either (Poggio, Motter, Squatrito & Trotter, 1985). Nothdurft and Li (1985) did not find any cells in Area V1 that responded to texture bars. The explicit analysis of the orientation and size of regions defined by color, motion, texture, and binocular disparity therefore probably occurs beyond area Area V1. At these higher levels the shape primitives available for each stimulus attribute limit and, in a way, identify the algorithms the visual system can use to represent shapes, to derive position-, size-, and orientation-invariant descriptions that form the basis for memory and recognition (Cavanagh, 1984, 1985).

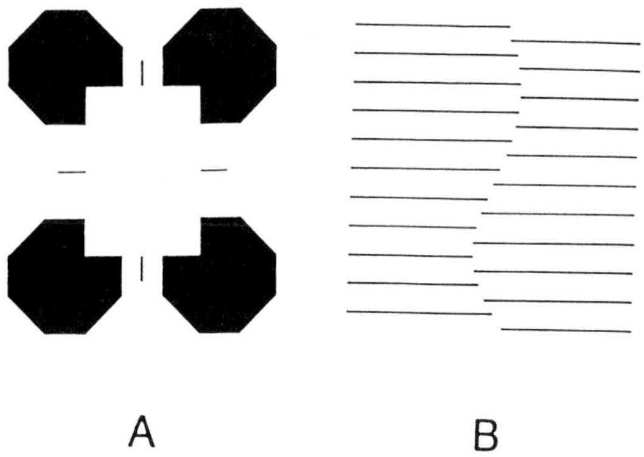

FIG. 10 Examples of subjective contours. (A) Brightness enhancement within a rectangular area delineated by subjective contours. (B) Subjective contour without brightness enhancement. From Kanizsa (1979).

B. Neural Coding of Subjective Contours

This section discusses the neural coding of subjective contours, as described by von der Heydt and colleagues (Peterhans & von der Heydt, 1989; von der Heydt & Peterhans, 1989a; von der Heydt, Peterhans & Baumgartner, 1984). The link between neurophysiological data and psychophysical observation is particularly close in this area, while subjective contours themselves reveal the algorithms employed by the brain in attempting to represent the visual world.

Contours can be perceived in the absence of any real edges or lines (Fig. 10). Such contours have been called "virtual," "anomalous," "illusory," "quasi-perceptual," "subjective," and "cognitive" (Schumann, 1900; Kanizsa, 1955, 1979; Lawson & Gulick, 1967; Coren, 1972; Gregory, 1972). The term "subjective" contours is preferred here because they have no direct physical analog in the stimulus, that is, a brightness step is perceived although there is no step in luminance. The ability to perceive such contours is likely to be useful under normal conditions of vision. Illusory figures, such as those in Fig. 10, demonstrate that the system has the means to reconstruct contours from cues other than luminance differences.

One difficulty in investigating subjective contours by recording from single cells is the interpretation of the response. Since these contours can only be generated by arrangements of ordinary lines or edges, how can we distinguish whether a neuronal response signals the subjective contour or the stimulus elements generating it? One possible approach is to use two abutting gratings as in Fig. 10B. In this way a vertical illusory contour can be produced by merely presenting horizontal lines. If a cortical neuron that is selective for vertical orientation responds to such a stimulus of purely horizontal lines, its responses can be presumed to relate to the perception of the subjective contour.

Figure 11 shows an example of responses of a single cell recorded in Area V2 of a rhesus monkey (von der Heydt & Peterhans, 1989a). The animal was trained to fixate a small target while the stimulus was presented near the fixation point. The cell responded to the abutting gratings (Fig. 11B) at the same orientation of the subjective contour at which the bar (Fig. 11A) was also effective. A continuous grating presented as a control elicited no response (Fig. 11C). Thus, one may assume that this kind of cell signals an illusory line and may actually mediate its perception although it is not physically present. Similar responses were found in about one-third of the

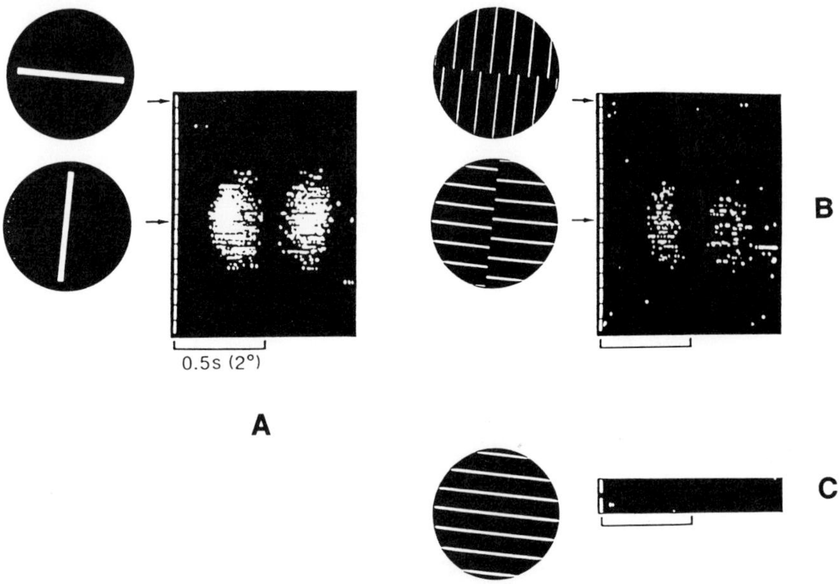

FIG. 11 Representation of subjective contours at the neuronal level. Responses of a cell in cortical Area V2 of an alert monkey. While the monkey was looking at a stationary fixation target, a light bar, or a subjective contour produced by abutting gratings, was moved back and forth across the receptive field at 16 different orientations covering 180° (only two are illustrated). The rows of dots represent the responses. (A) Bars elicited responses selectively at orientations near the vertical. (B) With abutting gratings, the cell responded according to the orientation of the subjective contour. It did not respond to the grating of switching phase (C). From von der Heydt and Peterhans (1989a).

cells in Area V2. Additional tests showed that the line ends by themselves were not effective stimuli; see Fig. 12.)

In a natural scene, when a number of lines terminate at a subjective border forming a straight line or a smooth curve, the border is usually perceived as the contour of an object. A possible inference is that the lines terminate because they are partially occluded by the object; the greater the number of aligned terminators the more likely a contour is present. The perception of subjective contours will therefore usually match the real contours of an object. The perceived contours become more salient as the number of terminators is increased (Fig. 12, top). No contour is perceived at the end of just one line; however, a weak contour begins to appear with three or four lines and becomes even more distinct with greater numbers. Apparently the perceived strength of the contour increases gradually with the probability of an occluding contour. The responses of a cell in Area V2 to such a stimulus is shown in Fig. 12. The increase in response parallels the perceptual salience of the contour.

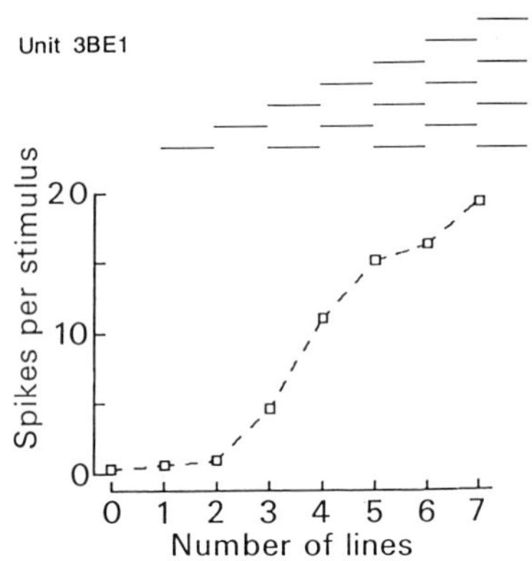

FIG. 12 The dependence of subjective contour and neuronal response rate of a cell in Area V2 of the monkey on the number of lines inducing the contour. In the experiment, the stimuli were centered over the cells receptive field. From von der Heydt et al. (1984). Copyright 1984 by the AAAS.

Neurons were also tested with other illusory figures, such as the well-known Schumann pattern (Fig. 13B), in which the subjective contours have orientations in common with the inducing elements. Here, it is necessary to distinguish between a neural representation of the subjective contours and the response to the edges inducing them. A possible solu-

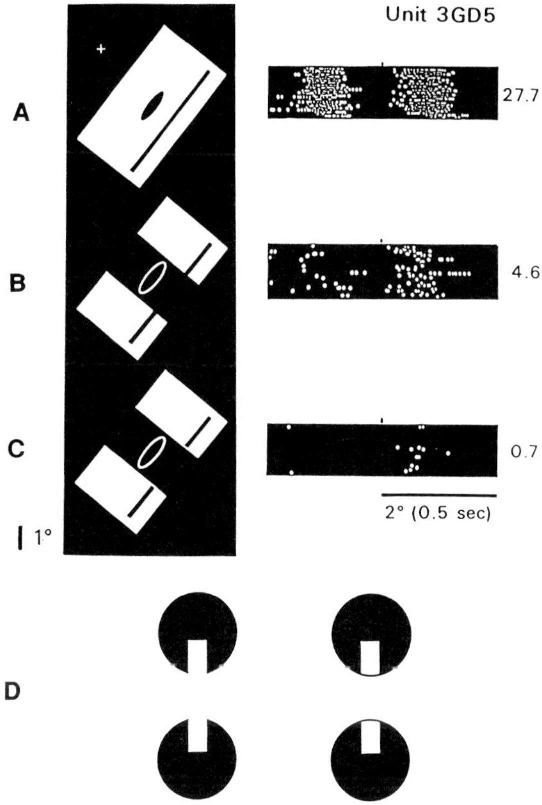

FIG. 13 Figure completion and the effect of closure in a cell of monkey Area V2. Ellipses indicate the cell's response field, i.e., the region outside which a bar evoked no responses, a cross marks the monkey's fixation point. (A) The responses to a moving light bar in a stationary dark rectangle, at the cell's preferred orientation. (B) When the central part, including the response field, was blanked out, the cell still responded regularly, although weakly, just as if a bar of low contrast were passing its response field. A moving illusory bar could be perceived crossing the gap. (C) When the ends of the bar were closed by thin lines, the responses were abolished just as the illusory bar disappeared (C). (D) Stationary figures that demonstrate a similar perceptual effect. The gap was 2° wide, the closing lines 2 minutes of arc. From von der Heydt, Peterhans and Baumgartner (1984). Copyright 1984 by the AAAS.

tion is to use a slightly modified figure which consists of similar elements but produces weaker or no subjective contours. Such a control figure is obtained by sealing off the ends of the upper and lower halves of a real bar with thin lines (Fig. 13C). Such closure abolishes the neuronal response and also eliminates the perception of the illusory bar (Fig. 13D). This result is particularly interesting, since it shows that very small changes in luminous flux made in the appropriate location can alter the neural response drastically. About one-third of the cells in Area V2 were found to signal subjective contours, whereas cells in Area V1 seemed to be "blind" to such contours and did not respond.

Many cells of V1 responded, of course, to the stimuli that produced subjective contours, but only if real edges or lines passed over the cell's response field at the preferred orientation. Thus, we can say that responses in Area V1 correlate with the perception of physically present contour, whereas many cells in Area V2 show an ability to construct or extrapolate contours in plausible ways, an ability which some have even deemed "cognitive" (Gregory, 1972; Coren, 1972).

Subjective contours have also been investigated in the cat visual cortex (Redies, Crook & Creutzfeldt, 1986). A border between abutting gratings similar to that of Fig. 10B was used. It was found to generate responses in complex cells of Area 17 as well as 18, but not in simple cells. The criterion was the continuity of the representation in a two-dimensional scanning plot of the responses. Whereas simple cells and end-stopped cells (if they responded at all) responded only to the line ends, complex cells brought out a continuous line. These results from cat Area 17 contrast with those from Area V1 in the monkey where orientation-selective cells in general did not respond at all to lines or patterns of lines orthogonal to the cell's preferred orientation (von der Heydt, Peterhans & Baumgartner, 1984). Nothdurft and Li (1985), using the same technique of analysis as Redies et al., found that complex cells in cat Area 17 do not make isoluminant texture borders explicit. With textures of short parallel lines, for example, the border between regions of different line orientation was not signaled as an edge or line would have been signaled.

If one can draw conclusions about cortical processing in humans from experiments in monkeys, the results described above cast new light on old questions of contour perception. First, the finding that cells in the primary visual cortex (V1) generally fail to signal subjective contours is contrary to the common assumption that a peripheral mechanism, such as lateral inhibition, plays a significant role in the perception of subjective contours (Brigner & Gallagher, 1974; Frisby & Clatworthy, 1975). It also makes it unlikely that subjective contours can be accounted for in terms of filtering out certain spatial Fourier components of the stimulus, as has been suggested by Ginsburg (1975) and Becker and Knopp (1978). Although the simple cells of Area V1 can be thought of as oriented spatial filters, they show no response to subjective contours. Furthermore, the neurons of Area V2 that do signal subjective contours are very sensitive to tiny changes in configuration (Fig. 13). They also respond vigorously to the border between gratings that is not represented in the Fourier spectrum at all. [Integrating the luminance along lines parallel to the border gives the same, constant value on either side of the contour; hence convolution with sinusoidal gratings of this orientation yields zero (see also Kelly, 1976; Parks & Pendergrass, 1982).] These findings are again hard to explain by the filter hypothesis.

Theories of subjective contours are often based on high-level inferences of occluding surfaces. Gregory (1972) and Rock and Ansom (1979) suggest that an occluding surface is hypothesized to simplify the interpretation of the stimulus. Such theories belie the fact that neuronal signals which might give rise to the perception of subjective contours are found as low as in Area V2, indicating that their perception need not be the result of higher level processing. The neurons in Area V2 are still mainly stimulus dependent, and the responses are stereotyped and reproducible, even in an alert animal. If the perception of subjective contours resulted from an attempt to reconcile the available stimulus with our perceptual postulate of it (Gregory, 1972), the observation that the strength of the illusion gradually increases with an increasing number of elements would be difficult to explain. Perceptual postulates cannot be gradual. On the other hand, neuronal mechanisms involving cooperative networks (Grossberg & Mingolla, 1985a,b; see Chapter 16, this volume) provide a plausible explanation for these phenomena. The finding that behaving cats might perceive illusory figures similar to the Kanizsa triangle (Bravo, Blake & Morrison, 1988) may also be interpreted as showing that cognitive processes need not be involved. Nonetheless, the possibility of top-down influences from higher areas cannot be ruled out completely.

To explain subjective contours in illusory figures, Peterhans, von der Heydt, and Baumgartner (1986) suggest a simple feed-forward mechanism that is compatible with the neuronal data and requires few assumptions. Their model assumes a convergence at the level of Area V2 of two parallel paths of computation, one for edge detection and one for detecting configurations formed by a series of terminators (e.g., line ends and corners). In this model, simple and complex cells constitute the edge-detecting path, while end-stopped (hypercomplex) cells contribute to the grouping path. A set of such receptive fields is lined up in a row according to the orientation signaled by the target cell, while the single fields are predominantly orthogonal to it (Fig. 14). This scheme explains, for example, the dependence of subjective contour on the number of lines (by summation in the grouping path) and the effect of closure (by the stimulation of inhibitory end zones). It also interprets the neurons with end-stopped receptive fields in a new way: their primary function would not be the detection of object features, but the evaluation of partially occluded patterns resulting from interposition (see also Redies, Spillmann & Kunz, 1984).

Several predictions follow from this model. Since the end-stopped fields of the grouping path are themselves orientation sensitive, the orientation of the inducing elements in subjective contour figures should influence the neuronal response. Subjective contours should be strongest when induced by orthogonal lines and less strong with oblique lines. This is indeed so (Fig. 15B; Kennedy, 1978). The perceived orientation of the subjective contours should also be biased toward an orientation orthogonal to the inducing lines. This is what one finds. The depth or overlay which is frequently perceived in subjective contour figures (Coren, 1972; Gregory & Harris, 1974; Coren & Porac, 1983) and the brightness enhancement in the

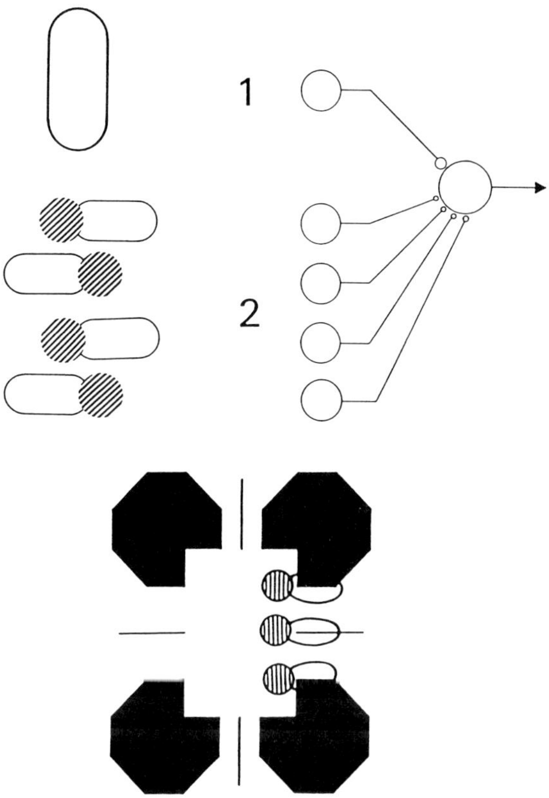

FIG. 14 A schematic representation of a neuronal mechanism that might underly the contour-related signals found in V2. A single cell of V2 is assumed to have input via two parallel paths, (1) from simple or complex fields ("edge detecting path"), and (2) from a set of end-stopped fields ("grouping path"). Both sets of fields overlap on the same patch of retina. Pairs of end-stopped fields straddling the center are connected by multiplication (×) with the effect that at least two of the end-stopped fields have to be excited simultaneously to produce a signal at the output, and the results are summed together with the edge signal. The figure at the bottom shows how the grouping path may be activated by a figure eliciting the perception of a subjective contour. After Peterhans, von der Heydt and Baumgartner (1986).

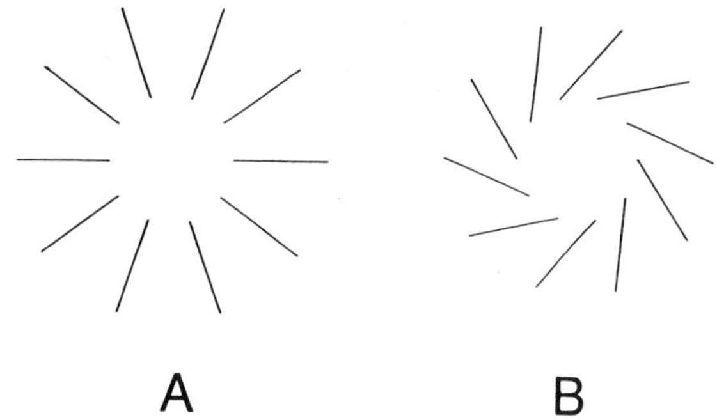

FIG. 15 (A) Subjective contours and brightness enhancement induced by line ends are most vivid when the contour runs at right angles to the lines; (B) with the inducing lines oriented tangentially there is no effect (Ehrenstein, 1941; Kennedy, 1978).

Kanizsa and Ehrenstein illusions (Fig. 10A and 15A) can similarly be explained by this hypothesis (von der Heydt & Peterhans, 1989b).

A neuronal mechanism derived from single-unit experiments with subjective contours can be interpreted as the computational solution to the problem of defining the contours in images of three-dimensional scenes without prior knowledge about the objects in the scene, a problem that can be solved only by exploiting the statistical properties of occluding contours. This hypothesis explains not only the perception of subjective contours, but also the brightness and depth illusions associated with them.

What does the visual system do with subjective contours once they have been extracted? There is a wealth of psychophysical evidence to suggest that they constrain many other aspects of perception such as stereopsis (Ramachandran, 1986a), apparent motion (Petersik, Hicks & Pantle, 1978; Ramachandran, 1985), and color (Ramachandran, 1987a,b). One wonders whether the many extrastriate visual areas (Van Essen, 1985) are somehow involved in mediating these interactions. Understanding the manner in which different visual "modules" interact is one of the great challenges for the future.

V. REPRESENTATION OF SHAPES

Once the visual scene has been parsed into the global areas that share particular features and that are likely to belong together as part of the same real objects, the three-dimensional shape of each area must be determined. Perceptual groups and areas can be defined by a number of stimulus attributes including luminance, color, motion, texture, and stereopsis, and the coding of shape might occur independently for each of these attributes. Using a variety of behavioral tasks, Cavanagh (1987, 1988) and colleagues explored the possibility that the analysis of each of these five attributes constitutes an independent "perceptual pathway." Cavanagh started from a larger set of potential pathways than is suggested by either physiological or neuropsychological data. Physiological studies show clear evidence for two independent streams, color/form and motion (Maunsell & Newsome, 1987) while neuropsychological reports of brain-damaged patients suggest only three physically separate and dissociable analyses, luminance (Rovamo et al., 1982), color (Damasio et al., 1980), and motion (Zihl et al., 1983). The five attributes that Cavanagh examined are meant to be exhaustive in that all other properties of the visual image (size, orientation, form, etc.) are properties of the spatial representations of one or more of these five attributes. Given that these attributes are only potential candidates for independent analysis, each of them was tested in several experiments for evidence of actual independence.

A. Evidence for Separate Pathways in Shape Perception

The first research on the perceptual capacities of individual pathways was the pioneering work by Julesz (1971) on images defined only by binocular disparity. [Prestriate Areas V3 and V3A may be involved in stereopsis (Zeki, 1979), possibly along with Area MT (Van Essen, 1985).] Julesz (1971) not only studied the sufficient conditions for the perception of depth in random dot stereograms, but, more importantly, he examined what qualities could be seen with images defined in this manner when no monocular cues were present. From Section II we know that the analysis of binocular disparity leads not just to the extraction of depth but also to the representation of the shapes of regions defined by their different depths. Julesz examined whether such shapes could produce classical visual illusions, identifiable letters, and various other perceptual phenomena. This approach has been extended to additional pathways, and comparisons have been made across these pathways (Cavanagh & Leclerc, 1989; Cavanagh, 1987).

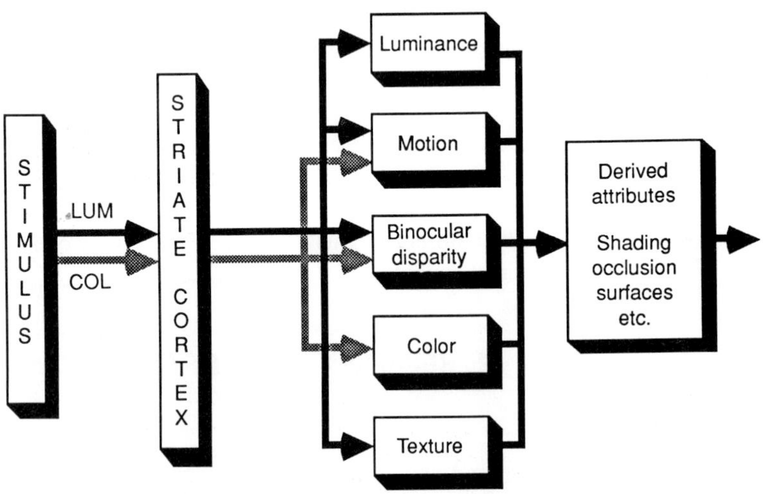

FIG. 16 Perceptual pathways in the visual system. Luminance (nonopponent) and color (opponent) pathways carry information from the retinal ganglion cells to the striate cortex where multifunction cells begin the analysis of orientation, motion, and binocular disparity. Beyond the striate cortex, information is routed to areas performing specialized analyses of various attributes such as color (Area V4; Zeki, 1978a,b) and motion (Area MT; Van Essen, 1985). Luminance, binocular disparity, and texture are other stimulus attributes that may receive specialized analyses in separate areas of extrastriate cortex. Each of these specialized areas generates a two-dimensional representation of the attribute being analyzed, contributing to an overall representation of stimulus shape. These independent representations may be followed by one or more high-level areas that recombine information from all attributes.

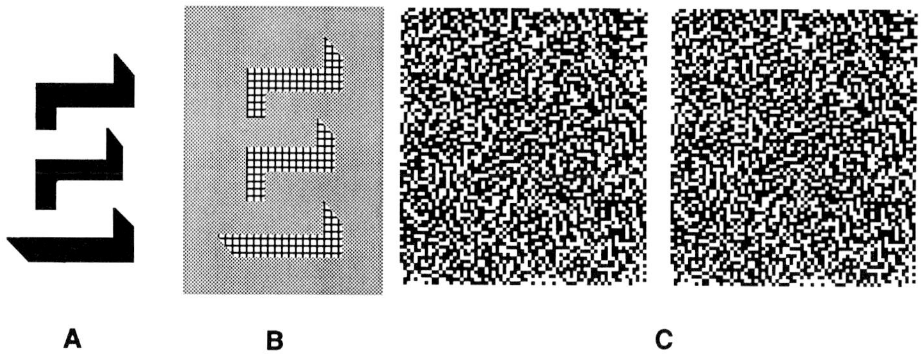

FIG. 17 Example of a shadowed block letter, E, represented by three different attributes: (A) luminance, (B) texture, and (C) binocular disparity. Most observers report the three-dimensional interpretation of the figure only for the leftmost stimulus defined by luminance. From Cavanagh (1988).

The studies described here examine perceptual pathways for five stimulus attributes (Fig. 16): color, luminance, texture, binocular disparity, and relative motion. To construct images defined by a single attribute, a black and white figure (Fig. 17A) was modified by replacing the black areas with, for example, a random texture moving in one direction, and the white areas with a similar texture moving in the opposite direction. Figure 17B,C demonstrates this attribute replacement for texture and binocular disparity.

In addition to the specialized analysis that is characteristic of each particular pathway, each possesses some degree of retinotopy in the underlying physiological structure (Maunsell & Newsome, 1987), and therefore each is inherently capable of representing two-dimensional contour. It is this common ground of two-dimensional shape representation that permits comparisons of coding and image analysis to be made across the pathways.

The first question addressed by these experiments is the type of shape coding that occurs at this low level. To segment image areas defined by a particular attribute, the visual system only needs to distinguish one region from another, which it could do very well by simply coding the value of the attribute (say, color) at each point in a retinotopic map (Fig. 18). We know, however, that in the case of luminance the visual sys-

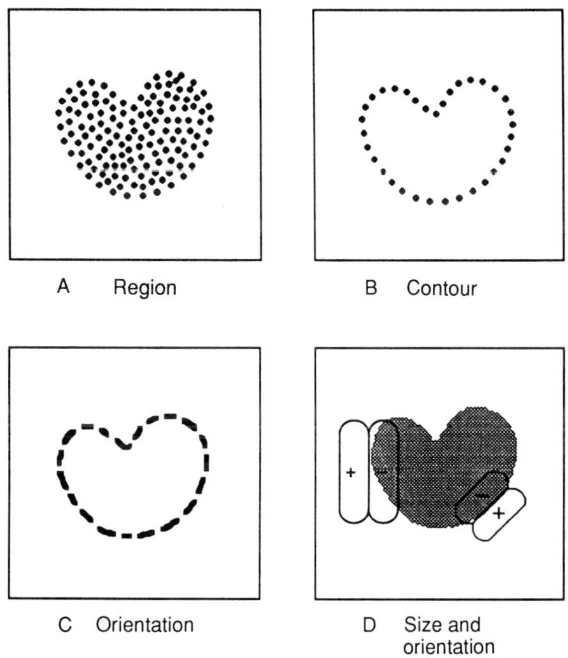

FIG. 18 Examples of the use of shape primitives to encode a two-dimensional region. (A) Point-by-point encoding of the attribute value preserves the region's shape. (B) Coding of only the region's contour preserves the shape and reduces the number of units needed to represent the shape. (C) Coding the contour with oriented tangents can improve the estimate of the region's outline if it is in a noisy presentation. (D) Overall shape can be decomposed into size- and orientation-specific units.

tem goes beyond this simple coding and extracts local structure (shape primitives) directly with cells that are selective to orientation and size (e.g., Hubel & Wiesel, 1968) and perhaps curvature (Dobbins et al., 1987). The visual system may use similar shape primitives for all attributes.

The second issue addressed by the experiments is the ability to use the two-dimensional shapes of regions defined by different surface attributes to infer three-dimensional object structure through cues such as shadows, occlusion, perspective, and contour junctions (Fig. 19). If this recovery of three-dimensional structure (three-dimensional shape from two-dimensional shape) is a higher level process that operates equally well on shape descriptions from any pathway, then the "shape from shape" approaches should work for two-dimensional shape defined by any surface attribute that the visual system can distinguish. For example, we should be able to interpret an ellipse as a tilted circle whether the ellipse is defined by color (red on green of equal luminance), by a random dot stereogram, or by luminance (black on white).

Finally, composite images were used to demonstrate the extent of cooperation between the pathways in producing geometrical illusions, stereoscopic depth perception, and apparent motion. These studies exploited the multiple pathways to localize various processes within the visual system. For example, if we can read a letter E whose horizontal bars are defined only by color and whose vertical bar is defined only by relative motion, then the identification process must have access to the combined information of the separate pathways.

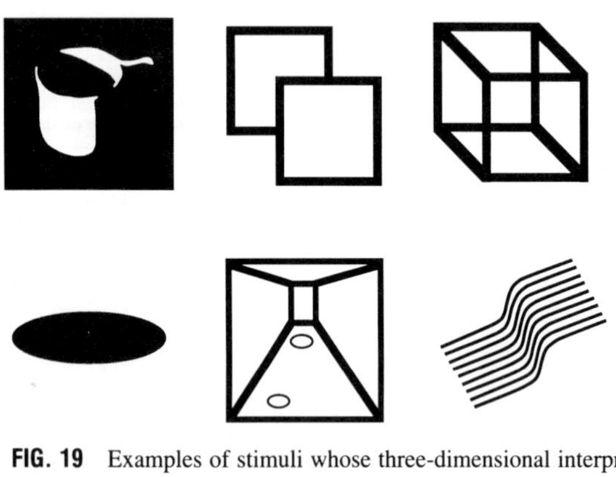

FIG. 19 Examples of stimuli whose three-dimensional interpretation is derived solely from two-dimensional shape cues. The examples do not have any gradient cues (shading, optical flow, or texture gradients) to convey three-dimensional information, but instead rely on shadows, occlusion, and perspective. Adapted from Cavanagh (1987) and Cavanagh (1988).

B. Use of Aftereffects to Infer Coding of Shape Primitives

When a stimulus sharing a particular property is viewed for some period of time, it induces an aftereffect which alters the threshold or the appearance of test stimuli viewed after the adaptation period. Figure 20 illustrates how adaptation to a fine grating makes a test grating appear coarser and vice versa. Similarly, adaptation to a grating tilted to the right from vertical makes a vertical stimulus appear to tilt in the opposite (to the left) direction and vice versa. Size (Blakemore & Sutton, 1969) and tilt aftereffects (Campbell & Maffei, 1971), as well as simultaneous induction paradigms (Georgeson, 1973; Klein, Stromeyer & Ganz, 1974), have been used to infer the existence of size and orientation coding in the luminance domain. The same procedures can be applied to stimuli defined by other attributes. Favreau and Cavanagh (1981) demonstrated that the color pathway has size-specific coding; Elsner (1978) showed a tilt aftereffect for equiluminous, colored stimuli; and Tyler (1975c) reported size and tilt aftereffects for random dot stereograms.

Using the size aftereffect paradigm, Favreau and Cavanagh (1981) induced simultaneous and opposite size aftereffects for color and luminance stimuli, suggesting these channels are separate. More recently they were able to make the same demonstration for the tilt aftereffect. It makes sense for the visual system to provide the color pathway with a rich set of shape primitives since shape analysis based on color information is frequently superior to luminance analy-

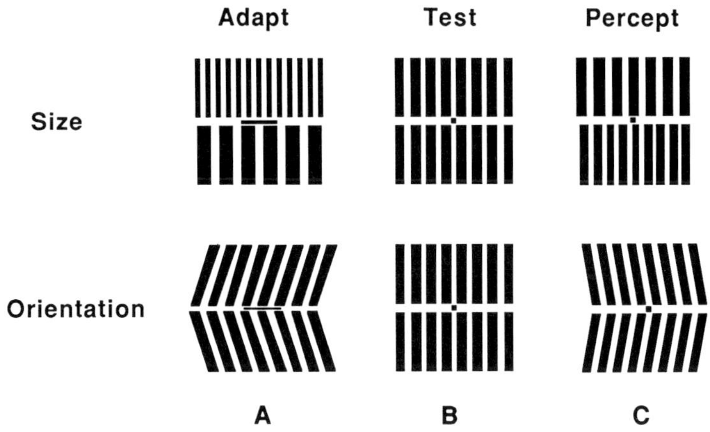

FIG. 20 Size and tilt aftereffects have been used to infer size and orientation coding in the visual system. Observers adapt to stimulus A for about 30 sec while scanning the central fixation bar. They are then asked to judge the relative size or tilt of stimulus B. Observers typically report that the central figures appear to have changed size (top) or tilt (bottom) as shown in C. From Cavanagh (1988).

sis. Color edges reliably move with the objects, while luminance edges are often confounded by the clutter of shadows unrelated to the objects across which they fall.

Tilt aftereffects were measured in each pathway using a standard induction and test procedure. Observers were first exposed to adapting gratings whose bars were tilted 15° from vertical and defined by relative motion. They were then presented with a vertical test also defined by relative motion (Fig. 20). When the test was presented, the observer matched its apparent tilt by adjusting a comparison stimulus presented in an unadapted region of the visual field. A tilt aftereffect of about the same magnitude was found for each type of stimulus. These data suggest that each pathway may perform a similar analysis of orientation.

The tilt or Zöllner illusion was also used to evaluate orientation coding in each pathway. In this illusion, parallel lines appear tilted away from crossing lines depending on the angle of intersection. This interaction has been claimed to result from inhibition between the orientation signals of the lines. If orientation coding exists for attributes such as color, texture, binocular disparity, and relative motion, then the illusion should persist when the stimulus is defined by each of these attributes. Indeed, the induced tilt was evident for all presentations and had approximately the same value, supporting the notion that orientation processing is ubiquitous in all pathways.

C. Visual Search in Separate Pathways

Evidence from visual search supports the inferences drawn from experiments using adaptation and aftereffects. Cavanagh, Arguin and Treisman (1990) used the search paradigm described earlier to determine whether size and orientation are privileged features, not only when defined by luminance differences, but also when defined in other pathways such as motion, color, and texture. Stimuli consisted of a large disk among small disks (size task) and a tilted bar among vertical bars (orientation task). They were defined by each of the five stimulus attributes. For the orientation task reaction time required to detect the presence of the target was independent of the number of distractors for all stimulus types except binocular disparity, indicating again that orientation may be a basic shape primitive in at least four of the five pathways tested. For the size task, reaction times were unaffected by the number of distractors for stimuli defined by luminance, color, texture, and relative motion but did show a significant increase for stimuli defined by binocular disparity (see also Nothdurft, 1985a,b). These data suggest that size coding may occur for four of the five pathways; however, further experiments may extend this to all five. In particular, experiments on size aftereffects by Tyler (1975c) do show adaptation for stimuli defined by binocular disparity, indicating that size is coded for this attribute. In summary, orientation and size coding appear to be very common in the visual system and may be used as shape primitives for each of the five attributes tested.

D. Shape Imaging Capacities of Individual Pathways

What are the elementary processes that underlie "shape-from-shape" inferences? Cavanagh (1987) has attempted to identify these processes by discovering the common aspects of a range of tests that *fail* in one pathway but not another. Tests are made with stimuli such as the Necker cube, perspective drawings, geometrical illusions, and subjective contours with each figure defined by a single attribute. Since the pathways other than luminance have poor spatial resolution (see Chapter 6, Fig. 7), it is necessary to use highly visible figures with no fine detail. Otherwise the inability to perform a particular task may be due simply to the reduced resolution or contrast inherent in a particular representation.

1. Figures with Explicit Contours

Information signaled by stimuli having explicit contours, for example, T-junctions indicating occlusion, was effective no matter which visual pathway was used to present them (Fig. 21). Simple, two-dimensional letter shapes could be easily identified, and objects defined by complete contours in line drawings involving occlusion and perspective gave rise to similar three-dimensional interpretations whether the line drawings were represented by luminance, color, or texture. When relative motion or random dot stereograms were used to present these same drawings, the depth suggested by two-dimensional occlusion and perspective sometimes conflicted with the depth indicated by the relative motion or binocular disparity used to present the figure. Many observers could see the depth implied by the drawing despite the conflict, although others could not. In cases where there was no conflict between the depth inferences in the picture and the depth used to present the picture (based on either relative motion or binocular disparity), the pictures were interpreted in the same manner as for luminance, color, or texture presentations. Shape information involving explicit object contours therefore appeared to be represented equally well in all of the five pathways. The depth and surface inferences based on these shape representations probably occur after the level of separate pathways and accept shape descriptions from any pathway. There was no indication that luminance information played any privileged role in these images.

2. Figures with Implicit Contours

The results for stimuli involving implicit contours were strikingly different. Figure 22 shows the two stimuli studied: subjective contours (Gregory, 1977) and shadows (Cavanagh & Leclerc, 1989). In both cases, a luminance difference was necessary between figure and ground for three-dimensional shape to be recovered. If the parts of the stimuli were presented without a luminance difference, they were interpreted as separate, unconnected islands of color or texture (see Liebmann, 1927). If a luminance difference was then introduced, the overall global organization of the stimulus became visible. Thus, the luminance pathway is essential for shadows and subjective contours, but it appears that it is the edges that are signaled at this low level and not the entire shadow region or subjective surface.

It might seem self-evident that shadows would require luminance information to be properly interpreted: a real shadow is always darker than the adjacent nonshaded region. Shadow analysis may therefore be part of the specialized processing in the luminance pathway. However, ignoring shape information in other pathways, the visual system must give up opportunities to reject areas as shadows because of "impossible" colors or inappropriate depths, motions, or textures. Indeed, observers saw depth in

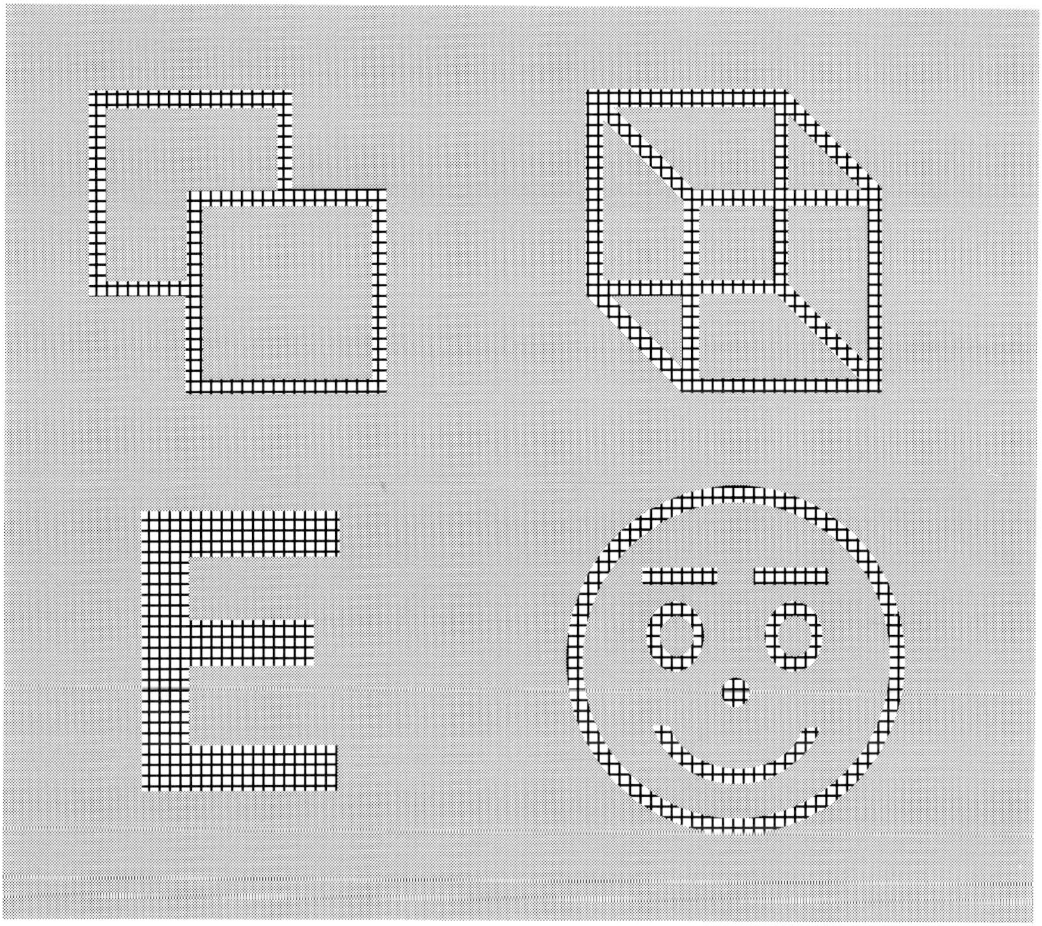

FIG. 21 Stimuli with explicit contours. The stimuli are defined only by a difference in texture and should be invisible if you squint your eyes. In a Necker cube perceived as a wire frame the background can be seen through the areas between the cube contours; in an occlusion figure consisting of one square covering one corner of a similar square, the areas between the contours hide the background. In general, the same perceptions are reported for these stimuli whether defined by luminance, texture, color, relative motion, or binocular disparity. However, large individual differences are sometimes found in the latter two cases. These occur when there are conflicts between depth suggested by the picture and depth defined by the relative motion or binocular disparity. From Cavanagh (1988).

shadow images even when they violated the color, depth, motion, and texture constraints of natural shadows (Cavanagh & Leclerc, 1989).

The coding of subjective contours by pathways other than luminance is doubtful. Brussell, Stober, and Bodinger (1977), Gregory (1977), and Prazdny (1985a) all report that subjective contours were visible only when there was a luminance difference between the regions defining the shapes. However, Kellman and Loukides (1987) and Prazdny (1987) were able to create subjective contours in the motion pathway using kinetic stimuli without any luminance contrast.

3. Illusions

Gregory (1977) evaluated several illusions for figures defined by color and Julesz (1971) for figures defined

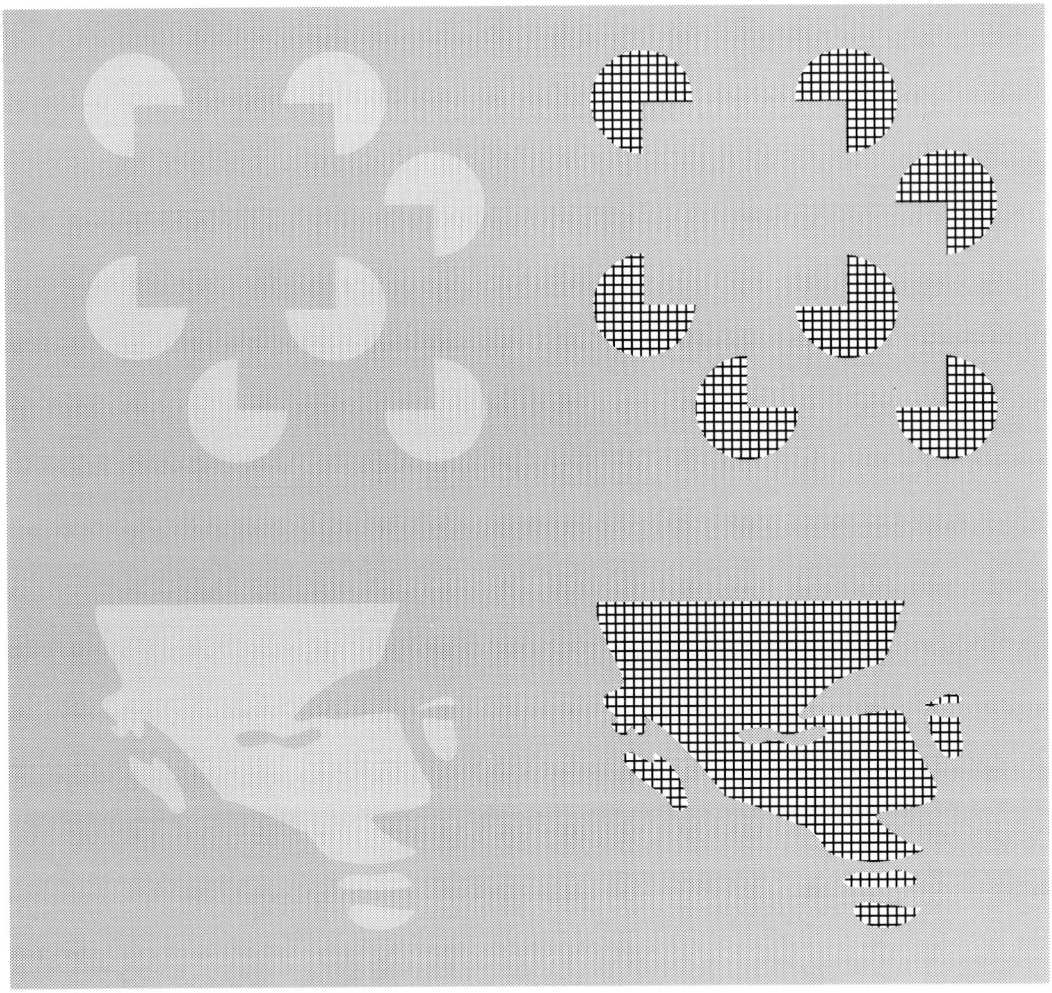

FIG. 22 Stimuli with implicit contours. Top row: subjective contours. When there is a luminance difference between the inducing elements and the background, subjective contours can be seen (left). When the same figure is presented without a luminance difference (right), subjective contours are weak or absent. Bottom row: shadows. Many of the contours in the figure (left) are shadow contours, not object contours, and many of the object contours, both external and internal self-occlusions, are implicit. The interpretation of the figure as a face changes when no luminance difference is present (right). The interpretation of surface relief due to shadows occurs for stimuli defined by luminance and not for stimuli defined by texture (shown here), color, relative motion, or binocular disparity.

by binocular disparity. Both report that the illusions remain undiminished with two exceptions, the café wall illusion and Fraser spiral, which Gregory discusses in detail. The strength of two additional illusions that Cavanagh tested also remained undiminished. In the Ponzo illusion a horizontal bar which appears closer also appears shorter than an equally long bar which appears to lie farther in the distance and in the horizontal–vertical illusion, a vertical line appears longer than an equally long horizontal line. Both illusion figures were presented in each of five stimulus dimensions (luminance, color, motion, binocular disparity, and texture), and both illusions showed the same strength for all presentations. The perspective and spatial scaling processes involved therefore appear to operate on shape codes that are available in each pathway.

E. Interpathway Cooperation and Localization

Interocular transfer and dichoptic viewing are useful techniques for localizing processes in vision, identifying whether the locus of origin of a given effect precedes or follows the emergence of binocular units. The multiple pathways of the extrastriate cortex may provide a similar opportunity. If certain analyses of shape operate only within independent pathways whereas other higher level analyses can operate on information from any pathway, the identity and locus of visual processes can be revealed using "composite" stimuli where different components of the stimulus (adapt and test, or inducing and test elements) are defined by different attributes. If, for example, the orientation analysis that underlies the tilt illusion occurs only within each pathway, adaptation to tilted lines defined by texture should induce an apparent tilt in a test line also defined by texture, but not in a line defined by relative motion (Fig. 23). On the other hand, if depth from perspective is a high level process, the impression of perspective should be produced even by the relative angle between two lines defined by different attributes. Experiments of this type can provide guidelines for the processing hierarchy of the visual system. Specifically, a perceptual effect that is preserved in a composite stimulus is necessarily located at some stage beyond the independent pathways. They may be localized beyond the prestriate cortex where information from all the pathways is accessible and integrated (Fig. 16). An effect that does not survive in a composite image must therefore be located in one or more, but not all, of the independent pathways.

1. Illusions

Three illusions, horizontal–vertical, perspective (Ponzo), and tilt (Zöllner), were tested with composite figures. With two exceptions (color and stereo could not be combined because red–green anaglyphs were used to present the random dot stereograms), all possible combinations of five attributes were applied to these figures. There were 23 different versions, 5 "within" figures with both the inducing and the test portion of the illusion figure defined by the same attribute, and 18 "between" figures in which the two components were defined by different attributes. A "between/within" ratio was computed by dividing the average strength of each illusion for all "between" figures by the average strength for all "within figures". A value of 1.0 for this ratio indicates that the processes responsible for the illusion had access to a combined shape representation, whereas a value less than 1.0 indicates that the processes responsible must, at least in part, be located in the segregated pathways so that the integrated figure was unavailable to them.

Both the horizontal–vertical and Ponzo illusions had between/within ratios very close to 1.0, indicating that the processes underlying the illusions had access to an integrated image. Processes involved in spatial scaling of horizontal and vertical dimensions and scaling size with distance (the perspective cue in the Ponzo illusion) should be expected to operate on an integrated image since they must deal with scenes made up of objects defined by an arbitrary assortment of attributes. For the Zöllner illusion, on the other hand, the ratio was significantly less than one, implying that the orientation coding underlying this tilt illusion occurs independently in each pathway: a composite figure would therefore produce a weaker illusion than one defined by a single attribute (Fig. 23). The ratio was, nevertheless, also greater than zero, indicating that there is some interpathway interaction for orientation coding or alternately some orientation coding in a common high level representation.

2. Motion

Apparent motion can be perceived between two shapes defined by different stimulus attributes (Cavanagh, Arguin & von Grünau, 1989). Ramachandran, Rao, and Vidyasagar (1973a,b) reported earlier that motion can be seen between two patches defined only

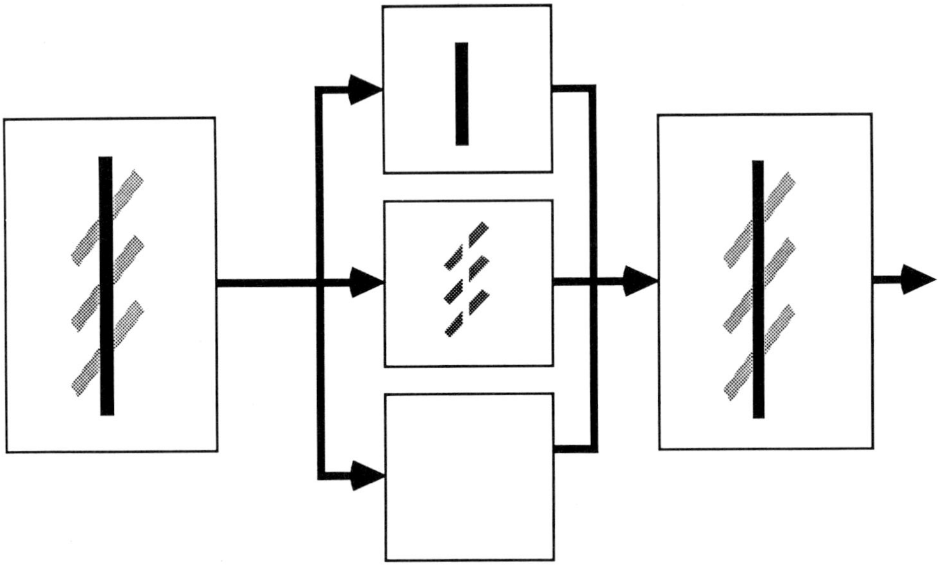

FIG. 23 Composite stimulus for inducing the tilt effect. Inducing bars are defined by one attribute and the test bar by another. On the left the stimulus is represented as a whole in the first cortical area, V1. However, at this level, no cells code for the orientation of bars defined by texture, relative motion, or binocular disparity (as a random dot stereogram). Therefore, no inhibition between orientations could be expected to produce the apparent tilt at this level when these attributes are involved. Similarly, in the center, the inducing and the test lines are represented in separate cortical areas (pathways) and thus have little opportunity to interact. Finally, on the right, in a representation where the individual attributes are recombined, a tilt illusion could occur if orientation is coded there.

by texture. Similar demonstrations have been made for stimuli defined by color (Ramachandran & Gregory, 1978) and binocular disparity (Julesz, 1971; Prazdny, 1986a,b). The demonstration that motion can be seen equally between patches defined by *different* attributes indicate that this motion process must have access to an integrated image. The strength of the motion, as measured by the maximum displacement over which the motion could be seen, was similar whether the two patches were defined by the same attribute or by different attributes.

3. Stereo

Similar studies of stereograms, where the figure presented to each eye could be defined by the same or different attributes, showed different and sometimes conflicting results. Binocular disparity between the monocularly visible patches seen by both eyes did produce a vivid impression of depth if the image in each eye was defined by the same attribute whether it was color, luminance, texture, or relative motion. Similar data were reported by Ramachandran, Rao, and Vidyasagar (1973a,b) and by Lee (1979). However, when different attributes were used in each eye, Cavanagh found that no depth was visible. This is not simply a matter of binocular rivalry; the images of the two eyes are also rivalrous in their luminance detail when both are defined by, say, relative motion, and yet depth is perceived in that case. Cavanagh concluded that, unlike the motion process, binocular disparity cannot operate on composite stimuli combining attributes across the eyes.

On the other hand, Ramachandran et al. (1973b) reported that one can obtain stereopsis by fusing a luminance border from one eye with a disparate texture border or chromatic border from the other eye, implying that different types of contours or edges may eventually be processed by a single mechanism in the brain that is indifferent to the manner in which the contour is constituted. Ramachandran et al. suggest that the purpose of such a mechanism would be to signal the presence of occlusion borders in the visual image and that there could even be a "channel" somewhere in the brain that is specialized exclusively for this role.

F. Conclusions on Separate Pathways Coding Shape

The studies reviewed here show that perceptual pathways can be probed with stimuli defined by luminance, color, relative motion, texture, and depth. Aftereffect, illusion, and visual search paradigms demonstrate that orientation coding is used for all the attributes. For the four attributes where evidence was available, size coding was also used. Simultaneous and opposing aftereffects showed that there are functionally independent streams of processing for luminance and color and that both perform similar analysis of size and orientation. The shape information available in each pathway was sufficient to support three-dimensional interpretations of images involving explicit contours but not for images involving implicit contours, namely, subjective contours and shadows. These images therefore appear to depend on a particular process or shape code available only in the luminance pathway. Composite images showed that the processes underlying perspective, the scaling of horizontal versus vertical dimensions, and form-based motion have access to high level representations where information from all the attributes is recombined. In contrast, orientation coding underlying the tilt illusion appears to be based in the individual pathways although some orientation coding may also occur in a high level representation. Finally, although depth could be perceived from form-based binocular disparity for each attribute, there is some doubt whether it could be achieved when the same form was defined by different attributes in each eye.

VI. PERCEPTION AND IDENTIFICATION OF OBJECTS

Once objects have been delineated by early processes of feature-based segregation and boundary formation, they must be *identified* as known individuals or instances of a familiar category. Identification seems to involve the use of two different strategies. The first is based on the use of particular, salient cues that directly label the object rather than on elaborate processing of all its parts. The second strategy allows us to extract spatial *relationships* between features (i.e., what is above, what is below). It is this second process that enables us to recognize pumpkin faces and snowmen in spite of locally misleading salient features (such as a carrot used for a nose). There is evidence that the two processes can be dissociated in visual agnosia (Humphreys & Riddoch, 1987) and in certain visual illusions such as the Thatcher illusion (Thompson, 1980). A frowning upside-down face is seen as a face because of the spatial relationships between features but it is seen as smiling because the features themselves are processed separately and can act as inborn ethological releasers.

A. Feature Integration

In most cases, object identification depends on comparing a complex conjunction of features to a stored representation. It is of interest to investigate how the visual system codes conjunctions, given the evidence for modularity of feature analysis described in Section II.

One important observation suggests that conscious experience and voluntary behavior necessarily depend on these later stages of perceptual representation. Although there is evidence that the analysis of color, motion, orientation, and other properties is modular at the early stages of coding (see Sections II, C and V), it is difficult for subjects to access separately the output of one module in order to control behavioral responses, while suppressing the outputs of other modules coding different properties of the same perceptual object. The Stroop test (Stroop, 1935) is a well-known example of such interference: In naming the colors of the ink in which words are printed, subjects are considerably slowed down if the words themselves are the names of other colors. The natural process of perception unites the outputs of the color and shape modules before they become available to introspection. In a task such as the Stroop test, in which the two modules evoke conflicting responses, a clear failure of selective attention is observed. We can select one object rather than another, but not one property of an object while excluding another property of the same objects (see also Kahneman & Chajzcik, 1983; Treisman, Kahneman & Burkell, 1983).

On the other hand, in tasks designed to tap the earlier stages of visual coding, the evidence suggests dimensional separation and modularity. In section II, we reported a number of results suggesting failures to conjoin or integrate different features: areas containing elements differing only in conjunctions of features do not spontaneously segregate or form perceptual boundaries, and targets in visual search are detected in parallel only when they have some unique defining feature not shared by the distractors. In this section the conjunction process is examined in more detail, together with the conditions under which features can be interrelated and structured to define perceptual objects.

Experiments on texture segregation suggested that elements are initially grouped within perceptual dimensions, forming, for example, a color map, an orientation map, a motion map, but not across dimensions. Thus, an element located between two groups and sharing a different feature with each group is less conspicuous and more often overlooked than an element with a unique feature (Treisman, 1982). A red O between a group of blue O's and red X's would be grouped with the red X's in the color map and with the blue O's in the shape map, and it would not appear at this level of processing to have an identity of its own. Targets in visual search tasks that are defined only by conjunctions of features (like the red O in the above example) are usually found through a serial process of checking and rejecting the nontarget items or distractors (Treisman & Gelade, 1980). The search time increases linearly with the number of distractors in the display, suggesting that attention must be focused to each item in turn in order to conjoin features correctly. The serial process could not be attributed to the heterogeneity of the distractors, because a target with either of two unique features (e.g., green or S) among the same heterogeneous distractors was detected in parallel. If the distractors were spatially grouped into homogeneous clusters (Fig. 24), search appeared to be serial across groups. However, the

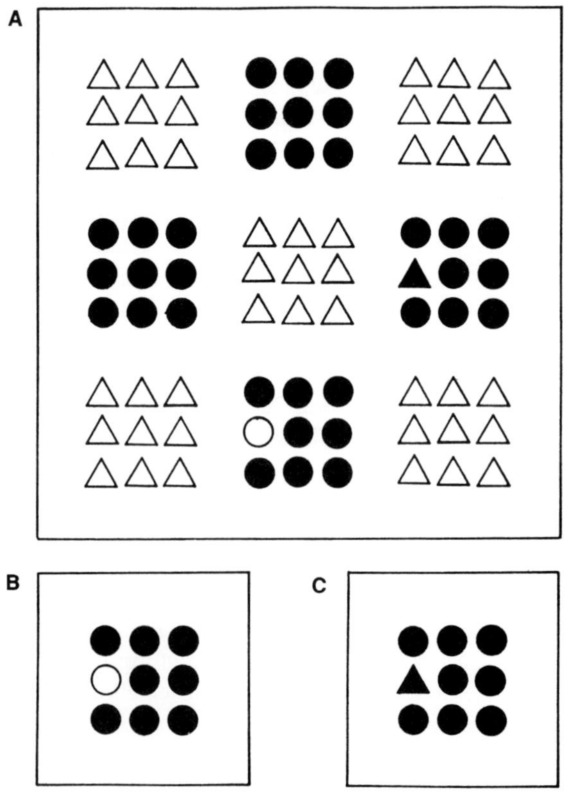

FIG. 24 (A) Display in which search for a conjunction target (e.g., a white circle or a black triangle) appears to be serial across groups but parallel within any one group. The items within each uniform group can receive divided attention, because within the group the target is defined by a single feature and will pop out, as it does in B and C. From Treisman (1985).

items within each group were checked in parallel (Treisman, 1982). In effect, the target could be distinguished from the distractors within any group on the basis of a single distinguishing feature. Similar results have been found with conjunctions of color with shape (curved versus angular as in O versus N or vertical versus diagonal components as in X versus T) and with conjunctions of parts of shapes (e.g., R's among P's and Q's).

Figure 25 shows the model proposed by Treisman (1986a,b) as a first attempt to account for the contrast between single features and conjunctions of features. The modular feature maps (as discussed in Section II) are linked to a master map representing their spatial locations. Attention is represented by a "spotlight" or a "window" (Kosslyn, 1987) selecting the features represented in a subarea of the master map. The features in this preselected location are integrated to form a unitary representation specifying their structural relations. The attention window is adjustable in size, depending on the precision required. Thus, when distractors are grouped into homogeneous clusters, the attention window can be set to accept each cluster as a whole. In a search task, attention scans the master map until all the distractors have been rejected.

The model distinguishes a representation of space (the master map of locations) from a representation of the features (e.g., color, orientation) that occupy locations in space (the feature map). As already men-

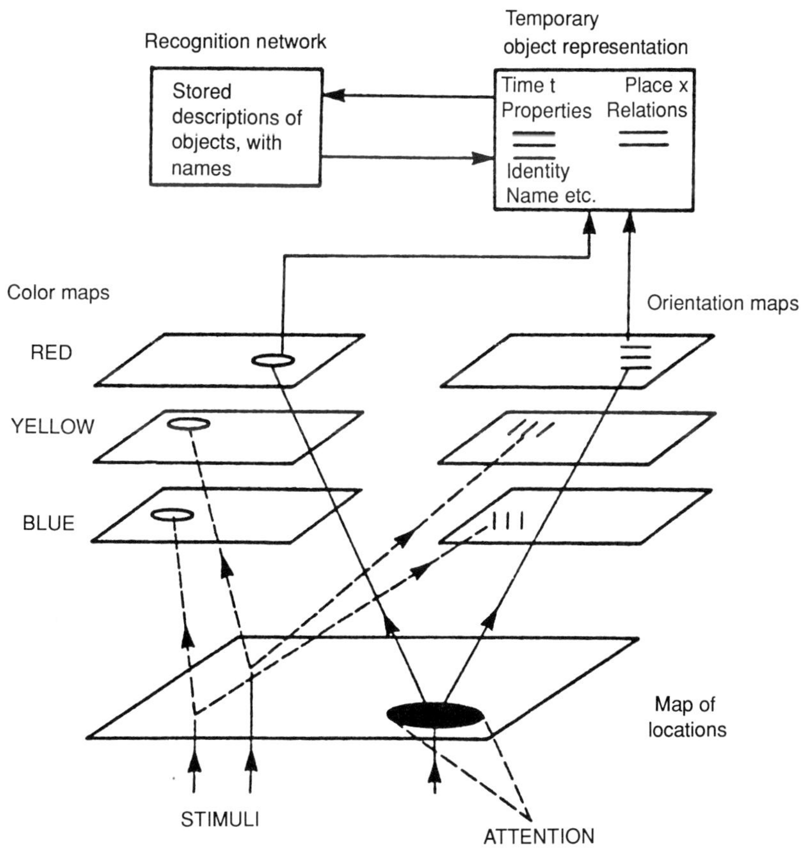

FIG. 25 General framework relating hypothesized feature maps to a master map of locations through which focused attention serially conjoins the properties of different objects within the scene. See text for details. From Treisman (1988).

tioned in Section II, a similar where-versus-what distinction has been drawn by neuroscientists (Mishkin, Ungerleider & Macko, 1983). Mishkin et al. have traced two separate pathways in the brain, one through the posterior parietal area, which appears to deal with spatial discriminations, and one leading to the inferotemporal cortex, which appears to deal with object recognition. Lesions to each pathway lead to quite different behavioral deficits. Other researchers have linked the parietal areas to spatial attention. For example, parietal lesions in human patients have been shown to lead to "neglect" of contralateral space (Jung, 1974; DeRenzi, 1982). Neurophysiologists (e.g., Robinson, Goldberg & Stanton, 1978; Mountcastle, Andersen & Motter, 1981; Wurtz, Goldberg & Robinson, 1982) have identified single units in the posterior parietal lobe of monkeys that respond only when the monkey attends to the stimulus. It is not inconceivable, then, that the parietal areas might play a role in integrating information relating to different attributes of objects, by controlling a serial scan of the locations in which they appear. A related hypothesis was proposed by Crick (1984), who attributed the selective and integrative role of the attention spotlight to facilitating bursts of activity from the pulvinar. The lateral pulvinar has strong connections to Area 7 of the parietal cortex, and cells in these areas appear to respond in similar ways to visual properties and to manipulations of attention (Robinson & Petersen, 1984).

Quite recently, however, the generality of the behavioral results with conjunction targets in visual search has been questioned. Nakayama and Silverman (1986) found that when the features defining a conjunction target are highly discriminable, the slope relating target search time to the number of distractors may become quite shallow (less than 10 msec per item) or even flat. This result suggests that conjunctions of features can sometimes be detected when attention is spread over several items at a time, or even over the whole display. The parallel detection of such stimuli is usually associated with a phenomenological impression of clear segregation between the two sets of distractors; these often appear to be in separate depth planes.

Treisman (1988) suggested that, with highly discriminable features distinguishing the two sets of distractors, attention can be directed to homogeneous subgroups of items as a whole (i.e., parallel access), even when they are spatially intermingled with other items. In terms of the framework in Fig. 25, this could be achieved by preselecting one complete set of distractor locations in the master map through inhibition (or activation) from the feature map that has this attribute. For example, if the target is green and horizontal among red horizontal and green vertical distractors, the locations of all red items might be selectively inhibited in the master map of locations, leaving activity mainly or only in the locations of the green items. These could then be checked with divided attention, since any remaining horizontal item would have to be the target.

Wolfe, Franzel, and Cave (1989) proposed a similar model and reported two new pieces of supporting evidence. (1) A target defined by a triple conjunction that differed in *two* features from each distractor was found more quickly than either a triple or a double conjunction that differed only in one feature from each distractor. For example, a large red cross gave very rapid parallel detection among large green circles, small red circles, and small green crosses. This would follow if inhibition coming from two feature maps could summate to reject each distractor location more effectively than inhibition coming from only one. (2) A target defined only by the spatial arrangement of its parts (e.g., a target T among distractor L's), could not be detected in parallel. This would follow from the hypothesis proposed, since neither feature of the distractors could be inhibited without also rejecting the target.

B. Temporary Object Representations

At the final stage of perceptual processing, objects are identified by matching them to stored descriptions of familiar objects. Many models of perception have equated "seeing" with "identifying" an object (LaBerge, 1975; Shiffrin & Schneider, 1977; Johnston & Dark, 1982). Identification is said to occur when the "nodes" standing for the object and for its properties are activated in a recognition network. The same idea appears in the physiological theories that equate perception with the activation of single "grandmother" cells (Barlow, 1972b) or assemblies of cells (Hebb, 1949). Recently discovered cells responding selectively to faces (Perrett et al., 1982) could be an example of such a perceptual model, at least for these highly significant biological stimuli.

However, in addition to the activation of nodes mediating recognition, one can argue for the existence of temporary object representations (see Fig. 25) that assemble the feature information in the correct structural relations and mediate "seeing" or perceptual experience (Treisman & Schmidt, 1982; Kahneman & Treisman, 1984). It is quite possible for us to "see" an unfamiliar object for which no prior representation has been established. We are also quite capable of seeing multiple replicas of an identical object when they are present, although each replica may take a measurable time to set up. The perceptual system must therefore form representations of "tokens" as well as of types. It must allow us rapidly to form one or many identical temporary representations of any arbitrary and unfamiliar conjunction of features in a visual field which may also contain a large number of other objects with potentially interchangeable properties. Moreover, it must be able to retain the perceptual identity and continuity of an object representation even when the object moves or changes its perceptual appearance.

Little research has been devoted to understanding these representations that presumably mediate our conscious experience. The separation of tokens (temporary object-specific representations of currently present perceptual objects) from types (the long-term stored representations abstracted from past experience and used for object recognition or labeling) has so far not found any physiological correlate.

C. Object Identification

The final issues, on which very little is known, concern the relationship between the temporary object representations and the stored descriptions to which they are matched (Fig. 25) as well as the matching operation itself. The object representations should, of course, specify three-dimensional solids in a three-dimensional spatial field rather than two-dimensional images. Their properties will therefore belong to a different vocabulary from the features of the image that reflect their real world origins only indirectly. Whether the features which are initially entered into the temporary object representations are the features of three-dimensional surfaces or whether the mapping is achieved only with focused attention once the features have been conjoined is still an open question. It seems plausible, however, that the visual system has evolved to extract information, even at the earliest stages, in a form which specifies the external world. Thus, rather than coding the properties of the retinal image as a physicist might (specifying the wavelength, the intensity, and the geometrical properties of the two-dimensional projection), the visual system may code such properties directly. Examples may be the gradients of texture and of motion that specify three-dimensional shapes and surfaces (Gibson, 1966; Braunstein, 1976) or the motion of edges in opposite directions that specifies "looming" in an approaching object (Regan & Cynader, 1979). Although these properties depend on relations across space and time, they need not be treated as conjunctions; specialized detectors may have evolved to code them directly. Such dynamic or relational properties actually appear to be detected and used earlier in infant development than static properties (Owsley, 1983; Kellman & Loukides, 1987).

Marr (1982) suggested that the representations which form the basis for perceptual recognition should be object centered rather than viewer centered. In other words, their descriptions should be independent of the viewing angle, distance, and illumination. The relations between the parts should be specified relative to the intrinsic axes of the object itself rather than of the visual field of the viewer. It is interesting to note, however, that the representation which we consciously experience as seeing is not object centered. Instead, perception is egocentric. Although the perceptual constancies of size, shape, brightness, color, and motion reduce the variations in the retinal image due to distance, three-dimensional tilt, line of sight, and illumination, they do not usually eliminate them completely. Moreover, we do not "see" the backs of objects or fill in occluded parts, although in most cases we easily infer them and are aware of their existence. Of course, our current spatial relation to the object is often as relevant to us as its identity; it determines our motor behavior in grasping, navigation, and so on. This may explain why conscious perception seems to represent both in an uneasy compromise that is neither completely viewer centered nor completely object centered. Whether the same compromise is present in the functional codes that represent the objects or whether those are fully object centered, leaving separate codes to specify the viewing conditions, is not known.

VII. PHYSIOLOGY OF VISUAL ATTENTION

Visual perception depends not only on the retinal image and its cortical representation but also on the focus of attention. We usually look at what we are interested in so that our direction of gaze coincides with our direction of attention in space. However, if needed we can also dissociate fixation from attention by attending to an event in our peripheral visual field without directly looking at it. The eye movement required to bring the fovea into register with the peripheral target is called a saccade. Saccades usually take 200–300 msec before they are initiated, a latency that is highly dependent on the stimulus conditions and state of attention.

The modulation of visual perception by attention has been studied in psychophysical as well as physiological experiments in man and monkey. The results obtained from single-cell recordings in various areas of the brain are described first. Neurophysiological studies of attention were only made possible by the pioneering work of Evarts (1966) in the motor system. He combined microelectrode techniques with psychological test procedures. Wurtz (1969) adopted this technique for the visual system and also precisely controlled the position of the eye. This was done by implanting a magnetic search coil (Robinson, 1963) in the eye or by using infrared light reflected from the cornea (Bach, Bouis & Fischer, 1983). All studies were done in the awake behaving monkey. Extensive reviews on the preparation of visually guided saccades (Fischer 1987) and on the relationship between saccades and visual attention (Fischer, 1986; Fischer & Breitmeyer, 1987) are available.

The basic idea in all studies on the effect of visual attention on single-cell activity is that the cell's response to a given stimulus can be modulated by the behavioral circumstances under which the stimulus occurs. Because it is impossible to know whether or not the animal is attending to the stimulus, one must rely on a motor reaction by the animal as a measurable response that can be related to the particular stimulus used.

Whereas in many psychophysical studies a manual response such as a key press is used, most studies in monkey have employed the oculomotor reflex, that is, the onset of a saccadic eye movement in response to a peripheral stimulus. In this way one can be sure that the stimulus that is viewed is also being attended to. The disadvantage, however, of this technique is that any modulation of a visual response in conjunction with a saccade may reflect the motor preparation of the eye movement rather than an effect of attention per se. In order to be sure that a given effect reflects attention only, one has to ascertain that the neuronal response can be obtained without a temporal change of the physical stimulus and without an accompanying motor response. We next describe a number of tasks that allow effects of visual stimuli, oculomotor occurrences, and attention on single-cell behavior to be assessed separately.

A. Experimental Tasks

1. Fixation Task

The first step in all experiments on the neurophysiology of the visual and oculomotor systems is to teach

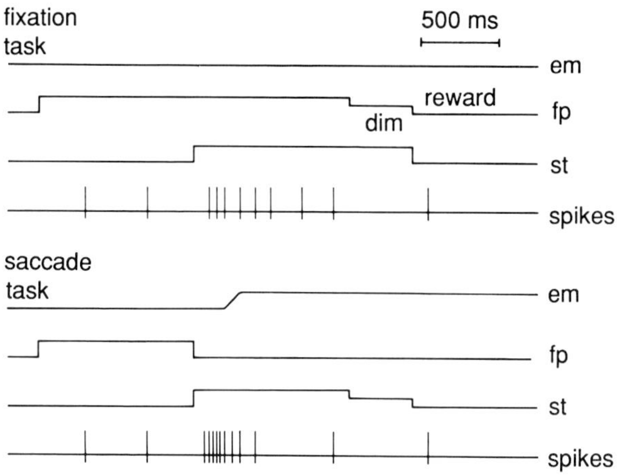

FIG. 26 Schematic illustration of the fixation task and the saccade task. The traces are identified as em (eye movement), fp (fixation point), and st (stimulus). The lowest trace (spikes) indicates the impulse activity of a single cell: in the fixation task the cell produces a moderate number of extra spikes after stimulus onset. In the saccade task, the same cell produces a burst of spikes. This response modulation is called the enhancement effect.

a monkey to fixate in a given direction. For this purpose a small fixation point is used (Wurtz, 1969). The animal quickly learns to look at the fixation point because he is rewarded each time he detects a mild dimming of the fixation light. The monkey signals the dimming by manually activating a switch. Following the detection and reward, the fixation point is extinguished, and a new cycle of fixations begins. In this way, up to 2000 fixation periods, each 2 to 8 sec long, may be obtained every day. This task is schematically illustrated in the top half of Fig. 26.

2. Saccade Task

During the fixation task, the fixation point is switched off and a new stimulus appears without delay in the monkey's peripheral field of vision. This stimulus has been positioned to project into the receptive field of the neuron from which recordings are made. The animal quickly learns to change his direction of gaze when the luminance of the new stimulus is turned down, and he will soon respond to the dimming of the peripheral light the way he responded to the fixation point before. The neural response to the onset of the peripheral stimulus (when placed in the cell's receptive field) will precede the beginning of the eye movement and may therefore reveal important cues to the processes occurring during the preparatory period. This saccade task is schematically illustrated in the bottom half of Fig. 26.

3. Delayed Saccade Task

To avoid confounding the occurrence of the saccadic target and the preparation of the eye movement, Fischer and Boch (1981b) introduced the delayed saccade task. In this task, the new stimulus appears before the fixation point is turned off so that any neural response elicited by the stimulus occurs well before the animal begins to prepare his saccade.

4. Suppressed Saccade Task

The suppressed saccade task is identical to the delayed saccade task with the only difference that the animal is required to suppress his eye movement to the new stimulus; he keeps looking straight ahead in the direction of the fixation point even after it has already disappeared (Fischer & Boch, 1985). A modification of this task is the blink task (Richmond, Wurtz & Sato, 1983). Here, the fixation point is temporarily turned off and a probe stimulus is flashed into the receptive field during this blink. Thereafter, the fixation point reappears, dims, and the animal is rewarded for pressing a bar upon the detection of the dimming.

5. Peripheral Attention Task

The peripheral attention task is similar to the suppressed saccade task except that here the fixation point remains visible while dimming occurs in the peripheral stimulus (Wurtz & Mohler, 1976a).

B. The Enhancement Effect

The enhancement effect was first reported by Goldberg and Wurtz (1972) for neurons in the superior colliculus nucleus. Figure 26 shows that during the fixation task the cell responds to the onset of a light placed in its receptive field with a moderate number of spikes distributed over the entire stimulus interval. However, during the saccade task, the same cell responds with a sudden burst as the stimulus now becomes the target for the saccade. The response is clearly enhanced. Note that the enhancement occurs already before the eyes begin to move, that is, at a time when the retinal image is still the same as in the fixation task. This effect has been attributed to the focusing of the animal's attention on the fixation point and its subsequent shift to the peripheral stimulus as the new target (Wurtz & Goldberg, 1972; Wurtz & Mohler, 1976a).

When a control task was introduced in these experiments, it became clear that the enhancement effect observed in collicular cells as well as those of other brain structures cannot always be attributed to attention. Instead, this effect is often related to the preparation of a motor response or to the transition from active to passive fixation.

C. Cortical and Subcortical Structures for Visual Attention

Possible candidates for the control of attention may be found by examining the anatomical pathways that connect the visual (afferent) system with the oculomotor (efferent) system, that is, the retina with the oculomotor nuclei. The most prominent structures are (in this order) the lateral geniculate body, superior colliculus, striate cortex (Area V1), prestriate cortex (Areas V2 and V3), prelunate cortex (Area V4), the cortex hidden in the superior temporal sulcus (Areas MT and MST), inferior temporal cortex (Area 22), posterior parietal cortex (Area 7), frontal eye fields (Area 8), and prefrontal cortex (Area 46). Figure 27 shows the location of the cortical areas in a side view of the left hemisphere of the rhesus monkey. Transections through the frontal and occipital brain along lines A and B, respectively, are also shown.

Earlier work on cells in the superior colliculus nucleus, the frontal eye fields, and the posterior parietal cortex has been summarized by Wurtz et al. (1982)

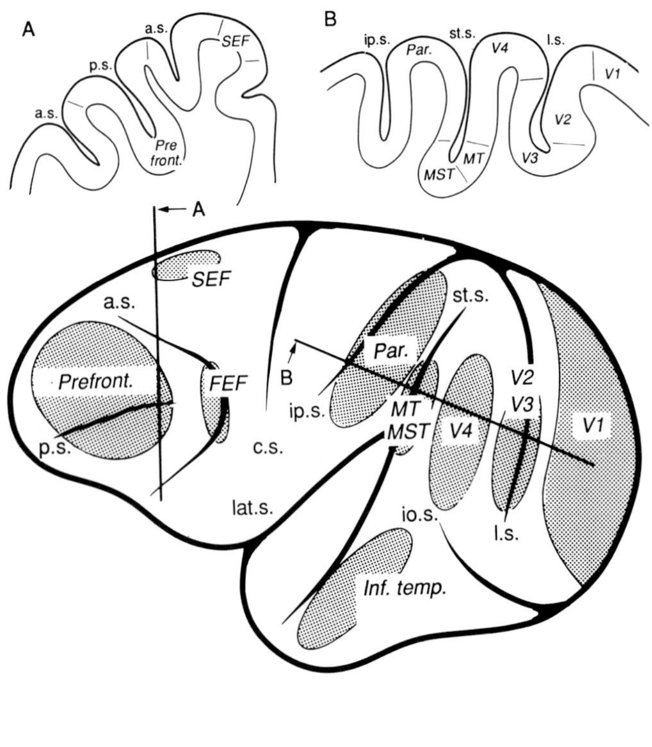

FIG. 27 Lateral view of the left hemisphere of rhesus monkey brain. Sulci are denoted by small letters as follows: ps., principal sulcus; a.s., arcuate sulcus; c.s., central sulcus; ip.s., intraparietal sulcus; lat.s, lateral sulcus; st.s., superior temporal sulcus; io.s., inferior occipital sulcus; l.s., lunate sulcus. Other abbreviations: Prefront., prefrontal cortex; SEF, supplementary eye field; FEF, frontal eye field; Par., parietal cortex; MT, middle temporal cortex; MST, medial superior temporal cortex; Inf. Temp., inferior temporal cortex. The transsections, made along lines A and B, show that many areas stippled in the lower part are, in fact, buried in the sulci and cannot be seen in a lateral view.

TABLE 1 Modulation of Neural Impulse Activity of Single Cells in Different Brain Structures as Tested with Different Tasks

Structure	Task[a] Saccade	Delayed saccade	Suppressed saccade	Peripheral attention
Superior colliculus	Selective (+)	(+)	Not tested	(−)
Striate cortex, Area 17	Nonselective (+)	Selective (+)	Selective (+)	Not tested
Prestriate cortex, Area V2	Nonselective (+)	(+)	(+)	Not tested
Prelunate cortex, Area V4	Selective (+)	Selective (+)	Selective (+)	(+)
Posterior parietal cortex, Area 7	Selective (+)	Selective (+)	Not tested	(+)
Inferior temporal cortex, Areas 21 and 22	Not tested	Not tested	(+)	(−)
Frontal eye fields, Area 8	Selective (+)	Not tested	Not tested	(−)
Prefrontal cortex, Area 46	Selective (+)	Selective (+)	Selective (+)	Not tested
Pulvinar cortex	Nonselective (+)	Not tested	Not tested	Selective (+)

[a]Plus (+), enhanced visual activity; minus (−), tested with negative results.

and Goldberg (1986). Here, new results are added and briefly discussed for each brain structure in which one of the above tasks has been used. For an overview, see Table 1.

1. Superior Colliculus

The superior colliculus consists of different layers of cells having visual and oculomotor properties. The cells in question are located in the intermediate layers. They show an enhancement effect concomitant with the saccade that brings the fovea in register with the image of the peripheral stimulus. The stimulus need not be visual; it can also be auditory (Jay & Sparks, 1987). This multimodality shows that the superior colliculus is involved in a sensory-to-motor conversion rather than in attentional mechanisms per se. However, motor commands are prepared and generated by this nucleus for those stimuli that have been selected as potential targets. It may therefore be assumed that the collicular cells are controlled by an attentional signal, even if this signal occurs together only with a saccade.

2. Striate Cortex

In the saccade task, a few striate cortical cells show enhanced visual responses. However, the enhancement is not spatially selective because it also occurs with saccades to targets located outside the cell's receptive field (Wurtz & Mohler, 1976b). In contrast, Boch (1986) found cells in striate cortex that were activated in the suppressed saccade task. Therefore, if striate cortex plays a role in visual attention, its contribution may be weak and of minor importance. Note that although electrical stimulation of striate cortex does elicit saccadic eye movements, cell discharges in that same area do not lead to saccades.

3. Prestriate Cortex

Cells in Areas V2 and V3 may also show an enhanced visual response in the saccade task, but again the enhancement is not spatially selective (Robinson, Baizer & Dow, 1980). The suppressed and delayed saccade tasks were used in a few cells (Fischer & Boch, 1985) with the result that even at this early stage of visual processing one can already find clear signs of extraretinal modulations related to visual attention and/or fixation.

4. Prelunate Cortex

In contrast to Areas V1, V2, and V3, Area V4 has been studied extensively. Many V4 cells show spatially selective enhancement in the saccade task (Fischer & Boch, 1981a). They are also activated prior to a saccade by a constantly illuminated stimulus in their receptive fields (Fischer & Boch, 1981b), in the delayed saccade task (Fischer & Boch, 1982, 1983), as well as in the suppressed saccade task (Fischer & Boch, 1985). Cells in Area V4 also differentiate between attended and unattended stimuli within their receptive field (Moran & Desimone, 1985). Furthermore, stimuli to which the animal has been "cued" elicit a response that is stronger than that when the same stimulus is uncued (Haenny, Maunsell & Schiller, 1988). In this experiment, the monkey is presented with a certain stimulus, the cue, to which he must respond if it recurs in the same trial. Other stimuli that might occur instead are uncued stimuli. The question of whether certain stimulus features, such as color and orientation, affect the selectivity of Area V4 cells still needs to be answered.

5. Posterior Parietal Cortex

For a long time, the parietal cortex has been considered a major source of attentional signals (Lynch, Mountcastle, Talbot & Yin, 1977; Robinson & Petersen, 1984). Parietal cells show a spatially selective enhancement effect which is independent of the type of motor reaction, be it eye movement or hand movement (Robinson & Petersen, 1984; Goldberg & Bruce, 1985).

Interestingly, cells in parietal cortex may be strongly activated by a visual stimulus placed in a (peripheral) receptive field while the animal attentively fixates the central fixation point. The response of these cells may be attenuated or disappear altogether if the same stimulus is used during eye movement or when the animal is not fixating (Mountcastle, Motter, Steinmetz & Sestokas, 1987). No difference of this kind has been found in prelunate cells, a result that has yet to be explained.

6. Inferior Temporal Cortex

Cells in the inferior temporal cortex may also be involved in attentional mechanisms. Most cells respond vigorously in the suppressed saccade task in which attention to the stimulus is not required (Richmond et al., 1983). This indicates that the absence as well as presence of a fixation point can modulate the visual activity both in inferior temporal and prelunate cortex. It is later shown that under similar conditions the monkey fails to produce short latency saccadic eye movements.

7. Prefrontal Cortex

Boch and Goldberg (1989) extended these studies to Area 46, a region located in front of the frontal eye fields (Area 8). Here they found neurons showing an enhancement effect in the saccade task. In addition, neural activity was increased both in the delayed and suppressed saccade tasks. Earlier studies using the delayed response task had already shown that neurons in the prefrontal cortex may be related to attention (Fuster, 1973). More recent work supports this notion on the basis of the differential responses in go versus no-go trials (Bakay, Pragay, Mirksy & Nakamura, 1987). These results further substantiate findings indicating that the neural activity in the frontal eye fields is closely related to the preparation of the oculomotor response (Bushnell, Goldberg & Robinson, 1981; Goldberg & Bushnell, 1981; Bruce & Goldberg, 1985).

D. Stimulus Selectivity and Receptive Field Properties

The concept of the receptive field of a retinal cell implies that a cell's activity can be modulated by a probe stimulus only if it is positioned in a restricted area of the retina and at a specific location. The concept does not specify any features the stimulus should have except that the probe must be small as compared to the receptive field size. The receptive field may possess an antagonistic center–surround organization, thus favoring concentric stimuli to produce a maximal response.

As one proceeds from the retina and LGN to higher cortical structures such as the prestriate and parietal cortex, the spatial requirements for a stimulus eliciting a neuronal response are largely the same. However, as the receptive fields become larger and less specific for physical stimulus properties such as form and color, other aspects of the stimulus become important. These aspects must be related to the behavioral context within which a certain stimulus occurs. This relationship has been demonstrated by Haenny et al. (1988) for cells in prelunate cortex. Area V4 cells may respond better to the presentation of a grating of one orientation than to the same grating presented with another orientation. Yet, if the animal is cued to the latter orientation the response is enhanced and may be stronger than the response to the "best" uncued orientation. Another aspect for V4 cells is the large size of their receptive fields as compared to the optimal size of the stimulus. Weber and Fischer have measured the distribution of optimal sizes of V4 cells. The same animal was then trained to make saccades to a constant small stimulus which thus became a revelant stimulus. When they repeated the measurement of optimal stimulus sizes, the same cortical area appeared to exhibit a preponderance of cells specific for small stimuli. Thus, cells in Area V4 do not seem to have fixed specificities but may change their responsiveness in accordance with stimuli in which they are "interested."

E. Conclusion

Table 1 depicts the different tasks used to study cells of the different brain structures. With the exception of prelunate cortex, none of the areas has been studied using all tasks. Nevertheless, it has become clear that the superior colliculus and the frontal eye fields, even though they may receive a signal for attention, are closely related to the initiation of a saccade without being purely of motor nature. In comparison, striate cortex as well as inferior temporal cortex seem to be more involved in the analysis of sensory information. These findings imply that a voluntary change of the direction of gaze requires a release from attention. Conversely, during a state of peripheral attention, eye movements may be blocked (inhibited) because attention is fixed (engaged) to a certain part of the visual field.

The following section summarizes a number of new experiments on the initiation of saccades which show that disengagement, that is, the release from active (focused) attention, indeed enables the visual-to-oculomotor system to produce goal-directed saccades after extremely short reaction times.

F. Saccadic Eye Movements

A saccadic eye movement is a motor reaction optimally suited to study the mechanisms underlying visual attention. In the past, however, reactions of the hand or finger in response to visual stimuli have been used more frequently. This is mainly because it is easier to record manual reaction times than to accurately measure eye position and determine the latency for a saccade. The use of an infrared light-emitting diode and two photocells mounted on a simple spectacle frame provides an inexpensive and simple method for detecting horizontal saccades and for measuring saccadic reaction times with a precision of one millisecond.

1. Express Saccades

In 1967, Saslow demonstrated in human observers that the introduction of a temporal interval between the offset of a central fixation point and the onset of a peripheral saccade target (so-called gap trial) significantly reduced the saccadic reaction time (SRT) as compared to the case in which the fixation point remained on (overlap trial). The reduction consisted of an overall shift of the SRT distribution to shorter values. Fischer and Boch (1983) using gap trials in the monkey found that SRTs were reduced but, more importantly, two separate peaks occurred in the latency distribution, one at about 70 msec and the other at about 140 msec. Saccades contributing to the first peak were called express saccades (because of their extremely short reaction time) and those contributing to the second, fast regular saccades (Fischer & Boch, 1983). Slow regular saccades forming a peak at about 200 msec were only obtained in overlap trials.

The existence of express saccades in man was first reported by Fischer and Ramsperger (1984) who repeated Saslow's experiment. Saslow may have failed to find express saccades because he used large bin widths for analyzing his latency distributions. Figure 28 shows the distribution of saccadic reaction times for two human subjects. Bimodal distributions like these are easily obtained when the fixation point is turned off before the saccade target occurs.

The introduction of a temporal gap, however, is not a necessary condition for the occurrence of express saccades. In humans the instruction "Do not pay attention to the fixation point" is sufficient to allow for express saccades in overlap trials (Mayfrank, Mobashery, Kimmig & Fischer, 1986). In the monkey, regular daily practice using overlap trials also produces express saccades (Boch & Fischer, 1986). In both species, daily practice increases the percentage of express saccades and reduces their latency (Fischer, Boch & Ramsperger, 1984; Fischer & Ramsperger, 1986). The observation that saccadic reaction times decrease drastically following changes in instruction and after periods of daily practice has led to new concepts of visual attention and a better understanding of its relation to saccadic eye movements and fixation.

G. Attention and Reaction Time

The basic idea in relating attention to reaction time is that any change in the state of visual attention takes time which may or may not be included in the saccadic reaction. Posner, Cohen, and Rafal (1982) and Posner, Walker, Friedrich, and Rafal (1984) used key pressing as a motor reaction to study attentional effects in man. From their results they concluded that the attentional system can be in either of two different states: engaged or disengaged. This distinction holds also for saccades: express saccades are obtained in trials where attention is already disengaged from the

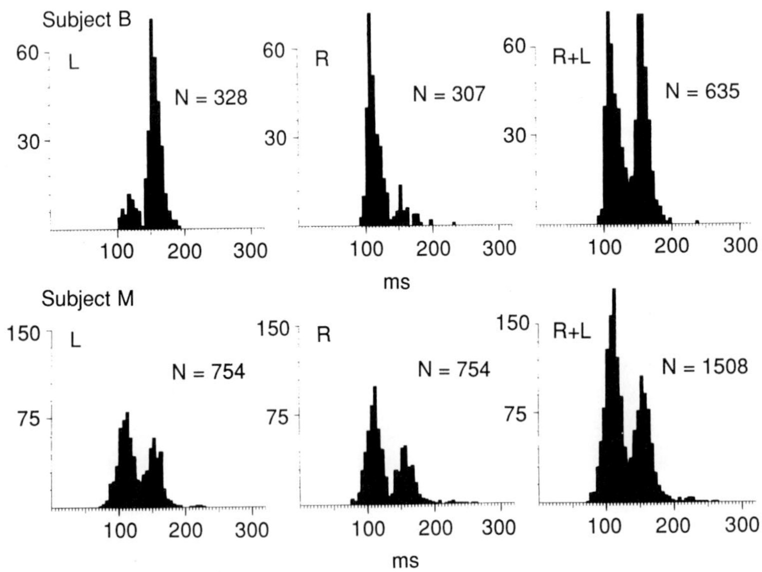

FIG. 28 Distributions of saccadic reaction times in humans. The results of two different subjects are shown. Ordinate: Number of saccades in a bin width of 10 msec; abscissa: saccadic reaction time. The saccade target occurred in random order at 4° to the left (L) or right (R) of the fixation point. The total number of saccades (*N*) is indicated in each diagram. The summed distribution for right and left directed saccades is clearly bimodal. Note the asymmetry in the response latencies of subject B for left directed versus right directed saccades. Saccades contributing to the first peak are called express saccades.

fixation point. On the other hand, reaction times are extremely long in trials where attention is still engaged. Engagement need not be in the location of the fixation point but can be anywhere in the visual field. Even if one attends to the location of the future target, SRTs will be long with express saccades virtually absent (Mayfrank et al., 1986).

It thus appears as though visual attention blocks saccades as long as it is engaged. In order to move the eye from one target to another, visual attention must be disengaged regardless of where in the visual field it is engaged. This interpretation suggests a cyclic mechanism governing vision with moving eyes under normal conditions (Fischer, 1987): As the direction of gaze changes due to saccades (i.e., every 200 to 300 msec), the state of attention also changes from engaged to disengaged. Each saccade is preceded by disengagement and followed by engagement. During periods of engagement visual information enters the afferent system, whereas during disengagement the next saccade is prepared by the efferent system.

H. Model for the Control of Saccadic Eye Movements

The fact that visual responses, saccades, and attention-related activity can be found in different cortical and subcortical areas and the multimodal distribution of saccadic reaction times have led to a concept of three loops that are involved in the control of vision and eye movements. Loop 1 would control the disengagement of visual attention; Loop 2 the decision to make a saccade; Loop 3 the computation of amplitude and direction. Figure 29 illustrates the loops and their functional interconnections. Although Fig. 29 suggests that each loop acts in parallel with the others, this is not necessarily so. To the contrary, each square may symbolize a logical AND-gate to ensure that all processes must have taken place before a saccade can be made. One may even postulate that processes involved in loops 1, 2, and 3 take place in a serial manner if one assumes that processes in loop 2 can be

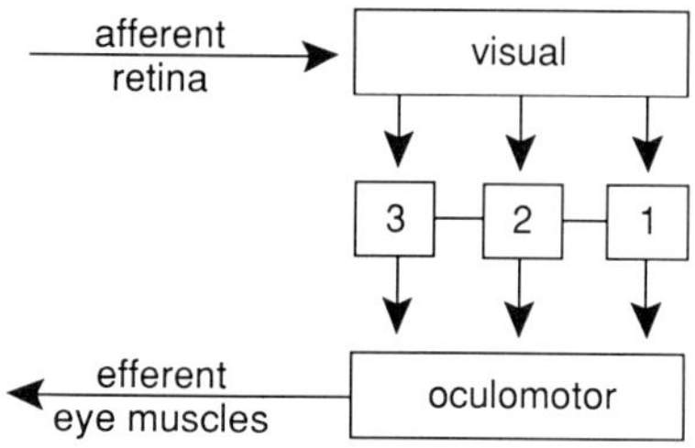

FIG. 29 Block diagram illustrating the three-loop concept for the control of eye movements by vision and attention. Loop 1 disengagement; Loop 2 decision; Loop 3 spatial coordinates.

started only after the processes in loop 1 have been completed and that processes in loop 3 can begin only after the processes in loop 2 are finished. Such a mechanism requires that all brain structures involved must function properly to generate a correct saccade. In view of this complexity one immediately understands why saccadic reaction times are so long (about 200 msec) in one condition and extremely short (about 70 msec) in another. It also shows how fixation may be achieved. Suppose the neural processes in one of the loops, let us say loop 1, cannot be completed as long as attention is engaged to a particular part of the visual field. In this case, saccades are arrested even if the object attended to is not being fixated. On the other hand, it assumes that if attention is disengaged the eye can execute a goal-directed saccade provided that the processes in the other two loops are completed.

The concept of the three loops is a functional, not an anatomical concept. Nevertheless one can attempt to identify different anatomically defined structures as contributing to one or the other loop as follows: (1) striate cortex and superior colliculus; (2) frontal cortex, in particular the frontal eye fields; (3) prestriate cortex and partietal cortex.

VIII. CONCLUSIONS

We are still in the very early stages of exploring the perception of form and relating it to the neuropsychological mechanisms of the visual system. In recent years many relevant discoveries have been made, but they chiefly emphasize the complexity of processing that must underlie the effortless experience of seeing. The broad picture seems to be one of initial analysis by a number of specialized channels or modules, and a subsequent coordination and integration of the information extracted.

Attention seems to play a central role, both in selecting the relevant object at any given time and in specifying its particular structured assembly of properties. Further issues for future research will concern the mechanisms of selection—whether attention acts by facilitating relevant stimuli or suppressing irrelevant ones; and whether it scans the visual field with continuous motion, as suggested by the frequently used spotlight and searchlight analogies; or whether it switches in discrete steps from object to object. These psychological debates may benefit from the accumulating evidence relating physiological recordings (e.g. Moran and Desimone, 1985) to behavioral tasks requiring selective attention.

The chapter opened with the example of a snowman seen against a blanket of snow. The evidence we have reviewed suggests that his features will be represented in multiple visual maps coding their color, location, orientation, and size, specifying boundaries and creating subjective contours where they are missing from the retinal image. How we reach, within a quarter of a second, our unified awareness, both of what he looks like and of what he is, remains a mystery which will challenge both psychologists and physiologists in future research.

ACKNOWLEDGMENTS

Preparation of this chapter was supported by grant number AFOSR 87-0125 to Anne Treisman from the Air Force Office of Scientific Research, Air Force Systems Command, USAF. Patrick Cavanagh received a fellowship from the Canadian Institute of Advanced Research and a grant from the Natural Science and Engineering Research Council of Canada. Rudiger von der Heydt was supported by grant number 3.939.84 from the Swiss National Foundation. Burkhart Fischer was supported by a grant from the Deutsche Forschungsgesellschaft (Sonderforschungsbereich 325, C5).

12

THE PERCEPTION OF STEREODEPTH AND STEREOMOTION
Cortical Mechanisms

David Regan, John P. Frisby, Gian F. Poggio,
Clifton M. Schor, and Christopher W. Tyler

I. BINOCULAR PROCESSING OF RELATIVE POSITION IN DEPTH

A. Introduction

It was realized long ago that, because the left and right eyes are set a little way apart, two points in the outside world that lie at different depths are separated by different distances in the left and right eyes' retinal images. In Fig. 1, for example, the distance d_L between the left eye's images of objects A and B is greater than the distance d_R between the right eye's images of the same two objects (d_L is the distance from b_L to a_L and d_R is the distance from b_R to a_R). This fact can be demonstrated by holding a three-dimensional object at arm's length, then alternately closing the left and right eyes.

First we should briefly define a few terms (vision specialists should skip the next few paragraphs). The relative binocular disparity of two object points is usually expressed as the angle corresponding to ($d_L - d_R$), that is, as the difference between angles $b_L B b_R$ and $a_L A a_R$ in Fig. 1. The disparity of point A is conventionally defined as zero so that in Fig. 1 the disparity of B relative to A is also the absolute disparity of B. The disparities of points closer than A are described as "crossed," and the disparities of points farther than A are described as "uncrossed." With the foveal centers pointed accurately at object A, the images a_L and a_R (and the images of all other objects with zero disparity) are said to fall on "corresponding points" with the same coordinates in both retinas. All points of zero horizontal disparity lie on a line that passes through point A in Fig. 1. By simple geometry (Ogle, 1950), this zero-disparity locus can be shown to be a circle called the Vieth–Müller circle (V–M in Fig. 2). However, simple geometry is not enough. The "horopter" is an experimentally measured locus, all points of which are subjectively judged to have the same visual direction in the two eyes (Fig. 2). [In point of fact, slightly different empirical horopters are obtained by different measurement techniques (Ogle, 1950). The reason for this plurality of horopters is not

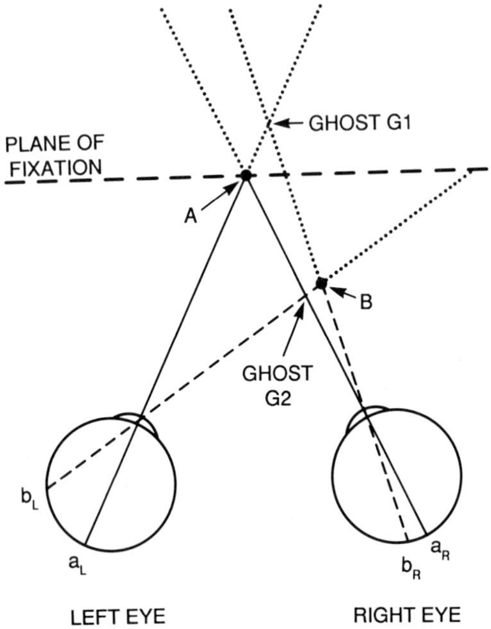

FIG. 1 Keplerian model of stereopsis and the correspondence problem. A and B are real targets. Suppose that they are identical vertical lines. The Keplerian model predicts that "ghost" images will be seen at G_1 and G_2. They are not seen. From Regan, D. (1989). *Human Brain Electrophysiology: Evoked Potentials and Evoked Magnetic Fields in Science and Medicine*. New York: Elsevier. Published with permission.

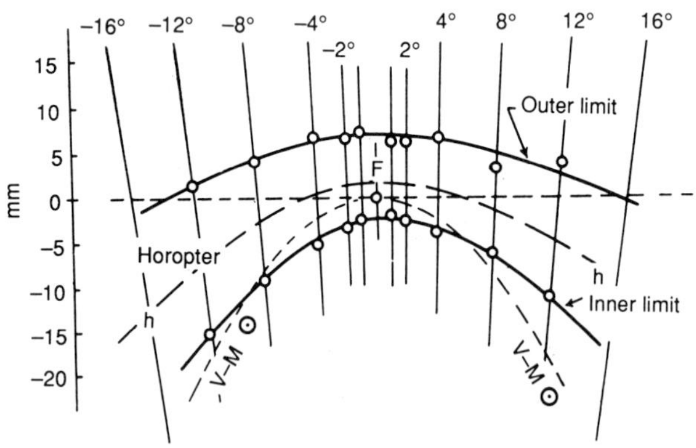

FIG. 2 Region of single binocular vision; the horopter and the Vieth–Müller circle. From Ogle, K. N. (1964). *Researches in Binocular Vision*. New York: Hafner. Published with permission.

understood.] Figure 2 illustrates that the empirical horopter departs from the Vieth–Müller circle. Figure 2 also illustrates that the left and right eyes' slightly different images can be fused to give a single fused percept, but that this binocular fusion is only possible over a limited range of depths. Points that lie within this region are said to have binocular disparities that "do not exceed the fusional limit," and thus fall within "Panum's fusional area." Points outside this region are seen as double.

Binocular single vision (i.e., fusion) should be carefully distinguished from stereoscopic depth perception. Stereoscopic depth can be experienced for objects that lie outside the fusion region of Fig. 2 so that they are seen in double vision. Conversely, some individuals with binocular single vision lack stereoscopic depth perception. This point is of clinical importance: a loss of stereopsis is only a minor inconvenience, whereas a failure to achieve binocular single vision (i.e., double vision) is a distressing handicap.

Figure 2 also brings out the important point that *depth is relative to the point of ocular convergence* so that disparities must be calibrated relative to the distance of the fixation point. The classic concepts mentioned above are discussed authoritatively in Ogle's book (Ogle, 1950; see also Ogle, Martens & Dyer, 1967).

The hypothesis that binocular disparity is the effective stimulus for depth sensation is credited to the astronomer Johannes Kepler. The demonstration that disparity alone can produce depth sensation was first provided by Wheatstone (1838) who constructed the first stereoviewer for the purpose of using line drawings as targets (because photography had not been invented yet), and he extended his demonstration to natural objects when (in 1852) stereophotography—already of excellent definition—was possible.

The Keplerian hypothesis, Richards' pool hypothesis, and Julesz' local–global distinction are three psychophysically based ideas that have strongly influenced the course of single-unit research. As was the case in color vision research, although psychophysicists were able to infer physiological facts long before physiologists were able to carry out experimental tests, psychophysicists also generated competing hypotheses that they were quite unable to reject until, after many years, the remarkable technical achievements of single-unit neurophysiology bestowed instant respectability to one of the competing psychophysical hypotheses, at the expense of others. We see below how the development of our present understanding of binocular vision illustrates the use of hypotheses that link psychophysical and physical data, the so-called psychophysical linking hypotheses (Brindley, 1960) or linking propositions (Teller, 1984, and Chapter 3, this volume).

B. The Keplerian Hypothesis and the Correspondence Problem

The Keplerian model of stereopsis is "merely an internal reflection of the external geometry of binocular parallax" (Richards, 1975). It can be taken to imply that, just as each orientation is represented by a specific cell or group of cells, so each disparity is represented by a specific cell or group of cells (Richards, 1975). The major difficulty with Keplerian-type models is the so-called correspondence problem. Figure 1 illustrates that the problem arises even for the simple case of two (identical) vertical lines at different depths, so popular in laboratory studies of stereoscopic acuity. Images (a_L a_R) of line A and images (b_L b_R) of line B are thrown onto the left and right retinas respectively. In practice, normally sighted people see what is actually there: two identical lines A and B at different depths. Within the Keplerian framework, this veridical perception means that the brain has first selected the corresponding images in the left and right eyes and then calculated the correct disparity [$d = (a_L - b_L) - (a_R - b_R)$]. But, because the four retinal images a_L, a_R, b_L, b_R are all identical, the brain has an immediate problem in selecting the corresponding images. The basic Keplerian model predicts that the identical images a_L and a_R are matched, thus assigning an object line to point A in the external world; then images b_L and b_R are matched, thus assigning an object line to point B in external space; then, in addition, image a_L is matched with the identical image b_R, thus assigning an object line to point G_1, and b_L is matched with the identical image a_R, thus assigning an object line to point G_2. But, in point of fact, we do not see these "ghost" lines at G_1 and G_2.

C. Julesz Random-Dot Patterns and the Sequence of Processing

The correspondence problem becomes critical when the visual system is confronted with a Julesz random-dot stereogram, because it is possible to match any given dot in the left retinal image with many alternative identical dots in the right retinal image. Thus, the brain's problem in assigning depth to any given dot in the left retinal image is that many different depth values are possible; the individual dot's disparity is multiply ambiguous. Nevertheless, the brain does solve this problem (Julesz, 1960, 1971), and solves it effortlessly, or so it seems when one sees a Julesz random dot figure floating in three-dimensional space. Figure 3 illustrates the principle of Julesz stereograms. Figure 4 is a special kind of random-dot stereogram (an autostereogram) that does not require any special equipment (Tyler, 1983).

Cyclopean random dot stereopairs differ from ordinary stereopatterns in that viewing the cyclopean pair with both eyes reveals a figure seen in depth that is invisible when viewed monocularly. With ordinary stereopatterns, on the other hand, the figure that appears in depth when viewed binocularly can also be seen monocularly, though of course not in depth (Julesz, 1960). Julesz' 1971 book gives many dramatic demonstrations of cyclopean depth.

Before Julesz illuminated this issue, it could be thought that the brain solved the correspondence problem for everyday scenes by first extracting objects from their backgrounds and only then matching

1	0	1	0	1	0	0	1	0	1
1	0	0	1	0	1	0	1	0	0
0	0	1	1	0	1	1	0	1	0
0	1	0	Y	A	A	B	B	0	1
1	1	1	X	B	A	B	A	0	1
0	0	1	X	A	A	B	A	1	0
1	1	1	Y	B	B	A	B	0	1
1	0	0	1	1	0	1	1	0	1
1	1	0	0	1	1	0	1	1	1
0	1	0	0	0	1	1	1	1	0

1	0	1	0	1	0	0	1	0	1
1	0	0	1	0	1	0	1	0	0
0	0	1	1	0	1	1	0	1	0
0	1	0	A	A	B	B	0	0	1
1	1	1	B	A	B	A	0	0	1
0	0	1	A	A	B	A	0	1	0
1	1	1	B	B	A	B	0	0	1
1	0	0	1	1	0	1	1	0	1
1	1	0	0	1	1	0	1	1	1
0	1	0	0	0	1	1	1	1	0

FIG. 3 Julesz random-dot stereogram. The stereopair consists of two random arrays of dots which are identical except that the central portion of one of the patterns is shifted to one side as illustrated by the A/B matrices. When one eye views the left pattern while the fellow eye views the right pattern and binocular fusion is achieved, the central area appears to be at a different depth to the surrounding dots. After Julesz, B. (1971). *Foundations of Cyclopean Perception*. Chicago: University of Chicago Press. Published with permission.

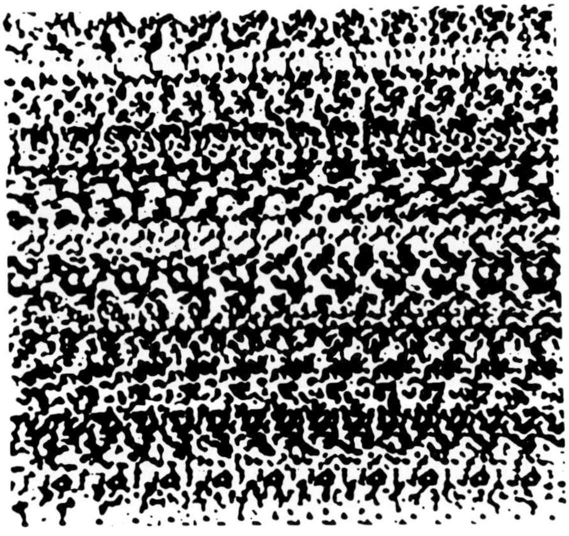

FIG. 4 Cyclopean depth perception in humans, This is a special kind of Julesz random-dot pattern devised by C. W. Tyler and J. J. Chang. At 40 cm viewing distance, hold a finger about 10 cm above the page and fixate the finger continuously. The stereoscopic percept will gradually emerge in the plane of the finger, which can then be removed for free viewing. The three-dimensional percept is a stereograting with horizontal bars. From Tyler, C. W. (1983). Sensory processing of binocular disparity. In C. M. Schor & K. J. Ciuffreda (Eds.), *Vergence Eye Movements* (pp. 199–295). Boston: Butterworths.

the same details in the two retinal images. In this way the problem of deciding what should match what is largely avoided by assuming that object recognition precedes binocular comparison of the retinal images. By inventing the random-dot stereograms in which the object forms are *perfectly* camouflaged, Julesz (1960) demonstrated conclusively that this was not the only means for establishing matches, if indeed it was used at all. Experiments with random-dot stereograms strongly suggest that the correspondence problem is solved at an earlier stage in visual processing than object recognition: stereoscopic depth is easily seen in Julesz patterns, but no monocular information whatsoever is available about the surfaces that appear in depth during binocular viewing. Julesz' experiments justify the experimental strategy of treating stereopsis rather independently of other processes.

Julesz (1971) defined "global stereopsis" as the ability to see in relative depth the form and motion of a textured surface of random dots. He suggested that this large-field process evaluates all of the many possible matches between individual dots in the left and right eyes, then eliminates "false matches" and selects the most frequently occurring disparity in the stereoscopic pair of stimuli. Julesz' "global" stereoscopic processing is distinct from the "local" stereoscopic processing that computes the binocular disparity between local features in sparse contour patterns for which the matching ambiguities are insignificant.

D. Psychophysical Evidence on the Correspondence Problem

We have seen that the correspondence problem can be tackled using (a) global processing or (b) local processing of the array of disparities present in the stereoscopic images. Global processing is defined as involving some kind of neighborhood interactions between competing matches which culminates in the selection of "correct" matches. For example, selection of matches can be made on the basis of some type of minimization principle of the "energy" in the chosen stereoscopic surface such that smooth surfaces are preferred. Section V reviews that approach and vari ous other forms of global stereoprocessing.

In contrast to global processes, local processes operate independently of neighboring disparities. An example of local constraint occurs for ghost images such as those depicted in Fig. 1. To the extent that the physical objects lie in the frontal plane, the ghost images will fall in symmetrical pairs along the line of sight (Tyler, 1977, 1983). Thus, most ghost images would be eliminated by a local mechanism that prohibited depth perception of multiple images along a given line of sight. Disparity domain inhibition (Tyler, 1975a) is only one of several physiological mechanisms by which such a prohibition could be achieved, but the point is that a large degree of apparently global processing can result from a purely local process of disparity domain inhibition.

The presence of such local processes in human stereopsis can be inferred from the perception of dynamic random-dot displays (where the image is changing too rapidly to allow global processes time to operate). Tyler (1977) has shown that ghost images are equally invisible in such dynamic displays when an identical field of dots is presented to each eye. However, when the pattern is changed to become uncorrelated in the two eyes, so that the ghost images lose their symmetry along the line of sight, they suddenly become visible as a field of dynamic random depths. Thus, it seems that the key factor in hiding the ghosts is not the complexity (or "unsmoothness") of the image they form, but its symmetry around the horopter.

A second local process that could radically reduce the complexity of the correspondence problem and the detection of ghost images is the retinal orientation and size specificity of the elements performing the correspondence match (Marr & Poggio, 1979). The tuning of the receptive fields of such neurons prior to making the match can reduce the probability of spurious matches by orders of magnitude, to the point where negligible amounts of global processing are required to deal with this problem. The neurophysiological evidence for orientation and size tuning in disparity-selective cells is unequivocal (Poggio & Fischer, 1977). At the psychophysical level, extensive size selectivity has been shown for disparity processing by means of bar stimuli with difference-of-gaussian (DOG) luminance profiles (Schor & Wood, 1983). But orientation selectivity is not so evident psychophysically. For example, Mayhew and Frisby (1978) found that a stereo signal carried by an oriented texture and masked by a similar noise texture is not unmasked when the orientation of the noise is rotated as would be expected if oriented units were responsible for forming binocular matches. Mayhew and Frisby (1979a) also showed that, in principle, surfaces possessing steep variations in depth present severe difficulties for orientationally tuned filter models of stereopsis.

E. Physiological Evidence on the Correspondence Problem. I. Simple Line Stereopairs

One approach to the theoretical "correspondence problem" is to bring into consideration not only *how* the retinal image matching is done, but also *which* local features are matched. Early single-unit studies supported the view that the correspondence problem is solved by matching oriented edges within the receptive field of cortical neurons (Barlow, Blakemore & Pettigrew, 1967; Nikara, Bishop & Pettigrew, 1968). Barlow et al. pointed out that "the number of identical trigger features lying in the same appropriate region of each eye can safely be assumed to belong to the same object" (Barlow et al., 1967). This proposal may well be fairly adequate for many real-world scenes that involve nonrepetitive patterns, though it is difficult to see how it explains the absence of "ghost" images in the situation shown in Fig. 1. A further difficulty arises with random-dot stereograms where all features (dots) are identical (see below). Barlow et al.'s (1967) solution is to limit acceptable matches to within the size of the classical receptive field of cortical neurons. Depth perception with random-dot stereograms requires that very large areas of the visual field be taken into account (see below). Computational-based approaches have found that local processing is usually insufficient on its own, and introduce constraints such as smoothness on the possible surface (Marr & Poggio, 1979).

The first reports on binocular properties of single cells seemed to be consistent with a Keplerian model of stereopsis. It was claimed that cat striate cortex contained cells that were rather narrowly tuned to disparity and that different cells were tuned to different disparities (Barlow et al., 1967; Nikara et al., 1968). But then followed a period of controversy. Earlier findings were challenged by Hubel and Wiesel (1970a) who claimed that there are few disparity-tuned cells in the cat and monkey *striate cortex* (i.e., Area 17 or V1). According to Bishop and Pettigrew (1986), this controversy arose largely because, in the early work, qualitative methods (e.g., listening to spikes) were used in the attempt to solve problems that could only be solved by quantitative techniques. Later, quantitative studies on sheep, monkey, and cat (Clarke & Whitteridge, 1977; Poggio & Fischer, 1977; Von der Heydt, Adorjani, Hänny & Baumgartner, 1978) showed that striate cortex does contain disparity-tuned cells and that most prefer disparities of 0.5 deg or less. A second key issue in this controversy was the precise control of binocular convergence and ocular rotation. A major problem with anesthetized animals, this challenging requirement of precise stimulus control was successfully met by Poggio and colleagues who recorded from awake behaving monkeys (see below).

F. Physiological Evidence on the Correspondence Problem. II. Random Dot Patterns

Gian Poggio and colleagues found that neurons subserving Julesz' seemingly complex process of global stereopsis exist as early as V1 and V2 in foveal cortex of alert macaque monkey: of 230 neurons investigated, 20% responded to cyclopean random-dot stereograms (Poggio, 1984; Poggio, Motter, Squatrito & Trotter, 1985).

Poggio et al. (1985) found an important difference in responses to random-dot stereopairs and line stereopairs. Although disparity tuning was observed for both simple and complex cells when the animal was stimulated with ordinary line stereopairs, the cyclopean dynamic random noise stereopairs created a dichotomy: many complex cells responded to cyclopean stimuli, whereas only very few cells classified as simple did so. According to Poggio and Poggio (1984), the complex cell has "the unique capacity of solving the correspondence problem by responding to the 'correct' binocular matches over the receptive fields in the two eyes." ["Correct" in this sense means to obtain the unique global stereopsis solution as defined by Julesz (1971) to the multiply ambiguous problem.]

A second important difference between responses to cyclopean and to ordinary line stereopairs is that some cells do not show the orientation and/or size tuning to the monocularly invisible cyclopean figure that is evident in their responses to the monocularly visible line stimulus (Poggio, 1984). On the other hand, there were important similarities between responses to ordinary and cyclopean depth stereopairs. The same two classes of "far/near" and "tuned" disparity-sensitive neurons were found with cyclopean stimuli as were found with line stereopairs, consistent with Richards' pool theory (see below). Intriguingly, a substantial number of neurons (about 30%) called "flat" neurons were not selective for disparity over a large range of disparities.

Poggio and Poggio (1984) sought to explain how some complex cells in V1 and V2 perform the formidable task of obtaining globally "correct" binocular correspondence. They pointed out that complex cells that are tuned to the depth of cyclopean random-dot figures must necessarily match the inputs from left and right eyes in a very precise and orderly manner. The neural organization for recognizing the globally "correct" binocular correspondence amid a large number of false correspondences can be imagined as sets of small subfields within the receptive field of one eye that were gated by a similar set of subfields located with appropriate positional disparity in the other eye. Poggio and Poggio cited the very precise and finely scaled retinotopic organization in striate cortical layer 4C as a possible basis for this precise binocular matching.

G. Richards' Pool Hypothesis

In 1970 Richards put forward the hypothesis that the human visual system contains three "pools": one for crossed disparities, one for uncrossed disparities, and one for near-zero disparities (Richards, 1970, 1971). According to Richards' hypothesis, a particular depth is signaled by the relative activity of crossed and uncrossed pools, rather than by a hypothetical neural element sharply tuned to one depth whose activity carries a unique "signature" of that particular depth.

Figure 5 shows the first evidence for Richards' pool hypothesis of stereoscopic vision: some "stereoanomalous" subjects lack stereoscopic vision for all crossed disparities, while uncrossed disparities are spared or vice versa (Richards, 1970, 1971). This evidence has been criticized on the grounds that fixation disparity could mimic the effect. A second piece of evidence is not open to this criticism: in the visual fields of many subjects there are restricted areas that

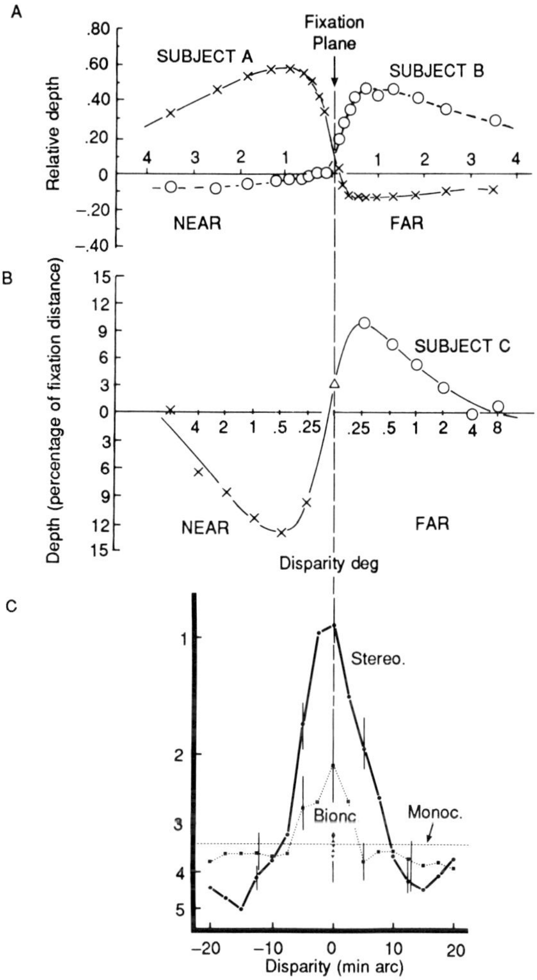

FIG. 5 Richards' pool hypothesis of stereopsis. (A) Subjective depth magnitude versus disparity for two stereoanomalous subjects. (B) Subjective depth magnitude versus disparity for a subject with normal stereoscopic vision. (C) Disparity thresholds in the immediate vicinity of the fixation plane ("stereo"). See text for details.

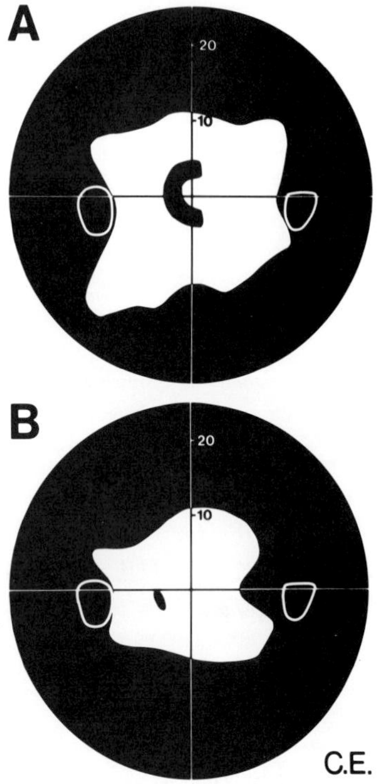

FIG. 6 Local specific "blindness" to stereomotion in humans. The black horseshoe-shaped area is absolutely blind to stereomotion, but static disparity thresholds and frontal plane motion thresholds are normal. The "stereoscotoma" is present for targets nearer than the fixation plane (A) but is almost absent for targets farther than the fixation plane (B). From Regan, D., Erkelens, C., & Collewijn, H. (1986). Visual field defects for vergence eye movements and for stereomotion perception. *Investigative Ophthalmology & Visual Science*, **27**, 806–819.

are selectively "blind" to stereomotion in depth. Figure 6 illustrates that these areas can be quite different for crossed and uncrossed disparities (Richards & Regan, 1973; Regan, Erkelens & Collewijn, 1986). Furthermore, Jones (1977) has shown that stereoanomalous subjects may retain normal stereoacuity for objects within a few minuntes of arc of the fixation plane.

Normally sighted subjects have both "far" and "near" mechanisms. The normal stereoscopic function in Fig. 5B can be approximated by subtracting the two curves in Fig. 5A. This is the evidence for Richards' hypothesis that the amount of perceived depth, and its sign (i.e., far versus near) are determined by antagonism between "near" and "far" mechanisms (Richards, 1970, 1975). This hypothesis can explain why the "ghosts" of Fig. 1 are not seen: the near and the far pools both respond to a wide range of different disparities, so they signal a weighted sum of all possible matches; multiple "ghosts" are not produced because the amount of perceived depth is uniquely determined by the *relative* activity of the near and far pools.

A third "pool" sensitive to the near-zero disparities is also included in the hypothesis. This pool accounts for our high stereoacuity near the fixation plane. (In addition, because the difference in slopes of the near and far processes in Fig. 5A is greatest at the fixation plane, the balance between the two processes is altered by a very small change of stimulus disparity.)

Figure 5C is one example of the body of psychophysical evidence (Ogle, 1950) that a "fine stereopsis" mechanism is active in and close to the fixation plane. Stereo sensitivity to relative depth was measured as follows. The subject fixated a pair of nonius lines (see Ogle, 1950) which (by definition) provided a fixed reference at zero disparity. The target oscillated sinusoidally backward and forward about some mean depth at a very low frequency (0.1 Hz). The subject altered the amplitude of the disparity oscillations to threshold. Stereo sensitivity was best (about 1 min arc) at zero disparity and fell to $1/\sqrt{2}$ of its maximum value at about 4 min arc on either side of the peak that is, at ± 4 min arc disparity (Blakemore, 1970; Regan & Beverley, 1973a).

H. A Physiological Basis for Richards' Pool Hypothesis

It was not until the formidable problem of recording from single cells in alert monkey trained to maintain accurate binocular fixation had been overcome that Gian Poggio and colleagues were able to provide a physiological basis for the pool hypothesis, and also resolve doubts about disparity coding in Area V1. They found that nearly 50% of neurons in striate cortex and an even higher proportion in V2 are sensitive to disparity (Poggio & Talbot, 1981; Poggio, 1984). Rather than finding neurons tuned to many different disparities as predicted by the Keplerian hypothesis, Poggio and colleagues reported just two classes of binocular cell in V1 and V2. The first class, corresponding to Hubel and Wiesel's (1970a) "binocular depth" cells, are tuned to disparity over a rather narrow range; most of these cells are excitatory ("tuned excitatory," Fig. 7A) and the rest inhibitory ("tuned inhibitory," Fig. 7B). The second class of cell, the so-called "near" and "far" reciprocally activated neurons, give excitatory responses over a wide range of disparities of one signal and inhibitory responses over a wide range of the opposite sign (Fig. 7C,D).

The links between human psychophysical data and the properties of individual neurons in monkey are impressively direct. First compare Fig. 5C with Fig.

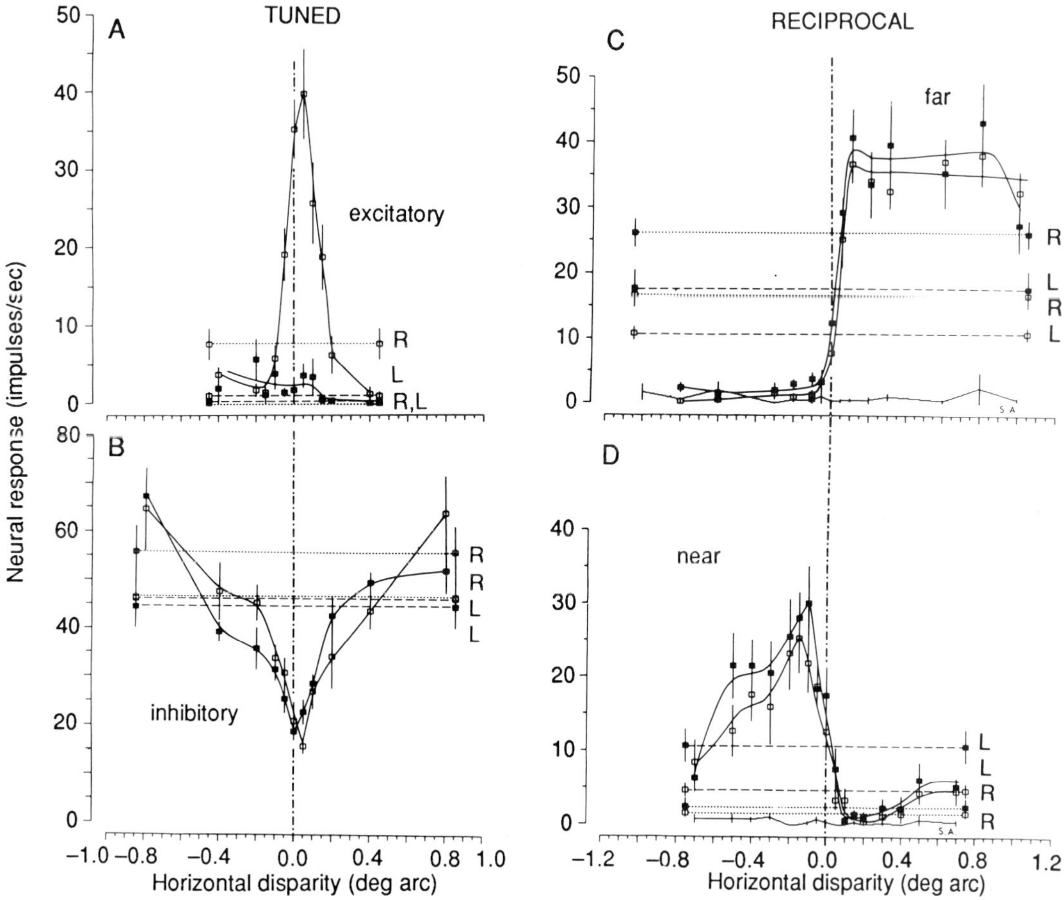

FIG. 7 The two classes of binocular neurons in monkey visual cortical Areas V1 and V2 are illustrated. A and B show cells that are sharply tuned for near-zero disparity in the immediate region of the fixation plane. C and D show the reciprocal "far" and "near" cells that respond best to moderately large disparities. Compare A with Fig. 5C and compare C and D with Fig. 5A. From Poggio, G., & Talbot, W. H. (1981). Mechanisms of static and dynamic stereopsis in foveal cortex of rhesus monkey. *Journal of Physiology*, **315**, 409–492.

7A. According to Poggio and Talbot (1981), "nearly all" tuned excitatory neurons peak within ±6 min arc of the fixation plane, and the mean tuning bandwidth is 10 min arc at $1/\sqrt{2}$ peak response for neurons in macaque striate cortex. This compares with the ±4 min arc bandwidth for the human psychophysical data (Fig. 5C).

Interestingly, human visual sensitivity to depth oscillations was considerably better than either binocular or monocular sensitivity when the target was no farther than 8 min arc from the fixation plane, but between about 8 and 20 min arc stereo sensitivity was actually *worse* than either binocular or monocular sensitivities (Regan and Beverley 1973a, see also Fig. 5C). This finding provides a second link between human psychophysics and monkey single cells: according to Poggio and Fischer (1977), inhibitory neurons in foveal cortex show maximum inhibition with ±6 min arc of zero disparity and *switch to facilitation* at disparities farther from the fixation plane (Poggio & Poggio, 1984).

According to G. Poggio, for many of these neurons disparity sensitivity for bar stimuli extends over a degree or so from the horopter. This accords well with Richards' psychophysical data (Fig. 5A,B). Both types of near/far neuron have a steep response gradient near zero disparity. Following Richards' hypothesis that disparity discrimination is determined by the relative activity of near and far pools (Richards, 1971), this finding is consistent with the well-established result that psychophysical disparity discrimination is best near zero disparity.

II. FIGURE–GROUND SEGREGATION BY DISPARITY ALONE

The main tool for the study of global processes in stereopsis is the random-dot stereogram. Julesz has applied this technique to a wide variety of problems (reviewed in Julesz, 1986). Here we consider the spatial properties of figure–ground segregation that is achieved by disparity alone.

The stereograting is a special kind of random-dot stereogram that was developed for this purpose by Tyler (1974). It is produced by spatial modulation of the disparity across the field of view (Tyler, 1974; Tyler & Raibert, 1975). An example of a stereograting is shown as an autostereogram in Fig. 4. (An autostereogram produces a cyclopean impression of depth without the need for a stereoscope or anaglyph spectacles; see Tyler, 1983.) Figure 4 illustrates that the modulation in depth is seen binocularly but cannot be seen monocularly.

Figure 8 shows a plot of disparity versus spatial frequency for just-visible depth corrugations. The curve shape resembles that of the threshold contrast sensitivity function obtained with a conventional sine-wave grating of bright and dim bars. But the whole curve is shifted leftward along the spatial frequency axis by about a factor of 10. In other words, spatial processing is about 10 times coarser for objects defined by disparity than for objects defined by lumi-

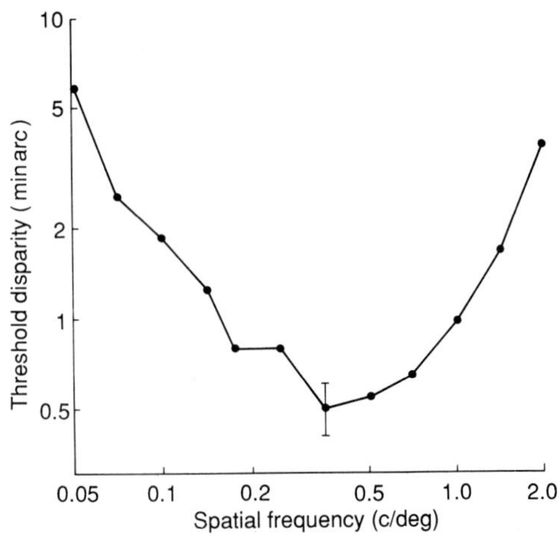

FIG. 8 Human disparity threshold versus spatial frequency for a stereograting. Ordinates plot the disparity difference between the "bars" of a stereograting for just-visible corrugations in depth. Abscissas plot the grating spatial frequency, namely, the number of cycles per degree of visual angle. (A cycle is one near plus one far bar.) A stereograting can be experienced by following the instructions to Fig. 4 above. From Tyler, C. W. (1983). Sensory processing of binocular disparity. In C. M. Schor & K. J. Ciuffreda (Eds.), *Vergence Eye Movements* (pp. 199–295). Boston: Butterworths.

nance. An interesting feature of Fig. 8 is the steep rise in threshold at the left side of the curve. This is consistent with the operation of cyclopean lateral inhibition (Tyler, 1983).

III. BINOCULAR FUSION AND DIPLOPIA

A. Panum's Fusional Area

As already mentioned, the classical view of binocular single vision is that a stimulus on one retina can be binocularly fused with an identical stimulus on the other retina over a definite range of position around the point of precise correspondence on the other retina. This range is called Panum's area. If the stimulus on the other retina is moved outside Panum's area, binocular single vision is lost and diplopia (double vision) ensues (see Fig. 2).

An assumption of this classical view is that each point on one retina has a *fixed* corresponding point on the other retina, and that Panum's area for any given pair of corresponding points is a fixed quantity. (Note that all the computational approaches to stereopsis published so far assume that corresponding points are fixed and also ignore the dynamics of Panum's area.) Both these physiological assumptions are challenged by recent evidence (see below).

The size and shape of Panum's area depends on the spatial and temporal parameters of the stimuli being fused. Tyler investigated the spatial aspects by presenting a sinusoidal wavy line to one eye to be fused with a straight line presented to the other eye. When the two lines were horizontal, so that disparity was vertical, Panum's area was comparatively independent of the period of the waves (Fig. 9B), but when the lines were vertical (Fig. 9A), Panum's area fell rapidly as the wave period was decreased (Tyler, 1975b). The maximum horizontal disparity could be as much as 1 deg when the wave period was 30 deg per cycle, but fell to 2 min arc when the wave period was reduced to about 0.3 deg per cycle. Tyler's finding showed that Panum's area is not a fixed property of a given retinal region.

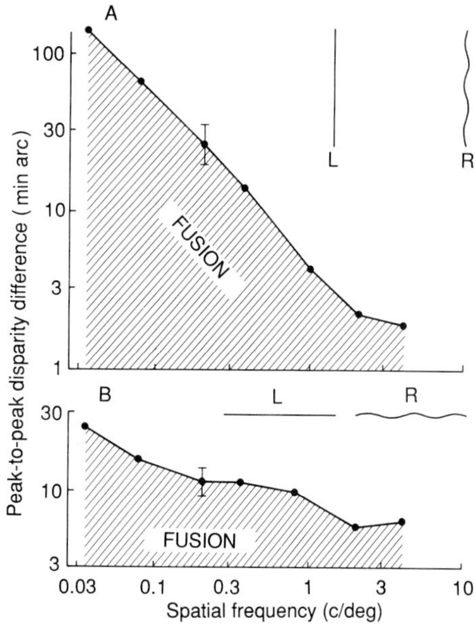

FIG. 9 Spatiotemporal properties of Panum's fusional area in humans. A and B depict the binocular fusional limit as a function of stimulus pattern. A straight line was presented to one eye and a wavy line to the other. Ordinates plot the maximum amplitude of the ripple before fusion collapsed, and abscissas plot the spatial frequency of the ripple. From Tyler, C. W. (1983). Sensory processing of binocular disparity. In C. M. Schor & K. J. Ciuffreda (Eds.), *Vergence Eye Movements* (pp. 199–295). Boston: Butterworths.

The temporal properties of Panum's area were investigated by Schor and Tyler (1981) who presented subjects with a pair of binocularly fused vertical lines, 0.5 deg on either side of the fovea, that were disparity modulated in counterphase. This technique effectively controls the effects of eye movements, since vergence tracking of one line would reduce its disparity excursion, but at the same time increase the excursions of the other line. The horizontal extent of Panum's area reached about 18 min arc for low temporal frequencies up to about 0.35 Hz, and then progressively decreased to about 3 min arc at about 5 Hz. As for spatial modulation, vertical disparities showed a different pattern of behavior. At low temporal frequencies Panum's area was only 6 min arc in extent

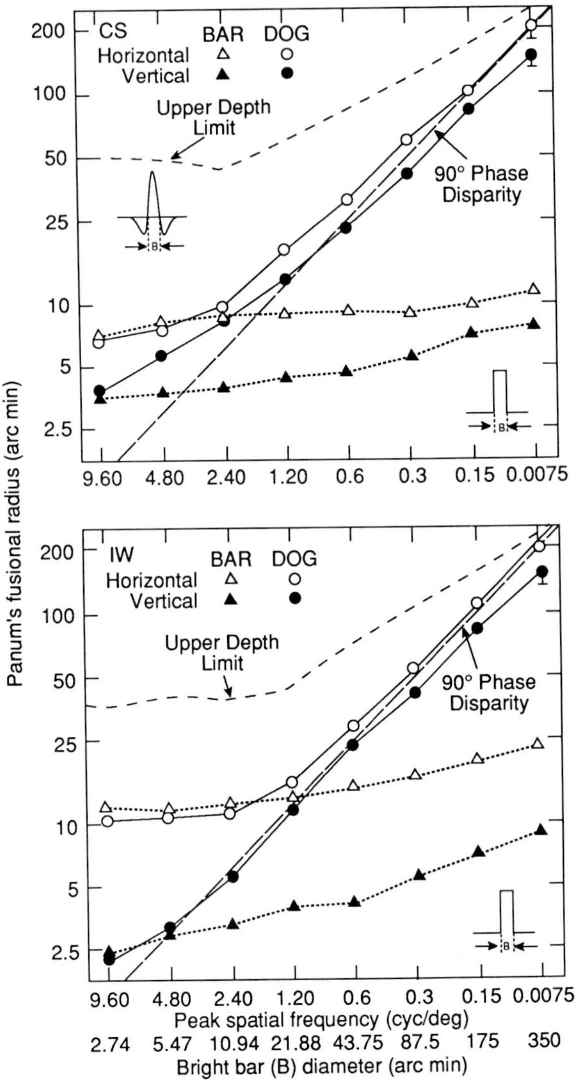

FIG. 10 Diplopia thresholds for two subjects are plotted as a function of bright bar width (BAR) and difference of two gaussian functions (DOG). Luminance profiles of these two test stimuli are inset below and above the data, respectively. A constant phase disparity of 90 deg is shown by the dashed diagonal line. Horizontal and vertical Panum's fusion ranges (solid lines) coincide with the 90 deg phase disparity for DOG widths greater than 21 arc min. At the broadest DOG width, the upper fusion limit equals the upper disparity limit for stereoscopic depth perception (bold dashed line). The standard deviation of the mean is shown for the broadest DOG stimulus. At narrow DOG widths, both horizontal and vertical fusion limits approach a constant minimum threshold. Panum's fusion ranges remain fairly constant when measured with bar patterns (dotted lines) and resemble values obtained with high spatial frequency DOGs. From Schor, C. M., Wood, I., & Ogawa, J. (1984). Binocular sensory fusion is limited by spatial resolution. *Vision Research*, **24**, 661–665.

and progressively fell to about 3 min arc at about 5 Hz. Thus, the shape and the size of Panum's area depend on temporal frequency.

Luminance spatial frequency is a third factor which influences the range of fusion for both horizontal and vertical disparities. Schor, Wood, and Ogawa (1984) stimulated fusion with band-pass filtered bars produced by a difference-of-gaussian luminance distribution. Bars with spatial detail centered about 2.5 cycles per degree (cpd) and higher yielded fusion limits of ± 10 arc min. However, the range of fusion increased proportionally with the spatial period of coarser fusion targets (Fig. 10). When filtered bars of 0.075 cpd were fused, the fusion range increased to 6 deg at the fovea. These results illuminate earlier reports by Richards and Kaye (1974) and Schor and Wood (1983) who found that the stereo threshold and the upper disparity limit for stereopsis also increased with bar width. These studies demonstrate a target size–disparity correlation that is consistent with Barlow et al.'s (1967) solution for limiting binocular matches, and that is predicted by the serial matching algorithm proposed by Marr and Poggio (1979) for stereopsis. It is important to note, however, that the size–disparity correlation is not present for moderate to high spatial frequencies (>2.5 cpd).

B. Physiological Evidence on Binocular Single Vision

Poggio, Gonzalez, and Krause (1988) investigated the physiological basis for binocular single vision by measuring single-cell responses to random-dot patterns of different disparities and degrees of binocular correlation. Over half the neurons in cortical Areas

V1, V2, and V3–V3A of the alert macaque were sensitive to binocular correlations. The proportion was similar in all three areas, even though the proportion of stereoscopic neurons is different in the three areas. Responses to uncorrelation extended the two-type classification of Fig. 7. It is the "tuned excitatory" neuron that most commonly responds to binocular uncorrelation while the other kinds of stereoscopic neuron (tuned inhibitory, near/far and flat) respond less commonly. Consider first the tuned excitatory neurons (Fig. 7A) with peak responses at very close to zero disparity (±3 min arc). Of the 34/52 that responded to uncorrelation, 100% responded with suppression. Figure 11 illustrates this pattern of response. Now consider the tuned excitatory neurons with peak responses at disparities greater than ±12 min arc. Of the 13/19 that responded to uncorrelation, 100% responded by activation. "Tuned excitatory" neurons peaking at intermediate disparities (+6 to +12 min arc and −6 to −12 min arc) showed mixed behavior, some being suppressed and some being activated by uncorrelation.

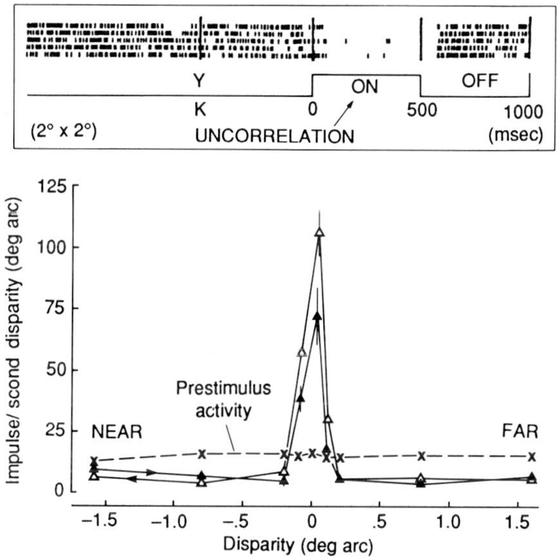

FIG. 11 Neurons near the fixation plane are strongly affected by correlation/anticorrelation. Data are for tuned excitatory neurons in Area V1 of monkey cortex with the peak response at zero disparity. The disparity sensitivity profile (bottom) was constructed by plotting the average impulse frequency within a time window of 300 msec centered on the discharge peak. Vertical bars indicate ±1 S.E.M. The stimulus was a bright solid bar subtending 1.7 × 0.2 deg. At top is shown the response of this neuron to dynamic random-dot correlograms. Each small line represents a neural spike. The dot pattern subtended 2 × 2 deg. From Poggio, G. F., Gonzalez, F., & Krause, F. (1988). Stereoscopic mechanisms in monkey visual cortex: Binocular correlation and disparity selectivity. *Journal of Neuroscience*, **8**, 4531–4550.

These physiological data parallel the shape of the human psychophysical "stereo" curve in Fig. 5C. Poggio (1989) suggests that the activities of the "tuned excitatory" neurons with the peak response at or close to zero disparity "may provide a reference for the stereosystem by signalling at all times the distance of convergent fixation, and may represent the essential neural substrate, for binocular single vision, carrying information for fusional mechanisms, both sensory and motor."

C. Binocular Vision during Head and Eye Movements

Dramatic reductions of stereo sensitivity to both static and dynamic variations in disparity occur when targets viewed are moved as little as a fraction of a degree, either in front or behind the fixation plane (Blakemore, 1970; Regan & Beverley, 1973a; Westheimer, 1979b; Badcock & Schor, 1985; see Fig. 5C). Consequently, optimal stereodepth sensitivity requires extremely precise control of disjunctive eye movements. Just how precise is the oculomotor control of vergence, and what effects do inaccurate vergence responses have on stereoscopic depth and sensory fusion?

During binocular fixation of a stationary target, ocular drifts and saccades are usually yoked corrections of versional errors (St. Cyr & Fender, 1969). However, unequal saccades can also correct vergence errors (Enright, 1984). During fixation, homologous features in the two retinal images are positioned over a range of disparities that can be as large as 0.25 deg, even while observers try to keep their eyes precisely aligned. There is no unique vergence angle within this range that can be identified as the optimal motor response that nulls out retinal image disparity. Accordingly, the accuracy of vergence response and the identification of corresponding retinal loci become a statistical problem. Accuracy of vergence is described in terms of variability and measures of central tendency. Riggs and Niehl (1960), St. Cyr and Fender (1969) and, more recently, Steinman, Cushman, and Martins (1982) observed fixational movements whose disjunctive component had standard deviations of 2–4 arc min. Clearly, this range is nearly an order of magnitude smaller than the threshold for diplopia (Panum's fusional limit), while at the same time it is an order of magnitude greater than the threshold for stereopsis. These movements are likely to limit stereo thresholds since displacement of a target by as little as 1 arc min causes a detectable elevation of stereo threshold (Westheimer, 1979b).

D. Accuracy of Vergence Tracking Eye Movement

Gain and phase plots of vergence responses to sinusoidally varying disparity have been used to describe the precision of vergence tracking eye movements. Such sinusoidal variations of up to 30 arc min in disparity occur normally during rapid voluntary head oscillation (Steinman et al., 1982). The frequency response for disparity vergence response to temporal disparity variations of small line stimuli has nearly unity gain and less than 25 deg phase lag for temporal frequencies up to 1.0 Hz (Krishnan, Phillips & Stark, 1973). However, the disparity vergence system is incapable of maintaining this tracking precision for more than 2–3 cycles as frequencies approach 1 Hz (Rashbass & Westheimer, 1961). In contrast, Erkelens and Collewijn (1985b) observed that the gain of vergence responses to large random-dot fusion patterns (30 deg rectangles) declined at temporal frequencies above 0.25 Hz. These gain reductions were accompanied by increasing phase lags that were well accounted for by an average delay of 210 msec. Parafoveal tracking of large targets is one factor which could contribute to the reduced gain of vergence responses at low temporal frequencies. Their large random-dot pattern stimulated the retina out to an eccentricity of 15 deg (Erkelens & Collewijn, 1985b). Vergence responses to disparity line targets presented only 3–5 deg in the parafovea have both reduced amplitude (Ludvigh, McKinnin & Zaitzeff, 1965; Ludvigh & McKinnin, 1966; Kertesz & Hampton, 1981) and lower initial velocities than vergence responses to foveal disparities (Schor, Robertson & Wesson, 1986). Hence the reduced gain of vergence responses to large targets could reflect the limited vergence tracking ability of the parafovea.

As the vergence stimulus amplitude increases, vergence responses to large random-dot patterns continue, even for absolute disparities beyond the fusion range (Erkelens & Collewijn, 1985b). However, when the random-dot pattern before one eye was replaced with a sinusoidal grating, the vergence responses to the nonfusible targets ceased. This result is in contrast to the step vergence responses to small nonfusible targets of dissimilar shape reported by Westheimer and Mitchell (1969). This discrepancy may be accounted for by different processes underlying transient and sustained components in disparity vergence (Jones, 1977) whereby transient vergence responds to targets of dissimilar shape, but sustained fusional vergence requires that similar patterns be presented to the two eyes.

In all the studies mentioned so far, the vergence system was driven by disparity changes alone. However, in real-world conditions, disparity changes are usually accompanied by size changes. Erkelens and Regan (1986) found that changing size alone can drive the vergence eye movement system (though rather weakly), and that vergence eye movements driven by a mixture of changing disparity and changing size are more precise and have less phase lag than when the changing size component of the stimulus is lacking.

It is often assumed that we can understand binocular vision adequately on the basis of experiments on subjects whose heads are immobilized (e.g., on a bite bar), and indeed all the experiments described so far have minimized head movements. Yet many people accompany their conversation by nods and other large-amplitude head movements, and ordinary walking is accompanied by considerable head movements. Normally sighted individuals do not lose fusion under these conditions, though whether stereoscopic vision (e.g., stereoacuity) is affected remains an open question. Furthermore, the world does not appear to move in depth when we move our heads, though this might be expected if head motion caused appreciable vergence eye movements. It is tempting to assume that eye position is automatically stabilized during head movements by visual feedback, or by vestibular feedback and possibly by connections from neck muscles to superior colliculus (Abrahams & Rose, 1975). Only recently has it become technically possible to measure with precision the stability of eye position during head movements. It turns out that binocular stabilization is so poor during moderate head movements that vergence changes of up to 1–5 deg can occur with retinal image speeds of up to 3 deg/sec without any disruption of binocular fused vision or any reported illusory movement in depth (Steinman & Collewijn, 1980; Patterson & Fox, 1984; Steinman, Levinson, Collewijn & Van der Steen, 1985).

The absence of illusory motion in depth can be explained straightforwardly. Humans are very sensitive to changing disparity when one object's disparity changes relative to another object's disparity. (Threshold for motion in depth is about 1–4 min arc/sec rate of change of disparity.) But we are much less sensitive to changing disparity when an object's absolute disparity changes and there is no reference mark in the visual field. Indeed, for an extended object we are *blind to changing absolute disparity* even at rates of several degrees/second, and no motion in depth is seen. Furthermore, vergence movements alone create no sensation of motion in depth, nor do they affect motion-in-depth sensation created by changes of relative disparity (Regan, Collewijn & Erkelens, 1986). Therefore, because vergence changes caused by head movements shift the entire retinal image bodily we would not expect to see any illusory motion in depth in real-world (extended image) conditions.

Whether the processing of static disparity is different under immobilized head and moving head conditions is less clear. Two sensory processes appear to preserve fusion during motor instability. The first is referred to as Panum's fusional limit. As described in Section III,A Panum's fusional limit varies with both the temporal frequency of disparity and the luminance spatial frequency of the fusion stimulus. Both of these factors influence the range of disparities tolerated during vergence tracking errors. Erkelens and Collewijn (1985b) found that with large random-dot patterns, fusion was limited by an upper velocity limit for changing disparity of 6–13.5 deg/sec. Using parafoveal line stimuli, Schor and Tyler (1981) found that fusion was limited by an upper velocity limit of only 0.15 deg/sec. The two studies also report marked differences in the disparity limits at low temporal frequencies. As reported in several studies (Fender & Julesz, 1967; Crone & Hardjowijoto, 1979; Hyson, Julesz & Fender, 1983; Erkelens & Collewijn, 1985a; Piantanida, 1986), the upper disparity limit with random-dot patterns is ± 2 deg. In contrast, the fusion limit with small line stimuli is only ± 30 arc min (Schor & Tyler, 1981). One reason for this discrepancy is that the upper disparity limit with random-dot patterns is based on a stereodepth criterion whereas fusion with line stimuli is based upon the perception of diplopia. It is well known that the upper disparity limit is larger for stereopsis than fusion (Ogle, 1950; Schor et al., 1984; Fig. 9). Indeed, individual dots within random-dot patterns appear diplopic at much smaller disparities than the upper disparity limit for stereopsis (Duwaer, 1983).

The extension of the upper disparity limit for stereopsis with random-dot stereograms is likely to be related to the broad spatial spectrum composition of these targets. As described earlier in this chapter (Section III,A), Schor et al. (1984) observed that both Panum's fusional limit and the upper disparity limit for stereopsis increase proportionally with the spatial coarseness or period of fusion stimuli to at least 6 deg of disparity at the fovea (Schor & Wood, 1983). Consequently, with moderate disparities (40 arc min) the low frequency components of a random-dot stereogram can be perceived in depth and fused while high frequency components are perceived diplopically. Ac-

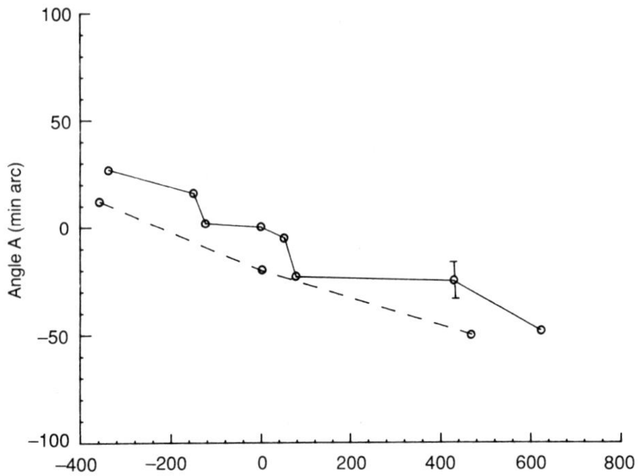

FIG. 12 Differences between subjective and objective measures of vergence error (Angle A) are plotted for two subjects as a function of the disparity stimulus amplitude. These differences are interpreted as a shift in binocular retinal correspondence that increases proportionally with the amplitude of the disparity vergence response.

cordingly, much larger vergence errors can be tolerated when fusing large complex targets composed of both low and high spatial frequency components than small targets with only high spatial frequency components.

A second sensory process that compensates for disparity vergence errors is a minor degree of plasticity of binocular retinal correspondence. Robertson and Schor (1986) and Kertesz and Lee (1988) observed differences between subjective and objective measures of vergence errors to disparity stimuli. Subjective measures are obtained by dichoptic nonius alignment, and objective measures are taken with the Stanford Research Institute (SRI) dual Purkinje eye tracker. The subjective method identifies retinal corresponding points using the identical visual direction criterion (Hering, 1879) which is more precise than fusion (haplopia criterion) or peak stereo criterion for measuring retinal correspondence (Ogle, 1950). When stimulating large amounts of disparity vergence (1–5 deg), subjective measures of vergence error are smaller than objective measures. Figure 12 is a plot of the difference between subjective and objective measures of vergence error for two subjects as a function of the amplitude of the disparity vergence stimulus. The differences (Angle *A*) increase proportionally with the amplitude of the vergence response. Robertson and Schor have suggested that these differences in subjective and objective measures can be interpreted as a shift in binocular retinal correspondence at the fovea of up to 0.5 deg. These binocular correspondence shifts could account for as much as 25% of the enlarged fusion ranges observed during inaccurate vergence responses to random-dot stereograms.

IV. BINOCULAR PROCESSING OF MOTION IN DEPTH AND MOTION PARALLEL TO THE FRONTAL PLANE

When an object moves toward the head the retinal images move in opposite directions and at the same time grow larger. Psychophysical experiments on human subjects have shown that either one of these two retinal image correlates of real motion is a sufficient stimulus for motion-in-depth perception. [However, the human visual system processes the two stimuli differently, and rather independently (Regan & Beverley, 1979).] By using a pair of cathode ray tube

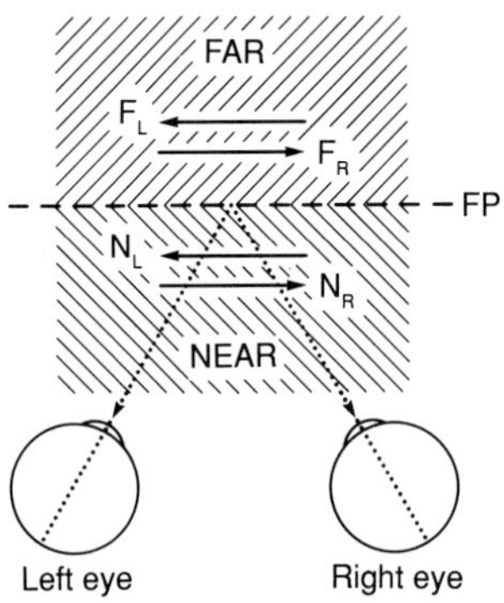

FIG. 13 Four disparity-coded channels for left–right motion in humans. The hypothesis depicted is based on human psychophysical data. See text for details. From Regan, D. (1989). *Human Brain Electrophysiology: Evoked Potentials and Evoked Magnetic Fields in Science and Medicine* New York: Elsevier. Published with permission.

(CRT) displays or optical projectors, the left and right retinal images can be made to move in opposite directions without changing size. This creates a compelling impression of motion in depth even though no object actually moves in depth (Wheatstone, 1852).

A. Disparity-Coded Channels for Frontal Plane Motion: Psychophysical Evidence

Figure 13 illustrates the idea that the human visual pathway contains four channels for left–right motion, two for objects beyond the fixation plane (F_L and F_R) and two for objects nearer than the fixation plane (N_L and N_R). The experimental basis for this hypothesis was psychophysical: after adapting to a target rotating clockwise in depth, subjects were less sensitive to clockwise rotation but, if anything, more sensitive to counterclockwise rotation (Regan & Beverley, 1973b). The same hypothesis can also explain the finding of disparity—specific motion aftereffects (Anstis & Harris, 1974).

B. Separate Psychophysical Channels for Motion in Depth and for Position in Depth

Before going on to discuss psychophysical and single-unit evidence on binocularly viewed motion in depth, it is helpful to review the graphical format in which the data are presented. The direction of motion in depth (in a plane containing left and right eyes) is given uniquely by the ratio of the left (V_L) and right (V_R) retinal image velocities. [In real-world conditions, however, an additional cue is usually available: the rate of change of size relative to the speed of translational motion. This cue alone is an adequate basis for discriminating different directions of motion in depth (Regan, 1986).]

In the polar coordinate system of Fig. 14 the left–

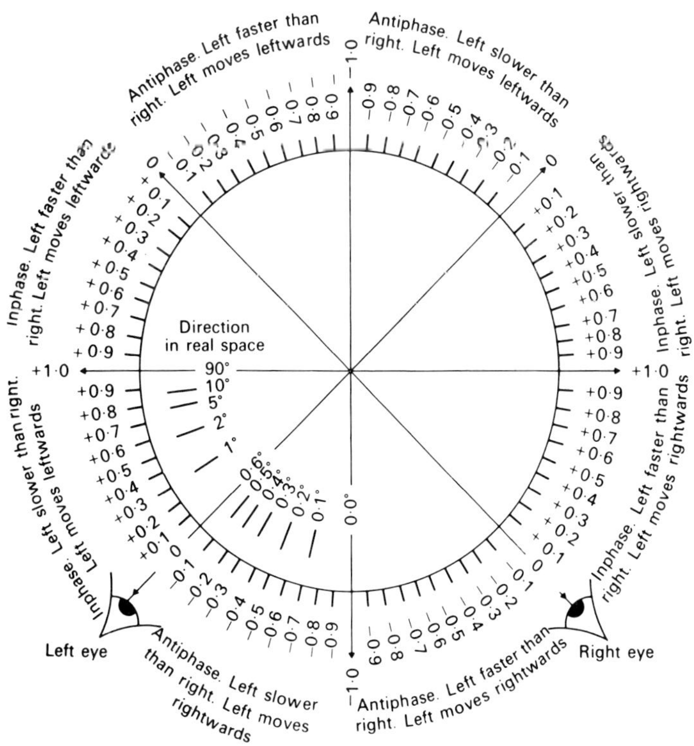

FIG. 14 Polar representation of stereomotion data. The ratio (V_L/V_R) is plotted linearly around the circumference of a circle, and the radial distance is proportional to psychophysical sensitivity, neural firing, visual evoked potential (VEP) amplitude. etc. Modified from Beverley, K. I., & Regan, D. (1973). Evidence for the existence of neural mechanisms selectively sensitive to the direction of movement in space. *Journal of Physiology*, **235**, 17–29, and Cynader, M., & Regan, D. (1978). Neurons in cat parastriate cortex sensitive to the direction of motion in three-dimensional space. *Journal of Physiology*, **274**, 549–569.

right image velocity ratio is plotted linearly around the circumference with the radial distance representing either psychophysical or electrophysiological response (Beverley & Regan, 1973; Cynader & Regan, 1978). The rationale is that the relative velocities of the retinal images are uniquely related to the direction of object motion in real space (for any given viewing distance) (Beverley & Regan, 1973). Figure 14 brings out the important point that the plot is highly nonlinear with respect to real space. In particular, the cone of directions intersecting the head is very much emphasized with respect to the rest of visual space. This is a straightforward geometrical consequence of plotting the velocity ratio. In point of fact, neural tuning to the direction of motion in depth can be so sharp that the tuning curve would appear as a thin line if plotted in real space coordinates (cf. Figs. 14 and 15).

In physics, velocity is the rate of change of position: one cannot travel at 100 km/hour for several seconds without moving from one place to another. It would be a mistake, however, to assume that the brain

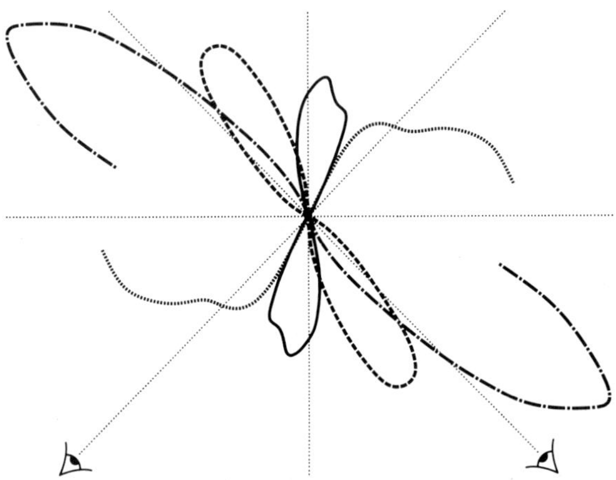

FIG. 15 Stereomotion channels in humans. Psychophysical sensitivities of the channels are plotted in the polar coordinates system shown in Fig. 14. From Regan, D. (1989). *Human Brain Electrophysiology: Evoked Potentials and Evoked Magnetic Fields in Science and Medicine*. New York: Elsevier. Based on data in Beverley and Regan (1973).

is modeled on elementary physics textbooks. There might be some advantage to processing velocity and positional information in parallel at some stage in the brain, and even of neurally representing velocity rather independently of position.

The first evidence that there are different channels for stereomotion in depth and position in depth was that adaptation to motion in depth reduces visual sensitivity to motion in depth without much affecting stereoacuity (Beverley & Regan, 1973; Regan, Beverley & Cynader, 1978). [The phrase "stereomotion in depth" is used to distinguish a sensation of motion in depth produced by unequal retinal image velocities in the left and right eyes from a similar sensation generated by a rate of change of retinal image size. The former can only be produced binocularly, while the latter can be produced either binocularly or monocularly.]

A subsequent and more compelling piece of evidence was provided by the finding that normally sighted subjects have areas of the visual field that are selectively "blind" to oscillatory stereomotion in depth and to unidirectional (ramping) stereomotion (Richards & Regan, 1973; Hong & Regan, 1989). Some of these stereomotion "blind spots," such as the one illustrated in Fig. 6, are quite specific: both stereoacuity thresholds and frontal plane motion thresholds are within the normal range in the stereomotion-blind area (Regan et al., 1986). Conversely, in other areas of the visual field the processing of static disparity fails, while depth oscillation thresholds are normal (Richards & Regan, 1973).

Stereomotion blindness is a subtle visual defect. Stereoscotomata seem invariably to spare the changing size system (Regan & Beverley, 1983b) so that in real-world conditions, sensitivity to motion in depth within a stereoscotoma is invariably present in some degree, supported by the changing size system (Regan & Beverley, 1983b). But, for geometrical as well as physiological reasons, the stereomotion system is more sensitive to small objects traveling fast along the line of sight than is the changing size system (Regan & Beverley, 1979). Therefore, motion-in-depth perception would fail only for that kind of target.

C. Psychophysical Channels for Motion in Depth Toward and Away from the Head

Psychophysical evidence that the human brain contains separate channels for stereomotion toward and away from the head includes the different critical durations for disparity pulses directed toward and away from the head (Beverley & Regan, 1974). Human evoked potential evidence was that both "far" and "near" pools had separate "toward" and "away" mechanisms (Beverley & Regan, 1973).

Threshold elevations were subsequently measured after adapting to 13 different velocity ratios (i.e., 13 different directions of oblique motion in depth). The data can be explained in terms of only four discrete pairs of channels tuned to different velocity ratios (much as color matching data can be explained in terms of only three color channels). Beverley and Regan (1973) proposed that "neural mechanisms 'tuned' to different right:left velocity ratios could provide a basis for sensing the *direction* in which an object moves in three-dimensional space." (This avoided the implication that ratio-tuned single neurons necessarily exist in the human visual pathway.) There are four channels for motion toward the head and four for motion away from the head. The psychophysical tuning curves are shown in Fig. 15.

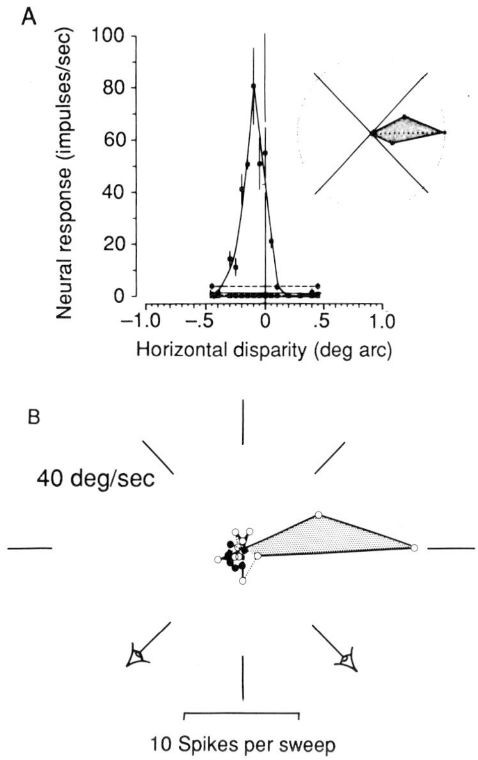

FIG. 16 Stereoscopic position-in-depth neurons in monkeys and cats. (A) firing response of an Area V1 cell in an alert, behaving monkey to a stimulus bar moved parallel to the frontoparallel plane. Interocular facilitation strongly enhances the response when the cell is located about 6 min arc from the fixation plane. The inset, plotted in the polar coordinates of Fig. 14, shows that this facilitation was strongest for motion accurately parallel to the frontoparallel plane. (B) Similar data for visual cortex Area 17/18 of an anesthetized cat. (A) From Poggio, G. F., & Talbot, W. H. (1981). Mechanisms of static and dynamic stereopsis in foveal cortex of rhesus monkey. *Journal of Physiology*, **315**, 409–492. (B) From Cynader, M., & Regan, D. (1978). Neurons in cat parastriate cortex sensitive to the direction of motion in three-dimensional space. *Journal of Physiology*, **274**, 549–569.

D. Physiological Evidence on Disparity-Coded Channels for Motion in the Frontoparallel Plane

As noted above, one type of cortical neuron in V1 and V2 (e.g., "tuned excitation") responds strongly to binocular stimulation over a narrow range of disparities. These cells are also tuned to the direction of motion in depth. Figure 16 illustrates that this class of cell creates its sharp tuning to motion in depth and to disparity by a powerful interocular facilitation (shaded area) that occurs when and only when (1) the left and right retinal images are moving in the same direction and at approximately the same speed, and (2) position disparity lies within some narrow range.

The stimulus used to drive Poggio and Fischer's "near" and "far" neurons shown in Fig. 7 was a line moving parallel to the frontoparallel plane. The directionally selective near–far neurons can therefore provide the four disparity–motion combinations (F_L, F_R, N_L, N_R) to explain the psychophysical finding of disparity-coded motion channels in human (Regan & Beverley, 1973b) diagrammatically illustrated in Fig. 13.

E. Physiological Evidence on Stereomotion Perpendicular to the Frontoparallel Plane

Some neurons in cat (Pettigrew, 1973) and monkey (Zeki, 1974) give strong unidirectional responses to leftward motion in one eye and to rightward motion in the other, so, if interocular summation is approximately linear, they respond to binocularly viewed motion in depth. A more interesting class of neuron is the kind whose binocular preference for motion in depth is sharpened or even created by a strongly nonlinear interaction between the two eyes. The binocular response of these cells cannot necessarily be predicted from their responses to monocular stimulation. Cynader and Regan (1978) found such cells in Areas 17 and 18 in cat visual cortex. Binocular inhibition to frontal plane motion created a sharp selectivity for directions of motion passing through or close to the head. Tuning could be very narrow: some cells responded strongly to a cone of directions only 1–2 deg wide, the remaining 358–359 deg range of directions producing comparatively weak responses (Fig. 17B). Similar cells are also found in Clare–Bishop Area (Toyama, Komatsu, Kasai, Fujii & Umetani, 1985).

Sharply tuned motion-in-depth cells are also found in monkey visual cortex. Figure 17A shows a motion-in-depth cell whose motion selectivity, according to Poggio and Talbot (1981), was created by a combination of interocular inhibition and excitation. The dashed and dotted arcs marked with triangles and circles show monocular responses of the left and right eyes, respectively; the binocular inhibition for motion parallel to the frontal plane is indicated by arrows. This binocular inhibition is also demonstrated in the upper response triplets for motion in the frontoparallel plane: the left eye gives a strong monocular response to leftward motion (L), and the right eye gives a strong monocular response to rightward motion (R), but these responses are suppressed during binocular stimulation (B). Motion in depth, on the other hand, produces binocular facilitation. The lower triplet shows that motion directly away from the eyes gives strong monocular responses from either the left (L) or right (R) eye alone, and the responses to binocular stimulation (B) are even stronger.

In both cat and monkey, motion-in-depth cells are much less selective for positional disparity than are the "binocular depth" cells (Cynader & Regan, 1978, 1981; Poggio & Talbot, 1981; G. Orban, personal communication, 1987) in accord with Cynader and Regan's suggestion that motion-in-depth cells and disparity-tuned cells might provide a partial physiological basis for the psychophysical motion-in-depth and position-in-depth channels reviewed above (Beverley & Regan, 1973; Cynader & Regan, 1978).

Pursuing this line of thought, the so-called hitting the head cells (Cynader & Regan, 1978) seem to be relatively rare (Poggio & Talbot, 1981). Perhaps this rarity might account for the frequency with which specific "blind spots" for stereomotion are found in normally sighted individuals. If, at best, very few hitting the head neurons serve any given point on the retina, it is easy to see how some retinal patches might have none at all as, for example, in Fig. 6 (in Hong and Regan's study only 6 of 21 subjects had full scotoma-free fields for oscillatory stereomotion).

The vergence eye movement system can also be "blind" to stereomotion in depth. For example, vergence eye movements could not be driven by a stimulus located within the behaviorally stereomotion-blind area in Fig. 6. On the other hand, conjugate eye movements could be driven from inside the stereoscotoma, and, correspondingly, the psychophysical threshold for frontal plane motion was normal. Thus, the vergence eye movement system and perception shared the same very specific local "blindness," suggesting that the common cause was a defect in the binocular processing of motion in depth (Regan, Erkelens & Collewijn, 1986).

F. Physiological Evidence on Oblique Stereomotion: Sharply Tuned Cells

In some cells, the nonlinear binocular interaction is strongest for some value of V_L/V_R other than $-(1:1)$ or $+(1:1)$ so that these cells will tend to prefer some

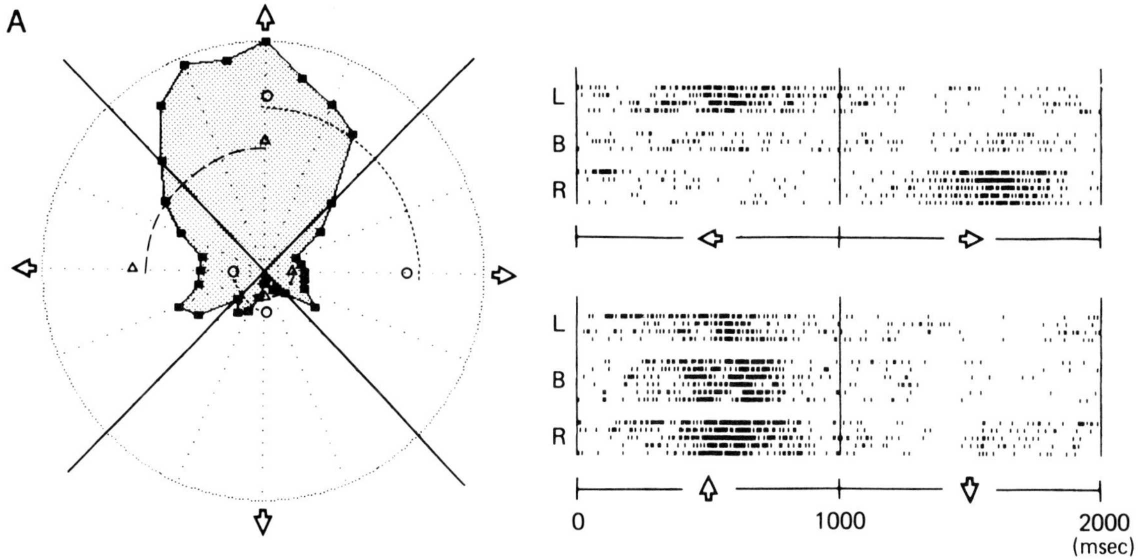

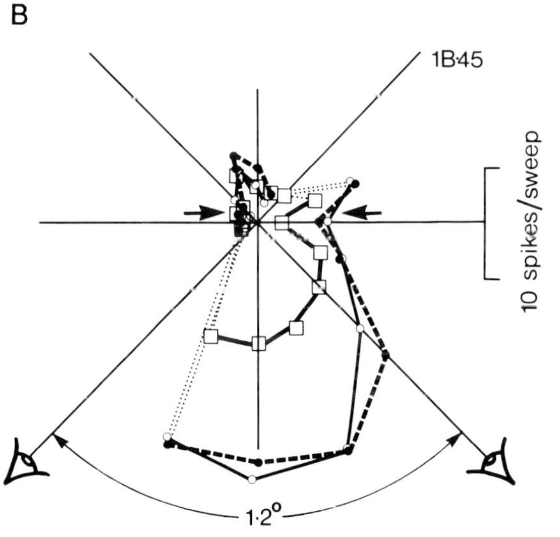

FIG. 17 “Hitting the head” neurons in monkeys and cats. Data are plotted in the polar coordinates system illustrated in Fig. 14. (A) The shaded area shows that the monkey neuron was tuned to the very narrow range of directions passing between the two eyes. Each dash in the right-hand graph represents an individual neural spike for binocular stimulation (B) and far left (L) and right (R) eye alone. (B) Polar tuning curves for a hitting the head cell in Area 17/18 of anesthetized cat visual cortex. The shape of the plot remains invariant as stimulus speed was successively doubled and quadrupled, consistent with the idea that the cell was tuned to the ratio of retinal image velocities. (A) From Poggio, G., & Talbot, W. H. (1981). Mechanisms of static and dynamic stereopsis in foveal cortex of rhesus monkey. *Journal of Physiology*, **315**, 409–492. (B) From Regan, D., & Cynader, M. (1982). Neurons in cat visual cortex tuned to the direction of motion in depth: Effect of stimulus speed. *Investigative Ophthalmology & Visual Science*, **274**, 549–569.

oblique direction of motion in depth. Cells of this obliquely tuned type were described in Areas 17 and 18 of cat cortex by Poggio and Talbot (1981). Obliquely tuned cells are not found in monkey Area MT (i.e., V5) (Maunsell & Van Essen, 1983b).

The direction of tuning to motion in depth remains precisely constant over a wide speed range in at least some of these narrowly tuned cells. Figure 17B shows a hitting the head cell that responded to a narrow 1.2 deg range of directions centered on a line passing between the animal's nose and right eye. This directional preference remained constant to within a few tenths of a degree as stimulus speed was doubled and quadrupled. The hitting the head cells of Fig. 17 correspond to the hitting the head psychophysical channels in human vision marked by the continuous line and heavy dotted line in Fig. 15, thus providing a second link between single neurons and human motion-in-depth perception.

Not all motion-in-depth cells are sharply tuned. Some neurons in cat and monkey cortex respond to a broad range of directions of motion in depth. Many of these broadly tuned cells are weighted toward motion in one quadrant of Fig. 14 even though they respond to motion in adjacent quadrants. These broadly tuned cells that prefer motion inclined to the frontoparallel plane correspond to the broadly tuned psychophysical channels for motion in depth marked by the dot–dash line and fine dotted line in Fig. 15, thus providing a third link between single neurons and human motion-in-depth perception.

Maunsell and Van Essen pointed out that there is in principle a possible artifact: If the stimulus bar were not accurately centered in the binocular receptive field, a classical binocular depth cell might be misinterpreted as a motion-in-depth cell. In the case of cat cortex, this impasse was resolved by Orban, Spileers, Gulyás, and Bishop (1986) who carefully repeated the experiment of Cynader and Regan, confirmed the existence of narrowly tuned, oblique hitting the head cells in cat Area 17/18, and showed that this selectivity is not an artifact of inaccurately centering the stimulus bar. The sharp tuning was preserved with the bar centered and (crucially) when the bar was decentered either closer or farther in depth (G. Orban, personal communication, 1987).

G. Relative versus Absolute Motion in Depth

When a stereoscopic pair of random-dot patterns is moved in antiphase on the two retinas and a stationary "landmark" is visible in the field of view, then a compelling impression of motion in depth results. But if all reference marks are removed, one is suddenly entirely blind to motion in depth no matter how large the change of absolute disparity. In other words, absolute change of disparity and absolute retinal image motion are quite ineffective stimuli for the stereomotion mechanisms. It would be interesting to know whether this is also true for hitting the head neurons.

V. COMPUTATIONAL THEORIES OF BINOCULAR VISION

A. Introduction

The opening section of this chapter reviewed psychophysical and physiological evidence on how biological vision systems might solve the stereo correspondence problem (defined as establishing correct matches between features in the left and right images in order to measure their disparity). Many computational studies of binocular vision have also grappled with this problem, not least because it is sufficiently well formulated to have permitted computational experiments. The goal of this section is to introduce biological scientists to the work they have done, both on that particular problem and on binocular vision more generally.

Most computational theories of the stereo correspondence problem have regarded it as requiring answers to two closely intertwined questions. The first is, What image features are to be used as so-called *matching primitives*? Typically, several different matches are possible for a given primitive, and so the second question that immediately arises is, What method can be found for resolving ambiguities in favor of the correct matches? The standard approach to answering the second question is to identify *constraints* which, as will become clear later from examples, are certain helpful aspects of the viewed world and its projection into stereo images. They are helpful because from them can be inferred *binocular matching rules* that eliminate false matches but preserve correct ones. In the computational literature on the stereo correspondence problem, unlike the psychophysical or neurophysiological ones that have also considered what constraints are available (see Section I), the value of any suggested constraint has to be tested by implementing its associated binocular matching rules in a computer vision program. This provides a brutally rigorous way of weeding out flawed ideas about constraints, or of refining valuable but rather vague notions into more precise formulations.

Facing up to the shortcomings of one's ideas via the discipline of computer implementation inevitably leads to an ever more thorough analysis of the nature of the task to be solved. At this top level of analysis, called by Marr (1982) the *computational theory* level, the questions constantly raised are twofold. First, what exactly is the goal of the computation? The answer to this is usually an abstract specification of a desired mapping from one kind of information to another, and often an ambiguity that must be resolved is identified. The stereo correspondence problem provides a good case in point: the goal is to take two stereo images and map them into a single representation that makes explicit the disparity of the various features in each image. And second, what method(s) can be devised for achieving the required mapping? The answer here usually has to do with identifying constraints flowing from the nature of the viewed world and its projections into images, or sometimes from the logic of the task, and demonstrating a method (often with a precise mathematical treatment) showing that these constraints are adequate in principle for achieving the desired mapping.

Testing the theory in a computer implementation requires attention to a second level of analysis, called by Marr the *algorithm* level. Here choices must be made about the particular input and output representations to be used and the detailed sequence of processing steps to be applied for achieving the required transformation. In short, issues at the algorithm level are concerned with achieving a practical implementation of the abstractly defined method specified in the computational theory. A third level of analysis concerns the *hardware*: How can the algorithm be realized physically? Here the considerations that arise often have to do with practicalities such as speed and shortage of memory storage, etc.

Marr (1982, p. 25) claims, "These three levels of analysis are coupled but only loosely: The choice of algorithm is influenced for example, by what it has to do and the hardware in which it must run. But there is a wide choice available at each level, and the explication of each level involves issues that are rather independent of the other two." This levels distinction is accepted without question in the design and analysis of man-made complex information processing systems. For example, ". . . in computer science . . . it is simply not feasible to describe a complex computation in terms of the events at the level of hardware. The technical language and formal principles that are relevant at the level of digital hardware are neither appropriate nor relevant at the level of algorithm . . . , and vice versa" (Stevens & Brookes, 1987, p. 18).

Nevertheless, neuroscientists do not always find Marr's three-levels distinction a comfortable one. This may be because neural structures genuinely require a quite different form of analysis, one in which perhaps the algorithm and hardware levels are inextricably bound up together. Also, it may be that a preoccupation with studying the neural mechanisms and phenomena of biological brains tends to lead naturally to a neglect of the computational theory level of task analysis, whereas this level is manifestly important when faced with the task of trying to build an "artificial brain" using computers. Yet another additional factor may be that the training and skills of biologists often make the computational literature rather inaccessible to them because of its mathematical leanings. Yet the bridge between the computational and biological literatures is now being traversed more and more often. Indeed, the term *computational neuroscience* (e.g., Sejknowski, Koch & Churchland, 1988) has been coined for the difficult but potentially richly rewarding enterprise of placing psychophysical and physiological knowledge about natural vision systems within a computational framework that provides a detailed analysis of the nature of vision task(s) being solved by those systems. One goal of this section is to promote those links in the field of binocular vision.

B. The Stereo Corrrespondence Problem

Numerous algorithms have been published in the computer vision literature, so much so that the stereo correspondence problem has been redefined as the problem of getting your own algorithm cited (J. Mayhew, personal communication)! As stated above, each algorithm seeks to exploit constraints for resolving matching ambiguities. These constraints are found by a careful analysis of the nature of the correspondence task, that is, by identifying what information is available that can be exploited for its solution. Each constraint has strengths and limitations for attaining the computational goal: the delivery of a *disparity map* representation in which matched primitives, usually representing *points* located on an object's edges or on its surface markings, are each given a disparity value. (Having identified the correct matches, subsequent processes then required to group the matched points into surface descriptions of some kind—see later.) Hence these algorithms typically have two distinct stages, (1) locating primitives in each image and then (2) matching them, although sometimes these stages can become closely intertwined as when disparity cues are used for obtaining surface descriptions directly without an intervening point-by-point disparity mapping stage.

1. Locating Primitives in Each Image

Because ultimately the goal is to deliver useful scene descriptions, primitives for stereo matching are chosen that stand in a close relation to scene entities such as surface markings or object edges (Marr & Poggio, 1976). Image point intensities, called pixels in the computer vision literature (cf. rod and cone activities), are generally not suitable as matching primitives because a given scene entity often produces pixels in the left and right images of rather different values, so any attempt to match left and right pixels of identical value is doomed. The pixel variation is due partly to various sources of noise but also to the fact that scene surfaces are usually at slightly different angles to the principal optical axis of each camera (or eye), so that the same scene entity reflects a somewhat different intensity into each one. It may be surprising to many readers unbruised by conducting computational experiments on vision that it is not satisfactory to choose as matching primitives "pixels of the same intensity," but, for natural stereo images of natural scenes, it is a fact. Edges are rather more directly related to scene entities than pixels, and so there has come about a plethora of *edge-based stereo algorithms*. Nevertheless, stereo correlation techniques based on matching left and right image patches of pixels can be useful in some circumstances; for example, they may be sufficient to support a fairly crude but useful stereo obstacle detection capability, or they may play a valuable role in "filling out" the typically sparse range maps provided by edge-based stereo algorithms.

2. Match Left and Right Image Primitives

As already noted, matching of left and right image primitives is done using constraints derived either from the geometry of stereo projection or from the nature of the viewed world. The constraints serve as reasonable assumptions that can be used as a basis for binocular matching rules for resolving the stereo ambiguity problem.

C. Constraints Arising from the Geometry of Stereo Projection

Exploiting the geometry of stereo projections requires calibration of the stereo camera rig. This fact is easy to overlook if attention is restricted to artificial images such as random-dot stereograms. For the latter, knowledge of which region to search in one image for the match of a primitive identified in the other is given directly from the method used to create the stimuli. For example, the search can be restricted to equivalent rasters in the two images if the disparity shifts used in the creation of the stereogram have been made along those rasters. But in a practical computer stereo vision system it will rarely be the case that matches will lie on equivalent horizontal rasters in the two images. In fact, the match for a given point primitive falls on a line in the other image called its *epipolar line*, which is tilted out of horizontal unless the eyes

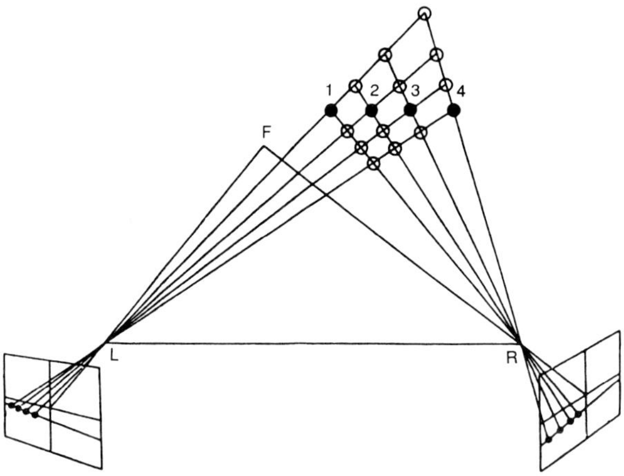

FIG. 18 Epipolar geometry and the stereo correspondence problem. In the imaging geometries with which we are concerned, the optical axes of the left and right imaging devices (LF and RF, respectively) lie in a single plane and thus intersect at the fixation point F (possibly at infinity). Consider the plane, denoted 1LR, formed by a single point in that space, labeled 1, and the optical centers of the two imaging devices, L and R. The plane 1LR is said to intersect the two image plates along a pair of epipolar lines. Furthermore, as a result of the fact that all points along 1L and all points along 1R are (by definition) limited to lie in the plane 1LR, all possible ghost matches associated with the point 1 must also lie in that plane and therefore project to a single pair of epipolar lines. The same is also true for all and only all other points that lie in that same plane, for example, points 2, 3, and 4. In short, matching points can only be found along a corresponding pair of epipolar lines. The possible ghost matches that exist in this case are shown as open circles, with filled circles portraying the physically existing points that give rise to them. From Pollard, S. B., Mayhew, J. E. W., & Frisby, J. P. (1985). A stereo correspondence algorithm. *Perception*, **14**, 449–470.

are fixated on a very distant object (which produces parallel principal axes, or so-called orthographic projection). Figure 18 illustrates so-called epipolar stereo geometry; note that epipolar lines in fact come in left–right pairs, which define all the potential matches of the points lying on them.

Working out the location of the epipolar line for a given primitive requires a solution to the nontrivial problem of knowing the spatial relationships between the two cameras, as well as facts about focal length, optical centers, etc. In all, camera calibration typically involves solving 12 free parameters! The usual approach in computer vision is to infer most of them from the projections of an accurately measured test object (e.g., Tsai, 1986), but complications arise if the camera geometry is variable (i.e., capable of taking on different fixations, vergence angles, etc.). The equivalent mechanisms in human vision are unknown, but the fact that we can adjust, given time, to perturbations imposed by various distorting lenses shows that they are adaptive in character, suggesting that a process of continual recalibration is at work.

Once the camera geometry is known, the *epipolar constraint*, as it is called (see Baker, 1982), reduces enormously the number of potential matches to be considered. Without the restriction to epipolar lines, the stereo matching problem becomes the motion matching problem in which searches for matches have to be made in all directions, that is, it becomes a two-dimensional search problem. But even given the epipolar constraint, errors in camera calibration and/or in image edge location may still make it desirable to search regions lying a little to either side of the predicted epipolar line.

D. Constraints Arising from the Nature of the Viewed World

The epipolar constraint is not in itself sufficient for solving the stereo correspondence problem. Resolving matching ambiguities *along* epipolars must be achieved using one or more additional constraints derived from assumptions about the nature of the viewed world. For example, if opaque surfaces can be assumed, then it is possible to exploit the fact that the order of primitives along an epipolar line in one image is preserved in the other image, the so-called *ordering constraint* (Baker, 1982; Arnold and Binford, 1980). This ordering property can be seen in the order of points along the epipolar lines in Fig. 18.

Another constraint, referred to briefly in Section I,

has been to assume that the visual world is made up of matter that is separated into objects whose surfaces are generally smooth compared with their distance from the viewer. In other words, the visual world is *not* usually made up only of a swarm of gnats. This is the *cohesivity constraint* of Marr and Poggio (1976). They used it to underpin their *continuity* binocular matching rule: *prefer possible matches that could have arisen from smooth surfaces*. Mayhew and Frisby (1981) used the same cohesivity constraint to justify a quite different matching rule: because cohesive objects generate surface edges and surface markings that are spatially continuous, *prefer matches which preserve figural continuity*. That is, give preference to any point-for-point matches which are part of an edge whose other component points also have matches, such that the whole forms a figurally continuous structure of points.

Marr and Poggio (1976) also identified the *uniqueness constraint*: a scene entity cannot be in two places at the same time; from this they derived the binocular matching rule: each item from each image may be assigned at most one disparity value. Marr and Poggio implemented their two matching rules in a cooperative network (see also the prior work of Dev, 1975, and its critical evaluation by Marr, 1982) whose nodes represented potential matches. Nodes exchange excitation if they have the same disparity, a form of mutual facilitation that gives preference to matches that could have arisen from frontoparallel planar surfaces (continuity constraint); inhibition is exchanged between nodes lying along the same line of sight (Fig. 18) which helps suppress more than one match for each primitive (uniqueness constraint). For a tutorial introduction to the Marr and Poggio (1976) algorithm, as well as an introduction to the computational approach in general, see Frisby (1979; Roth & Frisby, 1986).

A third constraint is that of *primitive similarity*, also termed *compatibility* by Marr (1982). The idea here, used widely in many stereo algorithms, is that correctly matching primitives will share certain stimulus properties such as contrast sign (e.g., a black-to-white edge point should not be matched with a white-to-black point), orientation (cf. Barlow's suggestion referred to in Section I), and color.

These are just a few examples of the constraints which have been used to solve the stereo correspondence problem. For extended reviews, see Marr (1982), Mayhew (1983), and Poggio and Poggio (1984). Before leaving this topic, however, a further constraint that here deserves special mention, as it was prompted directly from psychophysical studies, is the *disparity gradient limit* (Tyler, 1974; Burt & Julesz, 1980). Disparity gradient is a ratio defined as the disparity between two points divided by the distance between them. Steeply slanted surfaces give rise to steeper disparity gradients than gently slanting ones at the same distance (note that disparity gradient is scaled by I/d where I is the interocular separation and d the distance to the fixation point). To get a feel for disparity gradients, it is helpful to consider what happens when an opaque planar patch is made to slant more and more steeply by rotating it about a vertical axis: there comes a point at which one eye loses all sight of the texture on the surface because it is looking exactly along the surface. At that surface slant, for which the other eye can still "see" some texture because it is looking at the surface from a vantage point that is a little more "square on," the disparity gradient is 2.0, which is therefore the theoretical limit for disparity gradients between texture elements on opaque surfaces.

The so-called PMF stereo algorithm of Pollard, Mayhew, and Frisby (1985; see also Pollard, Porrill, Mayhew & Frisby, 1985; Pollard 1987) imposes a disparity gradient limit as a means of solving the stereo correspondence problem in a way which seems to subsume many other constraints (see also Prazdny, 1985b, for an algorithm based on the concept of disparity gradient). Thus the PMF algorithm uses a local neighborhood support scheme (cf. Marr & Poggio, 1976) in which neighboring primitives exchange facilitation only if they lie within a disparity gradient limit with respect to each other. The particular value chosen for the limit is not crucial although for values near 2.0 the disambiguating power of the limit is weak—ghost matches then receive as much support as correct ones (Pollard et al., 1985). It is interesting to note that the disparity gradient limit for fusion in human stereo vision was found by Burt and Julesz to be about 1.0, and this turns out to be quite a good value to use in PMF for many types of scenes. Here we have an unusually clear case of a psychophysical result leading to the design of a computer vision algorithm.

To understand what PMF is doing, it is helpul to note that imposing a disparity gradient limit amounts to enforcing a bound on the allowable degree of scene surface jaggedness. In so doing, using the disparity gradient concept breaks away from the restrictive notion of surface smoothness implemented by Marr and Poggio (1976). By insisting that only matches with the same disparity could exchange support they essentially imposed a disparity gradient limit of zero, which is another way of saying that surfaces "should be locally flat and viewed square on" if their elements are to be allowed to mutually facilitate one another. But it is evident from simple inspection of tufts of hair, bunches of flowers, etc. that human stereo vision can cope magnificently with scenes that are full of a wide variety of slants and depth discontinuities, scenes comprised of just about anything but even locally frontoparallel planar patches! Using a disparity gradient limit of around 1.0 is much less restrictive: for example, 1.0 is the maximum disparity gradient that can be generated between features on a planar patch viewed at a distance of 65 cm with an interocular separation of 6.5 cm and with a slant of 84°. The technical name for defining surface continuity in terms of a gradient limit is Lipschitz continuity. Pollard, Porrill, Mayhew and Frisby (1987) discuss formally the mathematical basis for using this notion of continuity in stereo algorithms (see also Trivedi & Lloyd, 1985).

E. The Coarse-to-Fine Matching Strategy

Coarse-to-fine processing is a commonly used technique in computer vision systems. It has been used for stereo matching in conjunction with one or other of the constraints referred to above (e.g., Marr & Poggio, 1979; Grimson, 1981, 1983). The key idea is that at a coarse image resolution (low spatial frequencies), there is little or no ambiguity problem for an edge-based algorithm because there are so very few "edges" to contend with. This enables a rough solution to be attained to the stereo matching problem in a given region without need of computationally expensive neighborhood facilitation–inhibition interactions, that is, no need for cooperative processes. The approximate coarse solution can then be used to guide the search for matches at a finer resolution (higher spatial frequencies) and so on in a coarse-to-fine sequence to the finest resolution required. Prazdny (1987b) has noted that this strategy relies on an assumption of spectral continuity.

Thus, coarse-to-fine fails if different spatial frequencies carry different depth information, as in images of transparent or lacy surfaces with mainly high frequencies lying in front of a background field of low frequencies. Here the outputs of a low spatial frequency channel would give no useful information whatsoever about the matches to be sought for the lacework. It is also of interest to note that Marr and Poggio's (1979) noncooperative algorithm of this type (which relied on vergence movements driven by coarser channels to bring finer resolution channels into their more limited disparity processing range) has been falsified as a model of human stereopsis by experiments showing that matches can be resolved over a greater spatial extent than that predicted by the Marr–Poggio theory (Mayhew & Frisby, 1979b). In short, it seems that human stereopsis really is cooperative, in the sense that it uses neighborhood relations between primitives to solve the stereo ambiguity problem, as Julesz (1971, 1986) has always claimed. On the other hand, and as reviewed earlier in this chapter, the link between spatial frequency and disparity range used by Marr and Poggio does seems to apply at the coarse end of the spatial frequency spectrum (Schor & Wood, 1983). But the very large disparities investigated in that study for low spatial frequencies (Schor & Wood, 1983) were much too big to arise naturally from scene depth variations in human vision, so the observed coupling may have more to do with maintaining eye alignment than with solving the stereo correspondence problem addressed by Marr and Poggio.

F. Interpreting Matches to Recover Useful Descriptions of Scene Geometry

A disparity map delivered by a stereo matching algorithm is not in itself particularly useful for controlling visually guided behavior. This point deserves considerable emphasis given the preoccupation in the literature with the correspondence problem. It remains true even if the disparities attached to matched features are translated into a depth map of how far away each feature is from the camera rig ("eyes") using geometry and knowledge of the viewing parameters of distance to fixation and angle of gaze (see later). What is required is that the disparity (or depth) data about individual features be interpreted to yield information about the scene in a form that makes explicit *useful descriptions of the scene geometry.* For example, if a robot is to pick something up, it needs visual information of a kind which can help it organize appropriate grasp movements such as "parallel plane faces bounding object M, with such and such size parameters, and with centers at 3D scene locations, etc.," or a description such as "*vertex* formed by regions *a, b, c* at 3D scene location *x, y, z* with such and such parameters of regions *a, b, c*, etc., etc." which could help it recognize one of its stored object models for which it has one or more pre-compiled grasp positions. For robotics vision systems, only when these kinds of geometric descriptions have been made available is it appropriate even to begin to talk about a 'solution to the stereo vision problem' (if indeed it is sensible to think of a single stereo problem).

Perhaps the simplest approach in the computational literature to acquiring useful scene geometry of this type is to group up connected edge points into strings (cf. Gestalt grouping) and then fit straight lines, circular arcs, etc to those groupings. This approach has been taken by Pollard et al., (1987), who used the resulting three-dimensional geometric entities for model matching. Those entities can also be used as the input for further stages of processing whose goal is to make explicit scene surface topology (i.e., labeling regions and their neighborhood relationships).

An alternative approach is to begin by reconstructing surfaces by interpolation between the sparse edge matches and then obtain descriptions of the properties (e.g., planar, quadratic) of surface regions so discovered. Grimson (1981) proposed a computational theory of surface reconstruction founded on the principle that the shape of the reconstructed surface should minimize variation in surface orientation, which is clearly a species of the surface smoothness constraint. One weakness of his scheme, as he was well aware, was that it attempts to smooth over genuine depth discontinuities, as when one surface occludes another. McLauchlan, Zisserman, and Blake (1987) attempted to overcome this limitation by finding where step discontinuities "should" be in the fitted surface, using an edge detector in much the same way as edges are found in the luminance domain. They then reran their surface reconstruction process but now minimizing variation of orientation within regions formed by the discontinuities, thereby avoiding unwanted interactions between different regions. The approach taken by Blake (1984; Blake & Zisserman, 1986a,b, 1987), and Terzopoulos (1984) is different in that surface discontinuities are found *during* the initial surface reconstruction process, by incorporating into the surface fitting equation a term which allows discontinuities to be fitted to the original data *if* the cost is worth paying because better smoothness is thereby achieved in regions lying in between the discontinuities. Such schemes are not without difficulties, however. For example, Blake and Zisserman's is liable on occasion to split up a smooth continuous ramp into a series of small steps. Terzopoulos also added the possibility of integrating into the surface fitting process information from other cues, for example, shading, motion, and texture (see also Kass, Witkin & Terzopoulos, 1987). These additional sources may provide information about the location of surface discontinuities (Barrow & Tenenbaum, 1978) as well as information about surface slants and tilts.

A quite different approach to interpreting matched disparity data is to treat them as a vector field and to find the deformation term of its partial derivatives which gives information about surface structure directly (Koenderink & van Doorn, 1978; Koenderink, 1986, provides a tutorial review). Space forbids an explanation of the technical details, but readers should be aware that this approach is being used to guide some current psychophysical studies of human stereo vision (e.g., Rogers & Koenderink, 1986).

Finally, it is worth mentioning approaches that attempt to obtain surface descriptions at the same time as solving the stereo correspondence problem. Pollard (1987) reports a version of the PMF algorithm in which potential matches "vote" for best-fit planar patches, an approach which he notes can be regarded as an implementation of some of the ideas of Koenderink and van Doorn just referred to. Hoff and Ahuja (1987) describe an algorithm that integrates processes of feature matching, contour detection, and smooth surface interpolation using a coarse-to-fine strategy (see also Kass et al., 1987).

G. Some Issues for Studies of Biological Binocular Vision Arising from Computational Investigations

1. Many Different Types of Stereo Matching

There seems no reason for believing in The One True Stereo Algorithm capable of dealing efficiently with all types of scenes and situations. Indeed, the reverse seems much more likely: different stereo mechanisms are designed for different circumstances and therefore exploit different constraints and strategies. There is a clear parallel here to the conclusion that human stereo vision is endowed with many forms of stereo mechanisms (Tyler, 1983; Regan and Beverley's work reviewed in Section IV; Ramachandran, 1986b). But if many different stereo mechanisms are to be incorporated into a stereo device, a critical research question then becomes one of controlling their operation and integration: When should each be applied, and how should their outputs be integrated?

2. Evolving Spatial Structures over Time

Many algorithms have been described for solving the stereo correspondence problem, for a wide range of natural and artificial images. Typically, however, the image data come from a single "stereo snapshot" (motion algorithms are rarely any better; their "temporal snapshot" is usually just two or three frames long). This neglects the fact that most scenes remain largely unchanged from moment to moment, offering huge potential for speeded-up stereo processing in eliminating the need to solve the stereo correspondence problem from scratch for all parts of the field of view at frame rate, even given a change of viewpoint (J. Mayhew, personal communication). Human vision is presumably endowed with such a capacity. At any rate, there are strong echoes here of the hysteresis effects studied by Fender and Julesz (1967) which suggest that human vision may utilize a dynamic memory buffer in a such a way that, once fused, elements can remain fused over much larger disparity ranges than are possible for initial fusion.

3. Possibility of Human Stereo Mechanisms That Integrate Matching and Surface Fitting

Mitchison and McKee (1985, 1987a,b) have reported experiments indicating that *un*ambiguous points at the ends of rows of ambiguous points can "pull" (cf. Julesz & Chang, 1976) intervening ambiguous points into interpolated depth positions that are inconsistent with any possible point-for-point matches. Such mechanisms might be particularly valuable for dealing with horizontal edge segments which cause edge-based stereo algorithms such major headaches. Horizontal edges are intrinsically ambiguous (infinitely many different depth variations are equally consistent with the left and right image data), and simple-minded edge-based stereo algorithms frequently choose bizarre matches. Smarter edge-based stereo algorithms (Porrill, Pollard, Pridmore, Bowen, Mayhew & Frisby, 1987) attempt to overcome this problem using some form of minimum depth variation interpolation between the unambiguous matches at the endpoints of the horizontal lines (reminiscent of Julesz', 1971, spring-coupled model of stereopsis; cf. also Mitchison and McKee). Even smarter computer stereo vision systems resort to more than two cameras! This is a commonly adopted tactic nowadays in many practical computer stereo vision systems, as the extra line of sight from a third camera solves at a stroke the customary stereo correspondence problem because the chances of ghost matches lying at the intersections of the lines of sight from all three camera positions is slight indeed (see, e.g., Faugeras, Ayache & Faverjon, 1986).

4. Cue Integration

The question of how to integrate disparity information with that from other cues has often been considered from a computational perspective (e.g., Marr, 1982; Kass et al., 1987), and of course that question has a long history of psychophysical studies (of which some recent stereomotion examples include the work of Regan and Beverly [Section IV]; Rogers & Graham, 1979, 1982). One current cue integration question worth mentioning here because it unites some computational and psychophysical studies is, Do texture boundaries help determine the loci of discontinuities in surface reconstructions from stereo? Human vision seems to do so. This has been shown using stereopairs of two planar surfaces forming ridge or step discontinuities in which the texture elements in the region of the discontinuity are present in one stereo image but are blanked out in the other (so that only monocularly visible texture elements are present in the region of the discontinuity; Buckley, Frisby & Mayhew, 1987; cf. Collett, 1985). Despite the lack of stereo cues in the region of the discontinuity, fusion of the stereopair results in a vivid surface reconstruction which uses the monocular elements to "cross the gap" in the stereo data. More importantly for the present question, if the monocularly visible elements possess a clear texture boundary, then a three-dimensional ridge or step discontinuity is seen in the monocular region whose locus follows that of the texture boundary, despite there being no stereo cues to the discontinuity. In short, the texture boundary, though only monocular, nevertheless helps shape surface reconstruction from the stereo data. Kass et al. (1987) report a computational scheme suitable in principle for integrating texture and stereo cues to achieve such a result.

A closely related question also creating interest at the moment psychophysically is that of the apparently crucial role of disparity discontinuities in surface perceptions from stereo. It has been claimed that for random-dot stereograms containing only disparity cues, surface perceptions seem to arise *after* disparity discontinuities have been detected. That is, disparity surfaces with constant gradient have been claimed to appear flat (Stevens & Brookes, 1987), with surface slant becoming visible only if there exists a zone where the disparities show nonzero second spatial derivatives (see also Gillam, Flagg & Finlay, 1984). Whether this surprising claim will survive the experimental assault which it is bound to receive is a moot point. Anstis, Howard, and Rogers (1978) have suggested parallels between disparity and luminance processing in that it is possible to obtain a Craik–O'Brien–Cornsweet (see Chapter 7, this volume) and other simultaneous contrast illusions in the disparity domain, though Stevens and Brookes challenge this parallel.

5. Role of Vertical Disparities for "Camera Calibration" in Human Vision

Mayhew (1982) has derived some remarkably simple and elegant equations for obtaining from vertical disparities the viewing parameters of distance to the fixation point d and gaze angle g (see also Longuet-Higgins, 1982; Gillam & Lawergren, 1983). Peek, Mayhew, and Frisby (1984) have demonstrated a computational scheme for exploiting those equations in which matched points vote for all the d and g parameters which could possibly have given rise to them and then a pair of d and g values is chosen that best satisfies all the data (a neat technique for solving Mayhew's simultaneous equations). It may be that human vision also implements the equations in that it is susceptible to a slant illusion known as the *induced effect*: if one eye's image of, say, a planar patch is vertically magnified then the patch appears rotated about a vertical axis, with the patch slanted toward the eye whose image is enlarged (Ogle, 1950). This result is as predicted by Mayhew's theory (Mayhew &

Longuet-Higgins, 1982; Frisby, 1984, provides a tutorial review), although observers do not often report an alteration in perceived distance or gaze angle (but note that the theory does not require the latter alterations in perception, just an alteration in perceived slant).

Porrill has extended Mayhew's equations to take account of cyclotorsion, predicted a new type of induced effect, and found it (Porrill, Mayhew & Frisby, 1987). This is not the only account of both the old and the new induced effects, however. Koenderink and van Doorn (1976; Rogers & Koenderink, 1986) also predict both effects from their theory of how surface slant can be obtained from the disparity vector field. Their scheme, however, also predicts yet another new induced effect but one which seems not to be observed in human vision (Porrill et al., 1987). The fact that vertical magnification produces slant illusions is strong evidence that human vision is sensitive to small vertical disparities (over the size range that occurs in natural viewing), but the issue of the use(s) to which they are put remains open.

6. Implications for Neurophysiology

Poggio and Poggio (1984) raise many issues relating to how neurophysiological studies of binocular vision might be profitably guided by computational considerations. One important question is, What exactly is the nature of the computation being performed by cells found to be selectively responsive to disparity? It is clearly not enough just to know that certain complex cells seem able to respond appropriately to random-dot stereograms. We also want to know *how* they come to have that sensitivity. Poggio and Poggio (1984) discuss various forms of correlation that they might be performing. One possibility that might repay investigation is to explore the extent to which the sensitivity of those cells is explicable in terms of the disparity gradient concept. Pollard et al. (1985) point out that their PMF stereo algorithm can be interpreted as effecting a correlation between images in which the figural distortions that characterize the differences between left and right stereo projections are not allowed to lower the correlation score. Do disparity-selective cells perform their correlation on a similar basis?

VI. CONCLUSION

The recent technical achievement of recording from single cells in the visual cortex of alert monkeys trained to fixate accurately gives a new precision of physiological stimulus control that has led directly to striking advances in our knowledge of binocular processing at the cellular level and revealed close parallels between human psychophysics and the properties of neurons in the visual cortex of nonhuman primates. After defining basic terms, this chapter compares human psychophysics and neurophysiology in the following contexts: (1) binocular processing of relative position in depth, (2) figure–ground segregation by disparity alone, (3) binocular fusion and double vision, and (4) binocular processing of motion in depth and of lateral motion. The final section reviews computational theories of binocular vision.

ACKNOWLEDGMENTS

D.R. acknowledges support from the Natural Sciences and Engineering Research Council of Canada and the sponsorship of the U.S. Air Force Office of Scientific Research. J.P.F. is grateful for the support from the SERC of the U.K. (Grant GR/D/1679.6). C.M.S. was supported by Grant EYO3532–06 and C.W.T. by Grants EY3660 and RR5566 from the National Institutes of Health. C.W.T. was also supported by the Smith-Kettlewell Eye Research Foundation. G.F.P. was supported by NIH Grant 5 RO1 EYO2966 and by a grant from the A. P. Sloan Foundation.

13

THE DEVELOPMENT OF VISION AND VISUAL PERCEPTION

Richard C. Van Sluyters, Janette Atkinson, Martin S. Banks, Richard M. Held, K.-Peter Hoffmann, and Carla J. Shatz

I. INTRODUCTION

This chapter discusses research on the development of the visual system in man and animals. In this work a variety of behavioral, physiological, and anatomical techniques are used to obtain information about the complex progression of events that characterizes the ontogeny of the mammalian visual system. One goal of this research is to uncover correlations between changes in the anatomy and physiology of visual neural pathways and the emergence of specific forms of visual behavior. It is hoped that more thorough investigation of these correlations will lead to the discovery of causal relationships.

This chapter describes findings in several areas of current research on visual development. This research spans an enormously broad area, yet our knowledge is still quite spotty. Whereas we know a great deal about certain selected phenomena, we know little, if anything, about many others. The peculiarities of this combination of "breadth and depth" of knowledge present a real challenge to those who seek to formulate unifying theories of visual development in humans and other animals.

Before we begin to relate neurophysiological data from animals to human visual development, we must first assess the role of nonneural factors in the development of visual behavior in infants. This is the approach taken in Section II, where we show that optical factors and changes in photoreceptor morphology can account for some of the reduced visual contrast sensitivity of infants compared to adults. In Section III, we present evidence of precortical and cortical neural contributions to several basic visual functions in infants. We examine data from studies of binocular vision and optokinetic nystagmus, and this serves as an introduction to the more detailed discussions of these topics that are presented in Sections IV, V, and VI.

One ultimate goal of researchers in this area is to relate the development of visual behavior to ontogenetic changes in the physiological properties of visual neurons. In Section IV, after giving a brief overview of the organization of the adult visual system, we show how this might be done by presenting a theory of binocular development together with some supporting research from neonatal animals. In Section V, we present a related neurophysiological theory of binocular development that specifically addresses stereopsis. This section focuses on some of the critical behavioral data on the development of human binocular vision and raises an important point: neurophysiological explanations must explain not only the form of development but also the timing pattern, especially any sudden changes in behavior that seem too rapid for neural growth models. In Section VI, we describe a different model relating neurophysiological development to the changes in the optokinetic reflex that underlie patterns of optokinetic nystagmus. We show how two neural characteristics, namely, genetic predispositions and feedback mechanisms, can be built into a model of neurophysiological development.

In summary, this chapter shows how research from several quite different approaches is converging toward a coherent explanation of human visual development. In some cases, our present understanding of the neural events underlying visual development in animals remains woefully incapable of providing plausible explanations for the remarkable changes in visual performance that occur in the first few months of a human infant's life. On the other hand, there are several instances in which related findings from various laboratories appear tantalizingly close to providing a firm understanding of the neural basis for a particular change in visual development. The neural data from animals allow psychophysicists to tie their models of human visual development more directly to known neural mechanisms. In addition, interesting new psychophysical tests in human infants have been spawned by theories of early neural development in animals. Finally, studies of visual development based on behavioral responses, such as preferential looking, optokinetic nystagmus, and eye movements, are providing a more detailed description of the form and timing of human visual development, thus guiding neurophysiologists in determining what to look for in neonatal animals. This beneficial interplay of data from human and animal studies of visual development is exciting to those of us working in this challenging area of neuroscience, and it is hoped that some of that excitement will be felt by the reader. For those who wish to read more about research on development of the visual system, a number of review articles are available (e.g., Dobson & Teller, 1978; Salapatek & Banks, 1978; Movshon & Van Sluyters, 1981; Werner and Lipsitt, 1981; Sherman & Spear, 1982; Mitchell & Timney, 1984; Boothe, Dobson & Teller, 1985; Teller & Bornstein, 1986; Teller & Movshon, 1986; Aslin, 1987; Banks & Dannemiller, 1987).

II. OPTICAL AND RETINAL FACTORS IN THE DEVELOPMENT OF HUMAN VISUAL PERFORMANCE

Many aspects of spatial vision improve significantly during the first year of life. A primary goal in studies of visual development is to understand the optical and neural underpinnings of these improvements. This goal dovetails nicely with the major question raised throughout this book, namely, How do neural factors combine to determine visual performance? In this spirit, the following section discusses how ocular and retinal maturation may contribute to the development of spatial vision in human infants.

It is well known that vision is quite poor in human neonates. Figure 1 displays contrast sensitivity functions (CSFs) measured behaviorally and electrophysiologically in neonates. A typical adult CSF is plotted for comparison. Contrast sensitivity is quite low in newborns; peak sensitivity is substantially lower than that of adults whether measured by forced-choice preferential looking (FPL) (Atkinson, Braddick & Moar, 1977; Banks & Salapatek, 1978) or by visual evoked potential (VEP) (Pirchio, Spinelli, Fiorentini & Maffei, 1978; Norcia, Tyler & Allen, 1986). One can also see that visual acuity in the first month of life is very limited, being roughly 25 times worse than that of normal adults (Dobson & Teller, 1978; Norcia & Tyler,1985).

An obvious question is, What optical and neural factors constrain newborns' acuity and contrast sensitivity to such low levels, and how do changes in

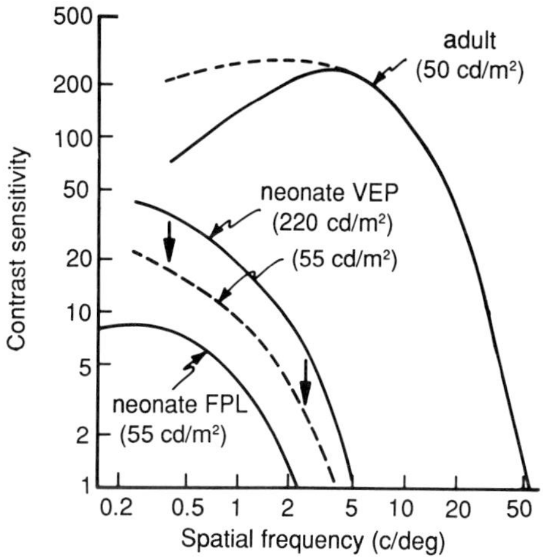

FIG. 1 Adult and neonatal contrast sensitivity functions. The curve labeled "Adult" represents data from Campbell and Robson (1968) that were collected at 50 cd/m². The curve labeled "Neonate FPL" is the 1-month data from Banks and Salapatek (1978). The FPL data were collected at a mean luminance of 55 cd/m². The curve labeled "Neonate VEP" is the 1-month data from A. Norcia (personal communication). The VEP data were collected at a mean luminance of 220 cd/m², so the function has been shifted downward by 0.32 log unit to indicate its expected location at 50 cd/m² (under the assumption that a square-root law holds).

these factors lead to age-related improvements in spatial vision? First, consider optical quality. Among the optical imperfections that could conceivably affect contrast sensitivity and acuity are spherical aberration, chromatic aberration, diffraction due to the pupil, and clarity of the optic media. The total magnitude of these factors, however, appears to be far too small in young infants to account for their sensitivity losses at such low spatial frequencies (see Salapatek & Banks, 1978, for details). The acuity and contrast sensitivity of neonates might be limited by another optical error, namely, inaccurate accommodation. This hypothesis is reasonable because accommodation, like acuity, improves notably during the first months of life (Braddick, Atkinson, French & Howland, 1979; Banks, 1980a,b). If accommodative error were an important limitation, one would expect neonates' acuity to vary with target distance. However, several investigators have shown that neonatal resolution does not vary with distance (Fantz, Ordy & Udelf, 1962; Salapatek, Bechtold & Bushnell, 1976; Atkinson et al., 1977). Thus, inaccurate accommodation also does not appear to be a significant limitation to neonatal acuity and contrast sensitivity. In other words, it is generally agreed that the quality of the retinal image exceeds the resolution performance of the young visual system (Salapatek & Banks, 1978).

By process of elimination, it can be concluded that receptoral and postreceptoral factors are primarily responsible for the poor performance of neonates. The retina and central visual system are immature at birth, but studies have found striking morphological immaturities in the fovea, particularly in the photoreceptors. Here the functional implications of such immaturities are addressed. More specifically, this discussion focuses on how much of the early deficits in visual acuity and contrast sensitivity can be explained by inefficient photoreception in the young fovea.

One current experimental approach to this issue (e.g., Banks & Bennett, 1988) uses the "ideal discriminator" developed by Geisler (1984). The ideal discriminator employs an optimal decision rule to discriminate stimuli on the basis of different effective quantum catches among photoreceptors. It therefore allows one to assess, without assumptions about subsequent neural mechanisms, the contributions of preneural factors to the detection and discrimination of spatial stimuli.

Before considering neonatal vision, it is worth noting that this approach has proved useful in another context. Banks, Geisler, and Bennett (1987) used the ideal discriminator to calculate the best possible contrast sensitivity the human adult fovea can have, given what is known about quantal fluctuations in the stimulus, the optics of the adult eye, and the size, spacing, and efficiency of adult foveal cones. They also included considerations of the functional summation area for gratings of different spatial frequencies (Howell & Hess, 1978). Figure 2 displays the CSF of the ideal adult observer for sine-wave gratings of a constant number of cycles. Different functions illustrate the contributions of various preneural factors. The function labeled "quantal fluctuations" represents the performance of an ideal discriminator with

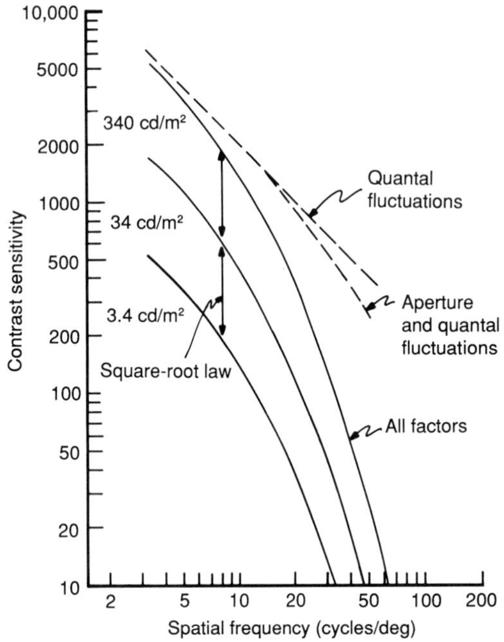

FIG. 2 Contrast sensitivity function of an ideal observer incorporating different properties of the human adult fovea. Contrast sensitivity is plotted against the spatial frequency of fixed-cycle sine waves. The topmost dashed curve shows the contrast sensitivity of an ideal observer limited by quantal noise, ocular media transmittance, and photoreceptor quantum efficiency. The slope of -1 is dependent on the use of sine-wave gratings of a constant number of cycles. Space-average luminance is 340 cd/m^2. The lower dashed curve shows the contrast sensitivity with the receptor aperture effect added in. Finally, the topmost solid curve shows the sensitivity with the optical transfer function added. The other solid lines represent the contrast sensitivities for mean luminances of 34 and 3.4 cd/m^2. From Banks, Geisler, and Bennett (1987).

no optical defocus and arbitrarily small and tightly packed photoreceptors. The function labeled "aperture and quantal fluctuations" represents performance when the photoreceptors are given the dimensions of adult foveal cones; comparing it to the curve above reveals the contribution of the receptor aperture effect. The solid lines represent performance with all preneural factors included; the differences between these functions and the one above represent the contribution of the optical transfer function of the adult eye. The solid lines represent contrast sensitivities at mean luminances of 340, 34, and 3.4 cd/m^2. As expected for ideal observers (Rose, 1942; Barlow, 1958b), these functions follow a square-root law: reducing mean luminance by 1 log unit reduces contrast sensitivity by 0.5 log unit.

Figure 3 shows ideal and empirically measured CSFs. The data points are contrast sensitivities from 5 to 40 cycles/degree for two adult observers who viewed the same targets that were presented to the ideal observer. As expected, contrast sensitivity declines monotonically from medium to high spatial frequencies, and sensitivity is greater for high than for low luminances. The solid lines are the three ideal CSFs of Fig. 2, shifted downward as a unit to fit the real observers' data. The lines fit the experimental data reasonably well. This similarity of shapes demonstrates that the high-frequency rolloff of the human adult's foveal CSF, for gratings with a fixed number of cycles, can be explained by the operation of preneural factors alone. This observation implies in turn that neural efficiency is constant from 5 to 40 cycles/degree for adult foveal vision. Note that the real and ideal CSFs are affected similarly by changes in mean luminance. This fact is important for the estimation of the functional losses associated with age changes in receptor efficiency.

The significant contribution of preneural factors to adult contrast sensitivity raises the question of how ocular and receptoral immaturities early in life might contribute to poor contrast sensitivity. Banks and Bennett (1988) conducted an analysis similar to that of Banks et al. (1987) for the human newborn. The only quantitative anatomical data on newborns concern foveal cones, so the analysis was restricted to this area of the retina in neonates. Unless otherwise stated, it was assumed that all factors incorporated in the ideal discriminator such as optical transfer and media transmittance (cf. Werner, 1982) are the same in newborns and adults. Thus, a comparison of ideal newborn and ideal adult performance is a measure of the contribution of morphological immaturities among foveal cones to visual deficits early in life.

Banks and Bennett (1988) used the best quantitative anatomical measurements available: those provided by Yuodelis and Hendrickson (1986). Figure 4 displays low-power micrographs of the fovea at birth,

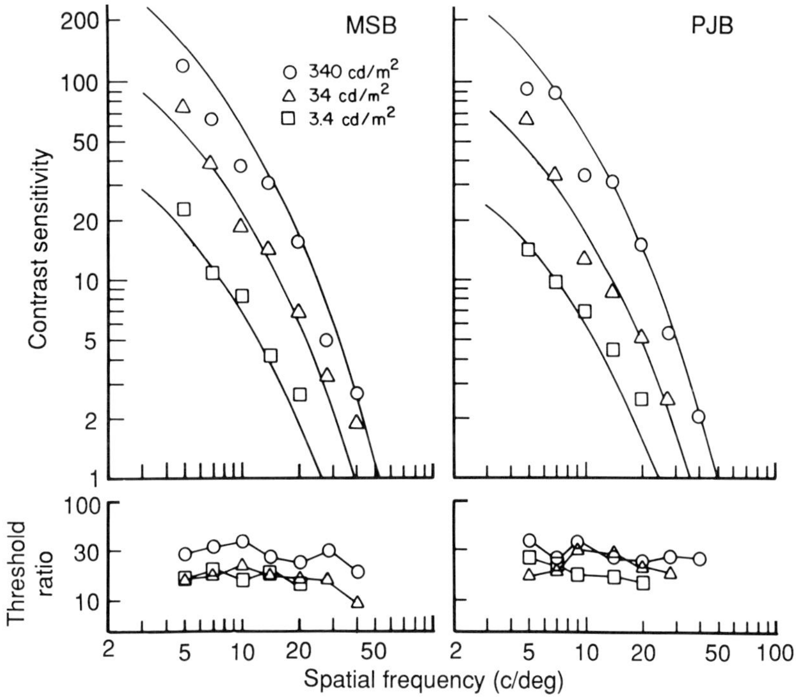

FIG. 3 Contrast sensitivity functions of two adult observers. The top graphs plot contrast sensitivity as a function of spatial frequency for the three luminance levels tested. The solid lines are the contrast sensitivity functions of the ideal observer (from Fig. 2), shifted downward by 1.33 log units for MSB and 1.43 log units for PJB. The bottom graphs plot threshold ratios as a function of spatial frequency. The ratios are the human observers' contrast thresholds divided by the ideal observer's thresholds. From Banks et al. (1987).

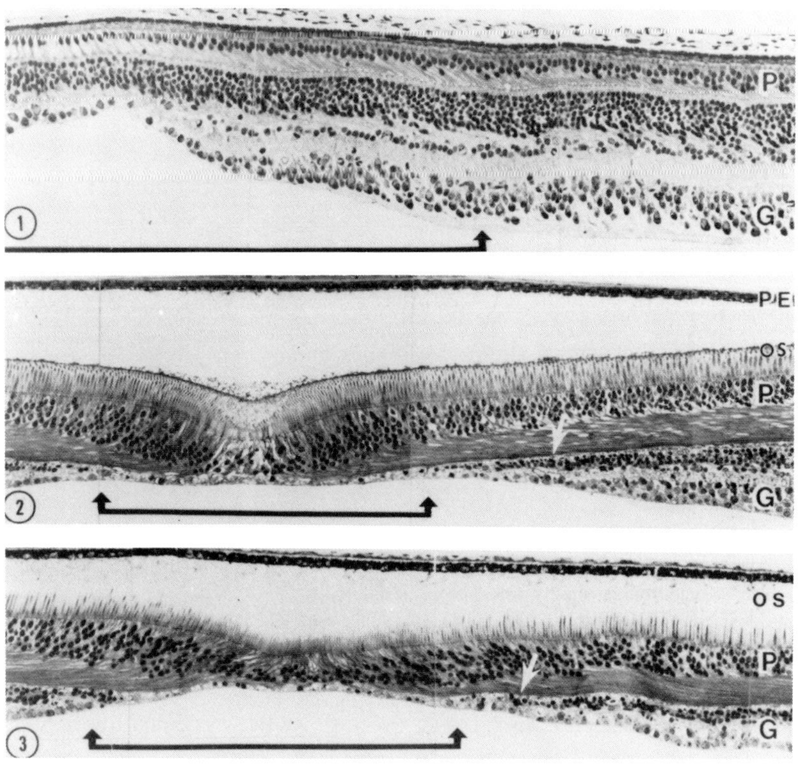

FIG. 4 Low-power micrographs of the human fovea at birth (1), 45 months (2), and 72 years (3) of age. The black lines and arrows mark the width of the rod-free foveola. Because at birth the foveola is very wide, only half of it is shown. The most central cone synaptic pedicles are indicated by a white arrow in (2) and (3). P, Photoreceptor nuclei; G, ganglion cell layer; OS, outer segments of photoreceptors; PE, pigment epithelium. From Yuodelis and Hendrickson (1986).

4 years of age, and adulthood. The black lines and arrows mark the rod-free portion of the retina, the so-called foveola. Note that the diameter of the rod-free zone, which is slightly greater than 5° at birth, decreases significantly during the next 4 years.

The individual cones in the young foveola are strikingly immature. Figure 5 shows this schematically for foveal cones at various pre- and postnatal ages. The anterior part of the eye is at the top of the figure, so light would enter the cones from above. The external limiting membrane is indicated by the horizontal tick marks. Notice how the cones of the newborn differ from those of a 4-year-old. The inner segment is much broader and shorter in the newborn, and, unlike its mature counterpart, the newborn inner segment is not tapered from the external limiting membrane to the interface with the outer segment. The outer segment is also much shorter than its more mature counterpart.

In mature cones, the inner segment captures light and, through waveguide properties, funnels it to the outer segment where the photopigment resides (Snyder & Miller, 1977). As light travels down the outer segment, several opportunities are provided to isomerize (i.e., bend, break, and eventually bleach) a photopigment molecule and thereby create a visual signal. Banks and Bennett (1988) examined how efficient the newborn's cones are at capturing light in the inner segment, funneling it to the outer segment, and producing an isomerization. They first estimated the effective collecting area of cones at different ages. The cone shapes they used to make these calculations are shown in Fig. 6. The dimensions are based on Yuodelis and Hendrickson's (1986) measurements. Banks and Bennett (1988) conducted separate analyses for cones in the central fovea and on the foveal slope because they differ morphologically. On the left is the model cone used for the central 250 μm of the neonate's fovea. The inner segment is not tapered. In the middle is the model cone used for the foveal slope. On the right is the cone used to represent mature central foveal cones. The slight taper of the mature inner segment facilitates its ability to funnel quanta to the outer segment.

Banks and Bennett (1988) used geometric optics and a ray tracing program to estimate the waveguide properties of newborn cones. Refractive indices were set to mature values. They found that in the neonate, cones do not act as effective waveguides. The reason is the following. The inner segment is short and much broader than the outer segment. Therefore, light rays approaching the inner segment wall at acute angles and reflecting off it cannot reach the outer segment. Varying the refractive indices and dimensions of the inner and outer segments within reasonable limits did not alter this result. The result held for both foveal slope and central cones. If the funneling property of the inner segment does not work, the effective aperture of newborns' cones must be the diameter of the outer segment itself. A similar conclusion was reached by a somewhat different route in a study by Brown, Dobson, and Maier (1987).

Taking the smaller size of the newborn eye into account, the angular diameter of outer segments is about

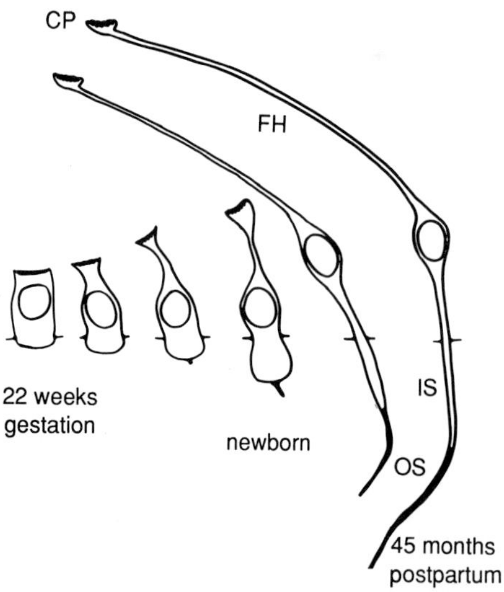

FIG. 5 Schematic drawings of foveal cones at different stages of development. From left to right, the ages represented are 22, 25, and 35 weeks postconception, birth, and 15 and 45 months after birth. The anterior part of the eye is above. FH, Fiber of Henle; CP, cone pedicle; IS, inner segment; OS, outer segment. From Hendrickson and Yuodelis (1984).

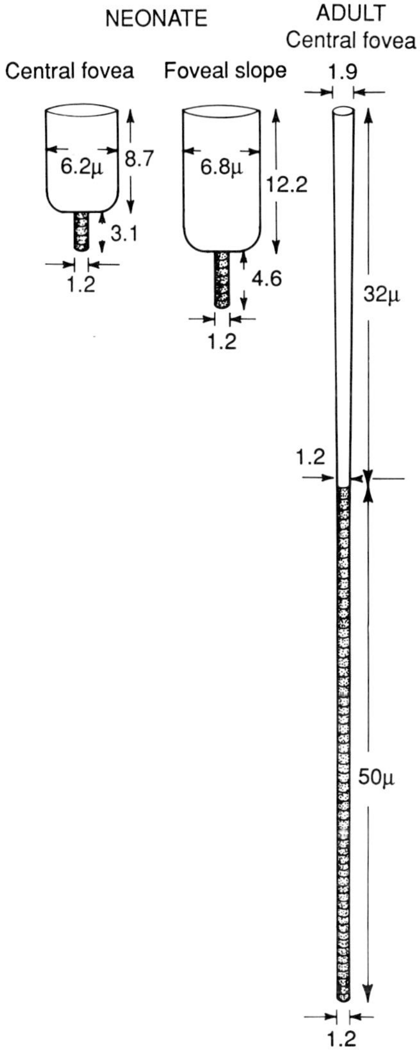

FIG. 6 Dimensions (in micrometers) and shapes used to model neonate and adult foveal cones. On the left is the model cone used for the central 250 μm of the neonate's fovea. The inner segment is not tapered, in accord with the observations of Yuodelis and Hendrickson (1986). In the middle is the model cone used for the foveal slope of the neonate. Again, the inner segment is untapered. On the right is the slightly tapered cone used to represent mature central foveal cones. From Banks and Bennett (1988).

0.35 min arc. The dimensions required to compute this value are given in Table 1. Banks and Bennett (1988) concluded that the effective aperture of neonatal central foveal cones is also about 0.35 min arc. Of course, the effective aperture of adult foveal cones is the inner segment, because it has an efficient waveguide. Thus, the aperture of adult cones is about 0.5 min arc. Therefore, despite their squat appearance, cones in the neonate are poor targets for incoming light.

The next factor Banks and Bennett (1988) considered was the efficiency of the outer segment. They did so by calculating the proportion of quanta incident on the outer segment that produce an isomerization, using equations described by Copenhagen and Owen (1976). The equations and relevant parameters are given in Table 2. It was assumed that outer segments in neonates and adults differ only in width and length. As shown in Fig. 6, the lengths of immature and adult outer segments differ substantially. For instance, in the central fovea, the ratio of adult to neonatal outer segment length is about 16:1. Intuitively, longer outer segments should provide more opportunities for a photon to produce an isomerization, and the equations bear this out. In Banks and Bennett's (1988) calculations, the 16:1 ratio in outer segment length produces about a 10:1 ratio in the number of isomerizations for a given number of incident quanta. The immature outer segments are a bit longer on the foveal slope, so the corresponding ratio of adult to neonatal isomerizations is slightly higher. These calculations mean that once quanta are delivered to outer segments, cones in the newborn are much less efficient than mature cones in producing isomerizations. The photoisomerization process is, like photon emission, a discrete (quantal) random process. The mean and variance of the Poisson statistics that are used to model such processes are equal, so the standard deviation is equal to the square root of the mean. Assuming that the appropriate measure of signal-to-noise ratio is the mean divided by the standard deviation (Green & Swets, 1966), the lower isomerization rate among outer segments in the neonate implies a lower signal-to-noise ratio than in the adult for a given

TABLE 1 Parameters Used to Compute Ideal Contrast Sensitivity

Factor	Source	Neonate central fovea	Neonate foveal slope	Infant (15 months) central fovea	Adult central fovea
Pupil diameter (mm)	Salapatek and Banks (1978)	2.0	2.0	2.5	3.0
Axial length (mm)	Stenstrom (1946), Larsen (1971)	16.6	16.6	20.4	24.0
Posterior nodal distance (mm)	From axial length ratios	11.7	11.7	14.4	16.2
Receptor aperture (min arc)	Miller and Bernard (1983), Yuodelis and Hendrickson (1986)	0.35	0.35	0.67	0.48
Receptor spacing (min arc)	Yuodelis and Hendrickson (1986)	2.30	1.66	1.27	0.58

TABLE 2 Outer Segment Efficiency[a]

	Specific axial density	Outer segment length (μm)	Relative number of isomerizations	Ratio to adult	Square root of ratio
Neonate	0.009	3.1	0.062	11.5	3.4
central fovea	0.014		0.095	9.0	3.0
Neonate	0.009	4.6	0.091	7.8	2.8
foveal slope	0.014		0.138	6.2	2.5
Infant (15 months)	0.009	22.5	0.373	1.9	1.4
central fovea	0.014		0.516	1.7	1.3
Adult	0.009	50.0	0.712	—	—
central fovea	0.014		0.855	—	—

[a]From Copenhagen and Owen (1976):

$$\text{Number of isomerizations} = (\text{incident quanta}/\mu\text{m}^2)\,(\text{effective collecting area})$$
$$\text{Effective collecting area} = IS \times F \times QE \times (1 - 10^{-SL})$$

where IS is the cross-sectional area of the inner segment, F the funneling efficiency from inner to outer segment, QE the quantum efficiency, S the specific axial density, and L the outer segment length. Holding IS, F, QE, and incident quanta constant:

$$\text{Number of isomerizations} \propto 1 - 10^{-SL}$$
$$\text{Relative number of isomerizations} = 1 - 10^{-SL}$$

number of incident quanta. In other words, for a given amount of incident light, the presence of a signal is harder to extract in the newborn from the pattern of isomerizations across the photoreceptor array.

Banks and Bennett (1988) next constructed receptor lattices such as those schematized in Fig. 7. They used Yuodelis and Hendrickson's (1986) data (see Fig. 4) to calculate the average spacing of cones in the newborn and adult fovea based on the assumption that newborn and adult foveal cones are arranged in a regular hexagonal lattice. Table 3 shows the resulting cone-to-cone distances (D) in minutes of arc. The corresponding Nyquist limits were calculated using the equation shown. The Nyquist limits, which represent the highest spatial frequency that can be resolved without sampling distortion (aliasing), are represented in the rightmost column of Table 3. The cone-to-cone separation in the center of the newborn

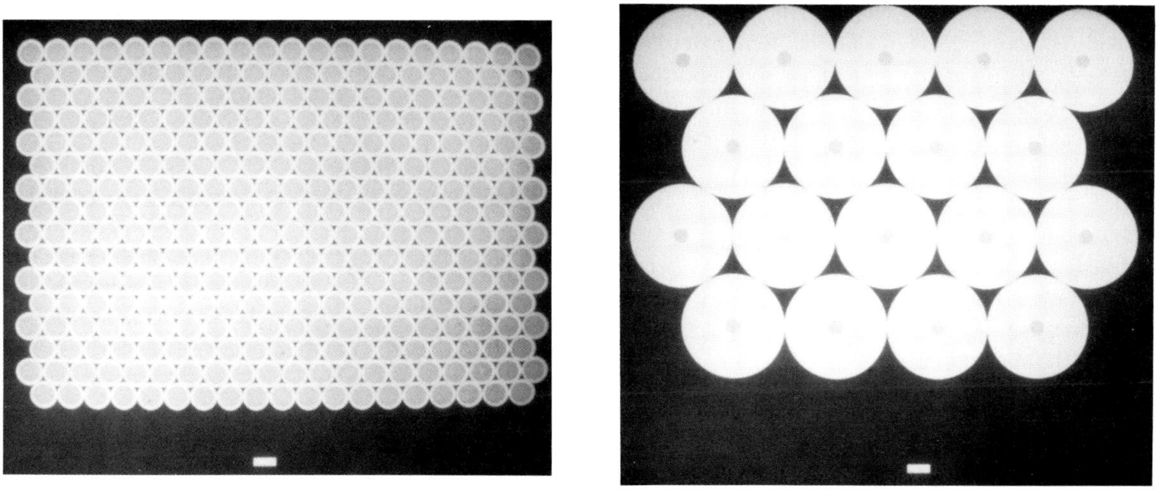

A B

FIG. 7 Schematics of the receptor lattices used in adult (A) and neonatal (B) ideal observers. The white bars represent 0.5 min arc. Light gray areas represent the individual cones; dark gray areas represent effective collecting areas. The effective collecting areas cover 65% of the adult central fovea but only 2% of the newborn central fovea. From Banks and Bennett (1988).

TABLE 3 Nyquist Limits[a]

	D (min arc)	Nyquist limit (cycles/degree)
Neonate central fovea	2.30	15.1
Neonate foveal slope	1.66	20.9
Infant (15 month) central fovea	1.27	27.2
Adult central fovea	0.58	59.7

[a]Assuming a regular hexagonal lattice:

$$\text{Nyquist limit} = \frac{60}{\sqrt{3}D}$$

where D is the center-to-center distance in minutes of arc.

fovea is about 2.3 min arc, which corresponds to a Nyquist limit of 15 cycles/degree. These values differ substantially from the adult values of about 0.6 min arc and 60 cycles/degree. Green (1970) and Williams (1985b; see also Chapter 10, this volume) have shown that adult grating acuity is similar to the Nyquist sampling limit of the foveal cone lattice. Thus, it is natural to ask whether a similar relationship is observed in newborns. The answer is evident from a comparison of Table 3 and Fig. 1. Although newborn Nyquist limits are much lower than in the adult, they are not nearly as low as the best grating acuities observed early in life. Thus, in newborns the Nyquist sampling limit of the foveal cone lattice far exceeds the observed visual resolution.

Figure 7A shows a schematic front-on view of an adult central foveal lattice. The dark gray areas represent the cone apertures, that is, the effective collecting areas. These are 0.48 min arc in diameter. Since the effective collecting areas cover about 65% of this retinal patch, roughly two-thirds of incident quanta should be collected within adult foveal cone apertures. Figure 7B displays the newborn central foveal lattice at the same scale. The intercone separation is about four times greater than in the adult lattice. Because the inner segments appear to be ineffective waveguides, the effective collecting areas represent the outer segments and are rather small. The collecting areas in this lattice cover only 2% of the total area. Consequently, the vast majority of incident quanta will not be collected within newborn cone apertures.

One can see from this analysis that the cone lattice

of the newborn fovea is quite inefficient in gathering and delivering quanta to the photopigment-laden outer segments. In addition the outer segments themselves are less efficient at absorbing the smaller number of quanta that arrive. Taking into account the age-related factors discussed here, the adult central foveal cone lattice should absorb about 350 times more quanta than in the newborn. Stated another way, if identical patches of light are presented to newborn and adult eyes, roughly 350 quanta are effectively absorbed in adult foveal cones for every quantum absorbed in newborn cones.

Banks and Bennett (1988) incorporated these neonatal cone lattices into their model of an ideal observer, one for the central fovea and one for the foveal slope. They used Geisler's (1984) SDE (Signal Defined Exactly) software for this purpose. Except for the spacing, aperture, and efficiency of photoreceptors, the transmittance of the ocular media, and the size of the eye, all other factors, including optical transfer were given adult values. Setting optics to adult values is reasonable because the optics of the newborn eye appear to be quite good, particularly in comparison to the observed visual acuity and contrast sensitivity in neonates (Salapatek & Banks, 1978).

Figure 8 shows the ideal contrast sensitivities which Banks and Bennett (1988) computed for fixed-cycle gratings at various spatial frequencies. The space-average luminance was 50 cd/m². Ideal CSFs are shown for an adult fovea and for the newborn on the foveal slope and in the central fovea. Ideal contrast sensitivity for the foveal slope in the newborn is higher than for the central fovea, because foveal slope cones are more efficient (Table 2). Most noteworthy, however, are the differences between adult and neonatal contrast sensitivity, which are substantial. For example, the ratio between adult sensitivity and neonatal central foveal sensitivity at 5 cycles/degree is about 19:1.

Of course, neither adults nor newborns are ideal observers, so one naturally asks whether these predicted differences in sensitivity can explain the differences observed between real adult and real newborn performance. If the visual systems of newborns and adults were identical except for the observed differences in eye size, and in cone aperture, efficiency and spacing, one would expect the neonatal CSF simply to be a shifted version of the adult CSF. To examine this idea Banks and Bennett (1988) compared empirically determined adult and newborn CSFs. Figure 9 displays an adult CSF at 50 cd/m² which is shown along with neonatal CSFs obtained at similar luminances with either behavioral (forced choice preferential looking) or electrophysiological (visual evoked potentials) methods. The vertical arrows indicate the shifts predicted from Banks and Bennett's (1988) analysis; they are the ratios of ideal adult contrast sensitivity divided by ideal newborn sensitivity at each spatial frequency. The ratios (and arrows) represent the information lost in the fovea of the newborn by inefficient quantum capture and photoisomerization.

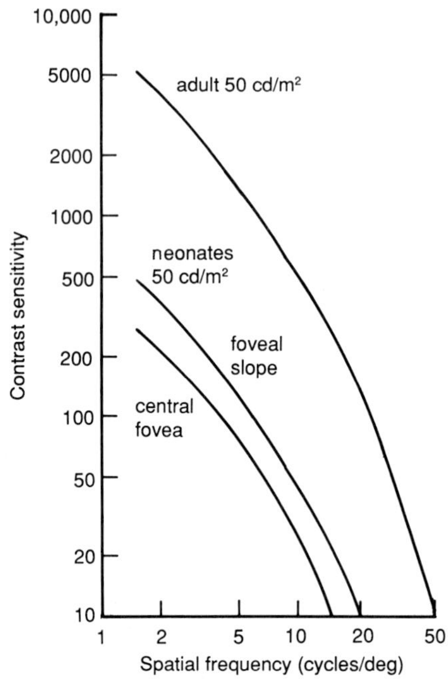

FIG. 8 Contrast sensitivity functions for ideal observers incorporating the preneural factors of the adult and neonatal central foveas and the neonatal foveal slope. As in Fig. 2, the stimuli were gratings of a constant number of cycles, in order to incorporate changes in summation area with spatial frequency. Mean luminance is 50 cd/m². The differences between adult and neonatal sensitivities are due primarily to the reduced quantum capture of the neonate's cone lattice. From Banks and Bennett (1988).

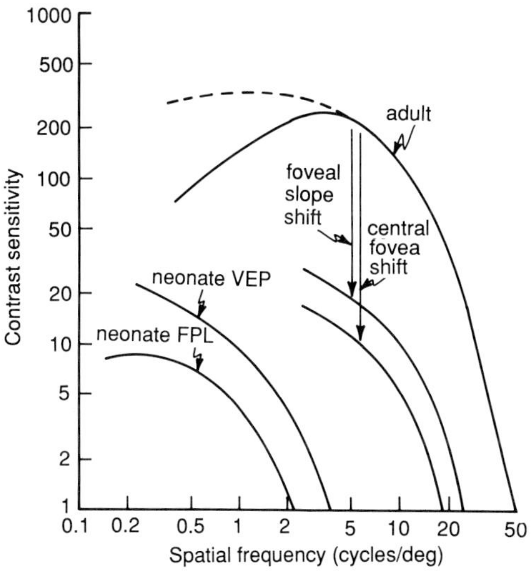

FIG. 9 Empirically determined adult and infant contrast sensitivity functions and the predicted loss of sensitivity caused by optical and receptoral factors. The curves labeled "Neonate FPL," "Neonate VEP," and "Adult" are from Fig. 1. Each vertical arrow represents the ratio of the ideal neonate sensitivity to the ideal adult sensitivity at each spatial frequency. The reductions in contrast sensitivity indicated by the arrows represent the effects of smaller image magnification, coarser spatial sampling by the cone lattice (two relatively small effects), and less efficient photoreception in the neonate. The curves at the bottom of the arrows are the CSFs one would expect if adult and neonatal visual systems were identical except for the preneural factors listed in Tables 1 and 3. From Banks and Bennett (1988).

If the visual systems of adults and newborns were identical except in eye size and cone dimensions, they should differ at each spatial frequency by about 20:1, as indicated by the arrows. The shifted function is not shown for spatial frequencies below 3 cycles/degree because lateral interactions among retinal neurons, a factor not included in this analysis, are required to explain the low-frequency rolloff of the adult CSF (Kelly, 1977). It is clear that the shifting accounts for a substantial fraction of the observed newborn–adult disparity, but not all of it. Therefore, additional factors must contribute to the newborn performance deficit. There are, of course, numerous candidates for these additional factors (inappropriate spatial and temporal summation, neural noise, poor motivation to respond, and so on).

Before ending this discussion, a caveat should be added. It is not clear which region of the retina infants actually use during contrast sensitivity experiments. Despite the fact that the fovea is very large at birth, it is possible that newborns' responses are primarily mediated by the parafovea or near periphery. It is also possible that newborns' parafoveal cones are more efficient than their foveal cones. Thus, the difference between predicted and observed contrast sensitivity might be greater than that indicated in Fig. 9. Unfortunately, this possibility cannot be evaluated because at present there are no quantitative data on young extrafoveal cones.

It can be concluded, therefore, that within the assumptions of the analysis performed by Banks and Bennett (1988), much of the spatial visual deficits observed early in life can be accounted for by immaturities in the morphology of foveal cones. In other words, a major constraint on spatial visual performance is the poor quantum catching and isomerization of the newborn's foveal cone lattice. The reduced sampling density of the young cone lattice is probably not an important limitation even to acuity, despite statements to the contrary (Jacobs & Blakemore, 1988). The receptor immaturities delineated here do not appear to account for all of the observed deficit in contrast sensitivity and acuity. To explain the entire developmental deficit, it is necessary to examine subsequent stages in the visual process. The development of some of these stages is discussed in the following sections of this chapter.

III. DEVELOPMENT OF PRECORTICAL AND CORTICAL VISUAL PATHWAYS IN HUMAN INFANTS

Three interacting changes have been proposed to take place during the development of human visual capabilities (Braddick & Atkinson, 1987): (1) sensory channels specifically tuned to particular visual attributes become functional; (2) attentional mechanisms develop in the active control of eye movements, so that the infant can direct focal attention at will; and

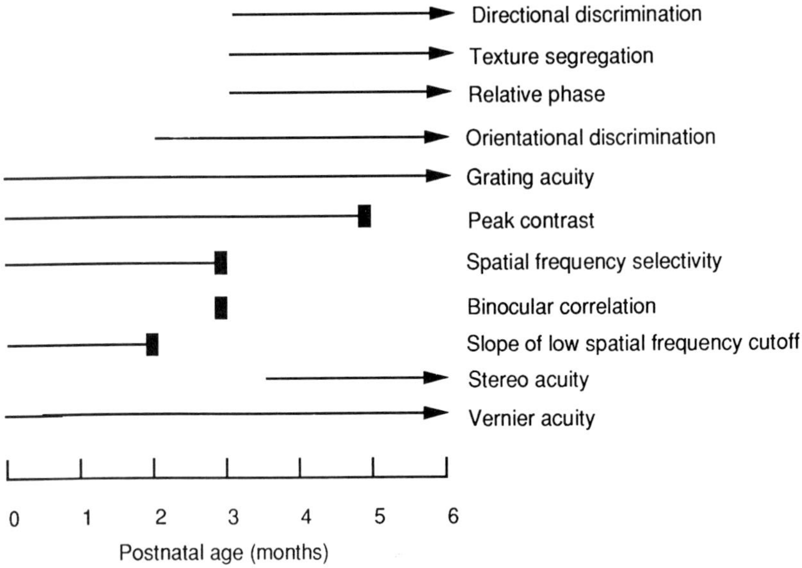

FIG. 10 Developmental timing of various visual functions in human infants. The beginning of each line marks the age of onset of the function concerned, with arrowed lines indicating continuing development. A rectangle indicates the age at which adultlike performance on a given function is believed to be attained.

(3) information becomes integrated across different sensory modalities, allowing object perception and scene analysis. This section presents a discussion of data on the development of selective channels and possible links between changes in behavior and underlying neural mechanisms.

Much of the research on infant visual development has concentrated on the development of sensory discriminations. Taking data from a range of different studies, Figure 10 illustrates a broad consensus view of the developmental timing of various visual functions. Figure 11 shows a similar view of changes in eye movement control that parallel the sensory development. At least crude forms of some visual attributes can be detected at birth, while others appear to be absent. The appearance of new attributes and improvements in selectivity occur over many postnatal months.

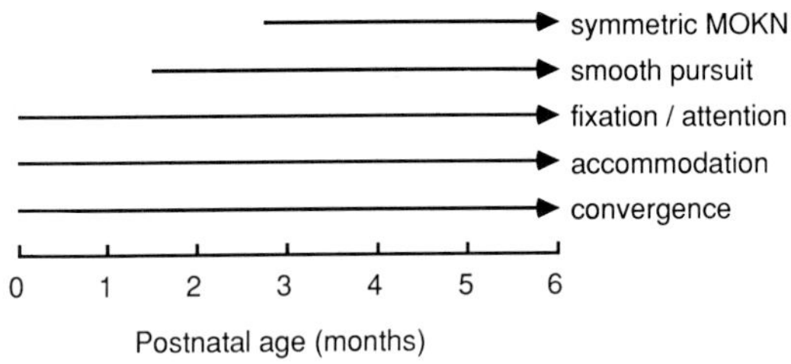

FIG. 11 Consensus view of the development of human eye movement control, with the same conventions as Fig. 10.

A. Spatial Detail

Detection of spatial detail (quantified in terms of grating acuity and contrast sensitivity) is an example of visual behavior that shows gradual improvement of performance postnatally. An initial, relatively rapid rate of development during the first few months is followed by a much longer period of more gradual improvement, so that adult values are not reached until possibly as late as 5 years of age. Although there are at present some discrepancies concerning the acuity of newborns (Dobson & Teller, 1978; Atkinson, 1984; Norcia & Tyler, 1985), it seems likely that many of these differences will be resolved when more careful comparisons are made across measuring techniques (Harris, Atkinson & Braddick, 1976). For example, it is likely that the forced-choice preferential looking (FPL) and visual evoked potential

(VEP) methods make different motor and attentional demands on the newborn. Behavioral methods, like FPL, appear to require somewhat more head and eye control as well as an orienting response. When VEP measures are used, care must be taken with spatiotemporal interactions and adaptation effects, which may affect thresholds differently depending on whether an investigator is using the sweep or the constant stimuli method (see Regan, 1980).

It is possible that acuity values obtained from different techniques may be limited by the capacities of different underlying structures. Working from anatomical and histological data (Yuodelis & Hendrickson, 1986), attempts have been made to pinpoint the limiting level, be it the structure of individual cones, their distribution in the retina, or postreceptoral sites (Banks & Bennett, 1988; Wilson, 1988; Section II of this chapter). At present it does not appear that any single mechanism can adequately account for the acuity limit at different stages of postnatal development. Rather, it is likely that both retinal and postretinal limitations are involved. Calculations that take into consideration optical limitations, such as depth of field, indicate that the poor acuities found in newborns are likely to be imposed primarily by receptoral and postreceptoral rather than (prereceptoral) optical limitations (Braddick et al., 1979; Banks, 1980a,b). On the other hand, if only a single orientation of grating is presented during testing, then regardless of whether VEP or FPL techniques are used to assess acuity during the first few postnatal years, the values obtained actually may be limited by optical blur, since significant astigmatic refractive errors are found in infants (Howland, Atkinson, Braddick & French, 1978; Mohindra, Held, Gwiazda & Brill, 1978).

B. Postnatal Cortical Development

A common approach to studying infant vision is to design stimuli specifically appropriate for activating particular neural populations. Positive visual responses, detected either behaviorally or electrophysiologically, can then be taken as an indicator of a functioning subgroup of cells or a particular pathway. Based on behavioral data from a number of studies, Atkinson (1984) has proposed a revised version of an earlier model (Bronson, 1974), in which it is hypothesized that newborn vision is controlled by subcortical pathways, and that a significant amount of human cortical development occurs postnatally. Behavioral findings that support this notion include (1) the poor ability to detect binocular correlation and disparity during the first few months of life; (2) the progressive loss of the markedly asymmetric (temporal to nasal) monocular optokinetic nystagmus (MOKN) that is present in newborns; and (3) postnatal development of the ability to respond selectively to stimulus orientation.

Additional, more tentative, support comes from (4) the inability of newborns to discriminate between patterns differing in relative spatial phase, or of "textons" (Atkinson, Wattam-Bell & Braddick, 1986; Braddick, Atkinson & Wattam-Bell, 1986); (5) the lack of sensitivity to direction of motion in the newborn (Wattam-Bell, 1987); (6) the similarities between the "externality effect" in newborn vision (Milewski, 1976) and "blindsight" following striate cortical lesions in nonhuman primates (Weiskrantz, 1986); (7) the finding that initially newborns make few, if any, smooth pursuit eye movements (Aslin, 1981; but see Kreminitzer, Vaughan & Kurtzburg, 1979; Hainline, 1984); (8) the marked improvement in the ability of infants to switch attention from one part of the field to another as they get older (Atkinson & Braddick, 1985; Braddick & Atkinson, 1987); and (9) in comparison to 3-month-olds, the reduced ability of newborns to detect stimulation of temporal versus nasal retina (Lewis, Maurer & Blackburn, 1985). Some of these behavioral findings are considered in greater detail below.

C. Binocularity

Signals from the two eyes first interact in the cortex. Probably the strongest body of evidence for the postnatal development of visual cortical function comes from studies of binocularity (reviewed by Braddick & Atkinson, 1983; Section V of this chapter). There is general agreement that by about 4 months of age most infants can discriminate the presence of binocular disparities (Atkinson & Braddick, 1974; Fox, Aslin, Shea & Dumais, 1980; Held, Birch & Gwiazda, 1980; Birch, Gwiazda & Held, 1983; Birch, Shimojo & Held, 1985), and infants become sensitive to the difference between binocular correlation and anticorrelation at a similar age (Braddick, Atkinson, Julesz, Kropfl, Bodis-Wollner & Raab, 1980; Petrig, Julesz, Kropfl, Baumgartner & Anliker, 1981). However, there has been no systematic comparison of correlation and disparity detection under the same conditions, nor has much attention been paid to the relatively wide range of individual differences found in onset times for both functions (ranging from 2 to 6 months).

It would be of interest to know whether there are any systematic relationships between the maturation of binocular function and the onset of sensitivity to other visual attributes. Such relationships might allow one to hypothesize about common pathways, or common precursors, for several aspects of visual function. A study of this kind compared the onset time of sensitivity to binocular correlation with the disappearance of asymmetrical MOKN, and with measures of visual acuity, longitudinally in a group of over 100 infants (Wattam-Bell, Braddick, Atkinson & Day, 1987). There was a moderate, but significant, positive correlation between the onset of sensitivity to binocular correlation and the onset of symmetric MOKN. The average ages at onset also were similar for these two visual capacities (15 and 13 weeks, respectively). On the other hand, neither of these onset times correlated significantly with visual acuity. In interpreting these relationships, it is important to bear in mind the differences between the techniques used (VEP for the binocularity measure, behavior for FPL visual acuity and MOKN). Nonetheless, the results suggest that development of a common, fairly specific population of cortical cells may be required for the pathways subserving binocularity and control of MOKN. On the other hand, the limits on visual acuity may be set elsewhere in the visual system, and this would explain why the development of acuity follows a different, more protracted, time course. The development of binocularity and pathways for MOKN is further discussed in Sections IV, V, and VI.

D. Orientation Sensitivity

Orientation selectivity is an important and well-established property of cortical neurons in nonhuman primates that is not found at earlier stages in the primary visual pathway (Hubel & Wiesel, 1977). A recently developed VEP technique can detect this selectivity in infants (Braddick, Wattam-Bell & Atkinson, 1986). The infant views a grating that changes in position (phase) on each frame and in orientation every third frame (see Fig. 12). A significant VEP, time-locked to the orientation changes, indicates that the infant's cortex has produced a response specific to ori-

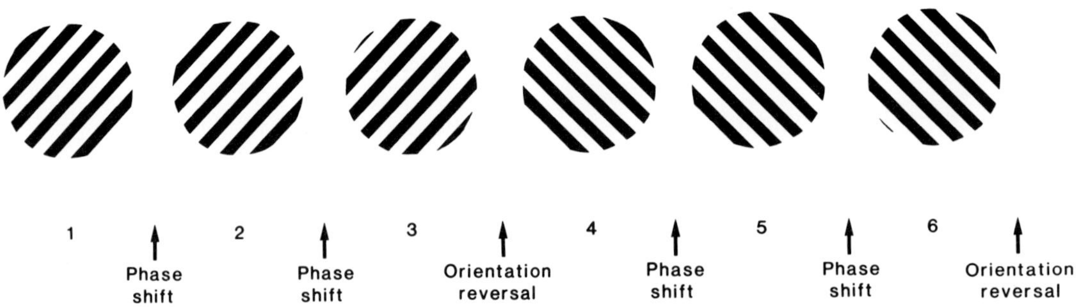

FIG. 12 Sample from the dynamic double orientation stimulus pattern. With each new frame the pattern undergoes a random position displacement (phase shift), and after every third frame its orientation is changed.

entation change and not just to local contrast changes. This orientation-specific VEP is usually first seen at around 6 weeks after birth, even though significant VEP responses to the appearance of a pattern can be recorded from infants' heads in the first few days of life. Figure 13 shows an example of an orientation-specific VEP response in a normal 7-week-old.

The postnatal onset of orientation-selective responses found with the VEP technique has been confirmed behaviorally (Atkinson, Hood, Wattam-Bell, Anker & Tricklebank, 1989) using the method of "infant control habituation." On successive presentations of a grating of a single orientation, the infant's looking time tends to decrease. When a criterion for habituation is reached, "test trials" are presented in which looking time is recorded for the familiar orientation and for a grating alternating in orientation. (All stimuli included the continuous position change as in the VEP stimuli.) A difference in looking times between the two stimuli indicates a discrimination based on orientation. Figure 14 shows the results for four different age groups. A significant orientation discrimination was found in the 5- to 6-week-old group but not in younger infants. This finding agrees well with the VEP results. It is unlikely that the failure of the younger groups is due to the cognitive and behavioral demands of the habituation task, because

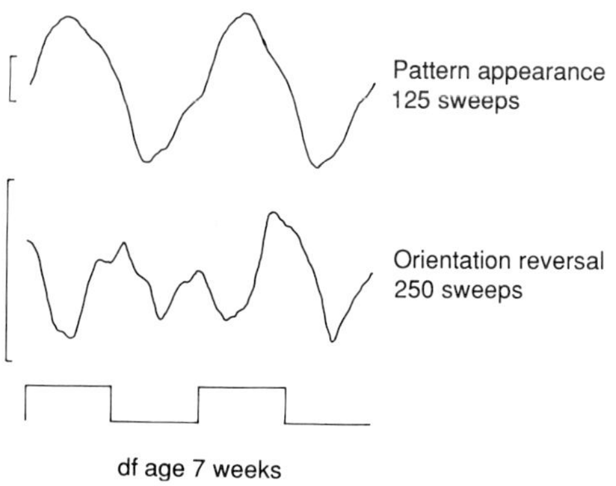

FIG. 13 VEP responses to pattern appearance and orientation change from a normal, 7-week-old infant. The bottom trace indicates the timing of the stimulus alternations (total duration 0.5 sec). Each record is the average of 125 or 250 responses. Vertical scale = 5 mV.

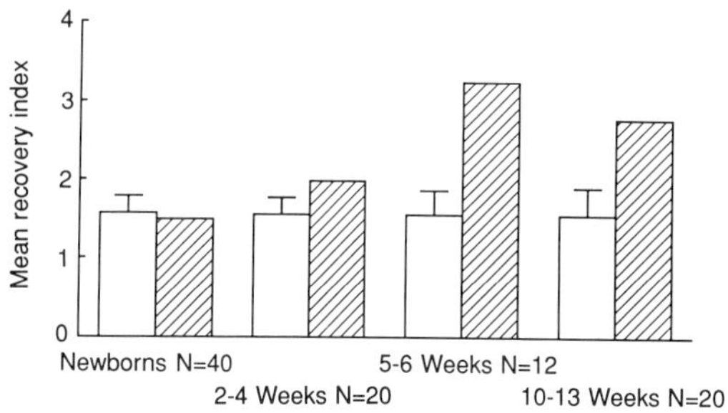

FIG. 14 Results from an experiment on orientation discrimination in infants, in which habituation was used as a control, for four different age groups. "Recovery index" refers to the looking time for novel versus habituated stimuli in test trials, normalized for each infant's looking time during trials where the habituation criterion was reached. The habituated stimulus was a dynamic grating pattern of a single oblique orientation displayed in randomly changing position ("jitter"). The novel pattern was a similar dynamic grating that also alternated in orientation between two obliques (as illustrated in Fig. 12). A significant difference in recovery index between novel and habituated stimuli indicates that the infants discriminated between them.

other visual discriminations can be demonstrated using the same method in newborns. An alternative explanation might be that the dynamic nature of the stimulus (continuous phase change) dominated the responses of the younger infants, masking any orientation discrimination ability they may have had. Further experiments are necessary to test this possibility. However, the striking consistency between the ages at which behavioral and VEP indicators of orientation selectivity appear suggests that both depend on cortical mechanisms that are immature at birth but become functional around 6 weeks later.

E. Directionality

Selective responsiveness to motion in different directions is another property that is common in visual cortical neurons but absent at lower levels in the primary visual pathway of nonhuman primates. Sensitivity to motion is often thought of as a very basic visual function, which might therefore be expected to emerge earlier in development than discriminations based on purely spatial pattern properties. The developmental course of direction selectivity can be studied by a VEP method quite analogous to that used for orientation (Wattam-Bell, 1987). The method tests for a VEP component that is synchronized with periodic up–down reversals in the motion of a random dot field. These direction reversals are embedded in a sequence of pattern changes, which ensures that any signal at the correct frequency must be linked to direction of motion and not simply to flicker or pattern change. Quite unexpectedly, the onset of directional selectivity on this measure (10–12 weeks of age) was found to follow rather than precede the onset of orientation selectivity. However, the onset is later for 20°/sec motion than for 5°/sec, raising the possibility that the use of still lower velocities might reduce the age at which directional responses can be measured.

As noted above, pursuit eye movements are largely absent in newborns, and it is likely that their control requires a velocity signal derived from directionally selective cortical neurons. (A VEP response might be associated with the occurrence of pursuit, but eye movement measurements suggest that this is not the basis of the directional VEP observed.) The optokinetic response, which is present at birth, also depends on direction-selective neurons. However, these are believed to be located in subcortical (pretectal) nuclei; apparently they do not generate a large enough response to appear in VEP recordings, at least at the reversal frequency employed (2 Hz). Thus, directionality provides another visual cortical function that emerges in the course of postnatal human development. The developmental sequence of orientation followed by directional selectivity may provide clues as to how these selective properties of visual cortex become established.

F. Shifts of Attention

Many of the neural mechanisms that control eye movements are subcortical. However, effective oculomotor behavior requires the selection of a target for fixation, as well as the ability to disengage attention from one object and switch to another (see Chapter 11, this volume). These abilities, which are likely to involve cortical control of subcortical oculomotor mechanisms, show striking changes in the early months of infancy.

Studies using techniques similar to those of clinical perimetry (e.g., Van Hof-van Duin & Mohn, 1986) show a rapid increase in the extent of the visual field from birth over the first postnatal year. Most studies have measured the probability of infants changing fixation from an attractive, centrally fixated target to a peripheral target, usually a single point of light. The detectability of such a target will, of course, vary with the infant's contrast sensitivity at various eccentricities. Thus, if the same target is used to reveal age-related differences in visual field size, any differences observed may reflect changes in overall contrast sensitivity and/or relative sensitivity between foveal and peripheral locations. The measure will also include a strong attentional component related to the ability to select and switch to a target, as discussed above.

Atkinson and Braddick (1985) attempted to isolate a number of these factors in a series of experiments on fixation shifts in young infants. When the target was a small patch of high-contrast grating presented either 15° or 30° to either side of an initial fixation light, they found marked differences in the latency and number of correctly directed fixations in 1- and 3-month-old infants (Atkinson & Braddick, 1985). At least two possible factors could be responsible for this difference. First, the stimulus would be expected to be nearer the threshold of detection, even centrally, for 1-month-olds compared to 3-month-olds. Second, the grating appeared in one of two bright patches located either to the right or the left of fixation, so that there was competition between a uniform bright field on one side and a patterned field (the patch of grating) on the other. This competition may have made it difficult for the younger infants to initiate or control their fixation shifts. In a second series of experiments, Atkinson and Braddick (1985) determined the threshold contrast required for a peripheral grating patch to elicit correctly directed fixations in 1- and 3-month-olds. When the stimuli were matched to the threshold for each group, they found that the latency differences in fixations between the groups were substantially reduced. However, if the competition between potential targets was subsequently increased (e.g., by keeping the central target on while displaying the peripheral target, or by presenting targets on both sides simultaneously), the performance of the younger infants was differentially degraded, implying that the development of attentional control mechanisms plays a significant role.

With more refined measuring techniques it may be possible to separate further the attention-getting from the attention-holding properties of visual stimuli, and thereby to improve our understanding of the infant's attentional mechanisms. For example, it will be important to determine how these mechanisms are distributed between subcortical, striate, and extrastriate areas. In this regard, it is interesting to note that the fixation behavior of 1-month-olds is similar in some respects to the behavior of patients with striate lesions (Forsyth, Barbur & Findlay, 1985) or nonhuman primates with parietal lesions (Mountcastle, 1978; Andersen, 1987). The development of controlled attention may well involve the interaction not only of striate cortex with subcortical centers but also of parietal and other extrastriate areas with each of these.

In conclusion, a variety of behavioral findings from infants are compatible with the view that at birth the visual behavior of infants is limited by photoreceptor immaturity and mediated in large part by subcortical structures. Cortically mediated visual behavior comes into play during the first 3–4 months. There are at least two aspects to this delayed onset of cortical function: (1) the selective responses of cortical neural systems to stimulus orientation, direction of motion, pattern properties, and binocular disparity become effective, and (2) cortical mechanisms for directing visual attention appear to establish control over the subcortical systems that execute eye movements.

IV. NEURAL FUNCTION IN THE DEVELOPMENT OF CONNECTIONS IN THE MAMMALIAN VISUAL SYSTEM

The mammalian visual system is an enormously complex, exquisitely organized structure, and the question arises, How does this elaborate system develop? This question is considered here by examining the formation of neural connections in the cat's visual system, and by referring to analogous development in nonhuman primates where possible. In particular, the development of the segregated pattern of eye input at the levels of the lateral geniculate nucleus and the primary visual cortex is examined in relation to the growing body of evidence suggesting that action potential activity both before and after birth is required for the segregated pattern to develop.

A. Overview of the Organization of the Adult Mammalian Visual System

The primary visual cortex of higher mammals (cats, monkeys) contains an orderly binocular map of the opposite half of the visual field (for review, see Hubel & Wiesel, 1977). This map arises from the partial decussation of ganglion cell axons from each retina in the optic chiasm: axons from the nasal half of each retina cross in the chiasm, while those from the temporal half remain uncrossed. Beyond the chiasm, the axons of retinal ganglion cells from the two eyes travel in the optic tract to the thalamus, where they terminate in a major visual structure, the lateral geniculate nucleus (LGN). The LGN consists of several cell layers interleaved by a fiber plexus. The axons of retinal ganglion cells from each eye terminate separately in alternate layers. This segregation of eye input can be demonstrated by injecting one eye with a tracer substance such as a tritiated amino acid. The tracer is taken up by ganglion cells in the injected eye, incorporated into protein, and transported by axoplasmic flow to their terminals within the LGN. When autoradiographic methods are then used to visualize the location of radioactively labeled axon terminals from the injected eye, terminals are localized in separate LGN layers. An example of the pattern of autoradiographic labeling ipsilateral and contralateral to an eye injection of [^{3}H]proline in the adult cat is shown in Fig. 15A,B.

Neurons in the LGN, in turn, send their axons to the primary visual cortex. The visual cortex, like neo-

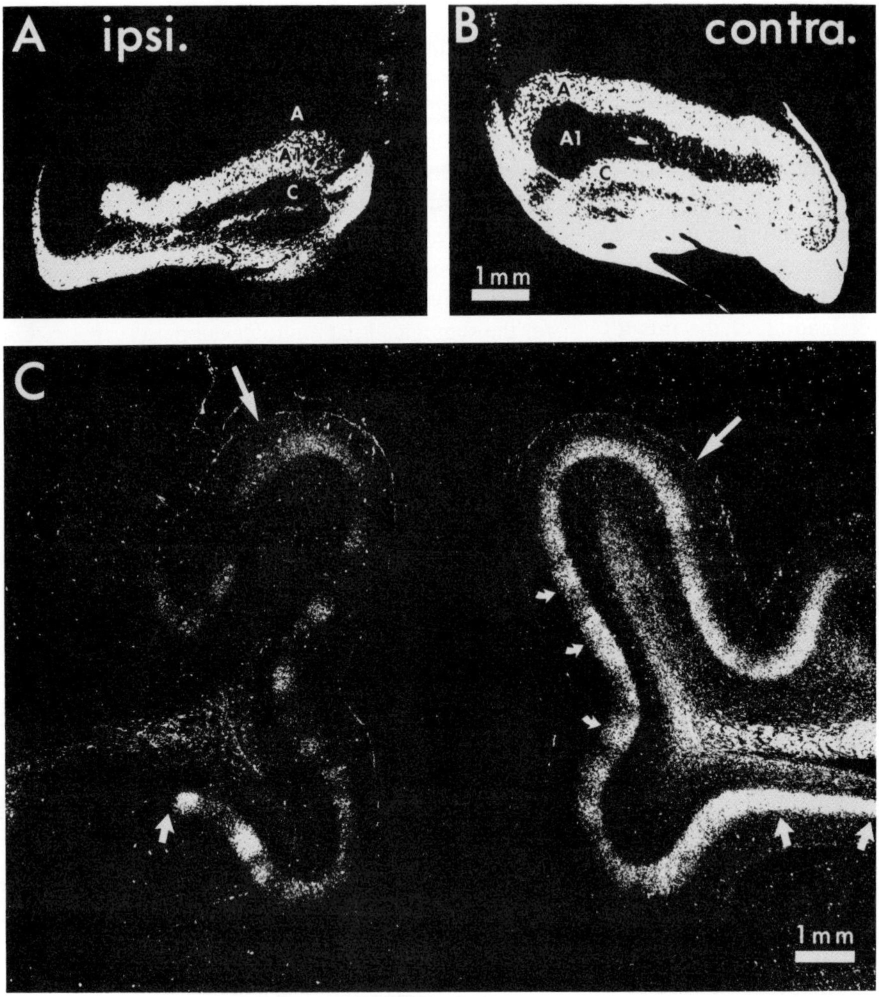

FIG. 15 Autoradiographs in which the distribution of exposed silver grains reveals the pattern of termination of ganglion cell axons in the LGN (A and B) and the termination of LGN axons in Layer IV of the cat's primary visual cortex (C), following an injection of [^{3}H]proline into the left eye. The photomicrographs were taken using dark-field optics so that regions containing silver grains appear white in this and subsequent similar figures. Note that within the LGN ipsilateral and contralateral to the eye injection, anterogradely labeled ganglion cell axons terminate in characteristic layers. Transneuronally labeled axons from the LGN terminate, in turn, in a band located in the middle of the cortex (Layer IV) that is rather patchy in appearance, especially in the hemisphere ipsilateral to the injected eye (C, left). From Shatz, Lindstrom, and Wiesel (1977).

cortex in general, is composed of six histologically distinct layers that are numbered I through VI from the pial surface to the white matter. The axons of LGN neurons terminate principally on the neurons of cortical Layer IV. Again it is possible to use autoradiographic labeling techniques to demonstrate the pattern of geniculocortical input to the visual cortex. When retinal ganglion cells transport radioactively labeled proteins to their terminals within the LGN, a small amount of labeled material leaks out of the terminals and is then available for uptake and transport by the LGN neurons. In this fashion, it is possible to label the terminals of LGN axons within the primary visual cortex by means of transneuronal transport (Grafstein, 1971). An example of the pattern of transneuronal labeling following an eye injection of [^{3}H]proline in the cat is shown in Fig. 15C. Radioactively labeled terminals are distributed in a patchwork fashion within cortical Layer IV. This experiment demonstrates another important feature of visual system organization: the inputs of LGN neurons representing each eye are segregated from one another into patches within Layer IV of the primary visual cortex. Thus, neurons within Layer IV of the primary visual cortex, like those within a given layer of the LGN, receive input from only one eye. The first binocular neurons are created when neurons situated in the other cortical layers receive connections from Layer IV neurons located both in right-eye and left-eye patches. It is this anatomical organization that gives rise to the system of ocular dominance columns within the primary visual cortex (Hubel & Wiesel, 1977).

Even from this cursory summary of visual system organization it should be clear that a considerable number of developmental tasks must be accomplished during the formation of the visual system. How are the inputs from axons representing the two eyes segregated from each other into layers within the LGN and into patches representing the ocular dominance columns within cortical Layer IV?

B. Formation of Connections during Development

To study the development of connections in the mammalian visual system, autoradiographic labeling techniques similar to those employed to reveal the pattern of connections in the adult visual system can be used, with the modification that fetal surgery must be performed in order to label connections at the earliest ages of interest. For example, in the cat, when tritiated amino acids are injected into one eye nearly a month before birth at embryonic day 40 (E40), the resulting pattern of autoradiographic labeling in the LGN indicates that layers have yet to form (Shatz, 1983). If a different label is also injected into the other eye, it is possible to demonstrate that ganglion cell terminals from the two eyes are intermixed within a good portion of the LGN at this age, as shown in the diagram of Fig. 16 (shaded areas). Between E40 and birth (E65), the regions of intermixing decrease as axons from the two eyes gradually segregate from each other and the eye-specific layers emerge. Thus, during development, connections from each retina initially are distributed diffusely throughout the LGN, and later they assume the adult laminar distribution by a process of segregation. A rather analogous process occurs during prenatal development in rhesus monkeys, where the segregation of axons from the two eyes begins some time after E80 and is complete by about E144, 3 weeks before birth (Rakic, 1977). While the time course of the formation of LGN layers

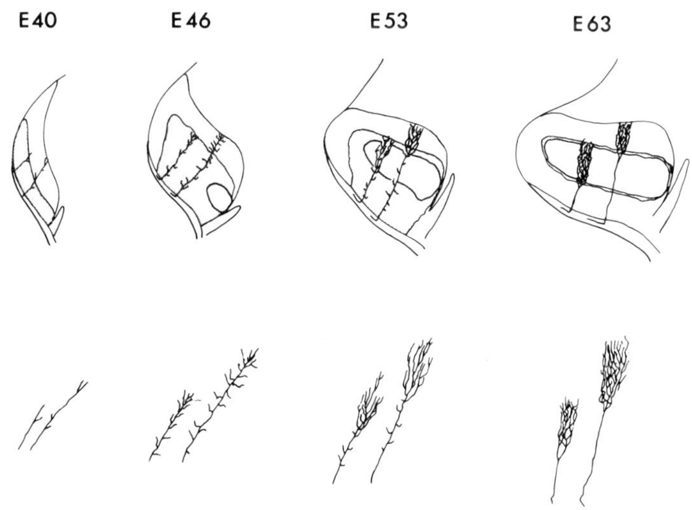

FIG. 16 Summary of the development of eye-specific layers within the cat's LGN. Shaded areas indicate regions within the LGN occupied simultaneously by ganglion cell axons from the two eyes. Diagrams below show the appearance of representative axons from the ipsilateral (shorter axon) and contralateral (longer) eyes at each age. Two days before birth (E63), the layers are clearly formed, with only a small amount of shared territory at the laminar borders; individual axons have terminal arbors restricted to the layer appropriate to the eye of origin and are smooth everywhere else. However, initially there are no layers. Note the hairy appearance of axons during the period of greatest intermixing of eye input (E46–53): axons from one eye have many side branches located in territory that will ultimately belong to the other eye. From Shatz and Sretavan (1986). Reproduced, with permission, from the Annual Review of Neuroscience, vol. 9. © 1986 by Annual Reviews Inc.

in the monkey is not known exactly, comparison between the two species suggests that this process requires roughly twice as long (e.g., 6 weeks) in nonhuman primates as it does in cat.

Further insight into the development of the LGN layers can be obtained by studying the changes in the morphology of individual retinal ganglion cell axons. This can be accomplished by using a special preparation in which the fetal or neonatal LGN is removed and maintained *in vitro* so that ganglion cell axons can be filled directly with tracers such as horseradish peroxidase that permit their shapes to be examined (Sretavan & Shatz, 1986). Results from such experiments, summarized in the bottom part of Fig. 16, indicate that when the LGN layers are clearly present (E63), ganglion cells have smooth axons that end in an extensive set of terminal branches restricted to the layer appropriate to the eye of origin. Initially (E40), growing axons from the two eyes are very simple, with a main axon shaft that ends in the specialized process known as a growth cone. During the period of segregation, however, axons have a hairy appearance and give off many side branches in regions that will later belong to the other eye (E46, E53). When these side branches are examined with the electron microscope, they are seen to make simple synaptic connections with LGN neurons (Campbell & Shatz, 1986). These observations suggest that during the formation of the eye-specific layers, ganglion cell axons from the two eyes may be interacting with each other by contacting common LGN neurons, a suggestion considered in more detail below.

A similar process of segregation occurs in the development of connections between LGN and visual cortex (see also Section V). Initially, LGN afferents representing each eye are uniformly distributed throughout Layer IV of the visual cortex, and it is only through a process of segregation that they come to form the patches characteristic of ocular dominance columns. This can be shown by means of transneuronal transport of radioactive materials following injection of one eye in neonatal cats, since the process of segregation at the cortical level occurs postnatally in this species (LeVay, Stryker & Shatz, 1978). In monkeys the same process begins prenatally about 3 weeks before birth but, as in the cat, is not complete until about 6 weeks postnatally (Rakic, 1977, 1981; LeVay, Wiesel & Hubel, 1980).

Figure 17 shows that at 15 postnatal days the pattern of transneuronal labeling within Layer IV of the cat visual cortex is uniform, indicating that LGN axons representing the two eyes are intermixed with each other. Consistent with this continuous labeling pattern, preliminary studies have shown that the terminal arborizations of individual geniculocortical axons in 2- to 3-week-old kittens are distributed over a much larger percentage of the cortex than in the adult (LeVay & Stryker, 1979). Segregation of the geniculocortical axons representing the two eyes proceeds during the next few weeks, and the adult pattern of labeling finally emerges in Layer IV (Fig. 17, 92 days). In fact, the degree of segregation within cortical Layer IV is probably achieved much earlier, by about 6 weeks postnatal, but is obscured in transneuronal autoradiographs like the one shown in Fig. 17, 39 days, owing to an artifact known as "spillover in the LGN," which is greater in immature animals (see LeVay et al., 1978, for details). A rough comparison between cat and monkey again suggests that the time course of segregation of geniculocortical afferents within Layer IV requires about twice as much time in monkey (9 weeks) as in cat (5 weeks).

What kinds of interactions are responsible for the process of segregation of axons within the LGN and Layer IV of the cortex? Many separate lines of evidence indicate that segregation is achieved through a process of synaptic competition between the axons from the two eyes for common postsynaptic target neurons, and that this competition requires the presence of functioning synapses. The original rationale for this idea came from studies of the visual cortex showing that if one eye is closed for even brief periods of time during the critical period of development after birth in cats or monkeys (a manipulation known as monocular deprivation), the patches occupied by geniculocortical axons representing the closed eye are much smaller, and those representing the open eye much larger, than normal (e.g., Wiesel & Hubel,

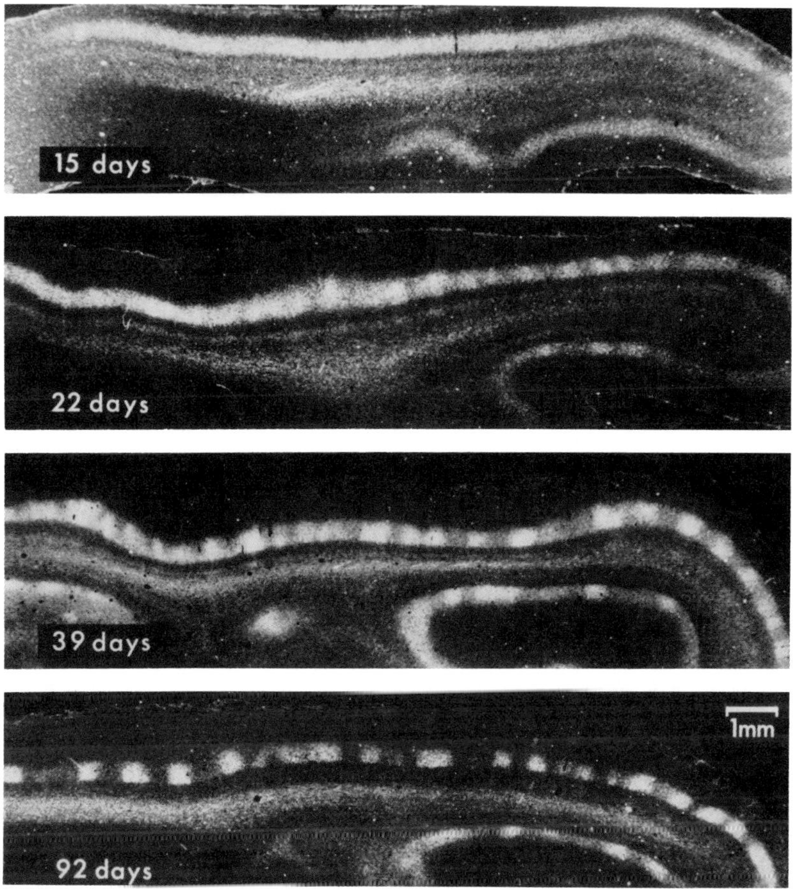

FIG. 17 Postnatal development of ocular dominance columns within Layer IV of the cat's visual cortex. At each age, one eye was injected with [^{3}H]proline, and the method of transneuronal transport was used to reveal the location of LGN axons representing the injected eye. At 2 weeks postnatal, there is a uniform band of label within Layer IV, indicating that LGN axons from the two eyes are intermixed with each other and that ocular dominance columns are not present. As segregation proceeds, the characteristic patches of label appear, so that the columns are clearly present by 92 days (compare with Fig. 15C). From LeVay et al. (1978).

1965; Guillery, 1972; Shatz & Stryker, 1978; LeVay et al., 1980; for review, see Movshon & Van Sluyters, 1981; Sherman & Spear, 1982). Since the first several weeks of the critical period coincide with the time during which the segregation of geniculocortical axons takes place, these observations imply that during the formation of ocular dominance columns, LGN axons from the two eyes may compete for territory within Layer IV of the cortex. The outcome of the competition, in turn, may be determined by the amount of stimulation, that is, through visual experience, received by the axons representing each eye. It is known that in neonatal cats LGN axons from the two eyes initially make synaptic contacts with common Layer IV cortical neurons, whereas in the adult the majority of neurons in Layer IV receive input from one eye only (LeVay et al., 1978, 1980). Thus, at the cellular level, competition might involve the formation and elimination of synaptic connections between LGN axons from the two eyes and Layer IV cortical cells, such that those synaptic contacts which are most active are retained while less active ones are eliminated (Hebb, 1949).

From the above considerations, it follows that pharmacological agents that block synaptic transmission, or that block neuronal activity in general, should prevent the normal segregation of LGN axons from the two eyes into ocular dominance columns. This prediction is borne out by the results of experiments in which the sodium channel blocker tetrodotoxin (TTX) was used to prevent action potential activity in retinal ganglion cells (Stryker & Harris, 1986). The experiment involved injecting TTX into both eyes of kittens between 2 and 8 weeks after birth, a time when the geniculocortical afferents would normally segregate. At the conclusion of the injection period, transneuronal labeling and microelectrode recordings were used to assess the consequences. The pattern of label within Layer IV was found to be continuous, and the majority of cells in Layer IV were found to be binocularly driven, consistent with the interpretation that segregation at the cortical level had been prevented. Further, that neuronal activity is instructive is suggested by experiments in which intraocular injections of TTX were made as before, but activity was artificially restored by implanting stimulating electrodes in the optic nerves or tract. Synchronous stimulation of axons from both eyes prevented segregation in the cortex, whereas asynchronous stimulation did not (Stryker & Strickland, 1984). Thus, the pattern of neuronal activity, rather than activity per se, plays an essential role in controlling the segregation of geniculocortical afferents representing the two eyes within Layer IV of the visual cortex.

The question arises whether a similar activity-driven competition between retinal ganglion cell axons from the two eyes could underly the formation of the eye-specific layers in the LGN during prenatal development. If so, such activity would have to arise spontaneously in the ganglion cells or perhaps early born interneurons, since photoreceptor outer segments are not yet present and therefore visually evoked action potential activity is not possible. The results of many studies are consistent with this suggestion. For example, not only are synapses from ganglion cell axons from the two eyes present in the LGN during the relevant fetal period, but also *in vitro* physiological experiments show that they are capable of functioning. Moreover, during the period of intermixing (E42–59) it appears that about 90% of the LGN neurons receive convergent synaptic inputs from both eyes (Shatz & Kirkwood, 1984; for review, see Shatz & Sretavan, 1986), whereas in adults LGN neurons receive input from one eye only.

While the above results indicate that all the machinery necessary for synaptic competition is present even prenatally, the question remains whether it is functioning via spontaneous activity from ganglion cells. If this is the case, then infusing TTX during fetal life might prevent the formation of LGN layers, just as blocking activity postnatally prevents the formation of cortical ocular dominance columns. To test this idea, osmotic minipumps containing TTX were implanted *in utero* at E42, before the onset of segregation within the LGN, and intracranial infusions were made for 1–2 weeks thereafter. The consequences of the TTX infusion were assessed by making intraocular injections of anterograde tracers and examining the morphology of individual retinal ganglion cell axons by means of *in vitro* horseradish peroxidase injections. One- or two-week infusions of TTX (but not control infusions of the vehicle solution alone) prevented the segregation of ganglion cell axons into the eye-specific layers without affecting the histological development of the LGN (Shatz & Stryker, 1988). Individual ganglion cell axons examined at E57 branched throughout the radial extent of the LGN without regard for laminar locations (Sretavan, Shatz & Stryker, 1989). These results indicate that action potential activity in the form of spontaneous activity very likely plays an important role in controlling the process of segregation of ganglion cell axons from the two eyes within the LGN.

Thus, neural activity, spontaneously evoked in the fetus and visually evoked postnatally, may be required for development of the sets of highly ordered connections that are characteristic of the adult visual system. If so, then it seems likely that the effects of abnormal visual experience (e.g., monocular deprivation, strabismus) also operate through competitive interactions between the two eyes which are mediated by the amounts and patterns of action potential activity, a suggestion that is considered more fully in Chapter 14 of this volume.

In summary, this brief consideration of the development of the mammalian visual system illustrates a number of features common to central nervous system (CNS) development in general. It is remarkable that in the formation of connections, for example, between retina and LGN and between LGN and cortex, the adult segregated pattern of eye input emerges gradually by means of the refinement of an initially diffuse set of connections. Refinement is known to occur elsewhere in the central and peripheral nervous systems such as at the neuromuscular junction, in the cerebellum, and in the auditory system. Just why this process occurs is unknown, but one possibility is that it is a genetically conservative way to achieve specificity in the nervous system. If each connection in the mammalian CNS were determined by a specific molecule or combination of molecules, the amount of genetic information required to wire up the brain would be enormous. On the other hand, molecular markers could be used to specify pathways for growing axons and their target structures, but the process of making the appropriate pattern of connections within the target could be specified by a few genes defining the rules of an activity-driven competition as discussed above. Neuroscientists currently know very little about those rules and nothing about the genes that code for them. However, the idea that similar competitive interactions might occur throughout the nervous system during development and that they might be under similar genetic control would considerably simplify the problem of establishing the enormous diversity and specificity of connections present in the mammalian CNS.

V. FUNCTIONAL CORRELATES OF THE SEGREGATION OF OCULAR DOMINANCE COLUMNS IN HUMANS

This section attempts to relate behavioral data on the development of binocular vision in human infants to neuroanatomical and neurophysiological data on the development of ocular dominance columns in the visual cortex of cats, monkeys, and humans. Evidence is presented showing that the onset of various binocular visual capabilities in infants and young animals is surprisingly rapid, and that these behavioral changes are coincident with neural changes in the striate cortex. This correlation has led to a model relating changes in cortical neural circuitry to the development of binocular visual behavior; this model has made some important predictions that were subsequently confirmed.

In the human infant, both electrophysiological (visual evoked potential) and behavioral (preferential looking) techniques have shown that perception of coarse stereoscopic depth and of binocular rivalry have abrupt onsets at about the same age, 3.5 months (Fox et al., 1980; Held et al., 1980; Petrig et al., 1981; Birch, Sandberg & Berson, 1982; Birch et al., 1985). Granrud (1986) has shown that the acquisition of stereoscopic depth discrimination in infants is accompanied by improved accuracy of reaching in depth. The onset of coarse depth discrimination is followed by a rapid increase in stereoacuity, which approaches adult levels within a few more weeks (Held et al., 1980; Birch et al., 1982). This sudden onset and rapid improvement stand in stark contrast to the development of grating acuity, which is present at the earliest age of testing (shortly after birth) and increases relatively slowly (Dobson & Teller, 1978; Gwiazda, Brill, Mohindra & Held, 1978, 1980). Vernier acuity develops more rapidly than grating acuity, but it is also measurable at the earliest age of testing (Shimojo, Birch, Gwiazda & Held, 1984). Why is the acquisition of binocular function distinguished from these other measures of visual function by being absent in the earliest months? One may suspect that some form of neural processing circuitry is simply not present in the neonatal nervous system, but becomes so in the course of normal neuronal development. Because we know so few details about the developing nervous system of the human infant, it is useful to consider analogous stages of visual development in other young animals for which more extensive data are available. The cat is one such animal, and, like humans and monkeys, it enjoys stereopsis.

Data on the acquisition of stereopsis and the development of stereoacuity in the cat are consistent with results from humans, but in cats these behavioral events take place a factor of three to four times earlier in life than in humans. The sensitivity to depth intervals, as tested behaviorally on a jumping stand by Timney (1981), rises rapidly during the fifth and sixth weeks of life. Binocular discrimination of depth intervals rises more rapidly and to a higher level of sensitivity than monocular discrimination. This difference provides grounds for claiming that the basis for the binocular discrimination is indeed stereopsis, since this function yields the more sensitive discrimination of depth.

Is there some event in the development of the cat visual system that parallels this abrupt change in visual capability? In particular, what neural event might correlate with the relatively late and rather sudden onset of the ability to process visual input for stereopsis based on retinal disparities? One might expect such a definitive behavioral marker to be accompanied by some distinctive change in the underlying neuronal substrate. Examination of such changes indicates that the anatomical segregation of ocular dominance columns in Layer IV of cat striate cortex approaches completion at about the same time as the behavioral changes are observed (e.g., LeVay, Stryker & Shatz, 1978, Section IV of this chapter). Moreover, Pettigrew (1974) has shown that single cells in the cat's striate cortex first respond to binocularly disparate stimuli—a prerequisite for stereopsis—at about the same age as stereopsis can be elicited behaviorally.

According to the fragmentary data that are available, the segregation of the ocular dominance columns in Layer IV of human striate cortex is completed between 4 and 6 months of age (Hickey & Peduzzi, 1987). What may be the significance of this segregation for binocular vision? Held (1985) has proposed a model (Fig. 18) that attempts to answer this question. In brief, prior to segregation of the ocular dominance columns, the overlap of the thalamocortical afferents from the two eyes in Layer IV of striate cortex causes a loss of eye-of-origin information. Therefore, the two monocular inputs cannot interact either in Area 17 or any other extrastriate visual area. This lack of interaction presumably precludes disparity detection and binocular rivalry during the early period of overlap. Only after sufficient segregation has occurred to allow preservation of eye-of-origin information can the subsequent interocular information processing take place.

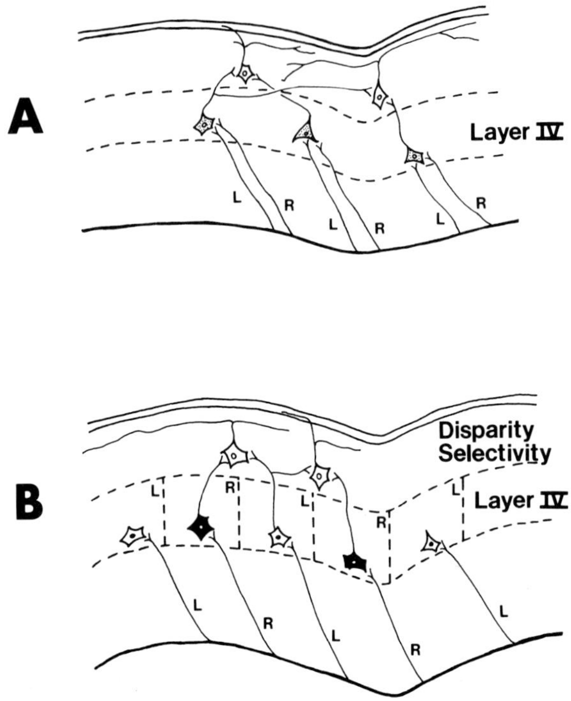

FIG. 18 Segregation of ocular dominance columns. (A) Geniculostriate afferents carrying signals from the right (R) or left (L) eye synapse on the same cells in cortical Layer IV, thereby losing information about the eye origin. (B) Geniculostriate afferents are segregated on the basis of eye of origin (R or L), and consequently recipient cells in Layer IV may send their axons to cells outside of that layer and synapse on cells which may be disparity selective.

The neuronal mechanism proposed in this model can be criticized on at least two counts. First, the process of anatomical segregation is not sudden. Can this relatively slow process account for the relatively abrupt onset of stereopsis? In response to this criticism, it is suggested that, as in the onset of many other forms of behavior, an underlying neuronal process that develops relatively slowly may at some point exceed an internal threshold, thereby allowing the sudden expression of a particular behavior. Moreover, it is recognized that while segregation of the ocular dominance columns may be a necessary condition for binocularity, it is not sufficient. Neuronal circuitry for analyzing the interocular differences also must be available. A second possible criticism is that some species, like the tree shrew, have stereopsis but do not have segregated ocular dominance columns. This criticism can be answered by assuming that different species have evolved different strategies for solving the same problem, and functional segregation of ocular inputs may be achieved by alternative anatomical layouts.

Apart from the validity of the specific neuronal mechanism, it is possible to test the functional implications of this model. What consequences might be expected to result from the absence of eye-of-origin information in prestereoscopic vision? The model suggests that inputs from the two eyes might be nonselectively combined in the single cortical representation of the images on the two retinas. Thus, if a vertical grating is presented to the right eye and a horizontal one to the left eye, the superimposed representation of the orthogonal gratings should appear as a plaid or grid figure. This suggests a simple test. It is known that infants prefer to look at a grid rather than a simple grating during the first 6 months (Fantz et al., 1962). Beginning at the age of onset of stereopsis, they also prefer to look at a binocularly fused rather than a rivalrous stimulus. If the orthogonal gratings yield the appearance of a grid by nonselective superposition, then they should be preferred to the fused (and therefore simple) gratings. However, if the orthogonal gratings should rival, they will not be attended to.

If the above reasoning is correct, then prestereoptic infants should prefer to look at orthogonal gratings, but their preference should shift to parallel gratings when selective binocular processing becomes available. Consequently, Shimojo, Bauer, O'Connell, and Held (1986) performed an experiment in which binocularly superimposed orthogonal grating stimuli were paired with binocularly superimposed parallel (hence fusible) gratings in a two-choice, preferential looking arrangement. The results showed that, following an initial preference for the orthogonal gratings of close to 100% during the first few months, there was a sudden shift to a preference of close to 100% for the parallel gratings. This shift occurred at about 3.5 months, the approximate age of acquisition of stereopsis, and was completed within an average time interval of 2 weeks for each infant. This result clearly confirms the abruptness of the transition to adultlike binocularity. It is also the first demonstration of a complete reversal of an infant visual preference. Finally, it confirms the validity of the model of the effects of segregation of the ocular dominance columns.

The very rapid increase in stereoacuity, following the onset of coarse stereopsis, may call for an explanation like that put forward to account for the rapid rise of vernier acuity during this period of infant development (Shimojo et al., 1984; Shimojo & Held, 1987). The achievement of hyperacute levels of resolution in both vernier detection and stereopsis occurs concomitantly. Both imply a rapid sharpening of spatial tuning as the result of the presumed growth of intracortical inhibitory connections. Alternatively, increased efficiency of cone photoreceptors in the retina could account for this phase of rapid development (see Section II).

VI. INNATELY SPECIFIED AND LEARNED COMPONENTS IN THE DEVELOPMENT OF THE OPTOKINETIC REFLEX

The optokinetic reflex (OKR) is a highly developed visuomotor reflex in which overall movements of the visual scene trigger a specialized form of eye movements known as optokinetic nystagmus (OKN). OKN is characterized by a series of smooth compensatory eye movements in the same direction as the movement of the visual scene (known as the "slow phase" of OKN), interspersed with rapid return eye movements in the opposite direction (the "fast phase" of OKN). The OKR is ubiquitous in the animal kingdom and in humans can be observed in the first days of life (see Section III). It is perhaps most easily observed by watching the eyes of someone who is riding in a moving vehicle and gazing at the scenery drifting by the window. By eliciting OKN, the OKR is constantly striving to achieve a stable retinal image of the moving visual world, an act clearly designed to facilitate resolution of the spatial details of moving stimuli by the visual system.

It is known that an essential component of the neural circuitry subserving the OKR is the pretectal nucleus of the optic tract (NOT), a small cluster of cells in the midbrain that relay signals related to movement of the visual image on the retina (Hoffmann, 1982; Precht, 1982). Comparative neuroanatomical studies in mammals have shown that while NOT cells receive projections both from the retina and from the visual areas of the neocortex, the proportion of visual input received indirectly from the cortex, as opposed to directly from the retina, increases as one ascends the phylogenetic tree. Studies of the development of the OKR in animals, and of the neural pathways that subserve this important visual reflex, have provided insight into the rules by which signals from the retina and visual cortex interact during development to give rise to the specific properties of neurons in the NOT of mammals.

This section presents a brief discussion of a proposed model (Hoffmann, 1987) that explains development of the OKR in various mammals in terms of specific interactions between an innately specified retinal component to the response properties of NOT cells and a later developing cortical component that is learned. The basic features of this model can be described as follows:

1. Axons from directionally selective retinal ganglion cells reach the NOT first during ontogeny. This projection is innately specified and can develop in the absence of visual experience.
2. Cortical projections to the NOT arrive later in development and are allowed to synapse onto NOT cells only if the signals they carry agree with those carried by the retinal axons. Normal binocular visual experience is critical for successful formation of this second set of connections.
3. After the corticopretectal projection has been established, retinopretectal connections gradually lose their influence over NOT cells, and ultimately they are replaced by the cortical projections.

As discussed below, this model of the development of the OKR can account for a variety of experimental findings, including (1) why the OKR normally is asymmetric early in development; (2) why, following lesions of the visual cortex in adult animals, the reflex becomes weaker and asymmetric in cats and monkeys and disappears in man; and (3) why monocular deprivation or strabismus during development leads to a loss of binocularity in the NOT and, as a consequence, to an impaired and asymmetric OKR.

A. Structural and Functional Organization of the Nucleus of the Optic Tract

Figure 19 summarizes current understanding of the overall organization of the neural pathways thought to subserve the OKR. As indicated in Fig. 19, there is an important difference between the visual response properties of neurons in the right NOT and those in the left: almost every cell in the right NOT prefers stimulus movements to the right, while those on the opposite side of the brain respond preferentially to stimuli that are moving to the left in the visual scene (Collewijn, 1981; Hoffmann & Schoppmann, 1981; Hoffmann & Distler, 1986). The output of the NOT neurons projects to at least three subcortical sites (not shown), the dorsal cap of the inferior olive, the nucleus prepositus hypoglossi, and the area of the nucleus reticularis tegmenti pontis (Precht, Montarolo & Strata, 1980; Magnin, Courjon & Flandrin, 1983; Lannou, Cazin, Precht & LeTaillanter, 1984). Each of these areas has been shown to contribute to the control of reflex or voluntary eye and head movements in different animals.

Single unit recordings from alert cats show that the discharge rate of NOT neurons depends entirely on

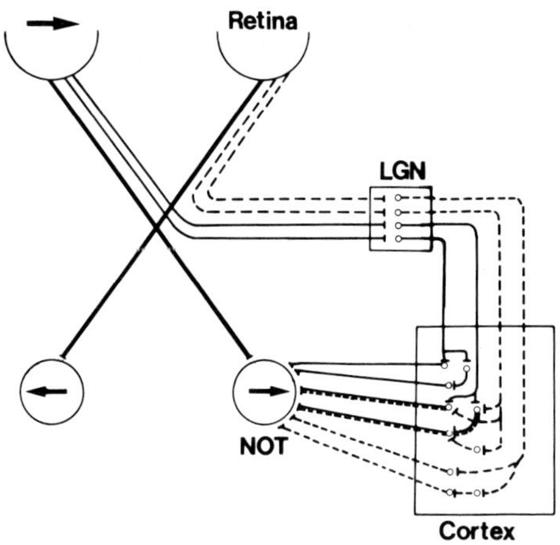

FIG. 19 Wiring diagram showing the connections from the retina to the NOT either by direct retinopretectal axons or by axons relayed through the LGN and visual cortex. Projections from the contralateral eye are shown by continuous lines, those from the ipsilateral eyes by dashed lines, and binocular projections by a combination of both. The arrow in front of the left eye indicates the horizontal preferred direction of stimulus motion (i.e., from temporal to nasal in the visual field) for on-center direction specific ganglion cells and for cells in the contralateral NOT. Cortical cells projecting to the NOT are direction specific (but all preferred directions are represented), and they can be activated by either eye alone or binocularly. The axons contributing to the NOT response have to be selected by an activity dependent process. From Hoffmann (1987). Copyright © 1987 John Wiley & Sons, Inc.

the extent to which movement of the retinal image of a drifting visual stimulus is incompletely cancelled by the compensatory slow phase of the OKR (Hoffmann & Huber, 1983). This residual motion of the retinal image is known as "retinal slip," and movement of the visual scene to the right results in a residual slippage of the retinal images that activates cells in the right NOT. Interestingly, electrical stimulation of cells in the right NOT elicits clear OKN eye movements whose compensatory slow phase is also toward the right. Thus, independent of whether neural activity is evoked by movement of the visual scene or by electrical stimulation, an increase in the level of activity in the right NOT over that in the left is always accompanied by OKN eye movements whose slow phase is to the right. Conversely, higher neural activity in the left NOT leads to OKN whose slow phase is to the left. Finally, as indicated in Fig. 19, in normally reared animals NOT cells can be activated by visual stimuli presented to either eye. It follows, then, that when the OKR is elicited by presenting a visual stimulus to only one eye of an alert animal (i.e., monocular OKR), the effectiveness of the reflex in minimizing retinal slip is about the same for horizontal movements of the stimulus in either direction.

B. Organization of the Input to the Nucleus of the Optic Tract

Several lines of evidence indicate that both retinal and cortical inputs play a role in determining the response properties of NOT cells (see Hoffmann, 1983, 1986, for reviews). The input to the NOT from retinal ganglion cells travels along slowly conducting axons. By this measure, these axons must originate from the class of retinal ganglion cells known as W-cells (Hoffmann & Stone, 1985). It would also appear that a subgroup of this class of ganglion cells, known as the direction selective, on-center cells, provides the major source of retinal input to the NOT. For example, the strong tendency for W-cells of this type to prefer horizontal movement of visual stimuli from temporal to nasal in the visual field corresponds well with the direction specificity of NOT cells. Furthermore, in decorticate cats, NOT cells retain their direction selectivity, and their velocity tuning curves very much resemble those of the direction selective, on-center W-cells. Finally, the relatively large size of NOT receptive fields could be the result of convergence of the inputs from several W-type retinal ganglion cells onto a single NOT cell.

Notwithstanding the presence of this retinal input from W-type ganglion cells, neurophysiological studies in adult cats and monkeys have revealed that the visual cortex normally exerts a strong general influence on the responsiveness of NOT cells, and that certain specific properties of the visual responses of these cells are critically dependent on cortical input. Thus, NOT cells in intact cats and monkeys exhibit direction specific responses over a wide range of stimulus velocities, including over 100°/sec. Also, many (in cats) or all (in monkeys) NOT cells normally can be activated from both eyes, whereas the direct retinal input to the NOT seems to come almost exclusively from the contralateral eye (Ballas et al., 1981; Hoffmann, 1983). Finally, bilateral lesions of the visual cortex in the cat result in NOT cells that are only weakly modulated by visual input, capable of being driven only by stimuli presented to the contralateral eye, and responsive only to stimuli moving at speeds less than 20°/sec (Hoffmann, 1981).

Several things are known about the properties of the cortical cells that give rise to the cortical projection to the NOT (for reviews, see Hoffmann, 1982, 1986). In the cat, the neurons in cortical Areas 17 and 18 that send axons to the NOT are pyramidal cells located in Layer V. These cells have quite large receptive fields (up to 5° in diameter), and they respond to moving bar stimuli as well as they do to drifting random dot patterns. All of these cells are direction selective to some degree, with preference for horizontal movements on average. They are sensitive to a wide range of stimulus velocities, and most respond well to speeds of greater than 20°/sec. Almost all of these neurons have receptive fields in both eyes, and they respond better to binocular than to monocular stimulation. Electrical stimulation in Areas 17 and 18 in the cat, or in Area V1, the middle temporal (MT), and middle superior temporal (MST) areas in the macaque monkey, is capable of activating cells in the NOT of these animals. Neurons in Areas MT and MST in the monkey are particularly sensitive to the movement of visual stimuli, and most are direction specific. Lesion studies have shown that Area MST appears to be involved in the control of the OKR in the monkey (Duersteler, Wurtz & Yamasaki, 1986).

C. Development of the Optokinetic Reflex

The model presented in Fig. 19 proposes that the receptive field properties of cells in the NOT are shaped by the interplay between retinal and cortical inputs during development. Figure 20 illustrates a possible mechanism by which selection of the appropriate retinal and cortical inputs to the NOT might be accomplished during development. Figure 20 incorporates some of the ideas discussed in Fawcett and O'Leary's

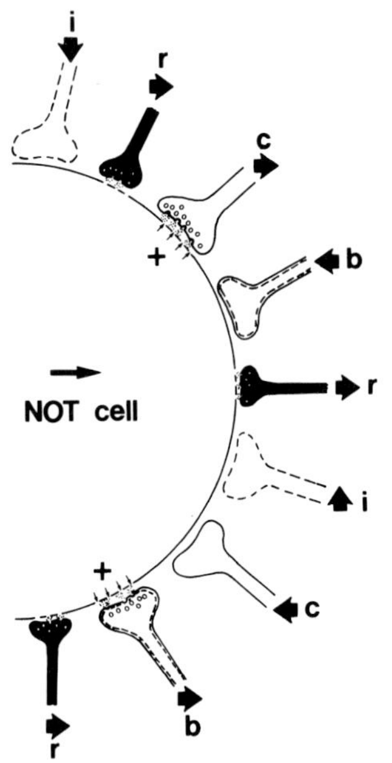

FIG. 20 Possible mechanism for the formation of direction specific connections in the NOT based on the assumption that survival of retinal or cortical projections or consolidation of their synapses depends on the availability of a critical amount of a trophic survival factor. This factor is released from the target cell in the NOT when it is strongly depolarized. The NOT cell responds preferentially to movements in the direction of the arrow, owing to a prespecified input from direction selective retinal ganglion cells with the same preferred direction of stimulus movement in visual space. This input arises mainly from the contralateral eye (solid terminals, r). Terminals from cortical axons (unfilled terminals), which increase their discharge frequency to movements in the preferred direction of the NOT cell, and which can be activated through the eye contralateral to the NOT, will receive enough survival factor to be sustained. The abbreviations c, i, and b signify corticopretectal axon terminals that can be activated exclusively through the contralateral, ipsilateral, or both eyes, respectively. Only synapses of c and b terminals, which code rightward movement, will be consolidated in the right NOT, and they are marked by a plus. From Hoffmann (1987).

(1985) summary of the role of electrical activity in the formation of topographic maps in the nervous system (e.g., Changeux & Danchin, 1976; Cowan & O'Leary, 1984; see also Section III). Its basic premise is that the survival or "consolidation" of synaptic inputs to NOT cells is dependent on the availability of a critical level of unspecified trophic factors. These factors are contained in the target cells of the NOT, and both the level and sites at which they are released are controlled by depolarization of the postsynaptic membrane. Retinal and cortical cells that have similar receptive field properties will tend to be activated simultaneously by visual stimuli, and the simultaneous activation of their presynaptic inputs to a NOT cell will cause the cell to be strongly depolarized. On the other hand, since retinal and cortical cells with dissimilar receptive field properties are unlikely to be activated simultaneously, their inputs to the NOT will be less effective in depolarizing the cells there. The presynaptic elements that discharge in synchrony with strong depolarization of the postsynaptic cell will receive more survival factors than inputs that are asynchronously active (Hebb, 1949), and they will therefore persist.

During early development, axons of the on-center, W-type retinal ganglion cells that respond preferentially to horizontal movement of stimuli from temporal to nasal in the visual field grow toward and ultimately terminate within the NOT. This growth is directed by as yet unidentified innate influences (for a review, see Shatz & Sretavan, 1986). The postsynaptic cell subsequently becomes strongly direction selective for global movement, or retinal slip, in the temporonasal direction. Thus, the cell will be strongly depolarized by stimulation of the contralateral eye with a target moving in the temporonasal direction, and it will remain uninfluenced by stimuli moving in the nasotemporal direction. At birth, direct retinal axons from the ipsilateral eye have a much weaker influence on NOT cells. Also, as has been shown for the rabbit (Oyster & Barlow, 1967), most retinal on-center, direction selective ganglion cells prefer horizontal stimulus movement in the direction opposite to that of the cells in the ipsilateral NOT. Thus, the weaker input from the ipsilateral eye will tend to be active when the target cells in the NOT are not being depolarized by their stronger input from the contralateral eye, and vice versa. As a result, the ipsilateral retinal input present at birth may even be weakened or eliminated during postnatal development. Development and maintenance of the retinal projection from the contralateral eye does not depend on visual experience, since deprivation does not alter this connection. For example, a clockwise or anticlockwise surgical rotation of the eye of a cat at birth results in a rotation of the preferred directions of the cells in the contralateral NOT by the same amount (K.-P. Hoffmann & M. Cynader, unpublished results).

While the genetically determined retinopretectal pathway is present at birth, the corticopretectal projection matures at about 4–6 weeks postnatally. The process by which the correct cortical axon terminals are selected by NOT cells depends on learning and may occur according to the following rule: cortical cells that are strongly activated by the contralateral eye and project to the ipsilateral NOT will have a higher probability of discharging their terminals in synchrony with the retinal inputs to the NOT cell than cells strongly activated by the ipsilateral eye. In addition, only those cortical cells whose preferred direction is similar to that of the retinal axons terminating on a target cell will survive. This is because only these "correct" corticopretectal synapses will be active during the intervals when the NOT cell is induced to release its trophic factors as a result of strong depolarization from its retinal input. This process will favor cortical axons carrying the same direction specific signal from the contralateral eye as the retinal axon. Other cells will be less successful depending on how much their preferred direction deviates from that of the retinal axons or how strongly they are influenced by the ipsilateral eye. Under the assumption that the activity of axons from the same retina is more correlated than activity arising from the two retinas, the ipsilateral retina will be connected to NOT cells only as an accompanist of the contralateral retina, through binocular cortical cells (Hoffmann, 1987).

After the corticopretectal connections have been established, the retinopretectal connections may gradually lose their influence and be replaced by cortical afferents. This process may occur to a small extent in cats, to a greater extent in monkeys, and almost completely in humans. So far, very little information is available on the development of this pathway in primates. However, the similarity in the ontogeny of the optokinetic reflex in cats and monkeys suggests that similar developmental mechanisms exist in all higher mammals, including humans.

In summary, the present model describes a sequence of neural events that seem to underlie the development of the OKR in humans and animals. This model provides possible explanations for several behavioral observations. For instance, the presence of weak and asymmetric monocular OKR in young infants (see Section III) would be due to the fact that early in life the OKR is dominated by monocular inputs from direction selective ganglion cells in the contralateral eye. The lack of effective driving of NOT cells by the ipsilateral eye and the progressive shift from retinal to cortical control of the OKR during development provide a possible explanation for why the reflex is much weaker and asymmetric in adult cats and monkeys, and absent in man, after loss of the visual cortex. This model also can account for the finding that the influence of the contralateral eye dominates even the descending cortical input to the NOT in normally reared cats. While all NOT cells receive cortical input, contralaterally dominated corticopretectal axons are selectively favored as a result of their higher correlations with the retinal input to NOT cells. In addition, the present model can explain why even in monocularly deprived cats the nondeprived eye is unable to take control of the ipsilateral NOT. The NOT cells are never sufficiently depolarized by the sparse ipsilateral retinal input during development, and the activity normally relayed by the more massive contralateral retinal input is rendered ineffective by eyelid suture. Finally, this model also provides a plausible explanation for why only contralateral retinal input controls the responses of NOT cells in cats reared with strabismus. In the adult, the only way for input from the ipsilateral retina to gain access to the NOT is through the descending projections of binocular cells in the visual cortex, and cortical binocular cells are rare in strabismic cats.

VII. CONCLUSIONS

The research described in this chapter spans the field of visual developmental neuroscience. Sections II and III deal with the remarkable changes in the visual capacities of humans that occur during infancy. These discussions of the development of human visual behavior are rich with references to basic neural data obtained from humans and animals. This interplay between behavioral and neural research is echoed in the following sections. Thus, Section IV describes the basic neural events that take place during development of the primary visual pathway in cats and monkeys, and Section V advances the hypothesis that in humans these same events underlie the onset of binocular visual behavior. Section VI describes a model for the development of optokinetic eye movement behavior in man and animals that is derived from a combination of behavioral and neural data from animals. The close relationship between behavioral data, which are often obtained from human infants, and basic neural data, which frequently come from studies of neonatal animals, demonstrates just how integral the overall theme of the present volume is to contemporary research on visual development. In fact, a large part of the current expansion of interest in this area of neuroscience certainly stems from the tantalizing nature of these correlations between behavioral and neural data.

ACKNOWLEDGMENTS

R. C. Van Sluyters is supported by research grants from the National Institutes of Health (NIH) (EY02193) and the National Science Foundation (NSF) (BNS-8418738), and by a CORE Facilities Support Grant from the NIH (EY03176). The research of J. Atkinson and the Visual Development Unit is supported by the Medical Research Council of Great Britain and the Regional Health Authority of East Anglia, U.K. The research of M. Banks is supported by a grant from the NIH (HD19927) and was done in collaboration with P. Bennett. Research reported from R. Held's laboratory is supported by the NIH (EY01191; EY02621; RR0747–18), and he thanks J. Bauer, J. Gwiazda, and F. Thorn for helpful comments on the manuscript. The research of C.J. Shatz is supported by the NIH (EY02858), the NSF (BNS58567221), and the March of Dimes and could not have been accomplished without the collaboration of Drs. P. A. Kirkwood, D. W. Sretavan and M. P. Stryker.

14

NORMAL AND ABNORMAL MECHANISMS OF VISION

Visual Disorders and Visual Deprivation

Anthony J. Adams, Ivan Bodis-Wollner, Jay M. Enoch, Marc Jeannerod, and Donald E. Mitchell

I. INTRODUCTION

Anomalies and pathologies of the visual system have, historically, provided the researcher with a form of noninvasive dissection of the structure and function of the normal visual system. Analysis of the abnormality in many cases aids the understanding of normal visual processes because disease produces conditions which are extremely difficult to reproduce in experimental animals. Studying impaired vision in patients may thus be considered a "reduced" version of studying vision in normal observers. In this case, alteration of function coupled with knowledge of the specific anatomical location or neurophysiological nature of the anomaly provides valuable insight into the normal role of a given mechanism.

There are classical examples of the use of inherited visual disorders to establish properties of the normal visual system. Perhaps the best known is the use of different forms of color blindness. Completely colorblind individuals, assumed to lack any functioning cones, were important in the establishment of the logarithmic relationship between rhodopsin concentration and visual sensitivity in the normal eye (e.g., Blakemore & Rushton, 1965a,b). Similarly, color defectives, presumed to have one less cone pigment than color normal individuals, for many years provided the best measures of the spectral sensivitivity of the cone receptors in the normal eye (e.g., Pitt, 1935).

Other pathological processes (infective, traumatic, toxic, neoplastic, and degenerative), especially if caught early in the course of the disease, are known to act at a specific locus or select neural "channel" within the retina and visual pathways. In some cases progression and/or remission of disease can provide a rare opportunity to identify and confirm presumed relationships between site and function. More recent examples of the use of visual disorders to probe the normal visual system, including the exploration of the role of specific neurotransmitters in the retina, are described in Section II,A and II,B of this chapter.

Another approach to the study of brain–behavior relationships has been to deliberately interfere with the process of normal neural development in the visual pathways in order to introduce changes in specific neural populations. Some of the links that can be drawn between the sequences of normal neural development at each level of the visual pathway and the acquisition of various visual capacities have been described in Chapter 13 of this volume. Complementing this work are studies of animals in which neural development has been modified by experimental manipulations of visual input, by early monocular lid closure or eye enucleation, or by lesions of certain central neural structures. Some of these conditions in effect result in a "reduced" visual system, that is, one that is lacking or has a substantially reduced population of neurons of a specific class. The results of these studies are discussed in Section II,C of this chapter.

Vision researchers have developed an impressive array of noninvasive tests to identify the site(s) or particular paths of visual processing; these have provided the clinician with important diagnostic and prognostic tools, as well as management information (e.g., monitoring the efficacy of new therapy). Some of these tests have shown foveal vision losses that were not apparent in clinical measures of central vision, such as visual acuity. Perhaps the best known of these tests is the measure of spatial contrast sensitivity which in some diseases has revealed loss of visibility for large, low contrast objects (low spatial frequencies) without any loss of visibility for small, high contrast objects (optotypes used on eye charts). Using these approaches, much has been learned about visual disorders and the nature of the pathological processes themselves (e.g., Parkinson's disease, diabetes, glaucoma, multiple sclerosis). Examples are described in Section III of this chapter.

Penetrating missile wounds of the brain, though tragic, have provided surprising insight into the way in which visual functions are organized at the cortical level. The extensive work of Teuber, Battersby, and Bender (1960), primarily on visual field defects, may be reviewed by those wishing to trace the history of studies on cortical mechanisms of vision. These studies provided the first detailed quantitative confirmation of expected visual field losses. They also showed that visual fields can be dissociated for color, size, flicker, and motion. For example, visual fields may be normal for one color and abnormal for others. In fact, this feature of dissociation was first demonstrated in patients with occipital injury; the patients showed dissociation of form and motion (Riddoch, 1917). Some researchers have seen these important studies as the precursor for investigations of what has come to be known as blindsight, where the functional visual field differs dramatically from the visual field for spots of light measured in perimetry. The issue of blindsight is taken up in detail in Section III,D of this chapter.

II. CONTRIBUTIONS OF ABNORMAL VISION TO UNDERSTANDING NORMAL VISION

A. Genetic Variations

A well-known example of an inherited retinal disorder used in the study of normal human vision is dichromacy, a particular form of color deficiency generally believed to represent a reduced form of normal color vision. Color defective dichromats (2% occurrence in males and 0.04% in females), whose cone photopigment complement is reduced from three to two, have played a central role in the understanding of the spectral sensitivities and dynamics of the cone pathways in normal eyes (e.g., Pitt, 1935). Spectral sensitivity for each cone type is difficult to determine in the normal eye because of the considerable overlap in spectral response. Studies in dichromats provided the first measurements, by retinal densitometry, of the kinetics and spectral sensitivity of cone photopigments in the human eye (Weale, 1965; Rushton, 1972). In the 1980s there have been exciting advances in the identification of genes that control the rod and cone photopigments, and again dichromats have played an important role in these studies. New approaches in molecular genetics have identified not only the chromosomal location but also the nucleotide sequence of each of the genes encoding human rhodopsin, as well as S, M, and L cone pigments (Nathans, Piantanida, Eddy, Shows & Hogness, 1986; Nathans, Thomas & Hogness, 1986).

Complete color blindness is rare (1/300,000) and is typically accompanied by severely reduced visual acuity (20/200 or less) and extreme sensitivity to light (i.e., photophobia). The complete achromat usually exhibits pendular nystagmus, which diminishes both with age and decreasing light level, and an extinguished photopic electroretinogram (ERG). The most common form, complete achromatopsia or rod monochromacy, is inherited as an autosomal recessive trait; for over a hundred years it has been believed to be due to the absence of functional cones. Consistent with this notion is the finding of a normal scotopic ERG and essentially normal funduscopic appearance. (For a review, see Sharpe & Nordby, 1989a.)

Apart from the need to help monochromatic individuals with their severely compromised vision (many are legally blind), the possibility that they represent an accurate model of a "pure rod" visual system makes these patients interesting from the standpoint of basic visual science. Rod monochromats have classically been used to study the relationship between rod photopigment (rhodopsin) concentration and sensitivity during dark adaptation. While in normal eyes higher cone sensitivity masks rod function during the first 10 minutes of dark adaptation (Fig. 1), in rod monochromats the threshold is presumed to be determined by rhodopsin alone and can therefore be measured over a wide range of rhodopsin concentrations.

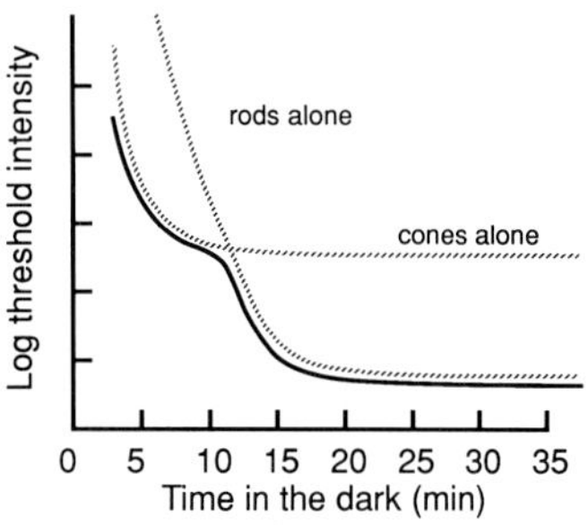

FIG. 1 Visual threshold during dark adaptation for the normal eye. Rod monochromats have curves similar to the "rods alone" curve.

An example of such a study is that of Hess and Nordby (1986a,b; see also Sharpe & Nordby, 1989b), who used the visual performance of their subject, a pure rod monochromat, to draw conclusions about the nature of normal rod spatial and temporal contrast sensitivities presumably in the absence of any influence from cones. Many putative rod monochromats can be shown to have residual cone function (e.g., Haegerstrom-Portnoy, Friedman, Adams, Schneck & Hewlett 1988), and all four eyes of rod monochromats which have been available for post-morten study had cones (Glickstein and Heath, 1975); for such eyes cone–rod interactions are possible. Nevertheless, interest in the putative rod monochromat lies in the fact that their post-receptoral cone influence is either absent or reduced, when compared to the normal trichromat. Such comparisons to the normal eye help to determine the importance of rod–cone interactions in normal vision function (e.g., Goldberg, Frumkes & Nygaard, 1983; Alexander & Fishman, 1984; Coletta & Adams, 1984; Buck, 1985).

B. Examples Involving Disease

1. Receptor Orientation

Psychophysical measures of light sensitivity can localize receptor function in the human eye, differentiate between functions mediated by rods and cones, identify the orientation of the receptors, and assess the degree to which they are uniformly aligned. How is this achieved?

Light entering the eye through the center of the pupil is more effective than light entering at a peripheral point near the edge of the pupil. This is called the Stiles–Crawford effect (1933) and it holds even though both pencils of light are focused on exactly the same point on the retina. The fact that the central (axial) rays of light can be about five times more effective than the peripheral (paraxial) rays is due largely to directionally sensitive photoreceptors which are oriented toward the center of the pupil. This property serves to enhance vision by minimizing the ef-

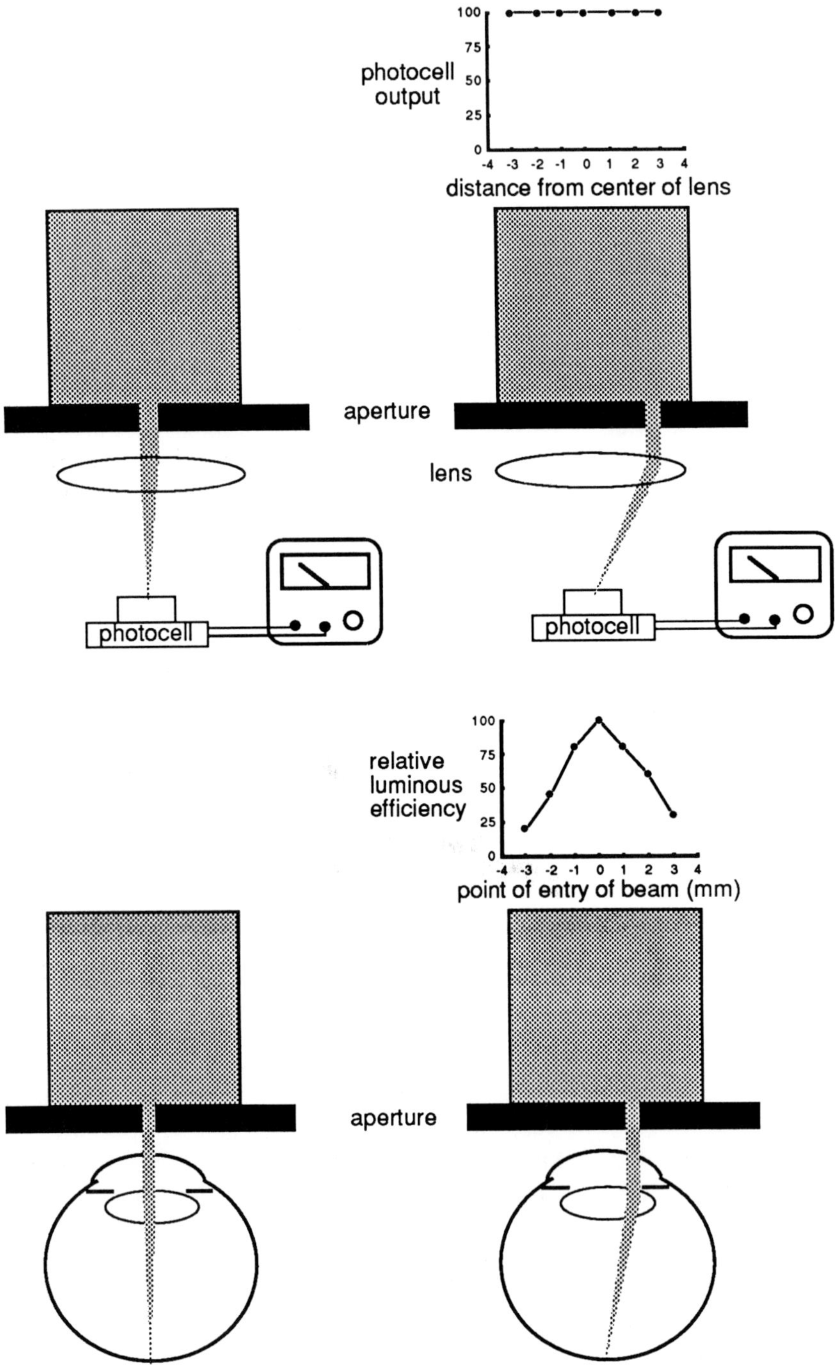

FIG. 2 Absence of directional sensitivity in a simple photocell (top). Directional sensitivity of the human eye (bottom). Adapted from Rodieck (1973). From The Vertebrate Retina by R. W. Rodieck. Copyright © 1973 W. H. Freeman and Company. Reprinted with permission.

fects of stray light. Studies have shown that we are born with well-aligned receptors (Laties & Enoch, 1971; Enoch & Tobey, 1981), which will regain their alignment even if misaligned by trauma (Campos, Bedell, Enoch & Fitzgerald, 1978). However, if the pupillary aperture is shifted toward an eccentric position, receptor orientation in the pupil plane will change toward the new center (Applegate & Bonds, 1981; Enoch & Birch, 1981). On the other hand, prolonged occlusion of light does not appear to be disruptive (Applegate, 1983; Enoch, Hamer, Lakshminarayanan, Yasuma, Birch & Yamada, 1987). These and other studies point to a genetically determined receptor alignment which is maintained by a positive phototropic mechanism and is resistant to at least 1 week of light occlusion.

Figure 2 shows how the directional sensitivity of the retina can be measured psychophysically; the resulting function shows both the location of the peak of the curve with respect to pupil entry and the change in sensitivity from the middle of the pupil to its edge. (The steepness of the parabolic function is a measure of receptor alignment.) The directional sensitivity, while being quite marked for cones, is much less so for rods when measured across the normal pupil entry (Van Loo & Enoch, 1975). The width of the function is influenced not only by the overall alignment of the receptors tested but also by the acceptance angle of the individual receptors (i.e., their numerical aperture). Insight into the degree to which the width of the function results from variations in receptor alignment, as opposed to the directional sensitivity of individual photoreceptors, has been sought through selective adaptation using different points of entry in the pupil (MacLeod, 1974).

Figure 3 illustrates two possible results of selective adaptation. If a broad Stiles–Crawford effect (SCE) were solely due to relatively large acceptance angles of the individual receptors (dashed curves on the left), projecting an adapting light through the center of the pupil should lead to an overall reduction in sensitivity. If, however, the broad function were due to "splaying" of the photoreceptors (i.e., individual receptors pointing in a variety of different directions), adapting to the same background light should lead to a selective loss of sensitivity for those receptors which are aligned toward the center of the pupil. In the normal eye little or no evidence for splayed receptors was found, suggesting that the receptors on a local patch of retina are aligned uniformly in the same direction (O'Brien & Miller, 1953; Makous, 1968; MacLeod, 1974). But how sensitive is such selective adaptation in detecting "splaying" of receptors?

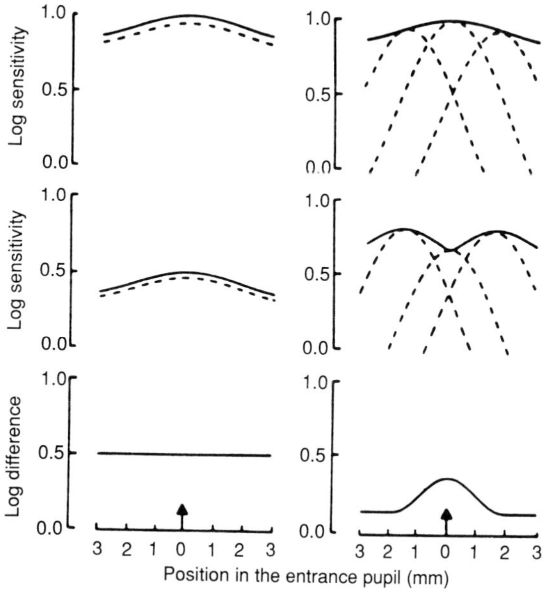

FIG. 3 Schematic representation of two possible outcomes of a selective adaptation experiment in subjects showing flattened Stiles–Crawford functions. (Left) Reduced directional sensitivity (top solid curve) due to individual cones with broad acceptance angles (dashed curve). Adaptation through the center of the entrance pupil (middle) leads to overall reduction in sensitivity. The difference between the top two functions is constant with position in the entrance pupil. (Right) Reduced directional sensitivity (solid curve) due to splayed photoreceptors with normal optical acceptance angles (dashed curves). Adaptation through the center of the entrance pupil (middle) leads to loss of sensitivity primarily in receptors aligned with the center of the entrance pupil. The difference function (bottom) peaks at the center of the entrance pupil. Arrows indicate pupil entry position of background light. From Birch and Sandberg (1982).

The study of two different diseases, retinitis pigmentosa and gyrate atrophy, helps to provide an answer. In each of these diseases the SCE has a broader function than found in normal eyes. Retinitis pigmentosa (RP) is a progressive degeneration of rod receptors leading to severe vision loss and blindness. Birch and Sandberg (1982) found that selective adaptation did not change the shape of the SCE function in RP patients. This finding is consistent with a broadening of the optical acceptance angle rather than a splaying of the receptors. In comparison, in gyrate atrophy, a progressive retinal and choroidal degeneration, selective adaptation yielded a substantial change in the SCE function, suggesting an increased splaying of receptors compared to the normal eye (Hamer, Lakshminarayanan, Enoch & O'Donnell, 1986). These studies show that the directional sensitivity of individual receptors or the degree of alignment of adjacent receptors (or both) can be altered by retinal disease involving the receptor layer.

2. Neurotransmitters: Parkinson's Disease

Parkinson's disease is relatively common, most frequently observed in the elderly, and generally accepted as a motor disorder resulting from a deficiency of the neurotransmitter dopamine. It is characterized by alternating tremor and rigidity. Changes in rigidity are thought to be a result of fluctuation in dopaminergic efficiency at the synapse. Patients have reduced sensitivity to visual contrast that may be related to the lack of dopamine (e.g., Bodis-Wollner & Yahr, 1978). In general, contrast sensitivity measures provide information not available in visual acuity measures. This is illustrated schematically in Fig. 4 by two observers, each with only a small and equal reduction of visual acuity (a factor of two), having very different contrast sensitivity functions, differing from each other by more than 20 times at medium and low spatial frequencies. Studies with Parkinson's patients have shown that contrast sensitivity may improve with dopamine precursor therapy (Bulens, Meerwaldt, van der Wildt & Keemink, 1986); in chronically treated patients, visual sensitivity changes in parallel with the effectiveness of the dopaminergic therapy at the synapse (Bodis-Wollner, Marx, Mitra, Bobak, Mylin & Yahr, 1987). Dopamine has been identified as a transmitter in the retina (Häggendal & Malmfors, 1965; Ehinger, 1983), and intracellular recordings (Piccolino, Neyton & Gerschenfeld, 1984; Teranishi, Negishi & Kato, 1984; Mangel & Dowling, 1985) suggest a dopaminergic feedback regulation at the level of the horizontal cells as a mechanism affecting the spatiotemporal tuning of individual cells. As such, studies of parkinsonian patients and appropriate animal models provide a better understanding of the role of dopamine in the normal visual pathways.

Riklan's report (1972) of reduced flicker sensitivity in parkinsonian patients was the earliest indication of vision impairment in these patients. Bodis-Wollner and Yahr (1978) subsequently reported abnormally delayed visual evoked potentials (VEPs), and they also observed that these latency changes correlated with the changes in rigidity ("on–off" syndrome). Parkinsonian patients under dopaminergic treatment showed a decrease in VEP latency, whereas psychiatric patients treated with dopaminergic blocking agents showed an increase (Bodis-Wollner, Yahr, Mylin & Thorton, 1982). Prolonged VEP latencies have also been found in rats that were treated with the dopamine antagonist haloperidol (Dyer, Howell & MacPhail, 1981). The results of this study suggest a retinal basis for the VEP delay since similar large delays could also be recorded from severed optic nerves.

Do Parkinson's patients have characteristic vision losses that provide specific information about the possible role of dopamine in the normal visual system? While visual acuity may appear clinically normal, spatial contrast sensitivity functions of parkinsonian patients have been shown to be abnormal (Kupersmith, Shakin, Siegel & Lieberman, 1982; Bodis-Wollner, Bobak, Harnois & Mylin, 1984; Regan & Neima, 1984). Most of the defect occurs in the peak of the contrast sensitivity function. When the patient has high dopaminergic efficiency, contrast sensitivity is pronounced; conversely, when dopaminergic efficiency is low, curves flatten out (Bodis-Wollner et al., 1987). The change in the spatiotemporal contrast sen-

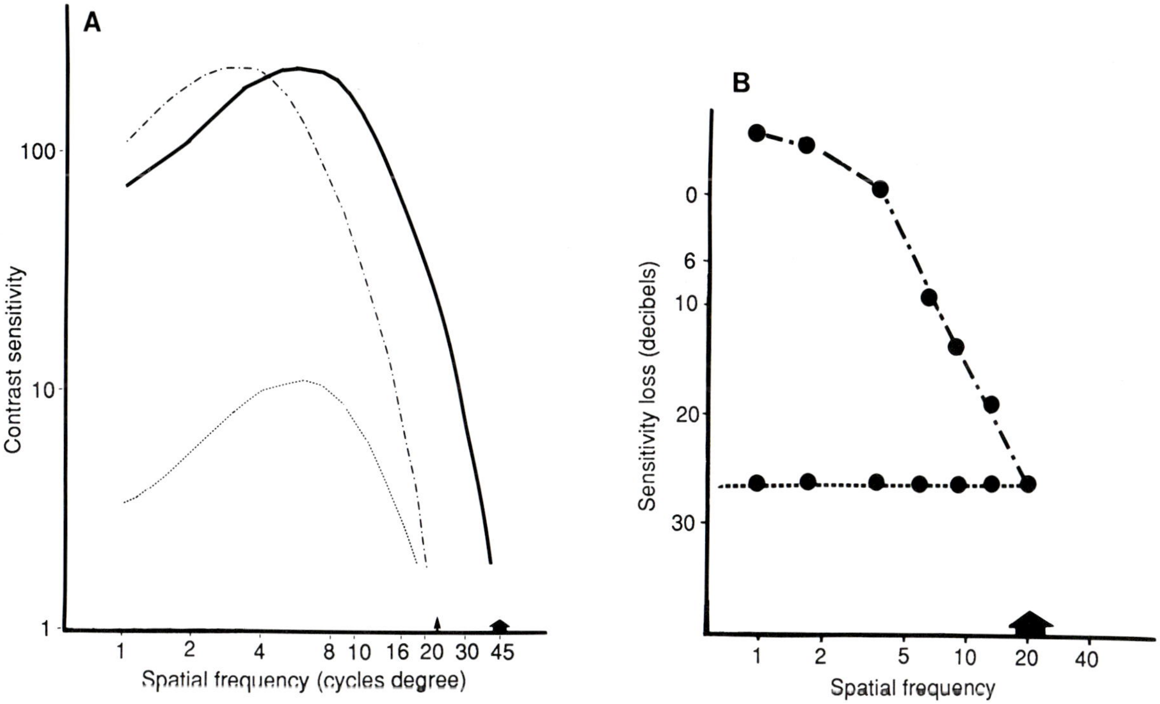

FIG. 4 (A) Normal contrast sensitivity curve (n = 10) shown with heavy line on logarithmic scales. The extrapolated highest frequency cut off (45 cycles/degree) represents the first detectable grating pattern at 100% contrast for observers with 6/6 vision and is shown with a broad arrow. A thin arrow at a cut off of 22.5 cycles/degree shows the extrapolated cut-off frequency for both contrast sensitivity curves illustrated with interrupted lines and is equivalent to a two-fold reduction in normal acuity to 6/12. The dash–dotted function results from a simple leftward displacement of the normal curve to lower spatial frequencies; the function with short lines results from a uniform sensitivity depression of the normal curve by a factor of twenty. The contrast sensitivity functions represented by interrupted curves are expressed as a ratio to the normal contrast sensitivity curve, and are expressed in decibels, at each spatial frequency. These visuograms, each for observers with 6/12 visual acuity, are quite different from each other and reflect very different contrast sensitivities for the two observers. (B) The dash–dotted lines represent the visuogram resulting from a leftward spatial frequency displacement of the normal curve; the dotted lines represent a downward sensitivity displacement of the normal curve. [Adapted from Bodis-Wollner & Diamond (1976)].

sitivity function appears to be characteristic of Parkinson's disease and is clearly not a simple change in visual acuity. Consistent with these findings are the earlier observations by Regan and Neima (1984) and Kupersmith et al. (1982) indicating that Parkinson's patients have reduced sensitivity for low contrast large Snellen letters as well as a loss of grating contrast sensitivity. Indeed, Domenici, Trimarchi, Piccolino, and Fiorentini (1986) have shown that dopamine agonists improve contrast sensitivity while shifting the peak of the contrast sensitivity function to higher spatial frequencies. Similar results were reported by Bodis-Wollner et al. (1987). The combined spatiotemporal frequency surfaces obtained with and without dopamine are represented in Fig. 5A,B. Figure 5C shows the difference between the two surfaces. This "difference surface" suggests that dopamine enhances peak contrast sensitivity while attenuating low frequency inhibition. It is thus possible that dopamine causes an overall change in the organization of the

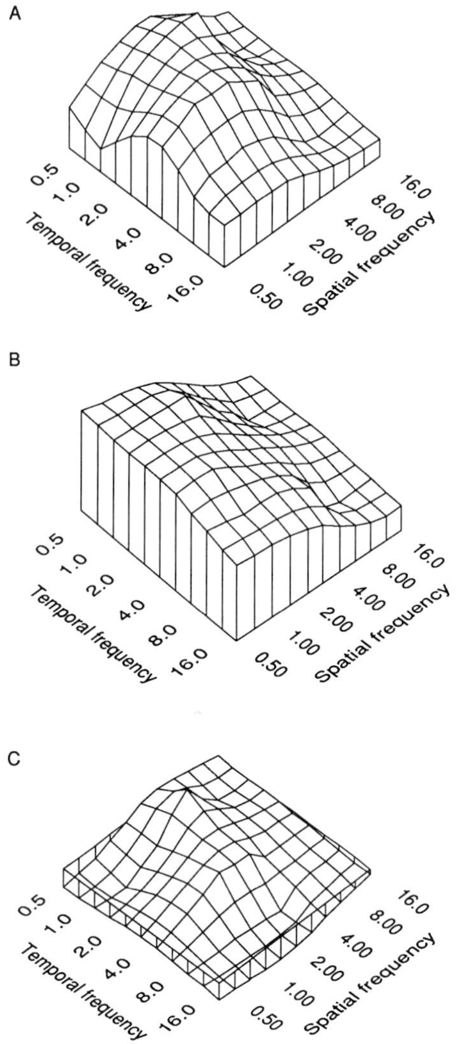

FIG. 5 Spatiotemporal contrast sensitivity surfaces for a parkinsonian patient suffering from the "on–off" syndrome. Snellen visual acuity was 20/20. (A) represents the patient's sensitivity during the on phase and (B) during the off phase. (C) shows the difference between (A) and (B). From Bodis-Wollner et al. (1987).

receptive field (as in dark adaptation) such that the center mechanism dominates over a weak antagonistic surround (Mangel & Dowling, 1985). Such a reorganization would certainly be expected to alter the spatial contrast sensitivity function.

For a better understanding of these results, studies of the effect of dopamine on neural circuitry will be needed to describe the role of dopaminergic transmission in temporal processing, along with details of the relationship between horizontal cells and feedback loops onto the receptors in primate retina. Additional studies on the relationship between adaptation and receptive field organization as a function of dopamine activity would also be useful.

C. Developmental Modifications of the Visual System

1. Modification of Neuronal Response Properties

From clinical experience with treatment of amblyopia (so-called lazy eye in which best-corrected visual acuity is reduced without evidence of eye disease), it had long been suspected that the central visual pathways possessed a degree of plasticity early in life that did not exist in adulthood. The first insights into the site and nature of this early plasticity were obtained by Hubel and Wiesel's pioneering studies. The first of these (Hubel & Wiesel, 1963) established that cells in the visual cortex of neonatal kittens displayed some, but not all, of the stimulus selectivity that characterizes cortical cells in the adult. Such cells are highly selective for stimulus orientation, direction of movement, and ocular dominance. Later work established that cells in neonatal kitten cortex become more selective only if the animal receives appropriate visual experience (e.g., Bonds, 1979); in animals reared in total darkness the selectivity of cells not only fails to improve but actually deteriorates (e.g., Blakemore & Van Sluyters, 1975; Buisseret & Imbert, 1976; Cynader, Berman & Hein, 1976).

(a) Monocular Deprivation. Wiesel and Hubel (1963a,b) examined the effects of selective rearing in experiments where the animal was stimulated in one eye only. This particular form of early monocular deprivation (by eyelid suture) resulted in widespread effects in the visual pathways and severely reduced the visual capacities of the eye that had been deprived of visual experience. In the lateral geniculate nucleus (LGN), the cross-sectional area of cells in laminae receiving input from the deprived eye had shrunk by over 30% relative to the laminae that receive input from the nondeprived eye (Wiesel & Hubel, 1963b). Subsequently it has been demonstrated that these morphological changes in the LGN are accompanied by substantial changes in the representation of the two eyes in the thalamic recipient zone in layer IV of Area 17; geniculate axons from the deprived eye occupied less than 20% of this zone while the representation of the nondeprived eye correspondingly expanded to include over 80% of the region.

Dramatic as these effects were, they were small when compared to the magnitude of the physiological changes observed in single-unit recording in layers other than layer IV in the visual cortex (Wiesel & Hubel, 1963a). Following several weeks of monocular deprivation in early life, virtually no cells could be excited by stimulation of the deprived eye. Figure 6 illustrates the distribution of ocular dominance among a large sample of cells recorded from Area 17 of normal cats, kittens in which one eye had been deprived by eyelid suture for several weeks, and kittens which had been subjected to artificial strabismus by cutting an eye muscle. Later work demonstrated that such biased ocular dominance distributions could be obtained after only a few days of deprivation in the fourth or fifth week of postnatal life, and that a few hours of deprivation at this time was sufficient to produce observable changes in ocular dominance (Freeman & Olson, 1979). Although the nondeprived eye appears to be the sole effective route for excitation of cortical cells in monocularly deprived animals, it is apparent that the nondeprived eye may retain some influence on these cells, particularly with relatively short periods of deprivation (Freeman & Ohzawa, 1988).

Comparable observations have been made in primates (for review, see Mitchell & Timney, 1984). The similar physiological results and the magnitude of the resulting behavioral deficit have led to the use of monocular deprivation in monkeys as an animal model of human amblyopia. In fact, one particular type of hu-

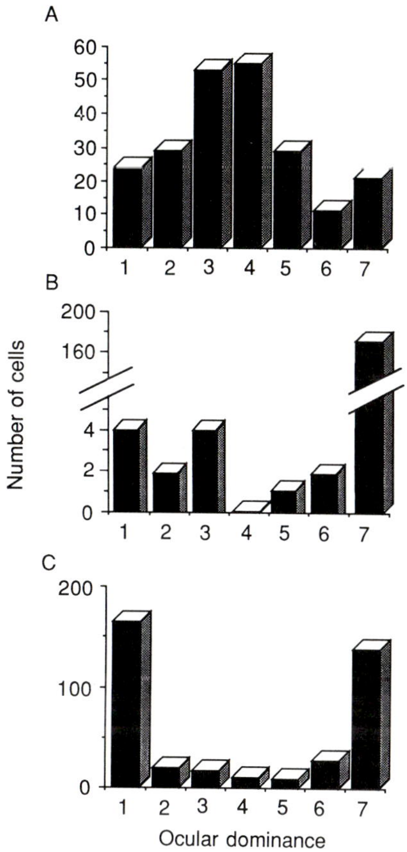

FIG. 6 Distribution of ocular dominance among samples of cells recorded in Area 17 as follows: (A) cells recorded from the visual cortex of a number of normal adult cats; (B) cells recorded from the visual cortex of five kittens that had been monocularly deprived by eyelid suture from the time of natural eye opening until recording at 8 to 14 weeks of age; (C) cells recorded from the visual cortex of four kittens reared with a strabismus induced by section of the medial rectus muscle of the right eye at 8 to 10 days of age. The cells were classified into seven ocular dominance groups according to the relative excitatory influence of the two eyes assessed monocularly. Cells classified as group 1 or 7 are excited exclusively from the contralateral (1) or ipsilateral (7) eye. The remaining groups are binocular: those classified as group 4 are influenced equally by the two eyes; cells classified as belonging to groups 3 and 2 show progressively greater bias toward the contralateral eye, while those classified as groups 5 and 6 exhibit increasing bias toward the ipsilateral eye. Total number of cells are given for each group. Adapted from Hubel and Wiesel (1965) and Wiesel and Hubel (1965).

man amblyopia, referred to as deprivation amblyopia (Von Noorden, 1967), can be caused by early monocular deprivation such as monocular cataract, severe corneal scars, or ptosis impeding pattern vision in one eye. Another form of human amblyopia, referred to as anisometropic amblyopia, is typically associated with an imbalance in the clarity of the two retinal images resulting from different refractive strengths of the two eyes.

(b) Sensitive Periods. The physiological and behavioral effects of monocular deprivation are observed only if the deprivation is imposed within a certain period of the animal's life. This has been called the sensitive period. The duration of the sensitive period in the kitten cortex begins in the fourth week and ends during the fourth month of life (Hubel & Wiesel, 1970b). Later studies found longer periods lasting until 8 or even 10 months of age (Cynader, Timney & Mitchell, 1980; Olson & Freeman, 1980; Jones, Spear & Tong, 1984). Figure 7 summarizes the results of one of these studies in which the sensitive period extended up to 4 months of age. This particular study employed a constant 10-day period of monocular deprivation that was imposed on different kittens at the ages shown. Note that the kitten visual cortex first becomes susceptible to the effects of monocular deprivation at 2 weeks of age. The effects are most pronounced at 4 and 5 weeks of age, but then begin to decline.

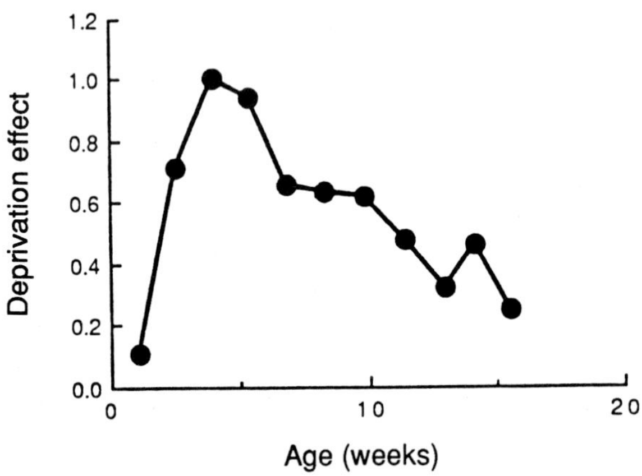

FIG. 7 Profile of the sensitive period for monocular deprivation in the visual cortex of kittens during the first 4 months. The data show the degree of functional disconnection of the deprived eye resulting from 10 to 12 days of monocular deprivation imposed on various kittens at the ages indicated on the abscissa. The effect of the period of deprivation is expressed by an index that is based on the proportion of cells dominated by the nondeprived (ipsilateral eye). Adapted from Olson and Freeman (1980).

Comparable experiments performed on macaque monkeys indicate that the sensitive period to monocular deprivation extends to well beyond the first year of life (LeVay, Wiesel & Hubel, 1980). However, in both cats and monkeys the sensitive period appears to be much shorter in layer IV of Area 17 than in other layers. This point is particularly evident for monkeys, where layer IV appears immutable beyond 10 weeks of age.

The demonstration of various sensitive periods during visual development has enabled a better understanding of the origin of human amblyopia. Although recognized and described by Leclerc (see Duke-Elder & Wybar, 1973) over two centuries ago, this condition could only be surmised as being developmental in origin on the basis of its frequent occurrence with various forms of unusual early visual input. Examples are strabismus (squint), anisometropia (different lens power), or monocular cataract (turbid or opaque lens), all of which result in discordant visual input to the two eyes.

Because the techniques used to study the duration and profile of sensitive periods in cat and monkey cannot be applied to humans, it is necessary to employ other, noninvasive methods to obtain information as to the length of the sensitive period in the human visual system. One attempt was made by Vaegan and Taylor (1980) who measured the visual acuity of children who had been deprived of patterned visual input in one eye for a period of time because of a dense traumatic cataract. Following surgical removal of the cataractous lens, the resulting aphakia was carefully corrected using a contact lens. The visual acuity determined immediately thereafter provided a measure of the effect of monocular deprivation during a particular period. Children who had acquired cataracts in the first 2 years of life suffered severe and irreversible loss of vision in the affected eye. In contrast, cataracts acquired after 9 years of age had negligible consequences, and children had normal visual acuity following removal of the lens. Although studies such as these do not pinpoint the site in the visual pathways where monocular deprivation exerts its effects on vision, the findings indicate that sensitive periods in the human visual pathway do not extend beyond about 9 years of age.

(c) Site and Mechanisms of Plasticity. A presumed locus of the effects of monocular deprivation was first suggested by Wiesel and Hubel (1965) who compared the physiological effects of monocular and binocular eyelid suture. They concluded that the effects of the latter were minor relative to the dramatic consequences of the former. They therefore proposed that the alterations induced by monocular deprivation were due to a process of competition between afferents of the two eyes at the cortex. Although effects of monocular deprivation can already be observed in the LGN, the primary site of binocular competition is in the visual cortex.

A physiological mechanism for synaptic modification has not yet been established. However, the observation that cortical connections will not be modified if the animal is lightly anaesthetized has prompted the hypothesis that some form of gating input from midbrain structures is required for synaptic modifications to occur (Singer & Rauschecker, 1982). Specifically, this finding suggests that a modification of ocular dominance in the cortex may depend on the release of various neuromodulators at terminals of fibers that innervate widespread regions of neocortex from various midbrain structures. Although the experimental evidence is still preliminary and controversial (Kasamatsu, 1986), claims have been made for involvement of noradrenaline, acetylcholine (Kasamatsu & Pettigrew, 1979; Bear & Singer, 1986), as well as NMDA receptors associated with membrane calcium channels in the changes associated with monocular deprivation (Bear, Cooper & Ebner, 1987). In general, there is growing belief that plasticity in the cortex depends on changes in neuromodulator or neurotransmitter receptor populations (distributions, number, or affinity) during development (Cynader & Shaw, 1986), which may in turn be triggered by unknown growth factors or cellular oncogenes.

(d) Recovery from Monocular Deprivation. The anatomical, physiological, and behavioral effects of early monocular deprivation are not necessarily irreversible since considerable recovery is possible if normal patterned visual input is restored to the deprived eye while the animal is still young. In cats, some visual, as well as physiological, recovery occurs after presenting normal patterns to the deprived eye (Mitchell, Cynader & Movshon, 1977). However, in order to promote recovery in monkeys it appears necessary to occlude the nondeprived eye at the time when visual input is restored to the deprived eye, a procedure referred to as reverse occlusion (LeVay et al., 1980; Blakemore, Vital-Durand & Garey, 1981). This procedure also promotes somewhat greater behavioral and substantially more physiological recovery in the visual cortex of kittens than that which occurs when the animal receives binocular visual experience during recovery (Mitchell et al., 1977; Mitchell, 1988a). The substantial (and sometimes complete) reversal of the physiological effects of monocular deprivation in Area 17 that can be induced by reverse occlusion was first demonstrated in a series of experiments by Blakemore and Van Sluyters (1974) in kittens, and by Blakemore, Garey and Vital-Durand (1978) in the monkey. Later work demonstrated that the physiological recovery induced by reverse occlusion is very rapid in both cats (Movshon, 1976) and monkeys (Blakemore et al., 1981). These studies broadened the concept of the sensitive period from an interval during which functional connections in the pathway could be modified by unusual visual input, to that of a period during which recovery from the effects of selective visual exposure (i.e., deprivation) is possible.

(e) Strabismus and Alternating Monocular Deprivation. Another way to alter the ocular dominance distribution of cortical cells was introduced by Hubel and Wiesel (1965) shortly after their pioneering work on monocular deprivation. Their objective was to alter sensory input by use of a procedure that would not exert any direct effects on the retinal image of one eye (as occurs with monocular occlusion). This procedure involved induction of strabismus. The idea of investigating the consequences of induced strabismus was raised by the familiar clinical observation that strabismic children, particularly those with esotropia (i.e., inward squint), frequently have poor vision in one eye (strabismic amblyopia) and also suffer from a loss of stereoscopic vision (Duke-Elder & Wybar, 1973). Hubel and Wiesel (1965) therefore misaligned the visual axes of the two eyes of kittens by cutting one of the extraocular muscles to produce a divergent strabismus (exotropia). Behavioral tests of the vision of four such kittens, as well as investigation of the ocular dominance distribution of the cortical cells, revealed no obvious imbalance between the two eyes. However, in striking contrast to normal animals, only a small proportion of cells could be excited by both eyes. The loss of binocular cells was even more evident following alternating monocular deprivation when each eye was occluded in turn for 24 hours. Again, each eye controlled about the same proportion of cortical cells, but very few cells could be excited by both eyes (Hubel & Wiesel, 1965).

Subsequent work performed on kittens and infant monkeys, in which strabismus was induced early in life, has produced a wide spectrum of findings (see Mitchell, 1988b, for a review). Surgically induced esotropia in both kittens and monkeys frequently, but not always, results in a shift of the distribution of cortical ocular dominance toward the nondeviated eye. Furthermore, most studies agree that there are dramatic effects of strabismus on the proportions of binocularly excitable cortical cells; they are substantially reduced in all forms of strabismus whether introduced surgically or optically (by prisms).

(f) Alteration of Other Response Properties of Cortical Cells. Two other properties of cells in Area 17, namely, their orientation preference and selectivity for a particular direction of motion, appear to be influenced by the nature of an animal's early visual experience. There is now good evidence that in deprived animals the distribution of preferred orientations of cortical cells is biased toward the particular orientation to which they were exposed. In the original experiments, kittens were reared in environments that contained contours of only a single orientation, but they were free to move their heads (see Mitchell and Timney, 1984, for a review). This obviously introduced some variability in the results. However, later studies using high power cylindrical lenses mounted in goggles and worn by the animals largely confirmed the initial findings. These studies reported strongly biased distributions of preferred orientations among cortical cells centered on the one orientation that was imaged clearly on the retina (Rauschecker & Singer, 1981).

Changes of directional preferences among cortical neurons have likewise been demonstrated by two different rearing procedures. The most pronounced effects were found in animals that had been reared from birth in an environment that was illuminated stroboscopically at a rate of 8 Hz. For humans, such an illumination eliminates the perception of smooth motion leaving the impression of a rapid succession of still pictures in which all perception of continuous motion is lost. Kittens reared in this environment demonstrate a nearly complete loss of direction-specific cortical cells without any effects on other cortical properties such as orientation selectivity (Cynader & Chernenko, 1976). An obvious change in the distribution of preferred directions in the visual cortex has been reported in kittens that were exposed early in life to objects moving in only one direction. Unidirectional rearing resulted in a nonuniform distribution with the preferred direction centered on the direction of motion experienced early in life (Cynader, Berman & Hein, 1975; Daw & Wyatt, 1976). Interestingly, the sensitive period for changing the directional preference of cortical cells is very much shorter than that for changing ocular dominance (Daw & Wyatt, 1976).

2. Alteration of Cortical Cell Responses and Perception

Studies of visually deprived animals have, for the most part, focused on the effects of various forms of early deprivation on cell populations, with the obvious functional alterations just described (Cleland,

Levick & Wässle, 1975). However, deprivation can also have other effects. For example, deprivation could increase the "noise" of individual cells thereby reducing their statistical efficiency (Parker & Hawken, 1985). In addition, it is known that deprivation decreases the sensitivity of cells so that they become more broadly "tuned" for stimulus features. Here, it is appropriate to begin with a discussion of the possible consequences of such changes for human perception.

(a) Alterations of Ocular Dominance. At first glance it is easy to relate the substantial shifts of cortical ocular dominance from the deprived to the nondeprived eye of animals to the clinical condition of amblyopia (particularly deprivation amblyopia). However, the connection between the two is not as simple as might be thought. Clinically speaking, amblyopia is defined simply as a loss of visual acuity without an organic cause, although the condition is characterized by a number of other sensory and motor impairments. There is no compelling argument that one can relate, a priori, the magnitude of the shifts of cortical ocular dominance to the magnitude of the loss of visual acuity in the affected eye. The same holds for the magnitude of the changes in the anatomical size of ocular dominance columns in layer IV of Area 17. Obviously, in the extreme situation where no cells can be excited through the deprived eye in Area 17 (and in other cortical areas as well), the deprived eye is functionally disconnected from the visual cortex and the animal would be expected to appear blind in that eye. However, in the more usual situation where the shifts of ocular dominance are not nearly so pronounced, there is no obvious way to predict the magnitude of the loss of visual acuity. This point will be made evident through a number of examples.

The first example is derived from experiments that were conducted in an attempt to optimize the extent of behavioral recovery from the effects of early monocular deprivation in kittens. Previous work (Mitchell, Murphy & Kaye, 1984) had shown that the recovery of visual acuity in the deprived eye during a period of reverse occlusion was rarely maintained once binocular visual input was introduced. On termination of the period of reverse occlusion, the visual acuity of the formerly deprived eye began to fall rapidly to low levels in only 2 weeks (Mitchell et al., 1984). At the same time, the vision of the other eye, which had been reduced during the period of reverse occlusion, did not recover to normal levels. The end result was often a condition of bilateral amblyopia (Murphy & Mitchell, 1987). In order to prevent these debilitating effects, Mitchell, Murphy, Dzioba, and Horne (1986) examined the effectiveness of various regimens of part-time reverse occlusion. In one such experiment kittens that had been monocularly deprived to 6 weeks of age were subjected to a 6-week period during which the initially nondeprived eye was occluded for only part of each day; thereafter both eyes were left open for the remainder of the day. Two of these regimens of part-time reverse occlusion, namely, 3.5 and 5 hours (equivalent to 50 and 70% of the 7 hours of total daily exposure), proved to be effective since both eyes eventually developed normal visual acuity, contrast sensitivity functions, and vernier acuity (Mitchell et al., 1986).

Composite ocular dominance distributions from samples of cells recorded in both hemispheres of the four animals are shown in Fig. 8 (Mitchell et al., 1986). Except for the results from one of the animals that received part-time reverse occlusion for 5 hours each day (C281), the ocular dominance distributions were quite abnormal. This was particularly true for animals C231 and C234 in which the initially nondeprived eye was occluded for 3.5 hours. In both cases the ocular dominance distributions were highly skewed toward the initially nondeprived eye, and the percentage of cells dominated by the initially deprived eye was low (11.2 and 11.8%, respectively). Yet vision in this eye was both normal and equal to that of the initially nondeprived eye!

A similar discordance between the vision of the two eyes and the proportion of cortical cells dominated by each eye has been reported in kittens which received a form of alternating monocular deprivation in early life where one eye was open for 8 hours on alternate days while the other was allowed only 1 hour of visual experience on subsequent days (for the rest of each day the animals were kept in total darkness). Follow-

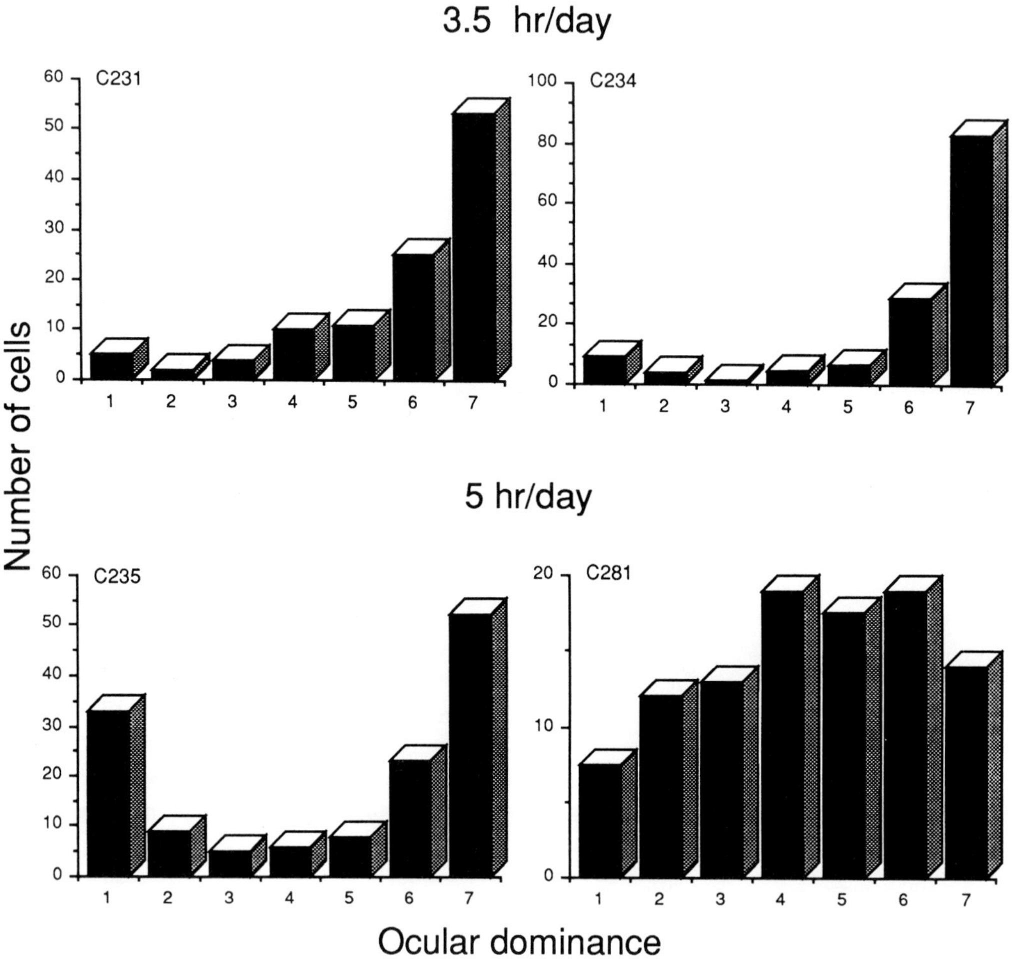

FIG. 8 Composite ocular dominance histograms derived from recordings made from hemispheres of four monocularly deprived kittens that had been subjected to two different regimens of part-time reverse occlusion. All four kittens were monocularly deprived by eyelid suture from the time of natural eye opening until 6 weeks of age at which time the eyelids of the deprived eye were opened. For the next 6 weeks the animals received only 7 hours of visual experience each day during which time the nondeprived eye was occluded by a mask for either 3.5 or 5 hours. Both eyes were open during the remaining period of daily visual exposure. All four kittens eventually recovered normal grating acuity, contrast sensitivity, and vernier acuity in the two eyes. Ocular dominance graphs are as defined for Fig. 6. Adapted from Mitchell et al. (1986).

ing such rearing, the two eyes developed equal and normal visual acuity (Smith, Holdefer & Reeves, 1982). By contrast, there was a substantial imbalance in the proportion of cortical cells dominated by each eye, with the 8-hour eye controlling the vast majority of cortical cells (Smith et al., 1982; Tieman, McCall & Hirsch, 1983).

These examples indicate that the ocular dominance of cortical neurons does not necessarily predict visual performance although there may be no discrepancy between proportion of cells and visual acuity (Smith, 1985). The behavioral capacity of the two eyes is, however, generally more likely to be related to the performance (i.e., the spatial resolution and tuning) of individual neurons, than to the fraction of cells responding to each eye (Giffin & Mitchell, 1978). Evidence for this conclusion has been provided by Blakemore (1988) from visually deprived monkeys in which simple measurements of ocular dominance of cortical cells were complemented by measurements of the spatial performance (contrast sensitivity functions for moving gratings) of individual neurons.

Not surprisingly, studies of the behavioral effects of early monocular deprivation have concentrated on the consequences for vision in the deprived eye. However, the enlarged territory in layer IV of Area 17 controlled by the nondeprived eye as well as the very high proportion of cortical cells in other layers dominated by this eye suggest that this eye might be capable of supernormal performance. A number of attempts have been made to demonstrate such supernormal vision, however, with mixed results. The earliest attempt (Freeman & Bradley, 1980) revealed supernormal vernier acuity in the nonamblyopic eye of human subjects as compared to the monocular performance of normal subjects. However, there is a strong possibility that this difference may be caused in part by lifelong practice effects. Indeed, a subsequent study of identical twins, one of whom had been monocularly deprived from birth as a consequence of a congenital unilateral lens opacity, revealed no evidence of enhanced performance in the nondeprived eye (Johnson, Post, Chalupa & Lee, 1982).

(b) Alterations in the Proportion of Binocular Cortical Cells. The drastic reduction of binocular cells in kittens or monkeys reared with artificial strabismus, or subjected to alternating monocular deprivation, might be expected to have severe consequences for binocular visual functions such as stereoscopic depth perception, binocular summation, and the control of vergence eye movements. Some evidence along these lines has been obtained; kittens reared in either manner exhibit severe deficits in depth perception consistent with a loss of stereopsis (Blake & Hirsch, 1975; Parkwood & Gordon, 1975), and infant monkeys reared with strabismus show no evidence of global stereopsis when tested with random dot stereograms (Crawford, Smith, Harwerth & von Noorden, 1984). However, it appears as though a reduction in the fraction of binocular cells need not necessarily imply a loss of binocular interactions. Quantitative tests of disparity tuning (Cynader, Gardner & Mustari, 1984) and of interocular sensitivity differences toward drifting gratings (Freeman & Ohzawa, 1988) reveal significant binocular interactions in cells considered purely monocular. The presence of such interactions provides a potential substrate for stereopsis despite a severe loss of cells defined as binocular by conventional tests of ocular dominance.

(c) Alterations of Orientation and Directional Preference. The changes in the distribution of preferred orientations that follow early exposure to contours of a single orientation are accompanied by only subtle meridional changes in visual acuity (see Mitchell and Timney, 1984, for a review). The magnitude of these perceptual changes in kittens reared in such a manner are comparable in magnitude to the meridional amblyopia found in humans with a history of uncorrected early astigmatism (e.g., Mitchell, Freeman, Millodot & Haegerstrom, 1973; Mitchell & Wilkinson, 1974; Gwiazda, Bauer, Thorn & Held, 1986). These results strongly suggest that meridional amblyopia results from a change in the distribution of preferred orientations and/or the spatial tuning width of orientation specific cells. These findings also imply that such cells play a role in the perception of oriented contours.

III. CONTRIBUTIONS OF VISION TESTING TO UNDERSTANDING ABNORMAL VISION

A. Role of Vision Testing for Understanding and Managing Patient Problems

When assessing visual disease, a number of questions need to be answered: (1) Where in the visual field does one examine the patient? (2) Did some other anomaly precede the manifest disease? (3) Which cell group is at risk? (4) How general is the pathological process? These are important but difficult questions to answer.

The vision researcher can contribute significantly to an evaluation of the natural history of the disease and to a determination of the efficacy of the therapeutic measures chosen. He can further assist in localizing, classifying, and delineating the parts within the visual system that are affected by the anomaly. Finally, he can help to understand inherited disorders and to specify the earliest changes in the disease or modest changes appearing in carrier states of inherited disorders.

1. Earliest Detection

The earliest changes occurring in a disease can often be defined by noninvasive means. Both diagnosis and prognosis are improved because the visual system is more intact in these early stages and can better respond to therapeutic intervention.

The traditional measures of vision function (visual acuity, visual fields) are most useful in documenting a patient's visual performance. However, they often fail to detect more subtle changes which are associated with early stages of eye disease. For many ocular disorders, early detection can have profound effects on the management of the disease, and consequently for its ultimate outcome. Three diseases are used to illustrate the need for early diagnosis and detection: diabetic retinopathy, glaucoma, and age-related maculopathy. These three diseases account for a significant percentage of all blindness. Each can be treated with considerable success in the early stages of the disease, and blindness can either be delayed or avoided. Yet in each of these conditions significant loss of vision can occur prior to loss of visual acuity (glaucoma and diabetes) or visual field changes (age-related maculopathy). Laboratory tests aimed at detecting visual changes in particular pathways have been increasingly applied and are beginning to find their way into the hands of clinicians who use them for early detection and diagnosis. Some of those tests are discussed in Section III,C.

(a) Diabetic Retinopathy. Diabetes is the leading cause of blindness in the 40–60 year age group and is fast becoming the leading cause of blindness around the world. In the last stages of the disease, retinopathy is common due to breakage of retinal blood vessels and subsequent bleeding into the vitreous body. The treatment of diabetic retinopathy has been aimed at retarding the progress and limiting proliferation of new blood vessels (Rand, Prud'homme, Ederer & Canner, 1985). Unfortunately, retinopathic changes seen ophthalmoscopically and capillary damage shown by fluorescein angiography may be relatively late manifestations of the vascular damage which affects the retina. Because of the devastating effects that diabetic retinopathy can have on vision, the identification of precursors to the breakdown of the blood–retina barrier would be highly desirable. Sadly, standard clinical measures of vision (e.g., Snellen acuity, visual fields) are quite insensitive in detecting vision change even *after* the onset of early fundus changes visible with the ophthalmoscope. However, color vision testing, as described later in Section III,C,3, has been used effectively for the early diagnosis of this disease.

(b) Glaucoma. Glaucoma is characterized by ganglion cell axon death typically caused by prolonged exposure of the eye to elevated intraocular pressure. The result is a loss of nerve fibers, observed as a change in color or shape of the optic nerve head and producing characteristic field defects in the peripheral retina. Clinical vision testing in glaucoma therefore involves the measurement of peripheral visual fields, the examination of the optic nerve head by ophthalmoscopy, the assessment of the iris–corneal angle by gonioscopy, and the measurement of intraocular pressure. However, there are so-called ocular hypertensive patients whose vision appears intact on visual field testing and whose optic nerve head by ophthalmoscopy appears equally intact; nevertheless, they too have visual changes as revealed, for example, by foveal contrast sensitivity measurements (Arden & Jacobson, 1978; Atkin, Bodis-Wollner, Wolkstein, Moss & Podos, 1979). The recent suggestion that a glaucomatous eye, with only mild or moderate visual field defects, may have lost as much as 50% of its ganglion cell axons at the optic nerve head

(Quigley, 1985) calls for early identification of the visual changes that precede axon death. Studies indicate that relatively early in the natural history of glaucoma there may be other changes of foveal functions (Atkin et al., 1979; Enoch & Campos, 1979; Tyler, 1981; Adams, Rodic, Husted & Stamper, 1982; Adams, Zisman, Rodic & Cavander, 1982; Airaksinen, Drance & Douglas, 1984; Anctil & Anderson, 1984; Adams, Schefrin & Huie, 1987; Adams, Heron & Husted, 1987c). Visual acuity changes in glaucoma typically occur only in the more advanced stages of the disease. Again, early, reliable, and valid detection of both foveal and peripheral vision function is needed.

(c) Age Related Maculopathy. Age-related maculopathy refers to retinal and choroidal degeneration in the macula common in the elderly. Age-related maculopathy is the leading cause of legal blindness in the United States after the age of 50. It may produce only minimal changes in visual acuity but relatively large changes in other vision function (e.g., color discrimination). The natural vision history of age-related maculopathy prior to visual acuity loss is not well documented, although individuals with drusen (small yellow spots visible with the ophthalmoscope) are known to be at risk (Gass, 1973; Chandra, Gragoudas, Friedman, Van Buskirk & Klein, 1974, Gregor, Bird & Chisholm, 1977; Sarks, 1980; Smiddy & Fine, 1984). Identification of the earliest changes, particularly of those that herald significant vision loss, is important in the treatment of this very common retinal disease.

B. Vision behind Ocular Media Opacities

Patients with corneal opacification, dense cataracts, and vitreal bleeding may have such reduced vision that estimating retinal and visual potential is, at best, difficult and possibly inaccurate. Yet tests are needed to help the clinician answer questions such as, Could the cataract (or other media opacity) account for the measured reduction in visual acuity, or is it also due to the presence of additional retinal disease? Could the surgeon expect a reasonable outcome if the cataract is removed? With the removal of the cataract, would the patient's visual field be adequate to meet the patient's needs? Do complications exist, and, if so, will they alter the probability of a successful surgical outcome? A number of approaches to measuring vision in the presence of opacities have been attempted. In general, they adopt one of the following strategies: (1) attempt to bypass the opacity (e.g., by interferometric fringes formed on the retina by focusing two coherent light beams into relatively clear portions of the lens; directing the light beam through a residual clear channel; using the visualization of entoptic phenomena); (2) develop tests that are relatively insensitive to either intensity or focused retinal imagery; or (3) identify changes in the normal profile of visual sensitivity across the retina.

(a) Retinal Images Bypassing Optical Media. Goldmann and Lotmar (1970) and, independently, Green (1970) demonstrated that a laser interferometer could be used to form sine-wave gratings at the retina behind cataracts, provided two clear areas could be found in the lens through the pupil. Cavonius and Hilz (1973) used a technique which also required a clear region in the pupil to present a target to the retina, by focusing the light source of the instrument into the pupil (Maxwellian view). This technique, like the laser interferometer, has found application in the clinical setting as the Potential Acuity Meter (Minkowski, Palese & Guyton, 1983). Each of these tests requires a clear window, relatively high luminance, and a large test pattern to be effective, although the latter may introduce ambiguity because such patterns simultaneously stimulate areas outside the fovea.

(b) Tests Resistant to Intensity or Blur. It has been known for some time that vernier tasks are relatively insensitive to light level and to blur (Stigmar, 1971; Westheimer, 1979b). Such hyperacuity tasks hold considerable promise for bypassing the effects of the ocular media and identifying the integrity of the visual pathways behind the opacity. Moreover, hyperacuity is highly dependent on retinal location, and, therefore, foveal and extrafoveal responses are easily identified (see Chapter 10, this volume). Clinical versions of these techniques have been developed (Enoch & Williams, 1983; Williams, Enoch & Essock, 1984). Hyperacuity paradigms (e.g., vernier acuity, stereoacuity, orientation discrimination, movement displacement thresholds) involve the relative localization of points in space (e.g., where is one object relative to another?) rather than the resolution of specific features (e.g., do you see one or two objects?).

Enoch, Williams, Essock, and Fendick (1985) have utilized one version of this task, the "gap test." As shown in Fig. 9, the shape of the measured vernier threshold versus gap separation curve is found to exhibit systematic changes in the presence of varying degrees of optical opacities. Gap size versus vernier acuity for cataract patients with normal visual acuity after cataract surgery provided the baseline data. The test was then applied to cataract populations to predict the outcome after surgery (Essock, Williams, Enoch & Raphael, 1984; Enoch et al., 1985). Retinal pathology was inferred when the minimum of the gap function was smaller than predicted by the cataract patient's visual acuity, i.e., the visual acuity loss for the patient was not entirely due to the cataract.

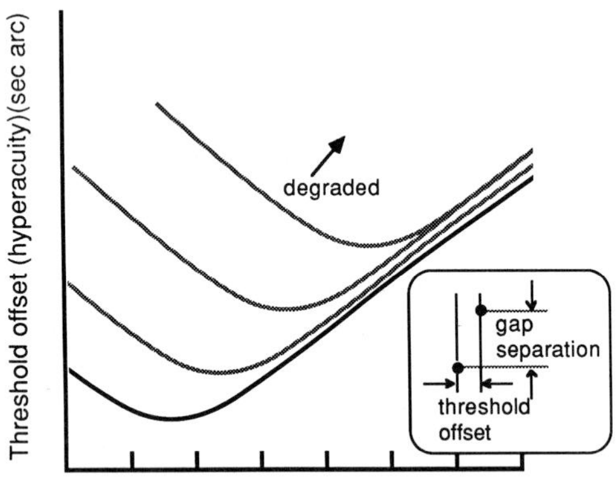

FIG. 9 Vernier acuity as a function of gap size for a series of degraded images. Individuals with poorer acuity due to cataract-induced image degradation have their best hyperacuity (lowest threshold offset) at larger gap separations. Copyright 1984, American Medical Association.

The presence of metamorphopsia (retinal image distortion) may be experienced by patients who exhibit certain forms of central retinopathy, choroidopathy, and/or a history of retinal detachment. Such distortion would provide a poor prognosis for patients considering cataract surgery. Again a hyperacuity task can be used to make predictions even in the presence of cataract. Traditionally, in the eye free of media opacities the metamorphopsia has been assessed using the Amsler grid (Amsler, 1947, 1949). More recently a relatively simple and rapid computerized video presentation of bright points of light has been used to detect metamorphosia behind cataract (Enoch, Baraldi, Lakshminarayanan, Savage & Fendick, 1988).

(c) Tests Exploiting Retinal Sensitivity Profiles. A third version of the vernier acuity task involves measuring these acuities across the retina. The comparison of visual function across the retina as a tool for identifying vision loss in the fovea is an important approach to bypassing effects due to ocular media. An example of its application for corneal scarring and cataract can be found as far back as the early 1970s (Spillmann & Roberge, 1972). In a more recent study, taking advantage of the robustness of hyperacuity tasks, vernier acuity was measured at several retinal eccentricities (Enoch, Williams, Enoch & Raphael, 1984; Essock et al., 1984). In this test, wide gap stimuli were used to examine three or five retinal loci, including fixation. Stimulus duration was within saccadic latency in order to prevent contamination by involuntary eye movements. Best performance was found to be centered on the fovea in the normal eye (Fig. 10).

This result is important from a clinical point of view because the rapid deterioration of vernier visual acuity with eccentricity produces a response function that is easily reproducible in a normal population. It is extremely sensitive to central retinal anomalies. (1) The presence and magnitude of the foveal peak in the response profile are indicative of maintained foveal function. (2) A deviation in the central retina of

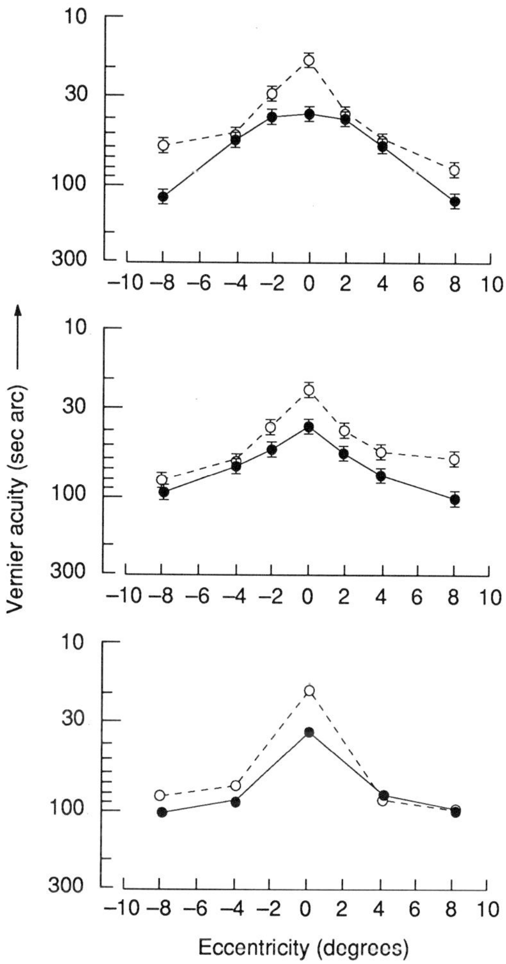

FIG. 10 Normal hyperacuity perimetric profiles obtained from three observers with varying amounts of image degradation. (a) Observer A: optimum refraction with no simulated opacity (open circles) and with ground glass simulating a 20/400 opacity (filled circles). (b and c) Observers B and C: no simulated opacity (open circles) and 20/200 simulated opacity. From Enoch et al. (1984).

the vernier response profile from its normal symmetric shape generally indicates the presence of a relative scotoma. (3) If the entire pattern is displaced to the side, the possibility of eccentric viewing must be considered. Enoch et al., (1985) provided examples of such curves obtained from testing of patients with retinal disorders behind cataractous lenses.

C. Psychophysical Approaches to Assessing Function of the Retina and Neural Pathways

1. Receptors and Photopigments

Burns, Elsner, Lobes and Doft (1987) reported a noninvasive technique for estimating effective cone photopigment density and kinetics; they used the technique to show that some diabetics require abnormally high light levels to bleach their medium and/or long wavelength sensitive cone photopigments. They attribute this to either a decrease in quantal catching efficiency or an increase in regeneration rate of the photopigments. The technique involves color matching of a mixture of red (650 nm) and green (546 nm) lights to a yellow light (589 nm). Color matching depends only on the spectral absorption properties of the photopigments involved; later neural processing cannot upset the match, only render the appearance of the match different. When the concentration of photopigment is "diluted" by bleaching, the changes in spectral sensitivity produce predictable changes in the color match. At high luminances more red is required in the match, and the increase is approximately linearly related to the change in photopigment concentration with bleaching (Burns et al., 1987). These measures of the optical density of the photopigments in eye disease provide an opportunity to identify anomalies restricted to the outer segments of the receptors. The development of such alternative methods to assess photopigment density and kinetics brings the measurement much closer to clinical application.

Receptor orientation and the degree of directional sensitivity (see Section II,B,1) of the cone receptors can also be assessed noninvasively (Stiles & Crawford, 1933). This has been used to identify progressive changes in receptor alignment and orientation in a wide range of diseases including retinal detachments (Enoch, Van Loo & Okun, 1973; Campos et al., 1978; Fitzgerald, Birch & Enoch, 1980), macular degeneration (Fitzgerald, Enoch, Campos & Bedell, 1979; Pokorny, Smith & Ernest, 1980; Applegate, Adams, Cavender & Zisman, 1987), choroidal atrophy (Bedell, Enoch & Fitzgerald, 1981), and retinitis pigmentosa (Birch et al., 1982).

More recently quantitative models have been developed to differentiate between receptoral and postreceptoral processes (Pugh & Mollon, 1979; Johnson & Hood, 1988). The Naka–Rushton function (see Chapter 5, this volume) has been applied to the electroretinogram (ERG) response amplitude in an attempt to identify the sites responsible for the sensitivity loss in central retinal vein occlusion. This retinal disorder is characterized by an impairment of retinal, but not choroidal, circulation because of a blockage of the central retinal vein. In some affected eyes new vessels will develop in the iris leading to the blinding condition of neovascular glaucoma. The ERG appears to be useful in identifying those eyes that are prone to developing neovascularization, allowing appropriate treatment to be considered in time (Johnson, Marcus, Elman & McPhee, 1988; Johnson & Hood, 1988). On the basis of their two-stage model for the Naka–Rushton function, Johnson and Hood (1988) believe that the sensitivity loss following central retinal vein occlusion occurs primarily in the photoreceptors.

(a) Retinitis Pigmentosa. Retinitis pigmentosa, an inherited disease characterized by progressive receptor degeneration (primarily of the rods), results in constricted visual fields and eventually reduced central vision and blindness. Vision researchers have applied a variety of techniques to determine the site(s) of the disorder. It has been suggested, from the symmetry of the field defects in each eye and their progression, that a retinal factor may be involved in the slowly evolving visual field loss (Finkelstein, Massof & Palmer, 1988).

Although retinitis pigmentosa is clinically described as a peripheral rod degeneration, psychophysical studies have also shown an early loss of foveal cone sensitivity (Sandberg & Berson, 1977; Young & Fishman, 1980, 1982). These losses were interpreted in terms of reduced cone pigment density. Fundus reflectometry suggested reduced rod pigment content (Highman & Weale, 1973; Ripps, Brin & Weale, 1978), and some advanced cases of retinitis pigmentosa have been shown to possess foveal photoreceptors which were shortened, twisted, and/or distorted (e.g., Szamier & Berson, 1977). Greenstein and Hood (1986) provide psychophysical evidence that the sensitivity loss is more likely to be due to a decreased responsiveness of retinal receptors than to a decreased ability of each receptor to catch light. ERG data suggest that, in addition to a loss of photopigment, an inner nuclear component may also play a role in retinitis pigmentosa.

(b) Night Blindness. Early studies of night blindness had suggested that the processes causing this disease were located in the rod outer segment and were related exclusively to the biochemistry of transduction. Later results, however, indicated that there was a surprisingly small degree of desensitization in human rods when they were exposed to intense light. More recently this position has received strong support from the single-cell recordings of primate rods by Baylor et al., (1984; Chapter 5, this volume). In fact, night blindness can occur as a result of changes beyond the receptor.

Studies of inherited night blindness illustrate the richness of the approaches in identifying the site(s) responsible for night vision symptoms in different diseases (Fig. 11). Patients with these inherited conditions have a variety of different bases for their common night blindness symptoms (Ripps, 1982). In the night blindness condition known as fundus albipunctatus (in which tiny white spots are distributed across the retina) the defect appears to be primarily due to an abnormality in the exchange of vitamin A between the rods and the retinal pigment epithelium during pigment regeneration, and not to a shortage of vitamin A (Carr, Ripps & Siegel, 1974). The disease is manifest as a delay in both pigment regeneration and visual sensitivity as well as a slow time course of the ERG "b" wave recovery. In the more common condition known as retinitis pigmentosa it appears more

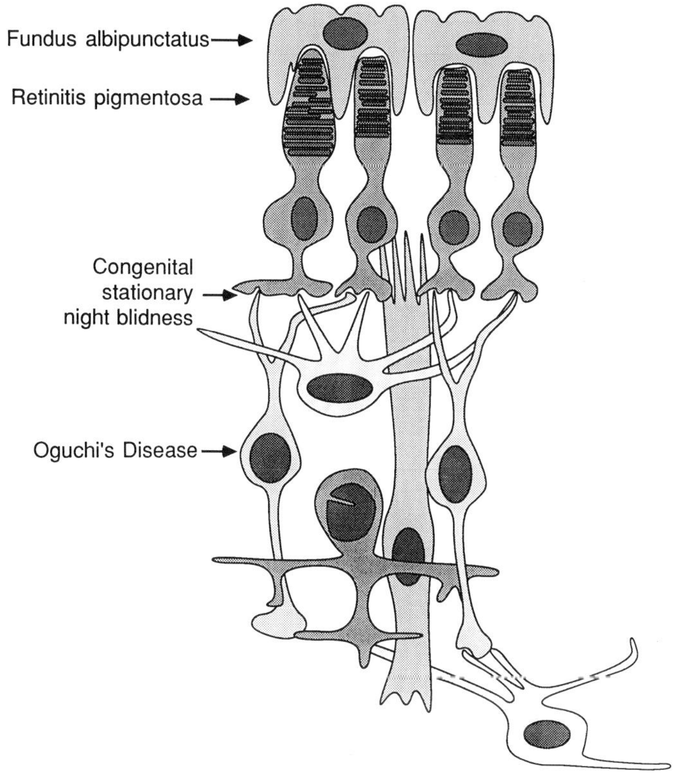

FIG. 11 Retinal sites that appear to be affected in night blindness disorders.

likely that a diminished rhodopsin content in the outer segment is the principal factor causing the symptom of night blindness.

In the third condition, congenital stationary night blindness, fundus inspection reveals no abnormality which would give a clue to the cause of the disease. After light adaptation, cone sensitivity recovers normally in the dark, but there is no rod phase seen in the dark adaptation curve. However, fundus reflectometry shows that the rhodopsin content of the rods and its regeneration in the dark are quite normal (Carr, Siegel & Weale, 1966). The ERG is abnormal with a reduced or absent "b" wave suggesting that in this disease the rod signals either are not reaching bipolar cells or are not received by them. In a fourth night blinding condition, Oguchi's disease which is characterized by a golden sheen in the light adapted retina, photopigment complement and recovery kinetics are normal. However, the slowed dark adaptation appears to be related to the delayed recovery (up to 4 hours) of the "b" wave of the inner nuclear layer, since there is a normal recovery of the receptor generated "a" wave of the ERG. It thus appears as though bipolar cells receive the rod signals but a postreceptoral anomaly limits recovery.

2. Layers of the Retina

A wide variety of noninvasive psychophysical and electrophysiological techniques have been developed to test specific layers of the retina. The human electroretinogram has long been used by many investigators and clinicians to distinguish between receptoral ("a" wave) and postreceptoral inner nuclear layer ("b" wave) function. The existence of a range of spatially induced sensitivity changes at some distance from the inducing light also allows separation of postreceptoral function. In particular, spatial sensitization functions for steady and intermittent backgrounds have been attributed to different layers of the retina (outer and inner plexiform).

One example of how changes in specific layers of the retina can be measured is provided by the series of tests known as "layer-by-layer" perimetry (Enoch, Fitzgerald & Campos, 1981). The layer-by-layer perimetric tests include a clinical adaptation of Westheimer's spatial desensitization–sensitization paradigm (Westheimer, 1965, 1967). In this paradigm, increment threshold for a small test spot centered on a circular background is measured as a function of background size. The result is an inverted U-shaped curve known as the Westheimer function. This has been interpreted as reflecting the center–surround antagonism of human receptive fields (see also Chapter 7, this volume).

In the clinical version of this test the luminance of the probe is held constant (at 0.8 log unit above the threshold measured on a uniform field) while the luminance of the background is varied until the test spot can just be seen. The result is a U-shaped Westheimer function. As background size increases, the luminance of the background required to render the test probe just visible first decreases (Fig. 12). This is analogous to the the normal "desensitization" effect and is due to spatial summation within the receptive field center. Beyond a particular background size, however, the curve reverses as more background luminance is needed to bring the test light to threshold. This is analogous to "sensitization" and is attributed to the lateral inhibition in the perceptive field surround. Because of the inhibition, increasingly larger backgrounds need to be more luminous to produce the same effect on test spot visibility. There is no further change in threshold once the outer limits of the perceptive field are reached. As a result, the curve levels off. The Westheimer function, also termed the "sustained-like" function because of the steady background used, thus characterizes the average spatial integration (excitation, inhibition) at a given locus of the retina. Pathological involvement of the inner retina, particularly the inner and outer plexiform layers, results in a marked reduction or absence of normal spatial sensitization. In such patients, an L-shaped response curve is obtained indicating the reduction or loss of lateral inhibition.

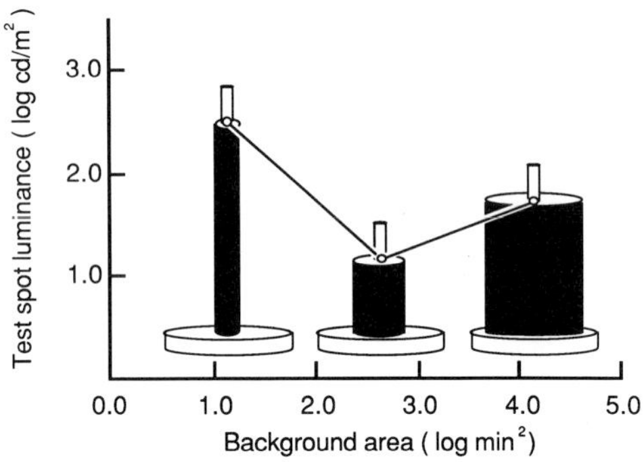

FIG. 12 The operationally defined "sustained-like" function. A variable intensity background (shaded) is varied in diameter in order to measure its effect on the visibility of a flashing test spot (central cylinder) set 0.8 log unit above its threshold on the surround alone, shown here as an open disk. Adapted from Enoch and Sunga (1969).

Another test in the layer-by-layer battery of tests is the "transient-like" test. It is based on the Werblin windmill paradigm (Werblin, 1972). Here, instead of a circular disk, a four-vaned windmill pattern (similar to a Maltese cross) is used for the background. Just as in the Westheimer function, the observer's threshold is determined by varying the luminance of the background until the test spot is just visible (Fig. 13). This is done for both a stationary windmill and a windmill rotating about the smaller test spot. In the normal eye it is found that the rotating windmill needs to be less luminous than the stationary one in order for the test spot to reach threshold. This result may be interpreted as an effect of motion induced desensitization.

The luminance difference between the two thresholds is typically of the order of 0.4 log unit in the fovea and increases with retinal eccentricity. As in the case of the Westheimer function, large abnormalities have been demonstrated in patients exhibiting inner

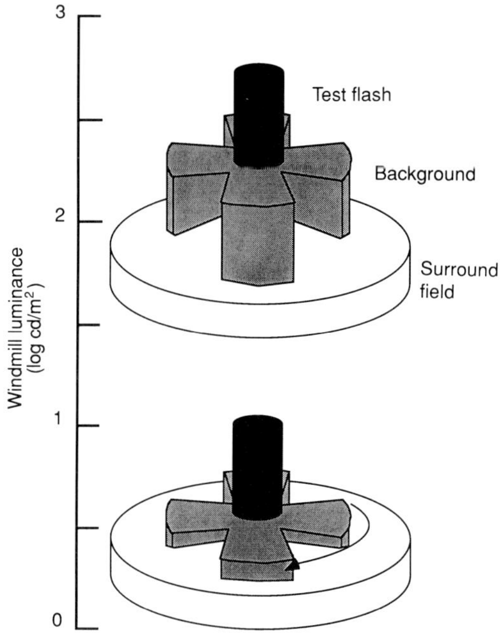

FIG. 13 The operationally defined "transient-like" function. A windmill pattern not rotating (top) or rotating (bottom) is presented. The luminance of the windmill is varied to determine threshold for a small, central flashing test spot. The luminance required is lower with the windmill rotating. From Enoch et al. (1981).

retinal pathology. However, unlike the sustained-like test, the transient-like test appears to be more specific for involvement of the inner plexiform layer of the retina. Both tests have been used to document the relative increase or decrease (during recovery) of pathological influences on retinal function (Enoch, 1978; Enoch, Fitzgerald & Campos, 1981).

Enoch and Campos (1979) conducted Westheimer (sustained-like) tests, along with kinetic perimetry and other psychophysical tests, in a large clinical trial repeated monthly over the course of a year on 49 patients with open-angle glaucoma and visual field loss. Significant changes of the Westheimer function were found in all patients. The curves reflected remissions and exacerbations of the disease. In patients tested with the Werblin windmill, the transient-like functions were grossly abnormal. The data suggest that a substantial portion of the inner retina and nerve fiber layer had been affected. Although abnormal sustained- and transient-like functions were generally found near nerve fiber bundle defects, they also occurred in areas beyond these boundaries (Enoch, 1978). These tests may be useful as predictors of future visual field abnormalities in open-angle glaucoma.

3. Pathways in the Retina

There is a great deal of psychophysical and physiological evidence to support the idea that at least two distinct and parallel visual pathways can be found, beginning early in the retina. (See Chapter 6, this volume.) These parallel streams have distinct properties defined by their responsiveness to different visual stimuli. Spatial, chromatic, and temporal parameters have been most useful in characterizing these paths. The same visual stimuli have been used to identify path-specific loss in a variety of diseases.

The use of colored backgrounds and test targets, designed to isolate pathways served by particular receptor types, has found broad application in both clinical and normal populations (Stiles, 1949; see also Chapter 8, this volume). Such techniques allow selective adaptation of certain visual pathways (e.g., chromatic versus achromatic) or selective isolation of nerve signals initiated by a single receptor type detecting such targets. Colored stimuli have allowed identification of very early vision changes in a number of retinal diseases and have even allowed specification of the particular cone pathways which appear to be affected. These more recent studies follow, in principle, the older use of color to clearly differentiate receptor function in measurements of dark adaptation; it is now commonplace for clinicians to use small red targets to isolate the initial cone function of a dark adaptation curve and large blue–green targets placed on the peripheral retina to identify rod function.

Colored backgrounds and test targets can be combined to isolate the pathways whose signals are initiated in one of three different cone types. For example, a bright yellow background selectively reduces the sensitivity of the medium (M) and long (L) wave-

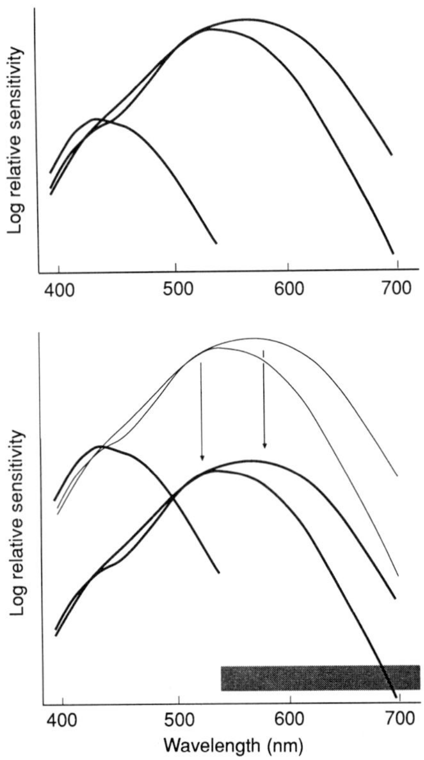

FIG. 14 Illustration of the spectral sensitivity of each of the three cone mechanisms (S,M&L from left to right), determined against a dim white background (top). Against a bright yellow background (bottom) the sensitivity of the medium and long wavelength sensitive cone mechanisms is selectively depressed, leaving the short wavelength sensitive cone mechanism to detect deep blue or violet test flashes close to threshold. Solid bar represents the wavelengths contained in the adapting background. Copyright 1987, American Medical Association.

length ("green" and "red") sensitive cones while leaving the short (S) wavelength ("blue") sensitive cones unaffected. Figure 14 illustrates that under such conditions a deep blue test flash (e.g., 440 nm) is detected only by the S cones. Laboratory studies have shown that with sufficiently intense yellow backgrounds and test flashes of sufficiently short wavelength, flash intensities of up to 100 times the test threshold are detected exclusively by S cones. Similarly, intense magenta (a mix of red and blue lights) and blue backgrounds can be used to isolate responses from the M and L cones, respectively (Wald, 1964; Marré, 1973).

It is now clear that many retinal diseases result in the selective loss of sensitivity for signals detected by the S cones (e.g. Adams, 1982a), whereas little or no loss of sensitivity is seen for the M and L cones when tested with bright magenta and blue backgrounds in the same subjects (Marré, 1973; Pokorny, Smith, Verriest & Pinckers, 1979). A number of studies have documented that there can be large sensitivity losses even in the absence of a visual acuity change in a variety of retinal vascular (Adams, 1982b, Zisman & Adams 1982, Adams, Schefrin & Huie, 1987) and degenerative diseases (Applegate et al., 1987; Eisner, Fleming, Klein & Maudlin, 1987; Haegerstrom-Portnoy & Brown, 1989), as well as disorders of the inner retina and optic nerve (Zisman, King-Smith & Bhargave, 1978; Adams, Rodic, Husted & Stamper, 1982a; King-Smith, Lubow & Benes, 1984).

The measurement of complete spectral sensitivity curves on each of these backgrounds is a time-consuming and difficult task, and it is often performed in the laboratory in complex Maxwellian-view optical systems, generally involving either a bite bar or chin rest with head restraints. For patient testing, Adams, Schefrin, and Huie (1987) have described a relatively simple clinical version of a test which can isolate S-cone sensitivity in less than 5 min and compare it, in that same time, to the sensitivity of the other two cone types. The test is designed to be essentially independent of differences in transmission through the pupil and ocular media from patient to patient and is little affected by refractive error and unsteady fixation.

The test uses a carousel slide projector to provide a four-alternative forced-choice presentation of blue or yellows spots against a yellow or blue background. It has been used to demonstrate that diabetics have a marked loss of S-cone sensitivity related to the degree of retinopathy (Witkin, Bresnick, Friedberg, Palta, Adams & Huie, 1986) and more specifically to the amount of edema in the retina (Adams, Zisman, Ai & Bresnick, 1987b). The test has also revealed significant losses in sensitivity for glaucoma patients across their entire central visual field (Heron, Adams & Husted, 1988), and even losses in ocular hypertensive pa-

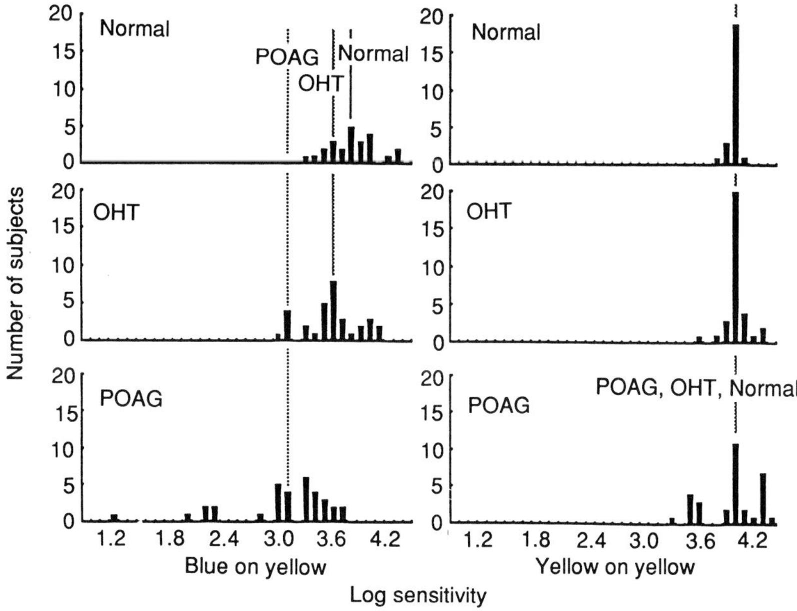

FIG. 15 Frequency histograms for log sensitivities to blue and yellow flashes (1°, 300 msec) on a 500 c/m² yellow background. Vertical dotted lines indicate log mean sensitivities for each group. Test sensitivities are shown for 33 patients with glaucoma (POAG), 32 patients with ocular hypertension (OHT), and 24 age-matched normals. As shown at right each group had the same sensitivity to yellow on a yellow background. At left the glaucoma group was about six times less sensitive (0.75 log unit) to blue light than the normal group and three times less sensitive (0.48 log unit) than the ocular hypertension group. These differences are statistically significant and easily identified clinically. There is also a statistically significant 1.7-fold (0.23 log unit) difference between the normal and ocular hypertensive groups. From Adams, Heron and Husted (1987).

tients whose other clinical vision measures are normal but whose intraocular pressure is elevated (Adams, Heron & Husted, 1987). This is illustrated in Figure 15 which shows differences in sensitivity between normal, glaucoma, and ocular hypertensive patients when measured with blue test flashes but not for the more traditional white flashes used in visual field testing. We show below how these tests have been useful in two diseases already described, diabetes and glaucoma.

(a) Diabetes. Many diabetics show large and specific losses of vision function prior to the development of retinopathy. In the early stages, these losses appear to be restricted to pathways carrying signals from the S cones (Marré, 1973; Adams, Zisman & Cavender, 1980; Adams, 1982a; Adams, Zisman, Rodic & Cavender, 1982b; Zisman & Adams, 1982). More specifically, there is evidence that this loss of sensitivity in the chromatic short-wave-sensitive pathways, prior to the development of retinopathy, may be a direct result of poor sensitivity control in the outer plexiform layer of the retina, where blue and yellow signals interact in the blue–yellow chromatic pathways.

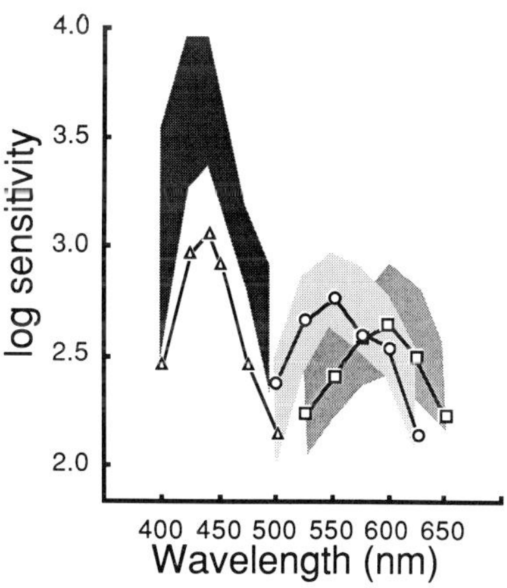

FIG. 16 Spectral sensitivities against bright yellow, magenta and blue backgrounds for 34 diabetics under age 40. Triangles, Against a 4.5 log troland yellow background (S cones); circles, 2.9 log troland magenta background (M cones); squares, 3.2 log troland blue background (L cones). Test spots (1°, 1 Hz) were flashed against 10° steady background after a 3-min adaptation to the background. Shaded areas equal 2 standard deviation zones for age-matched normals.

Figure 16 shows the sensitivity of a group of young diabetics whose vision was in other ways clinically normal. Note that there is a selective loss of sensitivity for targets detected by S cones on bright yellow backgrounds and little or no loss of sensitivity under conditions in which the same sized targets are detected against magenta and blue backgrounds (isolating M and L cones, respectively).

These same sensitivity losses for short wavelengths are also seen when flashes are presented against a bright white background designed to isolate detection by chromatically sensitive pathways (Fig. 17). Under these conditions the chromatic, not the achromatic, pathways are involved in detection (King-Smith, 1975; King-Smith & Carden, 1976). Again there is selective loss of sensitivity for S cones. These losses cannot be accounted for by changes in the ocular media (e.g., by increased yellowing of the crystalline lens). When test stimuli of the same size are flickered at 25 Hz and detection is based on detection of flicker, quite different spectral sensitivity is determined, and this appears to be due to detection by achromatic pathways (King-Smith & Carden, 1976). Diabetic eyes, in general, appear to have little or no loss of sensitivity for signals detected by this pathway (Adams, 1982a).

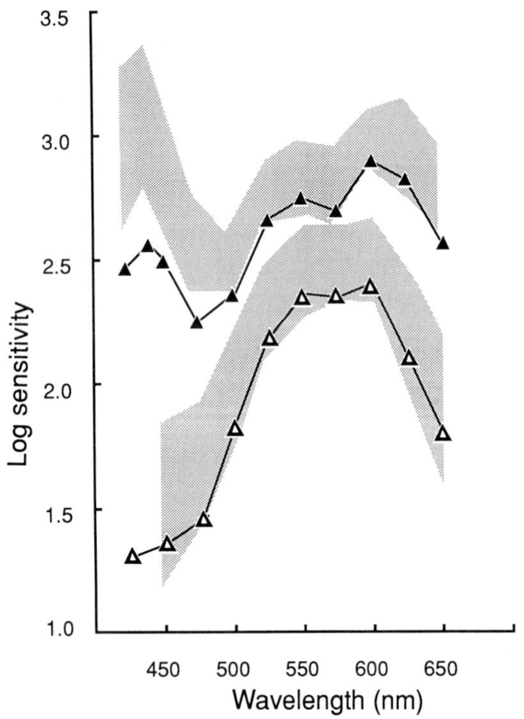

FIG. 17 Spectral sensitivity of 14 diabetics (mean age 25 years), with normal visual acuity (>20/25), for a 1° spot, flashed against a bright (3 log troland), 10°, white background. Open triangles, 25 Hz flashes. Filled triangles, 1 Hz flashes. Shaded areas equal 2 standard deviation zones for age-matched normals.

These data show that the sensitivity losses of diabetics evident in other functions (slow flashes on either a yellow or white background) are not due to the ocular media, since normal sensitivity at short wavelengths for flicker would not be anticipated if the eye contained a preretinal yellow filter. In fact the large sensitivity shifts seen in diabetics seem to be due, in part, to changes beyond the receptor (Adams, 1982a; Verdon, Adams & Haegerstrom-Portnoy, 1986).

Postreceptoral sensitivity losses may be among the earliest vision losses that can be detected in diabetes, preceding changes in the receptors themselves. What is the basis for this belief? Evidence for a postreceptoral component comes from the loss of sensitivity measured in two separate experiments. The first involves the measurement of the influence of the surrounding retina on S-cone sensitivity (Haegerstrom-Portnoy & Adams, 1983, 1988). Normal observers are more sensitive to a small test probe placed on a large yellow field than to one on a smaller field of the same luminance (Westheimer paradigm, Fig. 12). Since S cones absorb light appreciably only at wavelengths shorter than 550 nm, any changes in S-cone sensitivity against an expanded yellow background must be postreceptoral. Verdon et al. (1986) used this approach with diabetics and measured S-cone sensitivity on a large (2°) yellow (588 nm) field and on a small (35 min arc) yellow field. If diabetics had normal postreceptoral sensitivity control, they would be expected to show the same amount of spatial sensitization as the controls. Verdon et al. found, however, that three of the diabetics showed a slightly reduced sensitization effect; a fourth showed no effect at all (i.e., sensitivity was the same on both large and small yellow backgrounds). Thus, at least for some diabetics there is a sensitivity loss due to adaptation at a site beyond the receptor.

The second piece of evidence comes from unique green settings. The wavelength of unique green (having neither blueness nor yellowness) is thought to reflect the postreceptoral balance of signals from S and a combination of M and L cones. Consequently a reduced signal from either component receptor output would be expected to shift the wavelength of unique green. Schefrin (1989) measured unique green settings in diabetics with reduced S cone pathway sensitivity. With one exception, the four diabetics studied had unique green settings that were statistically indistinguishable from five normals. The equality of unique green between diabetics, who have S-cone sensitivity loss, and normals is consistent with a postreceptoral S-cone pathway loss. A selective loss of sensitivity within the S cones themselves would be expected to lead to a shorter wavelength unique green.

(b) Glaucoma. In primary open-angle glaucoma, a disease leading to characteristic or "signature" field defects, a different set of results emerges, suggesting quite different sites for the pathology. Here there is a selective loss of sensitivity for short wavelength targets accompanied by a loss of flicker sensitivity (Fig. 18). Thus, there appears to be a loss in both the chromatic and achromatic pathways, with a selective loss in the chromatic pathways involving only S-cone input (Adams, Rodic, Husted & Stamper, 1982; Adams, Heron & Husted, 1987c; Heron, Adams & Husted, 1988).

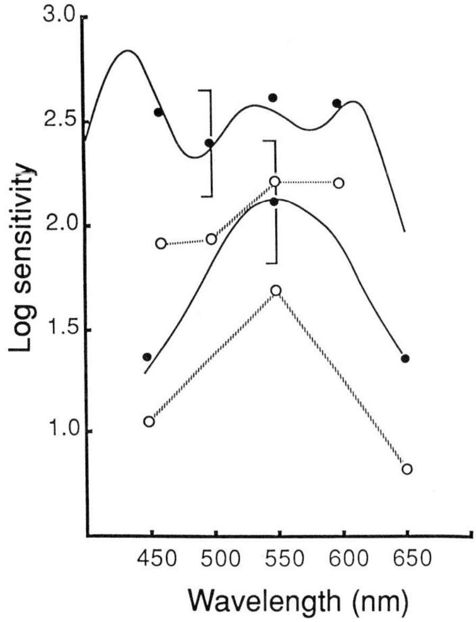

FIG. 18 Spectral sensitivity of 19 glaucoma subjects (mean age 52 years) and age-matched normals. Solid lines (through the normal data) represent results from a separate study of 11 young normals (mean age 24 years) under identical test conditions, except thresholds were determined at 20 nm intervals across the spectrum. Filled circles, means for age-matched normals; open circles, means for glaucoma subjects. Top solid line; chromatic increment thresholds for a 2° circular target flashed at 1 Hz on a 1270 photopic troland white background, foveally fixated; bottom solid line; achromatic increment thresholds for a 25 Hz test target under the same conditions. Error bars indicate ± 1 standard deviation for the normals (S.D. always less than 0.3 log units at each wavelength). Adapted from Adams, Rodic, Husted, and Stamper (1982).

4. Ganglion Cell and Visual Pathways

Although anatomical and physiological studies of primate retinas have suggested a clear dichotomy of ganglion cell types, with specific projections to the LGN (as described in Chapter 6, this volume), psychophysical or electrophysiological tests to isolate function at this level have been developed only relatively recently.

(a) Pattern Electroretinogram in Glaucoma. The pattern electroretinogram (PERG) is the retinal response, usually recorded with a contact lens electrode on the eye, to a phase-reversing patterned stimulus (Johnson, Riggs & Schick, 1966). The stimulus is often a grating or a checkerboard displayed on a television screen. The pattern elements (checks or bars) periodically reverse position, that is, they reverse in phase while a constant overall mean luminance is maintained. Responses can be analyzed only when the stimulus is focused on the retina and centered on the fovea during testing. It has been proposed that the PERG may result from changes in local luminance conditions within the retina (Spekreijse, Estévez & van der Tweel, 1973). ERGs elicited by flashes have been shown to exclude responses from ganglion cell layers. Indeed this has even been used to distinguish preganglion cell sites of anomaly from those with ganglion cell changes. Maffei and Fiorentini (1981) suggested that, in contrast to the flash unpatterned electroretinogram, the patterned electroretinogram specifically included activity at the ganglion cell layer. This method has since been used to identify a retinal component in conditions generally accepted to be due to anomalies at a higher, presumably cortical, level but suspected by others to involve ganglion cells (e.g., amblyopia).

The PERG has clinical value in monitoring inner retinal disease in patients with known preservation of the outer retina (Arden, Vaegan & Hogg, 1982). Abnormal PERG responses have been found in glaucoma, occlusion of the central retinal artery, optic nerve trauma, and in amblyopia. The PERG is a valuable tool in noninvasive functional assessment of the inner retina, though more research is needed on the cellular origin of this response.

Chronic open-angle glaucoma in the monkey was produced by laser damage to the trabecular meshwork (Gaasterland & Kupfer, 1974). In this monkey model, the course of visual changes accompanying both the glaucomatous disk atrophy and progressive intraocular pressure elevation have been followed using pattern electroretinogram measurements. The results obtained agreed with the human data: with progressing glaucoma, the ERG response to low spatial frequency patterns deteriorates when the temporal rate of modulation is around 6 to 8 Hz (Marx, Podos, Bodis-Wollner, Howard-Williams, Siegel, Teitelbaum, Maclin & Severin, 1986).

(b) Visual Evoked Potentials. An electroencephalogram (EEG) that is time-locked to a visual stimulus is called a visual evoked potential (VEP) or visually evoked cortical potential (VECP). It provides a diagnostic tool for the evaluation of patients suspected of suffering from demyelinating diseases and other forms of optic neuropathy. It is thought that the VEP recorded at the occiput (i.e., the back of the head) is dominated by responses from the foveal cones (Perry & Childers, 1969; Riggs & Wooten, 1972). The waveform of the VEP is variable and complex, consisting of a primary response, a secondary response, and an after discharge. VEP amplitude is affected by factors such as test stimulus image blur, binocular rivalry, stray light (although this problem can be minimized by the use of pattern reversal stimulation), and subject attention. It is of little use in the presence of ocular media opacities (e.g., Cracco & Bodis-Wollner, 1987). A delayed VEP is thought to suggest a slower conduction velocity in the demyelinated optic nerve (e.g., Parkinson's disease, multiple sclerosis). Experimental studies of rats and guinea pigs affected by demyelinating agents show that one major reason for a delayed VEP may be decreased conduction velocity in the central nervous system. Other clinical findings, however, imply other possible reasons, such as synaptic mechanisms (as in Parkinson's disease) or axonal pathology (as in glaucoma).

Using psychophysical and visually evoked potential (VEP) measurements on a patient, Bodis-Wollner (1981) reported the progression of rapidly evolving open-angle glaucoma. The data suggest that a VEP elicited by a low spatial frequency pattern, modulated at 8 Hz, may be affected prior to the conventional VEP, obtained at a lower flicker rate. Subsequent studies confirmed that the spatial frequency needs to be low and temporal frequency high for the electrophysiological diagnosis of glaucoma (Bobak, Bodis-Wollner, Harnois, Maffei, Mylin, Podos & Thornton, 1983; Wanger & Perrson, 1983, 1985; Porciatti & von Berger, 1984; Trick, 1985, 1986). Once again, it was found that a considerable number of ocular hypertensive patients show significant deterioration without development of optic nerve head cupping, optic nerve atrophy, and anomalous perimetric results.

Recall that low spatial frequency stimuli presented at medium to high temporal rates of modulation are useful in testing for visual damage in glaucoma (Quigley, Sanchez, Dunkelberger, L'Hernault & Baginski, 1987). The data suggest that glaucoma may affect predominantly the larger α-type or M type neurons feeding into magnocellular pathways at the LGN level. Visual acuity, on the other hand, is generally thought to be mediated by parvocellular neurons which may not be affected by the early glaucomatous process. This is consistent with the clinical observation that only in its advanced stages does glaucoma affect visual acuity.

(c) Multiple Sclerosis. Multiple sclerosis (MS) is a relatively common disease of the human nervous system. Its diagnosis for a long time depended on clinical observations alone. The demonstration that many patients have an abnormal VEP (Regan & Heron, 1969; Halliday, McDonald & Mushin, 1972) has significantly contributed to clinical diagnosis. At least 70% of MS patients have abnormal VEPs, and many of these show no evidence of any visual acuity change or history of retrobulbar optic neuritis, although both occur in a significant number of patients. The disease is characterized clinically by neurological symptoms and disabilities that may appear for a while and then disappear, while new ones appear immediately or some time later. This has made clinical diagnosis difficult. VEPs were (and are) helpful because the abnormal VEP latency remains all through these clinical changes. The abnormality typically observed consists of a delayed occurrence in the major positive peak of the VEP elicited by pattern reversal of a high contrast pattern such as a checkerboard.

The fact that many patients show abnormal VEP latencies has been attributed to the major pathophysiology of the demyelination. This might have been anticipated from the known properties of propagated versus saltatory conduction in nonmyelinated versus myelinated nerves. Further VEP abnormalities are not surprising since postmortem studies show that MS can affect any portion of the nervous system, and the optic nerves provide an especially vulnerable site.

The major positive component of the VEP, the so-called P100, is delayed or absent in 90% of eyes with optic neuritis. In patients with definite multiple sclerosis but without any optic neuropathy, the percentage is more than 70%. Even in 50 to 60% of patients in whom the diagnosis is considered "probable" the P100 is delayed or absent (Halliday, McDonald & Mushin, 1977). The effect of therapy in this disease has been evaluated in only a few studies. Since VEP latency changes little even while a patient may be spontaneously recovering, VEP amplitude rather than latency should be a better index of therapy. Indeed, pilot data from two patients (I. Bodis-Wollner, unpublished) show that VEP amplitude, not latency, responded to the therapy, suggesting that the steroids used may affect conduction block (such as edema) rather than improve myelination.

MS patients who complain of blurred vision, yet have normal visual acuity often show significant loss of contrast sensitivity (Bodis-Wollner & Diamond, 1976; Bodis-Wollner, Hendley, Mylin & Thorton, 1979). These defects in contrast sensitivity may affect only high spatial frequencies, or a narrow band of frequencies, or all spatial frequencies (Bodis-Wollner & Diamond, 1976). Regan, Silver, and Murray (1977) demonstrated that a good number of MS patients have contrast sensitivity deficits, either in one eye or both. These results support the concept of spatial frequency channels, derived by Campbell and Robson (1968) from psychophysical and physiological studies. Contrast sensitivity losses may also depend on pattern orientation (Regan, Whitlock, Murray & Beverley, 1980). This has been demonstrated in the VEPs of about 30% of all patients (Camisa, Mylin & Bodis-Wollner, 1981) and in a study comparing psychophysical and electrophysiological data (Kupersmith, Seiple, Nelson & Carr, 1984; Coupland & Kirkham, 1982).

However, the correlation between contrast sensitivity and VEP in multiple sclerosis is generally poor. Perhaps the poor correlation lies in the fact that while VEPs are tested at high contrast, contrast sensitivity is a measure of low contrast vision (Bodis-Wollner et al., 1979). Other psychophysical vision tests also correlate poorly with VEP and contrast sensitivity. For instance neither flicker sensitivity (Brussel, White, Bross, Mustillo & Borenstein, 1981/1982) nor delayed campimetry (Regan, Milner & Heron, 1976) correlate with either contrast sensitivity or VEP. Although it is true that multiple sclerosis may involve any part of the visual field, central vision is most commonly affected. Yet a unique spatiotemporal contrast combination characterizes the visual deficit in multiple sclerosis (Marx, May, Reed, Matteson, Van Dyk & Jayarman, 1984). For example, Medjbeur and Tulunay-Keesey (1985) found only three types of losses with ten MS patients. In most patients the greatest loss occurred for low to medium spatial frequencies at high temporal frequencies. In others, the deficit for high spatial frequencies increased and low spatial frequencies decreased with temporal modulation. The third type of deficit was made worse by any temporal modulation. This is consistent with the known pathology; the disease strikes haphazardly with respect to the time and site of attack in the nervous system.

In fact, whereas the major pathophysiology of multiple sclerosis consists of demyelination of central fibers, including the optic nerve fibers, much of what has been learned about visual dysfunction in multiple sclerosis also points to other effects. For example, in addition to myelin sheath damage, nerve cell death must ultimately occur. Ophthalmoscopic examination of the retina often discloses a loss of ganglion cell nerve fibers. Consistent with this clinical observation are results showing abnormal pattern ERG (PERG) amplitude in eyes of patients with multiple sclerosis (Bobak et al., 1983). PERG reflects the activity of retinal neurons with center–surround organization, probably ganglion cells. It follows that some of the visual loss in multiple sclerosis is likely to be caused by neuronal effects, rather than by long-standing demyelination.

There are additional challenges raised by studies of multiple sclerosis. The demonstration of orientation selective loss both by psychophysical and VEP methods (although not necessarily in the same patient) raises the possibility that they are due to cortical damage, since only cortical neurons are orientation selective. How could such a result be explained in a disease hitherto thought only to involve the myelin sheath of the optic nerve? Camisa et al. (1981) and Kupersmith et al. (1984) suggest that demyelination within the occipital cortex may account for orientation selective visual losses in multiple sclerosis. Gilbert and Wiesel (1983) have demonstrated axonal branching patterns of neurons within the visual cortex. These myelinated branches may be considered as bridges between columns responding to the same stimulus orientation but separated in the cortex by other columns responding to other orientations. Future psychophysical studies varying both orientation and retinal locus of the stimulus might provide an answer to this question.

D. Cortical Scotomas

Patients with cortical blindness, particularly those with blindsight, provide valuable insight not only regarding their functional condition, but also regarding the presence of auxiliary visual pathways in the normal visual system. In so doing they provoke reexamination of concepts of classical visual pathways.

1. Scotoma of Central Origin

Pathological destruction of visual cortex in man is classically thought to produce total blindness, except for pupillary response to light and very crude visual perception limited to sudden changes in illumination, a condition known in clinical practice as cortical blindness (e.g., Brindley, Gautier-Smith & Lewin, 1969; Jung, 1973). This conventional opinion, however, has been called into question, largely on the basis of experimental findings in monkeys. Although monkeys with striate cortex lesions appear to be profoundly impaired in their ordinary visual behavior, they are still able to generate motor responses for reaching objects moving across their visual field (Humphrey & Weiskrantz, 1967; Feinberg, Pasik & Pasik, 1978). In fact, these monkeys have considerable residual visual acuity, although their contrast sensitivity is severely affected (Miller, Pasik & Pasik, 1981).

The residual visual abilities have been attributed to activity of retinal ganglion cells surviving ablation of visual cortex. Transneuronal ganglion cell degeneration following lesion of the occipital lobe in monkeys is known to be incomplete. Van Buren (1963) observed, in one animal operated 4 years earlier for a right occipital lobectomy, partial degeneration of the ganglion cell layer of the left half of the two retinas. This finding was replicated and expanded by Cowey (1974) in one monkey with bilateral subtotal striate cortex ablation. After 7 years, and in spite of a massive numerical decrease predominating in the foveal region, ganglion cells were still present across the retina. In subsequent work (Cowey & Perry, unpublished, quoted by Weiskrantz, 1986), these remaining cells were found to be mostly of the γ and ε types, that is, cell types that project exclusively to the brainstem level. The amount of ganglion cell degeneration seems to depend on the age of the animal at the time of the operation. According to Dineen and Hendrickson (1981), degeneration may amount up to 80% of ganglion cells in animals operated at an early age, although it is reduced to about 15% in animals operated as adults. A similar pattern of retinal atrophy has been observed in man (based on fundus examination) following early cortical lesions (Hoyt, Rios-Montenegro, Behrens & Eckelhoff, 1972), but this finding has not been confirmed.

These anatomical findings represent a strong argument for the role of subcortical structures in mediating residual visual function in destriated monkeys. Mohler and Wurtz (1977) have shown that partially destriated monkeys, which were able to orient visually toward stimuli presented within their scotoma, lost this ability after subsequent destruction of the retinotopically corresponding zones of the superior colliculi. Thus, superior colliculi and possibly other brainstem areas that receive input from the retina may play a critical role either in mediating pure "subcortical vision" or in relaying visual input to other structures on which they project, including extrastriate cortex (for a review of these extrageniculocortical pathways, see Benevento & Fallon, 1975; Partlow, Colonnier & Szabo, 1977).

In man, clinical observations suggestive of incomplete or "relative" blindness within scotomas of cortical origin have been mentioned by several authors (e.g., Teuber et al., 1960; Williams & Gassel, 1962; see Weiskrantz, 1986, for review). However, systematic experimental evidence for residual visual abilities following lesions of the striate cortex was first reported by Pöppel, Held and Frost in 1973, followed by Weiskrantz, Warrington, Sanders, and Marshall (1974) and Perenin and Jeannerod (1975). All these experiments used a new methodological approach derived from studies in monkeys. In man, visual functions are commonly assessed by asking the subject whether or not he can "see" the stimulus. Patients suffering from a unilateral lesion of the visual cortex do not report seeing targets within the contralateral half of their visual field, that is, they lack the common subjective experience of "seeing." In contrast, monkeys, whose subjective experience is not accessible to the experimenter through language, are tested in a different way. Animals are trained to reach for targets or to point to which of two patterns they have selected. Pöppel et al. (1973) were the first to suspect that such behavioral responses could also be useful for testing visual capacities in man. Indeed, they asked their cortically lesioned subjects not to try to see stimuli that were presented within their scotomas, but rather to try to locate them by turning their eyes toward them. Pöppel et al. recorded eye movements, the direction and amplitude of which were weakly but definitely correlated with position of the targets. Because the subjects remained unaware of the stimuli, they subjectively experienced "guessing" rather than "seeing." This was a form of unconscious vision, later called blindsight (Sanders, Warrington, Marshall & Weiskrantz, 1974), where subjects abandoned their usual, perceptual, mode of visual detection and used an alternative mode based on a forced visuomotor response.

(a) Pointing within the Hemianopic Field. In the following, the motor responses obtained under such conditions are compared with those obtained from normal subjects. Data for this comparison are drawn from the study of residual vision in a group of six hemispherectomized subjects (patients in whom one hemisphere was surgically removed) operated at ages ranging between 6 and 9.5 years in five cases and at 17 years in one case (Perenin & Jeannerod, 1978).

In the experiment, subjects were placed at the center of a semicylindrical vertical screen, diffusely illuminated in the mesopic range. Targets were projected on the screen at subjects' eye level at 15°, 30°, 45°, 60°, and 75° on each side of the midline. Bright stimuli (a 6° × 8° horizontal rectangle, or a 2° to 3.5° diameter spot) presented for 100 or 500 msec were used as targets. Subjects, with head movements restrained, had to binocularly fixate a mark placed at the center of the screen. Central fixation was monitored by the experimenter by way of a television system. A warning tone was given prior to each stimulus presentation. The subject's task was to point rapidly with the arm at the target location, while keeping the gaze fixated at the center of the screen. This task was easily achieved for targets appearing within the normal half of the visual field, where the subjects could see the targets. For targets appearing on the hemianopic side, however, subjects were required to point immediately after the tone, at the point where they "guessed" the target had appeared.

Results from this experiment clearly showed that subjects did not point at random: pointing positions within the hemianopic field were definitely correlated with target positions. In the sessions where targets were presented for a short duration (100 msec), significant correlations were obtained in four of the five tested subjects. For target presentations lasting 500 msec, the correlation coefficients were significant in all six cases. One representative example is illustrated in Fig. 19.

The pattern of errors was consistent across all sessions. Subjects tended to overshoot target position for targets located within 30° from midline, although they systematically undershot targets located beyond that eccentricity. Increasing the duration of presentation of the targets (from 100 to 500 msec) tended to reduce the amount of this constant error without affecting the global pattern of error distribution. This effect is demonstrated in Fig. 20, which displays cumulated results from the six patients. Because these subjects were partly hemiplegic, they had to use their arm ipsilateral to the hemispherectomy (and, therefore, contralateral to their hemianopic field). This may have created mechanical constraints accounting for undershooting the most peripheral targets (e.g., beyond 60°). However, a similar pattern of undershooting was also observed in experiments with other patients where targets were localized by saccadic eye movements instead of arm pointing (Weiskrantz et al., 1974; Zihl, 1980).

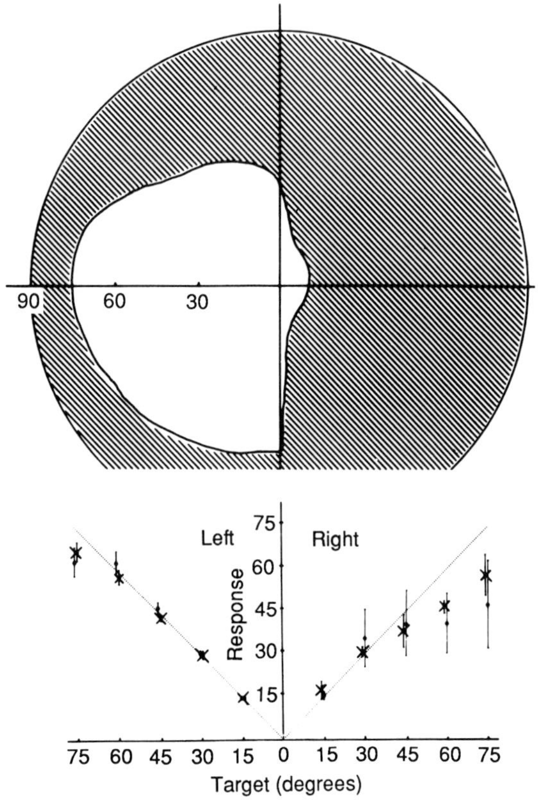

FIG. 19 Pointing directed at targets presented in the blind field in one subject with a left-sided hemispherectomy. (Top) Outline of the binocular visual field, as mapped with the larger and brighter (116′, 320 cd/m²) spot of the Tübingen perimeter. Targets were presented on the horizontal meridian at 15°, 30°, 45°, 60°, and 75° on each side of the vertical meridian. The targets were 8° square, striped patterns presented under bright illumination for 500 msec. Stripes within the pattern could be either stationary or moving. (Bottom) The plotted values each represent the mean of 10 responses. Crosses represent values when the stripes within the pattern were moving, while circles illustrate responses to stationary stripes. The experiment demonstrates that movement can slightly improve detectability of targets within the blind hemifield. From Perenin and Jeannerod (1978).

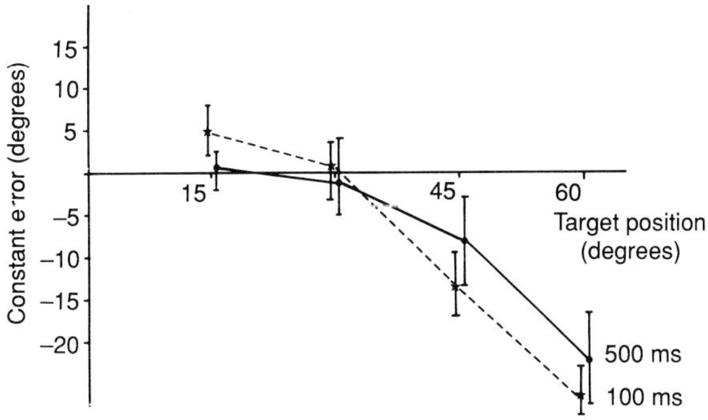

FIG. 20 Constant and variable errors of pointing movements executed with the hemianopic field in six hemispherectomized patients, plotted as a function of target exposure. After Perenin and Jeannerod (1978).

The demonstration of relatively accurate pointing in hemianopic fields has a number of important implications for the mechanisms that control both the initiation and the accuracy of visually goal-directed movements. The large errors made by cortically lesioned subjects in pointing toward their hemianopic field must be compared with those made by normal subjects. This comparison, however, can only be done with normal subjects pointing in a situation where control cues for the movement are reduced by the same amount. Examination of blindsight implies no conscious visual feedback from the moving hand, no reference signal from eye or head rotations toward the target (the subject has to fixate the center of the screen), and no information about target location during the movement (target exposure was limited to 100 or 500 msec in the experiments). Lacking such control cues, this situation results in large errors in normal subjects (Prablanc, Echallier, Komilis & Jeannerod, 1979). If the comparison is made for targets of the same eccentricities in both normal and hemianopic subjects, one finds that in the two groups the direction of errors is similar (i.e., overshoot for targets close to the midline and undershoot for more remote targets) and that the size of errors is of the same order of magnitude. The general pattern of responses to stimuli presented in the hemianopic fields of subjects with cortical lesions can therefore be regarded as only a slight exaggeration of the pattern of response of normal subjects.

These results on "blind" orienting and reaching stress the fact that movements can be initiated and executed with reasonable accuracy without a direct conscious representation of the goal. This is an example of the functioning of discrete neural channels subserving discrete behaviors, such as orienting or pointing. The lesion artificially splits behavior into modular units (in this case a cognitive unit and a visuomotor unit) which normally cannot be dissociated (Jeannerod, 1981). The fact that subjective experience is disconnected from information transfer and motor production mechanisms does not mean, however, that visuomotor channels make a direct transformation of visual input into motor output. The work of Zihl and Werth (1984a,b) has clearly shown that hemianopic subjects can be trained to improve performance (even though they remain unaware of the final result of their movements). Their two patients were required to direct their eyes where they guessed the targets had appeared. They first tended to make saccades of a rather constant amplitude without respect to target location. They were then informed that targets would appear at a different location each time, and that they should therefore shift their eyes by a corresponding amount. They were never informed, however, about the location of the target, nor about their localization performance. This "shaping" procedure, similar to that used in monkey training experiments, produced in the patients a clear and rapid improvement in performance (Zihl & Werth, 1984b). Thus, the internal "representational" mechanisms related to the process of motor learning can become accessible in a noncognitive mode.

(b) Pattern Recognition in Blindsight Patients. It might be asked whether blindsight is limited to the generation of visuomotor responses or whether it can also be demonstrated for other types of visual abilities. Indeed, it has been reported by several authors that patients with cortical lesions seem to be able to detect visual shapes within their scotomas. When tested with the forced-choice procedure, the patient of Weiskrantz et al. (1974) was able to discriminate simple shapes (e.g., O versus X, X versus triangle) or lines of different orientations (horizontal versus vertical), provided the stimuli were large enough. Shape discrimination was also reported by Perenin (1978), who found positive scores for simple shapes and line orientation in two out of six hemispherectomized patients, and by Ptito, Lassonde, Leporé and Ptito (1987), in two out of four. As a rule, those subjects who can discriminate shapes incurred their lesion early in life, whereas those who cannot incurred their lesion as adults (e.g., Perenin & Jeannerod, 1975; Barbur, Ruddock & Waterfield, 1980).

Shape discrimination within scotomas was also tested by using the paradigm of visual completion (Warrington, 1962). Torjussen (1978) found that three hemianopic patients presented with a luminous circle across their vertical meridian were, in fact, able to detect it as a complete circle, in spite of "seeing" only half of it, in a forced-choice situation. This did not occur if the stimulus was a half-circle presented within the intact field. In other words, these patients clearly detected the presence or absence of part of the stimulus within their scotomas.

These results raise the problem of the mechanisms for shape detection in patients with lesions involving the visual cortex. The contribution of associative visual areas, spared by the lesion and still visually integrated via retinal projections to the midbrain, has been invoked by Weiskrantz as a basis for true (though degraded) form perception (see Weiskrantz et al., 1974; Weiskrantz, 1986). It has been argued that this mechanism would not account for the results obtained in hemispherectomized patients, who underwent a complete hemidecortication on one side. Rather, in such cases, shape discrimination should reflect the capacity of subcortical pathways for visual detection and would rely on indirect cues, such as local differences in luminance or orientation of contrast (Perenin, 1978). One cannot exclude, however, the possibility that the intact hemisphere could play a role in detecting shapes presented in the blind hemifield. Ptito et al. (1987) have shown that hemidecorticated patients simultaneously presented with two shapes (one appearing in the blind field and the other in the normal field) could detect whether they were the same or different from each other. This result demonstrates that interfield comparison can take place in the absence of visual cortex on one side. Ptito et al. proposed the intertectal commissure (the commissure between the two superior colliculi) as a possible anatomical pathway giving the blind field access to the intact hemisphere. Such a mechanism was also suggested earlier by Pöppel and Richards (1974).

(c) Control Experiments. Blindsight is a controversial issue. Following the interpretation of Teuber et al. (1960) and Williams and Gassel (1962) for explaining residual vision in some hemianopic patients, it has been argued that subjects might be able to use light scattering from the targets into unimpaired parts of the visual field as a cue for detecting visual events occurring within the scotoma (Campion, Latto & Smith, 1983). There is no doubt that scattered light may be a problem in some of the experiments described above, particularly when bright targets and a high target to background contrast ratio are used. The argument thus is that intensity gradients resulting from stray light from the target into the normal field might have been used as a localizing cue. The validity of this argument can be dealt with in two different ways.

First, if scattered light were effectively used as a source of information, blindsight should be found in every tested patient. In fact, the amount of blindsight has been found to vary across patients examined in the same experimental situation. Blindsight is more likely to be present in young patients than in adult patients. Among adult patients, those with long-standing hemianopia are more likely to possess blindsight than those with fresh lesions (Perenin & Jeannerod, 1975; Hécaen, Perenin & Jeannerod, 1984). Because these differences between groups cannot be related to experimental conditions, they must pertain to specific characteristics of the groups, such as age, or type or extent of the lesion. This problem of poorer blindsight performance in certain patients, particularly in cases with lesions occurring late in life, is apparent even in the critical study of Campion et al.

(1983). These authors have reported on pointing performance in three hemianopic patients with lesions of the occipital lobe acquired in adulthood. Stimuli used as targets were as bright as those used in experiments made by previous authors, and they were presented for relatively long durations. Accuracy of pointing at targets presented within the scotoma was very poor in all three subjects, and the correlation between target position and pointing position was found to be clearly significant in one case only.

The second way to deal with the argument that blindsight is an artifact is to use specific tests for controlling the effects of scattered light. Normal subjects wearing goggles equipped with occluders masking half of their visual field (thus simulating a situation of artificial hemianopia) and tested in the same conditions as truly hemianopic subjects were not able to orient toward targets presented within their "scotoma" (Perenin & Jeannerod, 1983). Another control for the role of scattered light can be made in patients with a bitemporal hemianopia resulting from chiasmatic lesions. In such cases no blindsight is expected to occur, since all retinal projections subserving the temporal fields are blocked by the lesion at the peripheral level. Indeed, the two patients with bitemporal hemianopia examined by Perenin and Jeannerod (1978) were unable to point at targets appearing within their temporal scotomas. Finally, one of the most stringent tests for ruling out the influence of stray light is to plot the natural blindspot within the scotoma. As emphasized by Weiskrantz, who succeeded in doing this experiment in his patient, "a target light that cannot be detected by the subject when it is positioned on the optic disc cannot cause detectable stray light beyond a maximal angle determined by the distance between the edge of the target and the nearest region of sensitive retina" (Weiskrantz, 1986, p. 90). This angle can be estimated at 2° to 3°. Recent experiments also provided evidence for detection of very low intensity visual stimuli in hemianopic patients. Using a probabilistic method, Stoerig, Hübner, and Pöppel (1985) found evidence, in one patient, for discrimination between presence or absence of a 44″, 32 cd/m^2 spot presented for 200 msec within the blind field. Such a discrimination can hardly have been attributed to stray light from the target.

Scattered light is an unspecific factor common to all hemianopic subjects examined for blindsight. Therefore, there is no reason why it should not be used by all of them for detecting local differences in luminous flux and for directing movements at target location. By contrast, blindsight is a delicate effect revealing the residual activity of an impaired system, and there is no reason why it should be present in all hemianopic patients with cortical lesions.

IV. CONCLUSIONS AND DIRECTIONS FOR THE FUTURE

Altered visual systems, whether as a result of genetic variation, intervening disease, trauma or as a result of development in a modified or deprived visual environment, have been invaluable in determining the mechanisms involved in the normal visual system. Furthermore, experimental methods and instrumentation used in such cases have also made significant contributions to the understanding of disease processes themselves, as well as to the nature of developmental anomalies in reduced visual environments.

The variety of tools available to the researcher has increased greatly since the 1960s. For example, advances in extracting small signals from biological recordings and the introduction of computer controlled spatiotemporal processing of color on video displays have been important in the exploration of processing in the visual pathways. The introduction of nonlinear analytic techniques has provided new tools in dissecting "sequential" and "parallel" processing abnormalities in the human visual system. The 1970s and 1980s have also seen an impressive expansion of noninvasive, psychophysical approaches to identifying sites of particular vulnerability in visual processing. Numerous techniques now exist for identifying functional deficits in the ocular media, within the photopigments and receptors themselves, within the layers of the retina, and at geniculate and cortical levels.

ACKNOWLEDGMENTS

Supported in part by National Institutes of Health Grants EY 02271 to Anthony J. Adams, EY 03674 to Jay M. Enoch, and EY 01708 and EY 01867 to Ivan Bodis-Wollner, and Medical Research Council of Canada Grant PG-29 to Donald E. Mitchell. The authors thank Vasudevan Lakshminarayanan and Rolf W. Nygaard who provided considerable assistance with earlier versions of this chapter, and Wayne Verdon who critically reviewed the final version.

15

COMPUTATIONAL THEORIES OF VISUAL PERCEPTION

Robert Shapley, Terrence Caelli, Stephen Grossberg, Michael Morgan, and Ingo Rentschler

I. INTRODUCTION

The vast quantity of information about visual perception and its neurophysiological foundations is a problem both for experts and for newcomers to the field. The human mind needs some principles of organization, some theoretical generalizations, that compress the sheer weight of knowledge into more manageable concepts. The first part of this chapter, Section II–V, presents contemporary views on the problems with theories of spatial pattern perception, and some proposed formulations that clarify the theoretical issues. The second half of the chapter (Sections VI and VII) deals with models of form, color, and brightness perception that involve special-purpose neural networks. This chapter thus draws upon material in virtually all of the preceding chapters, except for those concerned with development and clinical applications. Ultimately, however, phenomena of development and abnormal vision may provide critical challenges for comprehensive models of human vision.

One of the interesting and unexpected points of agreement among many diverse theoreticians of vision is that a satisfactory account of visual perception demands consideration of the visual system as a *nonlinear system*. This conclusion follows from general arguments about information processing but also from specific functional characteristics of visual performance. For instance, the phenomena of masking of vernier acuity led Watt and Morgan, (1984) to propose a theory requiring a nonlinear transduction, *rectification*, of signals in the visual cortex before the positions of vernier lines were calculated. In a completely different context, Shapley and Gordon (1985) and Grossberg and colleagues (Grossberg and Mingolla, 1985a,b; Grossberg and Todorovic, 1988) observed that rectification or some similar nonlinear stage was required to explain contour perception. A third example of an appeal to nonlinear image analysis arises in the different accounts of the phenomenon of "pop out" or immediate recognition of the odd element in an array (see Chapter 11, this volume). Explanations of preattentive, rapid texture segmentation require either feature detection (Julesz, 1981; Treisman, 1982) or local energy computations (Caelli, 1985) that may be related to the rectifiers postulated by Morgan, Shapley, and Grossberg and their colleagues.

Another recurrent theme in vision theory is the idea of *parallel processing* by multiple, independent visual channels (see also Chapter 6, this volume). One aspect of parallel processing involves multiple spatial scales of analysis, or, equivalently, multiple spatial frequency channels. This idea is central not only to models of spatial vision, but also in other contexts where the independent, parallel computation of brightness and of bounding contour is an important theoretical novelty.

II. SPATIAL FREQUENCY CHANNELS AND THE FOURIER TRANSFORM THEORY OF VISION

Much of the theorizing about spatial vision since the 1960s has been influenced by the ideas of Campbell and Robson (1968) and colleagues who proposed that spatial patterns were analyzed into their spatial Fourier components and detected by specialized spatial frequency channels (see also DeValois and DeValois, 1988; Chapter 10, this volume). In order to place more recent theoretical ideas in context, we must briefly review the theories of spatial frequency channels and Fourier representations of visual patterns.

A. The Fourier Representation

Any real visual image is equivalent to a sum of sinusoidal grating patterns. This is the visual, spatial expression of Fourier's theorem which states that (almost) any waveform can be represented as a sum of sinusoidal waves. Thus, for any arbitrary one-dimensional luminance profile $L(x)$, the Fourier representation is

$$L(x) = \frac{1}{2\pi} \int_{-\infty}^{\infty} L(k)\, e^{ikx}\, dk \qquad (1)$$

The coefficients for each spatial frequency in the summation, $L(k)$, are the Fourier Transform of the original waveform $L(x)$. It is important to realize that in general $L(k)$ is a complex-valued function of spatial frequency k. That means $L(k)$ has a real and an imaginary part; it is usually represented as having an *amplitude* and a *phase*. Thus, in the literature, authors write about the amplitude spectrum and phase spectrum of spatial waveforms.

If there were neurons that were very finely tuned to spatial frequency, the visual system could extract the Fourier coefficients and represent spatial waveforms within the brain in terms of their amplitude spectrum. If, in addition, there were some way of calculating phase at each of the spatial frequencies represented in the amplitude spectrum, one could reconstruct each spatial waveform completely. The first condition, narrow spatial frequency tuning, has in fact been found in many neurons in the primary visual cortex of cats (Cooper & Robson, 1968; Maffei & Fiorentini, 1973; among many others) and of macaque monkeys (DeValois, Albrecht, & Thorell, 1982). Thus, there might well be a representation of the amplitude spectrum of visual images in the activity of the population of cells in primary visual cortex.

The representation of the phase spectrum is problematical. Spatial phase is encoded in the firing patterns of *simple* cortical cells in primary visual cortex, both in cats and monkeys (Movshon, Thompson & Tolhurst, 1978c; Pollen & Ronner, 1981; DeValois et al., 1982; Spitzer & Hochstein, 1985). However, in *complex* cells, spatial phase is encoded very poorly or not at all (Spitzer & Hochstein, 1985).

Explicit proposals that primary visual cortex (V1) computes the Fourier amplitude spectrum were made by Glezer, Ivanoff, and Tscherbach (1973) and Robson (1975). These ideas were implicit in the earlier research of Blakemore and Campbell (1969) and Graham and Nachmias (1971). They have formed the basis for many subsequent psychophysical investigations of spatial frequency channels, among them the papers by Graham (1980), Robson and Graham (1981), Caelli and Hübner (1983), Watson, Barlow, and Robson (1983), and Field and Nachmias (1984). An important qualification of the Fourier representation approach was included in Robson's (1975) proposal, namely, that Fourier amplitude spectra were only calculated over relatively small patches of the visual field. This proposal was intended to take into account the known large variation of visual properties with position in the visual field due to, among other factors, *retinal inhomogeneity*.

Localized Fourier-like analysis has been proposed to account for spatial pattern discriminations and hyperacuity (Wilson & Gelb, 1984; Wilson, 1986). The localization is accomplished by having spatial filters stationed at every retinal point. The Fourier-like analysis is accomplished by making the localized spatial filters moderately narrow in spatial frequency bandwidth and by postulating that there are several spatial filters with diverse spatial scales (optimum spatial frequency) at each position. In order to fit real data, it is important that the responses of each filter are passed through a static nonlinearity (simulated psychometric function) that is accelerating at low contrasts and decelerating at high contrasts. Pooling of responses of similar filters across space is required in order to account for spatial frequency discrimination. Pooling is done by taking the pth root of the sum of the p powers of all responses to be pooled. Thus, in Wilson and Gelb's (1984) model for spatial frequency discrimination, given any two patterns P_1 and P_2 the difference in response of the ith spatial frequency-tuned filter is given by

$$F_i(x) = F_i(P_1) - F_i(P_2) \tag{2}$$

and the pooled activity in one of the mechanisms is

$$F_m = [\sum_{i=1}^{n} (F_i(x)P]^{1/p} \tag{3}$$

The maximal response across the population of mechanisms determines which mechanism performs the discrimination.

III. PATTERN ACUITY AND HYPERACUITY

A central issue in contemporary models of spatial vision concerns the theoretical explanation for *hyperacuity*, the capability of human observers to make fine spatial discriminations on a spatial scale much smaller than the distance between photoreceptors in the retina. One possibility is that hyperacuity reveals the spatial scale of representation of visual position in the brain. An alternative view is that the hyperacuity limit depends on sensitivity and size of receptive fields but does not tell us about the representation of space in the visual system.

The view that hyperacuity reveals the spatial scale of visual representations derives from the scheme for spatial representation put forward by Marr (1982). According to this view, the major task of the visual system is to form a symbolic description of the outside world. In order to form this description, the visual system has to rely initially on the retinal image, the two-dimensional projection of light upon the back of the eye. One of the key ideas of Marr's theory of vision is that the first stage in vision is the formation of a symbolic description of the image itself: the so-called Primal Sketch. The Primal Sketch is a two-dimensional spatial description of the important structures in the image. The aim of this early symbolic process is to identify *features* of the image that are likely to be of importance in later scene-based analysis: features such as edges, bars, blobs, texture boundaries, corners. The Primal Sketch can be thought of as the internal representation of a cartoon of the image. Indeed, Marr (1982) adduced the fact that we so readily perceive meaning in cartoons as evidence for the existence of a natural counterpart to the cartoonist's symbols in the visual system.

Some important aspects of the Primal Sketch are the following: (a) The Sketch is symbolic. This statement is a little vague, but one can take it to mean that out of the practically infinite manifold of possible assertions implicit in the image, a symbolic process makes only a small number explicit, using a defined set of primitives (features) to do so. This relates to the next point: (b) The Sketch is inflexible. It is not adapted to symbolize any possible structures in the image. The sketch has available only a small set of primitives and is thus restricted a priori in what it can represent. This aspect of the Primal Sketch is challenged implicitly by evidence for plasticity of internal representations presented later in this chapter. (c) The Sketch is data-driven. It is not subject to top-down influences. This means that (linear or nonlinear) transducers transform the image to produce the outputs of early vision, the responses of filters or detectors for the primitives in the Sketch. When our cognitive processes fail to understand the logic of one of these early inflexible processes, we call the result an "illusion." An example of an illusion which probably originates at the Primal Sketch level is the Münsterberg illusion, shown in Fig. 1. The key to understanding the Münsterberg illusion is that bandpass, spatial-frequency filtering of the image produces locally tilted elements along the mortar lines (Grossberg & Mingolla, 1985a; Morgan & Moulden, 1986). These locally tilted components cause a global impression of tilt along the mortar lines, as in the Fraser effect, here illustrated in Fig. 2. (d) The Sketch represents spatially localized primitives. Spatial primitives in the Sketch are given a positional tag to locate them in the image. The tag is closely similar to Lotze's (1886) "local sign." It follows that the representational stages following the Primal Sketch must be able to interpret positional tags and use them to describe spatial relations.

To test the idea of a Primal Sketch we need to investigate the way in which human observers discriminate between and recognize simple forms and textures. Watt and Morgan (1983, 1984, 1985) have argued that pattern discriminations will be carried out with high acuity if they use the natural symbols of vision. Were this assertion true, one could discover the primitives of the Sketch (if such things exist; see Chapter 11, this volume) by comparing pattern dis-

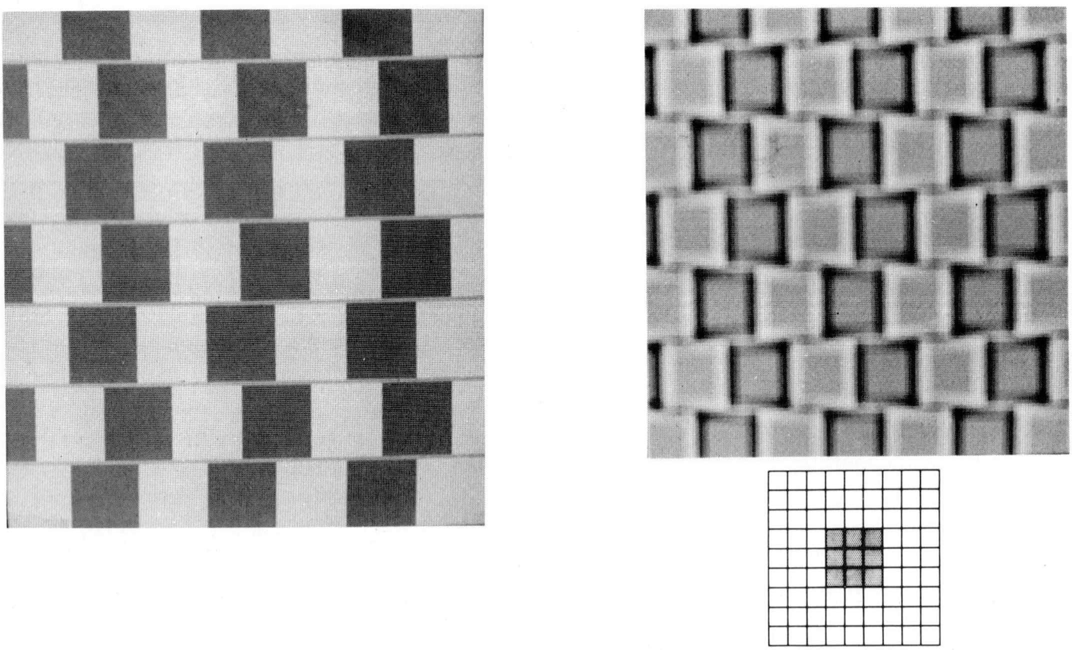

FIG. 1 At left is shown the Münsterberg or cafe wall illusion. The gray mortar lines are actually all horizontal (i.e., parallel), but they appear to be converging and diverging. At right is shown the results of band pass filtering the image with a Laplacian mask (inset). Note that filtering produces locally tilted elements along the previous mortar lines. From Morgan and Moulden (1986).

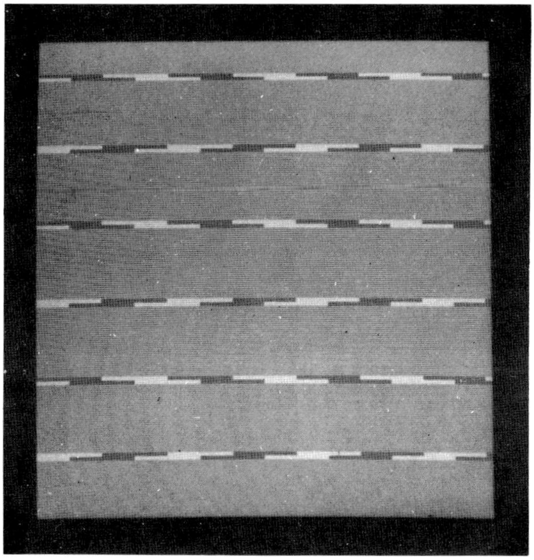

FIG. 2 A version of the Fraser twisted cord illusion, using phase-shifted rectangular elements instead of the usual tilted lines. If this stimulus is subjected to orientation filtering, it provides a maximal input to detectors tuned to orientations just off the horizontal. These local signals of tilt are apparently integrated to give an impression that the line is tilted as a whole, as in the Münsterberg illusion (Fig. 1).

crimination acuity for different spatial patterns. A useful class of pattern tasks for this purpose are "hyperacuities" (Westheimer, 1979a) such as vernier acuity or spatial interval acuity. For such hyperacuities, the minimum positional offset is an order of magnitude smaller than the distance between cone photoreceptor centers in the foveal cone mosaic. Hyperacuity tasks are useful for a number of reasons: thresholds can be measured by objective, forced-choice procedures; stimuli can be carefully controlled in contrast and spatial frequency content; and results are repeatable across observers both qualitatively and quantitatively.

It is possible that if we could understand how pattern acuity tasks are performed then we would be much closer to a viable theory of pattern vision in general. There is at present a sharp division between two theoretical approaches to the explanation of hyperacuity. One is the spatial primitives approach, exemplified in the literature by Watt and Morgan (1985). This theoretical position is the descendant of Marr's ideas about the Primal Sketch (Marr, 1982). The aim of this approach is to use hyperacuity data to constrain models of the early symbolic processes in vision, the local spatial primitives or features that are combined into the Primal Sketch. The emphasis in spatial primitive (feature) models is on the very restricted range of image variables which can be made explicit in the early stages of vision. In contrast to the spatial primitives approach are the models of Geisler (1984), Klein and Levi (1985), Parker and Hawken (1985), Wilson (1986), and Shapley and Victor (1986). Morgan mordantly refers to these theories as "Primal Soup" theories. He asserts that the original Primal Soup was an unstructured broth of amino acids and other useful things which evolved into life by aggregation and accretion. The proposed neural counterpart to this Primal Soup is the entire set of neurons in the primary visual cortex, each of which can be characterized by its spatial frequency and orientational selectivity. In models of pattern discrimination, such as that proposed by Wilson (1986), two patterns can be discriminated if they stimulate any subset of the Soup differently.

If two psychophysically discriminable patterns stimulate different populations of single units, it must be the case that at least one neuron exists which has a reliably different response to the two patterns. It ought to be possible to identify such units physiologically, and an impressive start in this direction has been made by Parker and Hawken (1985), who showed that single cells in monkey visual cortex should be able to respond to step changes in position of a bar within their receptive fields with a displacement hyperacuity threshold similar to that of a human observer. This prediction is based on the sensitivity of the most sensitive visual cortical cells to contrast reversal and on the small size of cortical receptive fields in the monkey (Parker & Hawken, 1985). If one asks how such a cell, or the class of neurons that it represents, should come to control the psychophysical discrimination, then one reaches the heart of the problem with Primal Soup theories.

No model of visual pattern discrimination, and certainly not the spatial primitives model of Watt and Morgan (1983, 1984), can deny that pattern discrimination thresholds are limited by differential neural activity. It is impossible that two patterns should be discriminated if they have identical effects on the brain, so if two patterns are discriminated, they must produce different neural responses. Theories such as Wilson's (1986) perform the essential function of trying to identify the subpopulation of units which limit performance. Using this approach one can answer such questions as, "Why is vernier acuity not better than 2 arc sec?" Geisler's (1984) ideal detector model addresses the same problem from the standpoint of photoreceptor mechanisms for differentiating stimuli. Shapley and Victor (1986) used a similar approach to demonstrate that positional hyperacuity was encoded in the impulse trains of retinal ganglion cells and was a natural consequence of linear filtering and a high signal-to-noise ratio. In fact, all of the Primal Soup theories point to the facts that pattern hyperacuities are limited by processing constraints in the visual cortex and that explicit signals for very small positional offsets in the hyperacuity range are present in the output of the retina. This is a complete turnaround from previous theoretical positions that postulated the need for central averaging and interpolation mechanisms to rescue miniscule hyperacuity signals lost in noise (Crick, Marr & Poggio, 1980; Barlow, 1981).

It can be argued that answering questions about the limits of hyperacuity falls far short of explaining how vernier or other hyperacuity judgments are made by the observer. The Primal Soup theories are not theories of explicit representation unlike, say, the Primal Sketch. The Primal Soup theories place no limits on what can and cannot be represented. Therefore they cannot be used to draw conclusions about many of the principal facts needed in an analysis of perception. Here we present these principal facts in the form of a series of assertions.

1. Observers Can Be Instructed How to Perform Pattern Discrimination Tasks

The point is simple and obvious but often neglected in theoretical analyses of pattern discrimination. Typical instructions might be: "I am going to show you two lines and I want you to tell me which one is longer by pressing the appropriate button on the response box." Subjects have no difficulty in understanding what these instructions mean, and they perform the task effortlessly. They do not need a long series of practice trials and they do not need feedback in order to achieve their best performance. Observers must therefore be basing their decisions on a visual representation of the pattern in which relations of length have been made explicit enough to be accessed through language.

How could this be done in the Primal Soup? The subject would have to discover that longer patterns stimulated one set of units and shorter another set. The problem of finding the right set of units would be hard enough if just two patterns had to be discriminated but it is even worse because:

2. Thresholds Can Be (and Usually Are) Determined Using a Range of Stimulus Values

The most commonly used methods of determining thresholds are derived from the Method of Constants. A range of stimuli is presented along some dimension and the subject must say whether each stimulus is "x" or "y." In the case of length discrimination, to continue the example given above, the question would be whether each stimulus is longer or shorter than the standard. If the observer were suddenly to be presented with a line longer than he or she had seen before, we can take it for granted that he or she would classify it unhesitatingly in a correct way. Thus, to explain pattern vision it is not enough to have a model that discriminates between patterns at threshold. The model must also explain how suprathreshold patterns are classified correctly and how novel stimuli can be recognized. In short, a complete model for pattern vision would have to explain how things look. This is exactly what Primal Soup theories fail to do. However, whether Primal Sketch theories explain pattern classification is unclear.

3. Pattern Acuity Judgments are Usually Directional

When observers discriminate between two lines of different length, they can say not only that they are different but also which one looks longer. Similarly, vernier judgments are made on the basis of the direction of the spatial offset. Any satisfactory theory should account for directional ability. The Primal Soup theories are usually not explicit about this ability to identify the directionality of the discrimination and what it would cost in terms of sensitivity. This is a crucial criticism since it indicates the computational incompleteness of most Primal Soup theories of pattern discrimination. However, a similar criticism could be directed at Primal Sketch theories.

4. Discriminations Are Hard if They Are Not Based on Natural Continua

This is a proposition for which there is little evidence, but it might be asserted anyway in order to indicate what the relevant evidence might be, as a guide to future research. Pattern discrimination tasks use natural categories, such as "larger versus smaller," or "shifted left versus shifted right." But if any arbitrary collection of filters can be grouped together for purposes of discrimination, it should be possible to construct an infinite set of discriminations which do not correspond to natural categories. An example would be a texture composed of a set of random-phase spatial frequency components in a passband defined by its center frequency and bandwidth. Suppose one finds that with textures which have a bandwidth of 0.5 octaves, two such textures can be discriminated when the difference in center frequency is 0.1 octaves. Consider now a set of ten such textures spaced 0.1 octaves apart from one another; we require the observer to respond "+" to even numbered stimuli and "−" to odd numbered textures. Since all members of the set are discriminable by definition, they all reliably stimulate different mechanisms, so it should be possible according to Primal Soup theories to give the mechanisms appropriate weightings to solve the discrimination. As another example, vernier offsets of less than 20 sec arc in either direction could be called "sheep" and those absolutely greater "goats." It is interesting to compare this prediction with the experiments by Rentschler, Hübner and Caelli (1988) on classifying mirror-symmetric Gabor functions described below. They found that with sufficient pretraining subjects could reach 85% accuracy at discriminating such "unnatural" patterns. They conclude from these experiments that there are adaptive spatial filters in the visual system that can be modified to allow "unnatural" spatial discriminations.

5. Patterns Can Be Described as Well as Recognized

Perhaps one of Marr's most valuable contributions to the theory of image interpretation was his criticism of the traditional emphasis on pattern "recognition." What matters about seeing the telephone is not that one can say "phone" but that one can say things like "it consists of two separable parts connected by a cord; one part is roughly oblong with depressions in it into which the other parts fit." Similarly, observers can look at a vernier target for the first time and *describe* it. It is hard to believe that the processes which are involved in making this explicit description are not also involved in vernier discriminations. However, this conclusion must be labeled conjecture rather than inference since there is little evidence at present that ties the visual processes involved in description with those responsible for pattern discrimination.

6. Localized Edges are Important in Pattern Acuity

This sounds like a glimpse of the obvious, but consider whether it ought to be true. If the image of a face has the phases of all its Fourier components jumbled, it will appear to be a mess, but it remains uniquely specified over a set of filters. Thus, it should remain discriminable from other faces treated in the same way, according to Primal Soup type theories. Using the same line of argument, one can imagine a set of one hundred faces the observer can discriminate and even name reliably.

The appearance of images is certainly influenced by their amplitude spectrum, and, consequently, altering the amplitude spectrum by filtering changes their appearance (Ginsburg, 1984). Harvey (1986) used a series of band pass amplitude filtered images of a human face to find the filtered face that most closely approximated the mental image of the face in memory. Using multidimensional scaling techniques, he concluded that visual memory behaves like a band pass filter, centered on 3.8 cycles per degree. with a bandwidth of 2.8 octaves.

The appearance of images is specified to a much greater degree by their phase than by their amplitude spectra. If an image is produced with the amplitude spectrum of an image A and the phase spectrum of a different image P, it will resemble image P rather than image A (Oppenheim & Lim, 1981; Piotrowski & Campbell, 1982; see also Fig. 3). The explanation is that the phase spectrum determines the spatial structure of a signal. There is evidence that the visual system's response to spatial structure is dependent on *local computations*: either local reponses to edges, bars, and blobs or local spectral energy in even and odd symmetric filters (e.g., Caelli & Moraglia, 1986). These may be two different verbal descriptions of the same computation. Whatever the nature of the local computation, it must depend on the positioning of Fourier components in the image and thus on their relative phase.

Primal Soup theories were designed to explain dis-

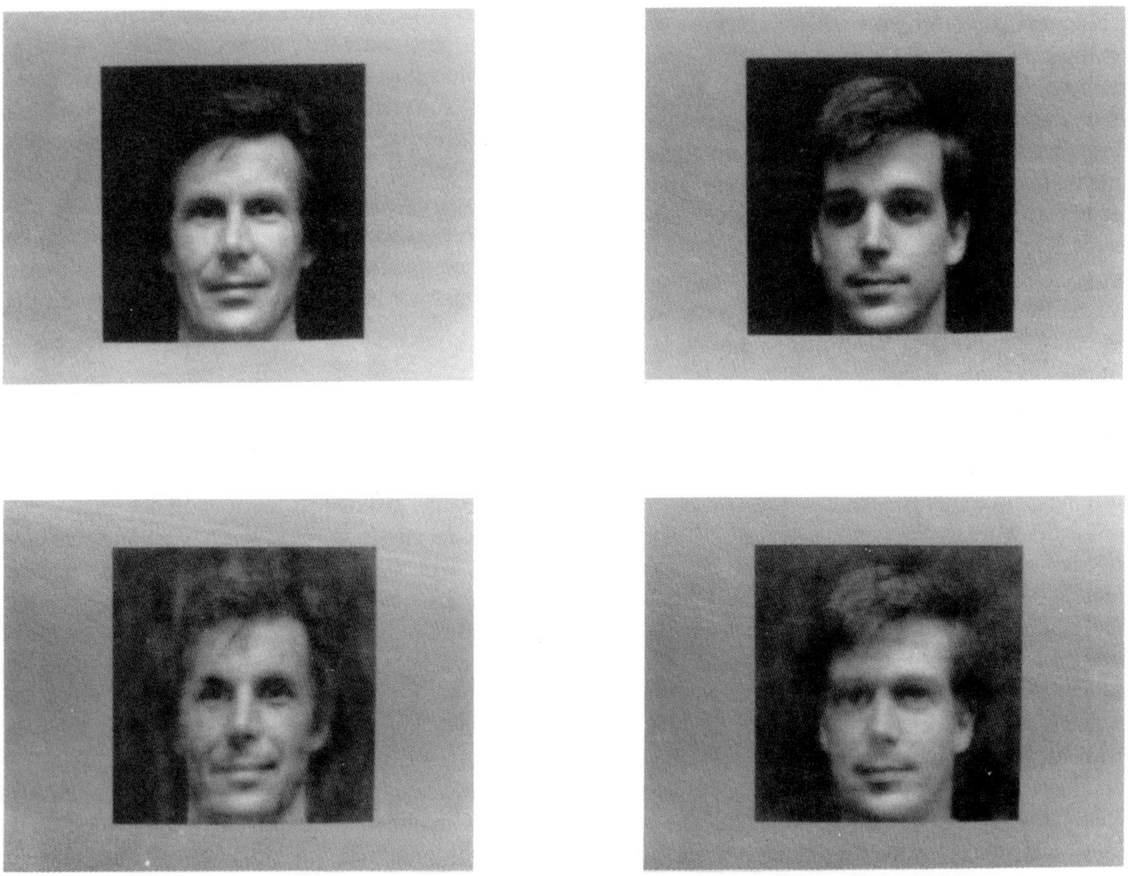

FIG. 3 Effect of scrambling amplitude spectra while keeping phase spectra unchanged between images. The top row of images comprises two different faces. In the second row, the images have had their amplitude spectra varied while keeping the phase spectra unchanged. A comparable distortion of phase spectra with no change in amplitude spectra produces unrecognizable faces.

crimination and hyperacuity, not appearance. These theories have demonstrated that discriminations and hyperacuity may be understood as threshold detection problems: threshold detection in the presence of a masking pattern, the discriminandum. They were not designed to handle appearance. The success of Primal Soup theories in accounting for hyperacuity performance reveals that the assumption that studying hyperacuity should lead to the mechanisms for producing appearance is not necessarily true.

IV. COMPUTATIONAL RULES FOR SPATIAL VISION

Modeling biological spatial vision in terms of selected signal types and system parameters is not entirely adequate. For example, though masking and adaptation studies show "tuning" to spatial frequency, orientation, and phase parameters of simple grating patches (e.g., Wilson, McFarlane & Phillips, 1983; Breitmeyer, 1984), these curves do not predict masking effects with more natural images. Repeatedly it has been found that the properties of *local image luminance profiles* are directly relevant in such tasks. Transform domain parameters (e.g., Fourier amplitudes and phases) are only predictive when they determine significant characteristics of the luminance profiles (Caelli & Moraglia, 1986). This is the reason that, in the development of models of spatial vision based on Fourier methods, there has been a progression from models in which spatial phase was not preserved to a model such as Wilson and Gelb's (1984) in which position information is retained.

What is required for an adequate paradigm for spatial vision is not details of psychophysical procedure, nor the enumeration of parameter tuning for postulated neural mechanisms, but, rather, *general computational constraints* that are necessary and sufficient to solve given perceptual tasks. This idea is reminiscent of Marr's (1982) parsing of computational vision into levels of description, the highest level of which is the computational theory. Work by Caelli (1988) and Rentschler et al. (1988) suggests that the type of detectors, their tuning characteristics, and use of detector responses by decision-making processes may be adaptive to the signal and task demands. Then the true *invariants* for visual information processing consist in the types of computations available.

One of the major tasks of the visual system, according to this computational paradigm for vision, is object and texture segregation. This means that the system must parse retinotopically registered, viewer-dependent projections of object-reflected light into parts which mean something to the observer. There may be a natural division of such segmentation mechanisms into two classes. These are often referred to as *boundary-extracting* and *texture-encoding* mechanisms in the literature on image processing. They register luminance information in terms of two components over a range of spatial scales. The boundary extraction processes are usually thought to be determined by threshold outputs of detectors with retention of contrast sign. On the other hand, the texture processing system is viewed as registering the energy of the outputs of filters (or detectors) at each position, producing a distribution of activity that does not encode the sign of the detector's reponse. Several authors have shown that energy response measures are more representative of human texture discrimination performance than are texton or feature detector theories (Laws, 1980; Ade, 1983; Caelli, 1985; Bergen & Adelson, 1988). We now compare and contrast these different approaches to texture segmentation.

The perception of textural segments involves the ability of observers to carry out a labeling process whereby each position is allocated to one of a number of textured regions. These regions are usually perceived as contiguous, so forming a complete covering of the image surface. The task of a complete model for texture segmentation is to produce an algorithm that reflects human performance on this task.

Theories of texture segmentation have varied, including statistical or global integrative computations (Julesz, 1981) to detector-based models based on notions of fixed, highly tuned filters or "textons" (Laws, 1980; Julesz, 1981; Treisman, 1982; Julesz & Bergen, 1983; Caelli, 1985; Bergen & Adelson, 1988) or adaptive filters derived from the second-order statistics of texture stimuli (Ade, 1983). Most current theories involve the notion of image decomposition by filters having point-spread functions of different shape, typically having center–surround (isotropic band pass) or orientation-specific even and odd symmetric profiles. However, the human visual system apparently does not use the outputs of such detectors in some texture segmentation tasks. This can be seen in Fig. 4 where two points are illustrated: (1) local orientation detection is clearly dependent on local contrast sign while (2) if local orientation is detected, the visual system is amazingly insensitive, in segmenting texture, to the sign of contrast. Such observations and others have led Caelli and colleagues to conclude that, in the texture mode, the appropriate filter output is energy or some other even nonlinear function of contrast and merely measures the magnitude of detector activity rather than its sign. The actual point-spread functions of the filters or detectors that are used for texture segmentation are still unknown.

One of the more serious logical errors in this area is the simple enumeration of filters or detectors in terms of apparently important components of texture micropatterns. For example, it is known that the crossing-line and end-of-line detectors are simply not necessary to produce texture discrimination in textures generated by Julesz (1981) and Treisman (1982) to confirm this claim. Detailed analyses of these textures demonstrate segmentability by simple

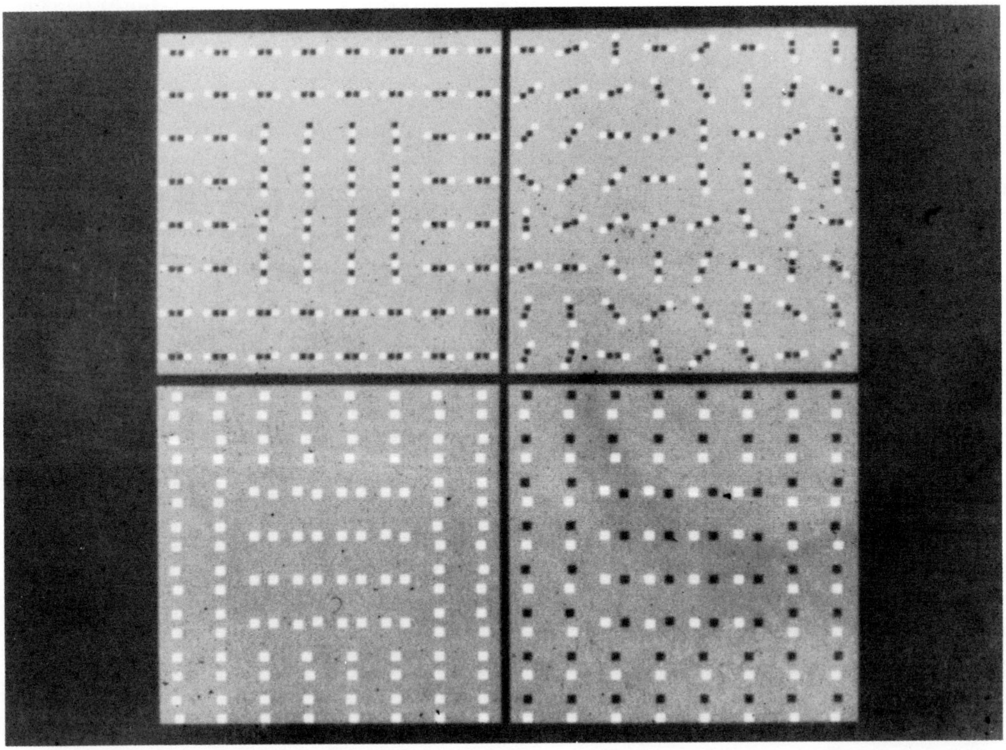

FIG. 4 The top row shows how orientation-specific texture segmentation is dependent on the local contrast of oriented dipoles. The bottom row shows that when sufficient orientation-specific micropattern differences are not present, contrast distribution differences are not sufficient to produce segmentation. From Caelli (1988), © 1988 IEEE.

orientation-specific, or even isotropic, band pass filters equivalent to retinal center–surround receptive fields (Caelli, 1985; Bergen & Adelson, 1988).

In order to understand the degree to which perceptual data tell us anything about the neural filters that allow humans to perform texture segregation, the filter design problem has to be considered in the context of the system's information processing characteristics. To do this we first note that texture segmentation involves the notion of region contiguity. That is, textures, or regions between texture boundaries, are perceived as regions where all positions are labeled as belonging to the same equivalence class. This constraint usually involves some form of *relaxation labeling* where the texture processing system aims at attaining contiguity by updating the labeling according to near neighbor labels—a form of cooperative processing.

Another consideration for filter design is the inherent redundancy in a large number of filters which, by virtue of spectral overlaps, have signal responses that are correlated. It is important to realize that the types of redundancies in detector outputs can be used to reshape current filter characteristics or to develop new detectors to capture the useful information in the texture statistics or luminance gradients.

To capture explicitly these principles of maximizing the spatial contiguity between texture boundaries and minimizing the number of functional detectors, the following associative-network equation has been developed by Caelli (1988):

$$A_i^{t+1}(x,y) = \frac{1}{\alpha\beta} \sum_r^{\alpha} \sum_s^{\beta} A_i^t\left(x + r - \frac{\alpha}{2}, y + s - \frac{\beta}{2}\right) + \sum_{\substack{j=1 \\ i \neq j}} w_{ij}^t A_j^t(x,y) \tag{4}$$

where $A_i^t(x,y)$ corresponds to the activity (energy) of detector i at position (x,y) and time t. The first determinant of the response is a simple linear version of relaxation where the response at position (x,y) to detector i is reinforced or inhibited as a function of the responses of the same detectors in its neighborhood. One neurophysiological basis for this process could be variable excitatory or activating links between cells in similar cortical areas having similar receptive field profiles where the strength of spreading activation varies directly with the cell's response. The second response determinant [the right hand term in Eq. (4)] contains the redundancy computation. Here the activity of detector i at position (x,y) is updated by the degree to which it is correlated over the textured regions with others at time t. This cooperative process has the effect of forming "attractors" in the detector space whereby detectors whose responses are correlated tend to become more correlated. This rather simple associative network demonstrates how many broadly tuned detectors can be adapted to signal characteristics so as to result in fewer, more appropriately tuned, and orthogonalized profiles.

Figure 5 shows examples of equilibrium ($t = 7$ iterations) results of this system using 24 Gabor functions as initial filter kernels. It is particularly important to note that the 24 detectors (only 12 are shown in Fig. 5) converged on one isotropic, low-pass profile that was sufficient to segment the center from surround regions, so producing contiguity of the texture regions. That is, what started off as a 24-channel model reduced to a single-channel model. In this model the decision process simply involves determining the degree to which detector outputs at each position differ, where the degree of difference indexes the degree of texture segmentability.

Figure 6 shows examples of four different textures segmented according to these principles. The results for column 2 correspond to zero associativity or independence of processing. Here, strength of segmentation closely corresponds to what is perceived both casually and experimentally (Julesz, 1981). Column 3 corresponds to classification strength as a result of filter update by the response correlations. Results here are compatible with those for the 24 channels. Thus, equivalent performance is achieved with a much more economical model. Column 4 illustrates what would happen if the filters had inhibitory connections during updating. It would not work. Inhibition in this context results in region differentiation, a result not consistent with the aim of extracting contiguous textured regions.

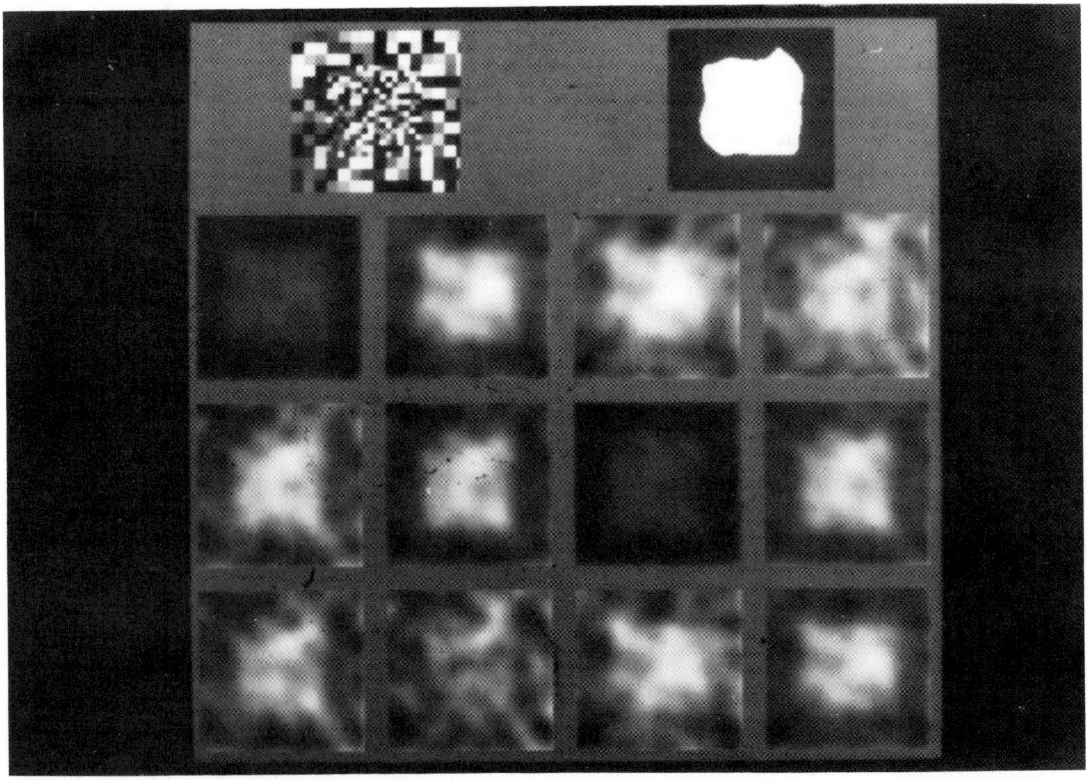

FIG. 5 Final activity profiles of 12 of 24 detectors used in a simulation of the associative processing algorithm in Eq. 4, in response to a texture varying in granularity. All of the detectors initially were two-dimensional Gabor functions but were modified as in Eq. 4 to become low-pass spatial filters. The test pattern is illustrated in the top left panel of the figure, and the texture segregation achieved by the adaptive filters is illustrated in the top right-hand panel.

Present attempts to understand vision in terms of filter theory usually result in hypotheses relating neurophysiology to psychophysics only if hypothetical filters are estimated to have similar values in the two types of tasks. This is not necessary since it is the algebraic form of the model and the proposed computations that are essential ingredients for the depiction of a model.

One final point should be made about the relationship between the computational mechanisms for the texture system and possible neurophysiological substrata. If we assume that the visual system has a "default" set of detectors tuned to, say, orientation and size, then what is claimed by Caelli et al., 1988 is that the type of information extracted from the response profiles either may modify the detectors or may cause new detectors to be produced. It may be that biophysical changes at the cellular level are involved in this modification process.

V. THE PATTERN RECOGNITION CONCEPT OF DIGITAL SIGNAL PROCESSING

The pattern recognition approach advocated by Rentschler et al. (1988) implies that objects are provided with a number of attributes, some of which constitute

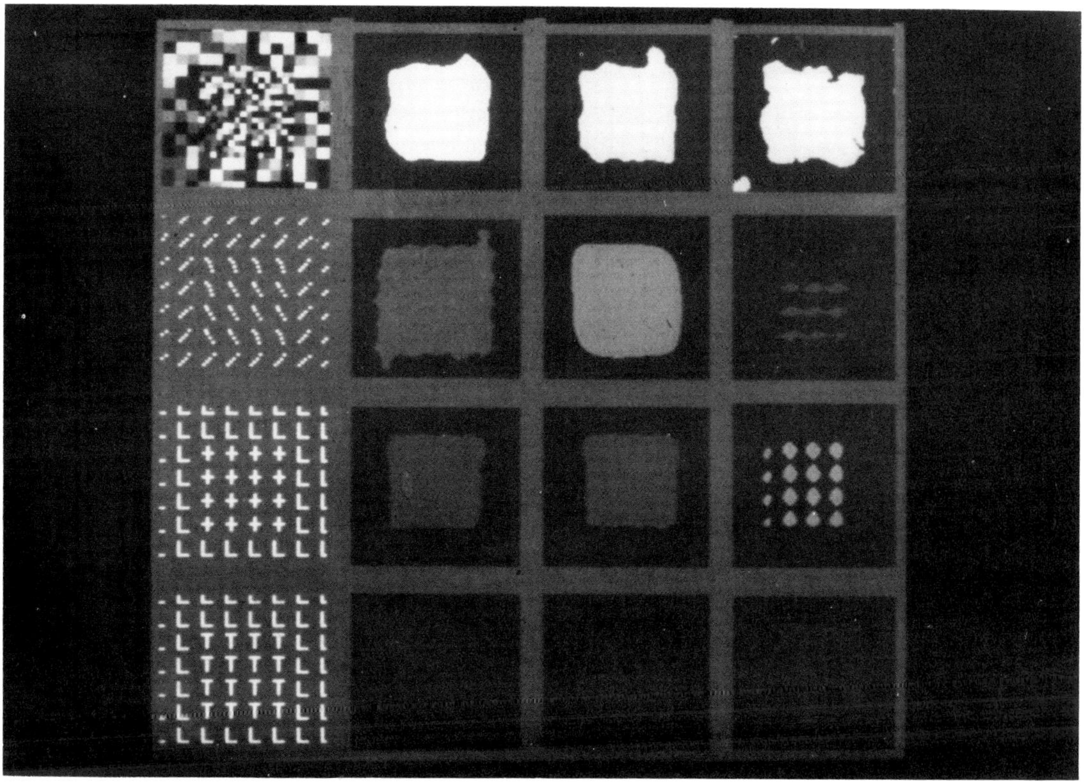

FIG. 6 Segmentation results for 4 textures (column 1) resulting from the outputs of 24 detectors with no associativities (column 2), with associativities (column 3), or with inhibitory mass action (column 4). For details see text.

the peculiarity of a specific object while others which may be called "features," determine the class to which the object belongs (Watanabe, 1985, Chapter 11, this volume). Pattern recognition begins with the observation of a number of variables that is usually quite large and ends with the determination of a single binary variable on which the membership of the given object to a certain class depends. It follows that *the reduction of variables* is essential for solving a problem of pattern recognition. The reduction of dimensionality is often done in several steps. One step may involve a transformation of variables with unimportant ones being rejected. This corresponds to the mapping of the original signal space onto a subspace of lower dimensionality (Watanabe, 1985). Classification, the last step of a pattern recognition procedure, consists of establishing a metric (a distance function) for that subspace and a decision rule for assigning the object to a certain class.

Let the input signal be a digital image composed of $N \times N$ picture elements (pixels). It can be considered as a vector in a vector space of $N \times N$ dimensionality, each pixel being a component of the signal vector. Usually this signal is subjected to an orthogonal transformation (e.g., the discrete Fourier Transform), but it is important to note that such a transformation does not alter the dimensionality of the signal. This implies that the application of a Fourier Transform per se cannot constitute a theory of visual pattern recognition. Feature selection, with the emphasis on dimensionality reduction, depends on an a priori decision, the usefulness of which can only be judged in terms of classification performance. The resulting signal space of strongly reduced dimensionality is called the feature space.

Pattern classes consist of a set of n feature vectors, or samples, and it is usually assumed that the latter form a cluster in feature space. During "supervised learning," the classifier constructs "class prototypes" as the mean of the feature vectors within a class. Thus, if we write a cluster as:

$$c_i = \{Z_{i1}, Z_{i2}, \ldots Z_{in}\} \tag{5}$$

then the class prototype will be:

$$Z_i = n^{-1} \sum_{j=1}^{n} Z_{ij} \tag{6}$$

After the learning period, classification is made according to which prototype is closest in feature space to the input pattern. This criterion depends on the metric assigned to the feature space. Below we discuss an experiment by Caelli and colleagues in which a Euclidean metric, namely, the square root of the sum of the squares of component differences between pattern and prototype, was used successfully in conjunction with a maximum-likelihood estimate to account for the decision behavior of human observers. In this case the probability for assigning pattern i to class k is

$$p(k|i) = \frac{(d_{ik})^{-1}}{\sum_{j=1}^{m} (d_{ij})^{-1}} \tag{7}$$

with d_{ik} denoting Euclidean distance between pattern i and prototype k. The number of classes is m. A non-Euclidean metric is also described below.

The critical issue about pattern recognition is the conceptual framework within which feature selection and classification are being performed, and not the type of representation of the $N \times N$ dimensional input signals (as spatial or spectral). Moreover, the success of a given solution in a pattern recognition problem does not imply uniqueness of the solution. Watanabe (1981) proved that a necessary, unique solution cannot exist. It follows that theories and results of experiments related to human pattern recognition can provide insight into possible strategies of visual information processing but cannot provide sufficient information about the actual implementation in terms of neural machinery.

A. Classification of Compound Gabor Signals: Evidence for Adaptive Filtering

In a first experiment, Caelli, Rentschler, and Scheider (1987) studied the classification of compound Gabor signals as used also by Caelli, Hübner, and Rentschler (1986) and Rentschler, Hübner, and Caelli (1988) in studies on gray-scale textures. Such signals have luminance profiles defined by

$$g(x,y) = e^{-r^2/\alpha^2}[a \cos(2\pi f x) + b \cos(2\pi \cdot 3fx + \phi)] \tag{8}$$

where α determines the space constant of the isotropic Gaussian aperture with

$$r = (x^2 + y^2)^{1/2} \tag{9}$$

The amplitudes of the first and third harmonics in the Gabor function were a and b, respectively. The phase angle of the third harmonic was denoted ϕ. Results from two experiments are shown where observers learned the classification of learning sets of 15 samples into three categories. The signals were generated on a display with 128×128 pixels, 8 bits per pixel. Variations of the signals were restricted to amplitude and phase of the third harmonic. Examples of such images are illustrated in Fig. 7.

A procedure of supervised learning was applied consisting of a variable number of learning units. One unit consisted of three presentations in random order with a stimulus duration of 200 msec. Following each stimulus presentation a number was displayed specifying the pattern as a member of a certain class. At the end of such a unit, the subject was tested as to how he/she was capable of classifying the samples of the learning set. Only one exposure per pattern was used here. If the individual did not reach a criterion of 100% correct, he/she had to undergo another learn-

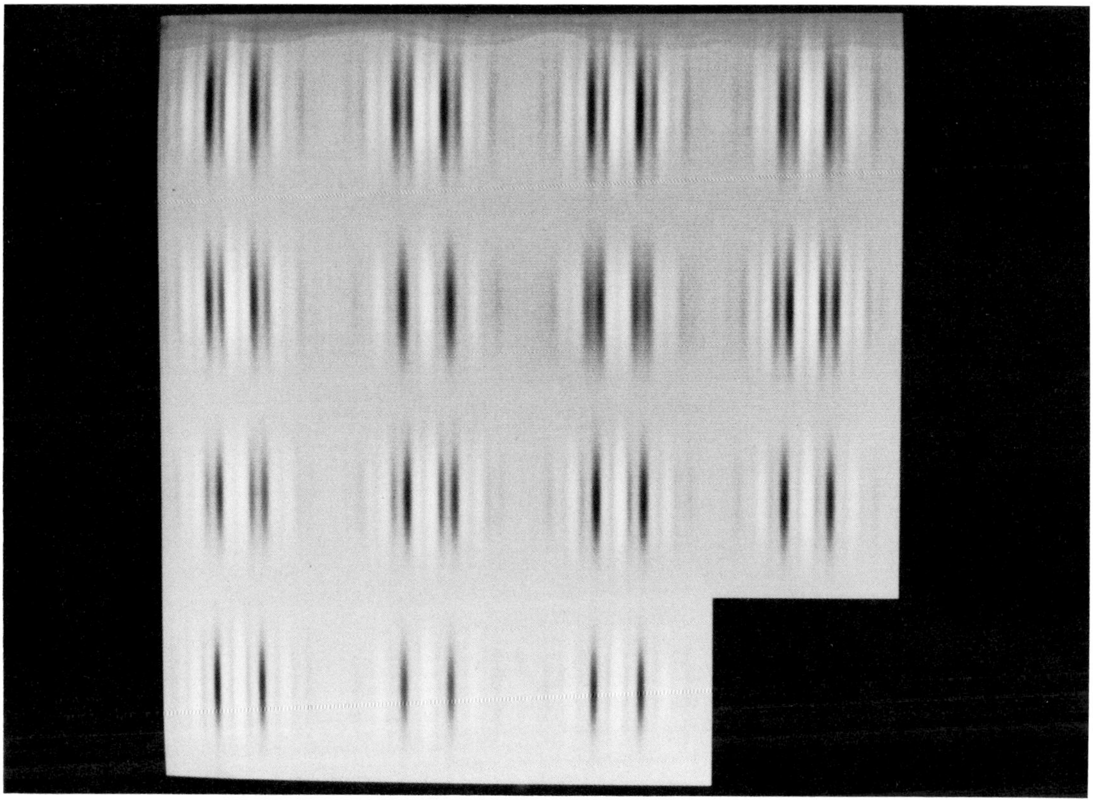

FIG. 7 Compound Gabor signals described by Eq. (8). Variations of the signals were restricted to the amplitude and phase values of the third harmonic.

ing unit, up to a maximum of 15 learning units. Cumulative confusion matrices over all stimuli and test runs were obtained for each subject. Figure 8 shows stimulus configuration 1 and the mean classification performance over four subjects.

The classification model used to account for these results was a least-squares minimum-distance classifier. It uses the Euclidean metric in feature space, but it is different from the regular minimum-distance classifier because it maps the feature space into a decision space, the dimensionality of which equals the number of classes used (for details see Ahmed & Rao, 1975). The feature space is the two-dimensional Cartesian coordinates of evenness and oddness of the third harmonic, that is, $x = b \cos \phi$ and $y = b \sin \phi$. The classification performance predicted by such a model is shown at the right of the Fig. 8.

The consistency between the observed and predicted classification data demonstrates the adequacy of feature selection and the least-squares minimum-distance classification model, involving a Euclidean metric in feature space, in predicting behavior. However, this solution may not be unique. There may be other ways of selecting features and classifying signals that lead to equally good predictions. What can be concluded is that the results cannot be explained on the basis of a fixed number of invariant "channels," or spatial filters. Rather, the view of class pro-

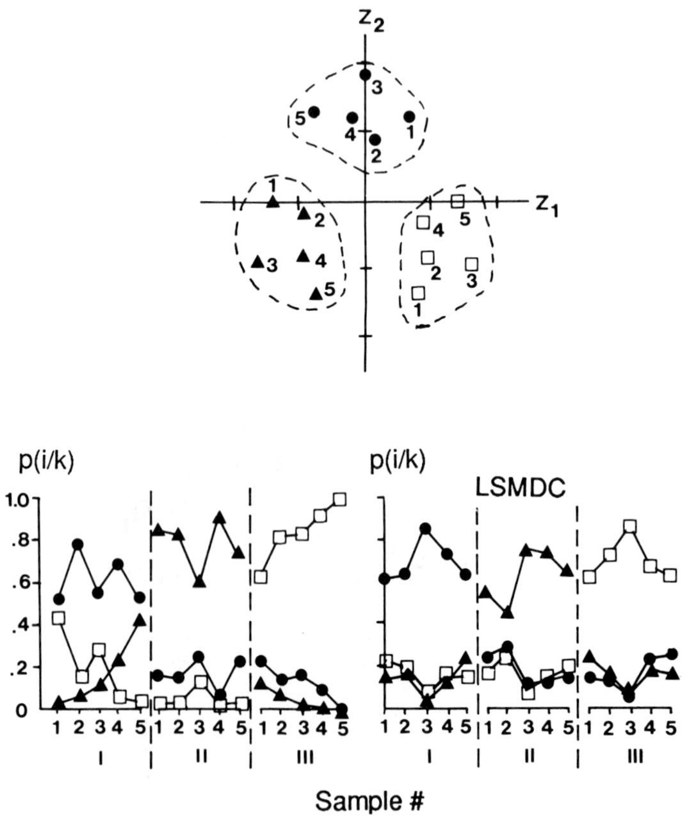

FIG. 8 Mean classification performance for four subjects on stimulus configuration 1 from the set of compound Gabor signals illustrated in Fig. 7 (upper left-hand panel).

totypes as exemplar images (see Watanabe, 1985, for a detailed discussion) which are matched with signals presented for classification is equivalent to defining them as adaptive filters.

B. Classification of Mirror Image Compound Gabor Signals: Evidence for Effects of Cooperativity

A specific property of the two-dimensional feature space of evenness and oddness is that signal pairs having the fundamental waveform in cosine phase with (x_i, y_i) and $(x_i, -y_i)$ coordinates only differ with respect to the sign of their oddness component and therefore have mirror image luminance profiles. Previously Rentschler and Treutwein (1985) have shown that, independently of scale, mirror image compound grating pairs are indistinguishable in extrafoveal vision. The same is true for texture pairs composed of such signals as micropatterns (Rentschler et al., 1988). Bennet and Banks (1987) have confirmed these findings and interpreted their results in terms of the four channel model of Field and Nachmias (1984). Their main conclusion was that odd symmetric channels do not exist in peripheral vision. What is particularly relevant for the present chapter is that mirror image gratings (Field & Nachmias, 1984; Rentschler & Treutwein, 1985) and compound Gabor signals (I. Rentschler, unpublished observations) are more difficult to distinguish in foveal vision as well. To pursue this issue, Rentschler et al. used the procedures described above to study pattern classification of compound Gabor signals with mirror image relationships.

Twelve signals, clustered into four groups and symmetrically located in feature space, were used throughout the experiment. Four of the signals (one in each cluster) had the same high amplitude of third harmonic, while eight of them (two in each group) had the same low amplitude. What is important to note is that each signal in the upper half-plane of feature space had its mirror image correspondent in the lower half plane (Fig. 9A). The influence of pretraining on the classification of mirror image signals was studied by means of the following protocol. (1) The four subjects of group 1 were initially trained to 100% criterion in classifying the twelve patterns into two classes that contained three pairs of mirror image signals each. These subjects therefore were not required to distinguish mirror image patterns during pretraining. (2) The four subjects of group 2 were initially trained to criterion in classifying the twelve patterns into two classes with the mirror images being in different classes. Thus, these subjects learned to distinguish mirror image signals. (3) A third group of five subjects received no pretraining. (4) In the main experiment, each of the 13 subjects was then trained to criterion in classifying the same twelve patterns into four classes thus distinguishing between mirror image signals.

The results of the experiment are quantified as confusion matrices (Fig. 9B). A diagonal confusion matrix means that no pattern is confused with any other; classification is perfect. In the actual results, subjects from group 3 (no pretraining) had nondiagonal confusion matrices. Furthermore, the confusion matrix was often asymmetric. For example, patterns from class I were classified as belonging to class IV more often than patterns in class IV were classified as belonging to class I. Unlike those from group 3, subjects in group 1 showed smaller off-diagonal elements in their confusion matrices, and subjects in group 2, who had learned to discriminate mirror image patterns during pretraining, had almost perfectly diagonal confusion matrices. In summary, with increased specificity of pretraining the confusion matrix tends to diagonal structure.

These results suggest that the idea of independent, fixed, and invariant channels, so popular in vision research, only applies to very specific situations where the brain is already highly adapted to that specific

A

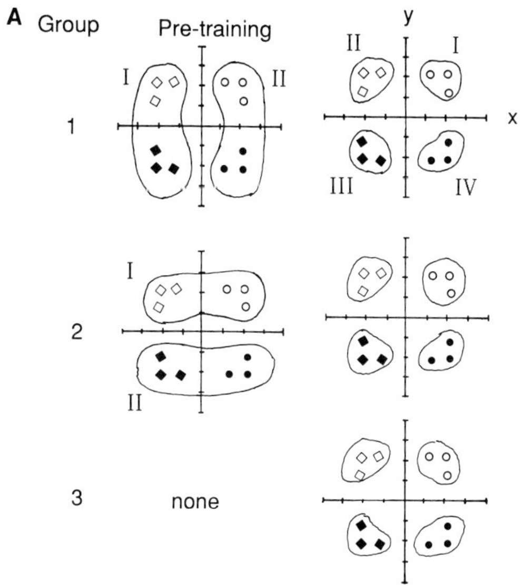

B

Group 1 (4Ss, $N = 364$)

.74	.06	.05	.15
.01	.78	.18	.03
.01	.31	.63	.05
.29	.02	.04	.65

Group 2 (4Ss, $N = 102$)

.85	.07	.01	.17
.06	.81	.12	.01
.01	.15	.82	.02
.13	.0	.05	.82

Group 3 (1S: $N = 138$)

75	.07	.0	.18
.02	.81	.09	.08
.01	.42	.44	.13
.51	.06	.04	.39

FIG. 9 Testing procedures and classification performance on the mirror image Gabor signals. (A) The task of the main experiment was to assign the twelve Gabor signals to four classes. The three groups of observers received different pretraining: Group 1 had to assign the twelve signals to two classes with mirror images belonging to the same class. Group 2 had the same task with the mirror images belonging to different classes. Group 3 had no pretraining. (B) Cumulative confusion matrices for the three groups.

task. It would be these specific states where the response to a certain class of signals, or objects, is adequately captured by determining the class prototype or (adaptive) filter. Visual psychophysicists may still wish to call such prototypes "channels." It is conceivable that these mechanisms are built up by synaptic modification as a consequence of learning. Yet, it may be that such channels have functional significance only in the brains of hard-working psychophysicists, or in the brains of their hard-working subjects. The inexperienced are more likely to use a "scatter brain" where the response to a signal consists of a distributed pattern of activity involving a whole ensemble of channels, prototypes, or neurons.

Summarizing these considerations, Rentschler et al. suggest that current models of spatial vision via fixed, invariant, and independent channels are inherently insufficient to explain visual pattern recognition. By definition, these concepts fail to capture active (i.e., signal dependent) processes of feature selection, and they are also inappropriate to examine the issue of cooperative interaction between filter mechanisms. On the other hand, standard procedures from computer pattern recognition can be adopted to investigate such problems in human vision.

VI. THEORIES OF THE NEURAL BASIS OF BRIGHTNESS AND FORM PERCEPTION

A. Relative Strength of Contrast and Assimilation in Brightness Perception

It seems that brightness perception is effortless, rapid, and simple; however, visual scientists have known for years that complex neuronal computations are required for satisfactory performance of this task (Jameson & Hurvich, 1959; Chapter 7, this volume). The visual system is not a photometer, and the perception of brightness is not simply a matter of counting photons. The primary determinant of brightness perception is local contrast, the local difference between luminances on either side of a boundary normalized by the (local) average luminance (Heinemann, 1955; Shapley & Enroth-Cugell, 1984). However, local contrast is not the only physical stimulus attribute that affects brightness perception. The spatial arrangement of nearby bright or dark objects, and the total amount of lightness and darkness in the local vicinity, may influence the apparent brightness of a test object in a way contrary to the effects of contrast. The psychobiological process that mediates this additive effect of local brightnesses has been called *assimilation* because it is similar to color assimilation (Hurvich, 1981). Assimilation is responsible for the filling-in of brightnesses from the borders of objects where contrast is computed. From comparison of psychophysical and neurophysiological experiments on brightness induction, Shapley and Enroth-Cugell (1984) and Reid and Shapley (1988) have concluded that local contrast is computed in the retina. Assimilation, however, is not seen in subcortical visual neurons and therefore must be a process that is introduced in the visual cortex, perhaps even at a higher level than Area V1.

Why is brightness perception so dependent on contrast, and why is there the additional process of assimilation that acts as a corrective to contrast? The key to understanding brightness perception is in comprehending the meaning of brightness constancy and how constancy results from response dependence on contrast.

Animals and men have evolved in a world of reflecting surfaces: water, earth, flowers, fur and skin and feathers. What characterizes a reflecting surface visually is its reflectance. The reflectance is determined by the physical properties of the surface of the object. The reflectance is more or less invariant with respect to illumination. The luminance of an object L_O is proportional to the product of the object's reflectance and illumination, thus

$$L_O = K \cdot R_O \cdot I \qquad (10)$$

We know from Wallach (1976) and others that over a wide range of illumination the brightness of a reflecting object does not change, even though its luminance may vary widely, and that the brightnesses of an array of reflecting surfaces are perceived approximately in the order of their reflectances. Land and McCann

(1971) went so far as to say that the visual system was designed to calculate reflectance. We now know that this is not correct, but it is on the right track. The visual system calculates contrast and from this derives relative reflectance, as shown below. Stockham (1972) has pointed out that, under natural conditions, illumination [I in Eq. (10)] is a slowly varying function of time and space, while reflectance is a rapidly varying function because of the reflectance borders (edges) between objects and their backgrounds. Thus, light adaptation and spatial filtering would tend to remove the slowly varying factor in the luminance signal in Eq. (10) and would make the visual system more dependent on the biologically relevant reflectance function.

The early stages of vision compute contrast not reflectance. What this means is that the response of retinal, lateral geniculate and some primary cortical neurons is proportional to contrast over a low-to-medium contrast range, and then may saturate at high contrast. This is indicated by the results in Fig. 10 which show response proportionality to contrast over a hundredfold range of luminances in cat retinal ganglion cells (R. Shapley & E. Kaplan, unpublished). This result was already adumbrated by the contrast sensitivity measurements of Enroth-Cugell and Robson (1966) who demonstrated invariance of the contrast sensitivity of cat retinal ganglion cells with background luminance over several log units of mean luminance.

An important feature of these results is that constancy of response with contrast is achieved for stimuli that activate only the center mechanism of the receptive field. This means that responsiveness of the visual system to contrast is not a result of center–surround interaction, or, in other words, of lateral inhibition (as in the standard textbook accounts, e.g., Cornsweet, 1970). Rather, the key to understanding dependence of response on contrast is to realize that contrast dependence is primarily a result of the automatic gain control that produces *light adaptation* (Whittle & Challands, 1969; Shapley & Enroth-Cugell, 1984; Chapter 5, this volume). The automatic gain control that regulates the contrast sensitivity of a receptive field center is localized to the center, and thus contrast is computed only locally (see Shapley and Enroth-Cugell, 1984, for a comprehensive review). An elementary calculation demonstrates how light adaptation yields dependence of neural reponse on contrast and therefore discounts the illuminant and produces brightness constancy.

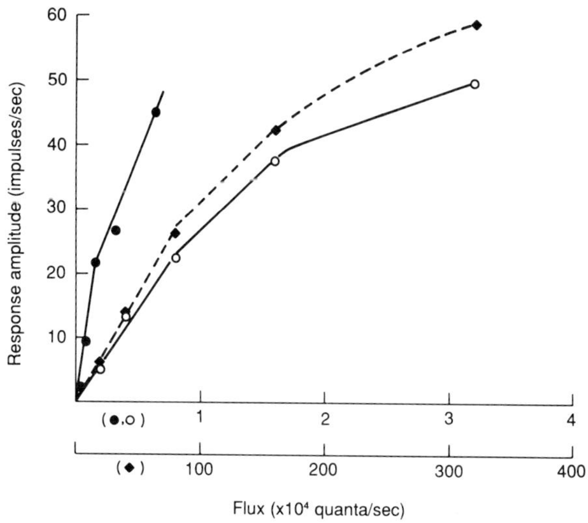

FIG. 10 Responses of an X-type cat retinal ganglion cell to drifting sine-wave gratings matched to the receptive field center, at three mean illuminances. Filled circles are responses to the gratings at the lowest mean illumination. Empty circles are responses to gratings around a mean illumination 10 times higher than the lowest. Diamonds represent responses to gratings at a mean illumination 100 times brighter than the second mean, and 1000 times brighter than the lowest. The diamonds are plotted on the lower axis of the abscissas, while the two sets of circles are plotted against the upper axis. Plotting the data in this way shows that, for empty circles and diamonds, responses are simply proportional to contrast (stimulus flux divided by mean or background flux).

Consider as an example a uniformly illuminated scene with an object on a background. The light from the object side of the border is $I \cdot R_O$ while the light from the background is $I \cdot R_B$ where I is the illumination. Contrast in this case can be defined as $(IR_O - IR_B)/IR_B$ which reduces to $(R_O - R_B)/R_B$. It is evident that contrast is independent of illumination. Now consider the response of a retinal neuron to the same object on the background. Retinal neurons respond to change as when the eye moves the receptive field across the border between background and object.

The effective stimulus in that case will be the difference between the light coming from the object and the background, that is, $IR_O - IR_B$. The response of the neuron will be the stimulus input multiplied by the gain of the input/output transduction. The gain, determined by the light adaptation mechanism, will be approximately proportional to $1/IR_B$. Thus, the response of the neuron will be proportional to $(IR_O - IR_B)/IR_B$, the contrast. And the neural response will also be proportional to $(R_O - R_B)/R_B$ when the illumination is factored out of the fraction. Thus, neuronal response will be proportional to contrast and independent of illumination. Objects of a given reflectance will look equally bright against the same background because they have the same contrasts. Notice that all these statements hinge on the claim that gain is reciprocal with illumination, that is, Weber's law. This law only holds in a limited range of mean illuminations (Shapley & Enroth-Cugell, 1984). When neuronal responses do not follow Weber's law, they also no longer are dependent strictly on contrast and invariant with illumination. This is particularly true at low luminances, as can be seen in Fig. 10. A strong prediction is that brightness constancy will fail when Weber's law does, and this prediction has been confirmed (Heinemann, 1955).

B. Contrast vs. Reflectance: Simultaneous Contrast

Shapley and Reid (1985) showed that it is contrast and not reflectance that the visual system is computing by confirming and extending classical studies on "simultaneous contrast." An example is the elaboration of the classic picture of equally luminant circles on a nonuniform background, as in Fig. 11. Figure 11 shows twelve equally luminant circles placed on rectangular stripes that vary in luminance. This could be interpreted as a scene with twelve equally reflective disks placed on a cloth with twelve different rectangular regions of reflectance. If the visual system is computing local contrast, then the disks should all look different in brightness because their contrasts are not all the same. If the visual system were computing

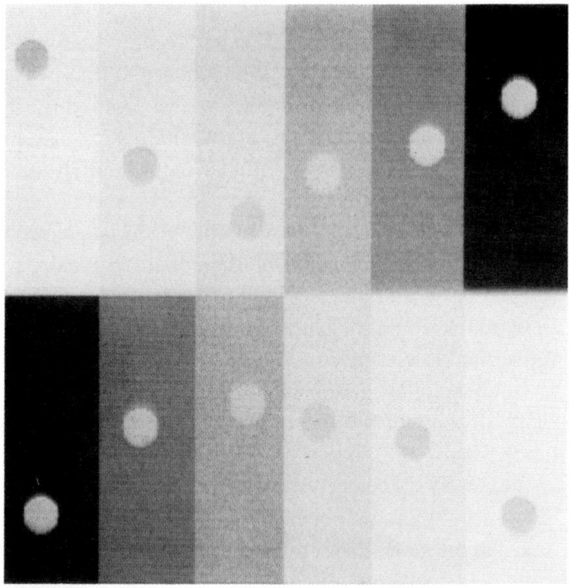

FIG. 11 Twelve equiluminant circles on a nonuniform background look different in brightness. From Shapley (1986).

reflectance as Land and McCann (1971) suggested, then all the twelve disks should look the same shade of gray. It is obvious that they look different, and so at least qualitatively the quantity computed is closer to contrast than to reflectance. Land and McCann (1971) anticipated this refutation of their theory (the 1971 Retinex) in a footnote to their paper in which they asserted that pictures such as Fig. 11 were unnatural because the objects were completely surrounded by their backgrounds. This argument has little merit since in nature isolated objects on backgrounds are the rule rather than the exception. But, accepting the Land and McCann argument as valid for the moment, we can put it to the test by constructing a "Mondrian"-like pattern that Land and McCann consider more natural and by looking again at equally reflective objects on nonuniform backgrounds. This is shown in Fig. 12. It can be seen that the circle and square though equally luminant are not equally bright. An explanation is that neurons are computing local contrast and the visual system is basing its estimate of brightness on contrast-dependent neural re-

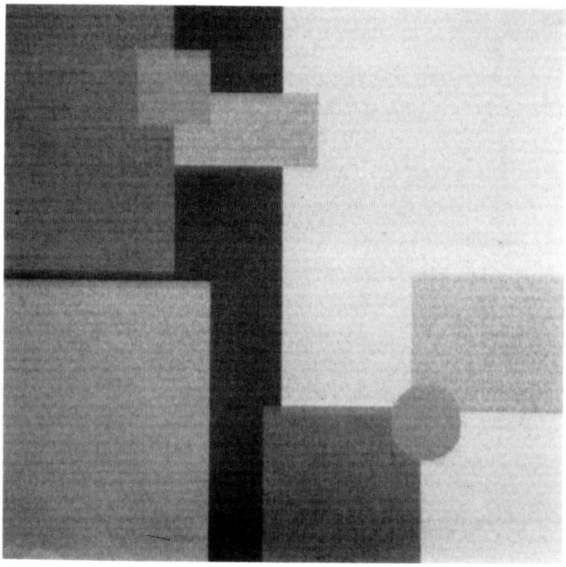

FIG. 12 The square (upper left) and the circle (lower right) are equiluminant but look different in this "Mondrian-like" pattern because the average local contrasts around their borders are quite different. From Shapley (1986).

sponse. Reid and Shapley (1988) have measured the magnitude of this brightness induction in Mondrian-like patterns, and it is virtually identical to that seen in more conventional displays such as Fig. 11.

C. Contrast and Assimilation

Besides local contrast, another component of the brightness computation is assimilation, the additive effect on brightness of an object produced by the brightness of its background. Previously, it has been hard to separate assimilation from contrast because backgrounds have been made brighter and darker by varying their luminances, and this has affected border contrast as well as background brightness. Shapley and Reid (1985) and Reid and Shapley (1988) have used a different approach by varying the brightness of an outer surround so as to vary the brightness of an inner surround by induction while its luminance remained fixed, as in Fig. 13. The inner circles in Fig. 13 are equally luminous, and they lie on annular backgrounds that are equally luminous (though slightly less luminous than the small circles). The outer background is a gradient of luminance such that one annular background appears brighter than the other. As a consequence, the circle on the brighter background appears brighter only by assimilation since its luminance and its *local contrast* are identical to that of the darker circle.

The magnitude and spatial dependence of assimilation were measured by Reid and Shapley (1988) who showed that assimilation was usually weaker than contrast and that it waned with distance. This can be expressed formally as follows. Consider two spots labeled T for test and C for comparison, surrounded by two regions S_T and S_C, respectively, and these in turn surrounded by an outer background B as in Fig. 13. The contrast between T and S_T is denoted C_T and between target C and its background as C_C. Reid and Shapley propose that to compute the brightness of

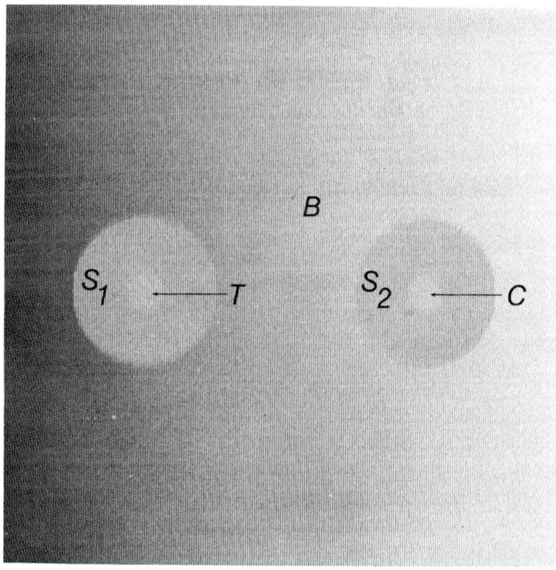

FIG. 13 Two equiluminant circles T and C placed on two equiluminant annuli S_1 and S_2 which look different in brightness because of the luminance gradient in the outer surround B. The inner circles T and C appear different in brightness because of assimilation. From Shapley and Reid (1985).

spots T and C, the visual system does the following: contrasts of the outer surround with the two annuli, C_{S_T} and C_{S_C} respectively, are multiplied by an assimilation weighting factor, which depends on distance between the borders of the spot and the annulus, and then added to the local contrast around the circle. Thus,

$$B_T = C_T + \alpha C_{S_T} \quad (11)$$
$$B_C = C_C + \alpha C_{S_C}$$

The assimilation weighting factor, α, is unity at zero distance and declines to half at a distance of approximately 0.33 degree visual angle (Reid & Shapley, 1988). It is interesting that the Retinex theory (Land & McCann, 1971; Land, 1983) implicitly included an assimilation term that was unity in value, independent of distance (see Reid & Shapley, 1988, Appendix). In such a theory, brightness is a truly global computation since contrast at any border anywhere adds in with equal weight to all others. It is this global nature of the Retinex that endows it with the capability to calculate reflectance, and causes it to compute that objects of equal reflectance are equally bright, regardless of nearby surroundings. Visual neurons and human observers perform a much more *local computation* in order to calculate brightness. Assimilation can be seen as a weak corrective to the visual system's sole reliance on local contrast, but it is not strong enough to overcome the "illusions" in Figs. 11 and 12. The neural implementation of assimilation may be by lateral interactions between cortical neurons as suggested by Reid and Shapley (1988) and included in a formal neural network treatment by Grossberg and Todorovic (1988; see below).

D. Nonlinearity in Boundary Detection

One of the most surprising recent developments in understanding visual form perception is the finding that fundamental neural mechanisms of pattern segregation are essentially nonlinear because these mechanisms ignore the sign of the contrast. The discussion above demonstrates that the signed contrast is crucial for perception of brightness. The sign of the contrast is what separates dark (negative contrast) from light (positive contrast). If, as we now find, form perception depends on a mechanism that ignores sign of contrast, then form and brightness must be computed by separate neural circuits with different rules. This realization has emerged from recent work on texture segmentation, described above, and also from experiments on interpolated or "subjective contours" (Shapley & Gordon, 1985, 1987). The theoretical development of the two-mechanism idea is discussed in detail in Section VII. At this point, we discuss the experimental evidence from interpolated contours.

The best way to understand the evidence from interpolated contours is to see it (Fig. 14). In Fig. 14 there is a circular object on a shaded background. In fact, the luminance in the background is a linear gradient with position, and the mean luminance of the gradient is precisely in the middle of the picture. The luminance within the circular object is also a linear gradient, but increasing in the opposite direction from that in the background. Again, the average luminance of the circle's gradient is reached in the middle of the picture. Along the line down the middle of the picture, luminance is constant. There is no objective border down the center line. In fact, the luminance contrast between object and background are below threshold for several lines on either side of the middle of the picture, as can be verified by the reader by occluding the right- and left-hand sides of the picture leaving a blank zone down the middle. In spite of the absence of the segregating border when viewed in isolation, when the entire picture is viewed the border is completed or interpolated between regions in which it is visible and across regions where it is invisible on its own. This is an example of a subjective contour (Petry & Meyer, 1987). What is most fascinating about Fig. 14 and similar pictures is that the interpolated border links regions of *opposite* sign of contrast.

Various lines of evidence indicate that interpolated borders are caused by neural mechanisms of border detection that are the first stage in form perception (see Chapter 11, this volume). Shapley and Gordon (1987) have offered perceptual evidence on the contrast and spatial dependence of border interpola-

FIG. 14 A circular object that illustrates nonlinear border interpolation. The background region consists of a one-dimensional luminance gradient that has its mean in the middle of the picture. The interior of the circular region also is a luminance gradient with the opposite sign of that of the background, also going through its mean luminance (the same mean as the background) in the middle of the picture. Thus, there is no luminance border down the middle of the picture, yet one sees an interpolated "subjective" contour between regions of opposite sign of contrast.

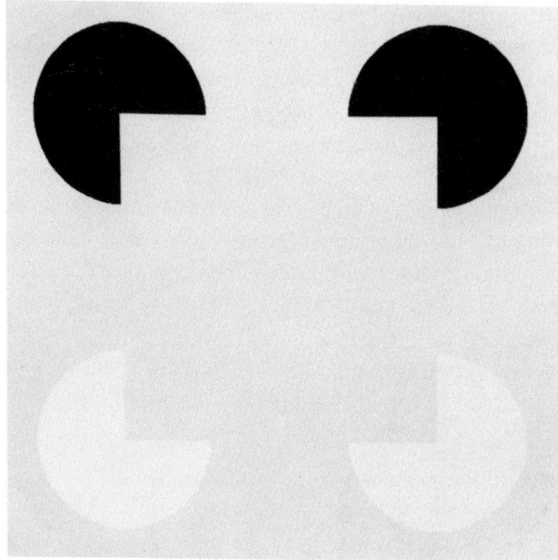

FIG. 15 A Kanizsa square, formed by inducing figures that alternate in sign of contrast. The subjective contours perceived are as strong as those seen with inducing figures of the same sign of contrast, again revealing that the contour sensing process does not respect sign of contrast. From Cohen and Grossberg (1984) and Shapley and Gordon (1985).

tion that implies a hard-wired neural mechanism as opposed to the cognitive mechanisms proposed by Prazdny (1983) and others. The crucial feature of such a border detector is its independence of the sign of contrast, implying an even-order nonlinearity such as rectification or squaring (energy calculation) before signals are combined. Thus, form depends on the magnitude of contrast at a border, while brightness depends on the sign. Another demonstration of the importance only of contrast magnitude and independence of interpolated borders on sign of contrast is offered in Fig. 15, which is a Kanizsa square with inducing figures of alternating sign of contrast (Shapley & Gordon, 1985; see also Cohen & Grossberg, 1984, for a similar picture). The illusory percept is as good as in Kanizsa figures of the same sign of contrast.

VII. NEURAL NETWORK MODELS OF PREATTENTIVE VISUAL PERCEPTION: EMERGENT SEGMENTATION AND FEATURAL FILLING-IN

Grossberg (1984) has developed a neural model for preattentive visual representation of three-dimensional form. He observed that the visual system uses multiple types of locally ambiguous information about edges, textures, shading, multiple spatial scales, and stereopsis to achieve this representation. The representation allows hyperacute spatial resolution and percepts of brightness and color that discount variation in illumination. Understanding how this happens is one of the outstanding problems in vision science.

Two types of visual process play a fundamental role: emergent boundary segmentation and featural filling-in. Grossberg's neural network theory attempts to explain how these processes work (Cohen & Grossberg, 1984; Grossberg, 1984, 1987a, 1987b, 1988; Grossberg & Mingolla, 1985a, 1985b, 1987; Grossberg & Todorovic, 1988). This theory describes neural processing rules for a boundary contour system (BCS), which generates preattentive three-dimensional emergent segmentations, and a feature contour system (FCS), which discounts the illuminant and regulates featural filling-in of brightness and color signals (Fig. 16).

The neural network model for the BCS and FCSs is illustrated in Figure 16. This is the simplified version

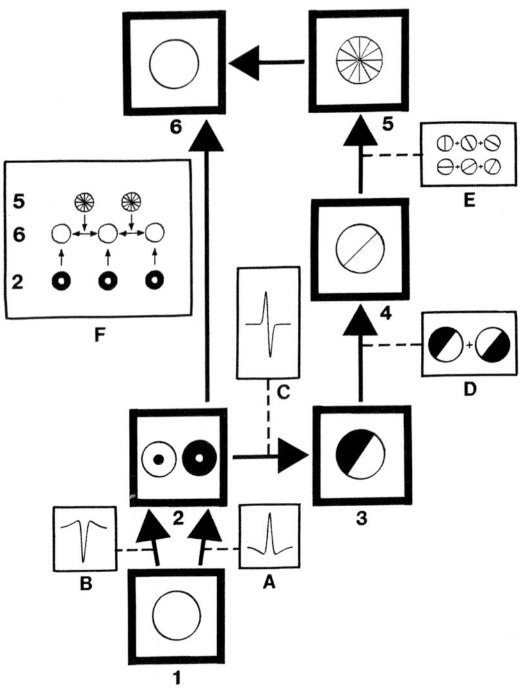

FIG. 16 Overview of the neural network model of Grossberg and Todorovic (1988). The thick-bordered rectangles numbered 1 through 6 correspond to the levels of processing within this simplified model of the FCS processing. The symbols inside the rectangles are graphical mnemonics or icons for types of computational units residing at that level. Arrows depict interconnections between levels. Inset F illustrates how the activity at Level 6 is modulated by outputs from Levels 2 and 5. See text for additional details.

of the full model and is taken from the paper by Grossberg and Todorovic (1988). There are six levels to the neural network model. Level 1 is simply the stimulus distribution sampled on a discrete lattice. Level 2 includes center–surround spatial filters within the FCS constructed so that they do all the work of the retina: spatial filtering and automatic gain control to achieve Weber's law. Levels 2 feeds into both BCS and FCSs. Levels 3, 4, and 5 are within the BCS. Level 3 is a grid of orientation-sensitive neural elements that retain sensitivity to the sign of contrast. These could be thought to be representative of the ensemble of simple cells in Area V1 of the cortex. The elements of Level 4 are orientation-sensitive but contrast sign-insensitive neurons and are thought to correspond to cortical complex cells. Level 5 cells are proposed to be a sheet of neurons that integrate signals from Level 4 "complex cells." The Level 5 cells are the BCS units. Level 6 is composed of a syncytium of cells within the FCS. Any point in this syncytium receives input from a small group of center–surround units from Level 2. Signals from corresponding points in Level 5, the BCS, can reduce diffusion of signals within the Level 6 syncytium by inhibitory gating. Therefore, a BCS signal creates a barrier to filling-in at its target cells. The map of activity across the Level 6 FC syncytium constitutes the internal representation of the visual field in the model although there is some input to the object recognition system (ORS) directly from the BCS and FCS. The network equations for each of the levels in the model are given in the Appendix of the paper by Grossberg and Todorovic (1988). They suggest that the FCS may receive input from the "blob" system in V1 cortex, while the BCS may get its input from the hypercolumn system.

A. Elementary Properties of Boundary Contour and Feature Contour Interactions

The BCS and the FCS were originally introduced to account for paradoxical data concerning brightness, color, and form perception, including the percepts of illusory contours. BCS signals are used to synthesize boundaries, whether real or "illusory," that the perceptual process generates. FC signals initiate the filling-in processes whereby brightness and colors spread until they hit either their first boundary contour or are attenuated due to spatial spread.

The BCS is insensitive to sign of contrast as evidenced by Fig. 15, discussed earlier (Cohen & Grossberg, 1984; Grossberg & Mingolla, 1985a,b; Shapley & Gordon, 1985, 1987). A color and brightness system, such as the FCS, must remain sign-sensitive. In Fig. 15, two vertically oriented and spatially aligned edges generate an intervening visual boundary across a region that has no color or luminance contrast. The boundary completion propagates *inward* between pairs of inducing elements and is *oriented.* On the other hand, many experiments discussed below indicate that color and brightness signals (produced by hypothesis by the FCS) diffuse outward away from scenic edges in an unoriented manner to "fill in" regions with their own featural quality (Krauskopf, 1963; van Tuijl, 1975; Yarbus, 1967).

The BCS can be used for texture segmentation, as for example in the case of Glass patterns (Glass & Switkes, 1976; Fig. 17). These texture boundaries may be "invisible but recognizable," that is, boundary signals may excite the BCS without having the FCS indicate that they are bounding regions of differing color or brightness.

The presence within the FCS of different filled-in signals on opposite sides of a boundary is, according to Grossberg's model, necessary for sustaining the perception of figural form. Object recognition can, however, be based on signals from the BCS and FCS to the object recognition system (ORS), which Grossberg postulates is a higher stage that integrates the signals from BCS and FCSs, as illustrated in Fig. 18A,B.

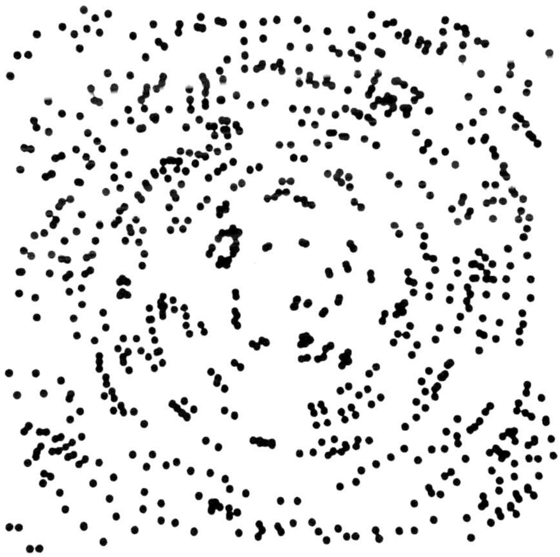

FIG. 17 A Glass pattern. The emergent circular pattern is recognized although it is not "seen" as a pattern of differing contrasts. From Glass and Switkes (1976).

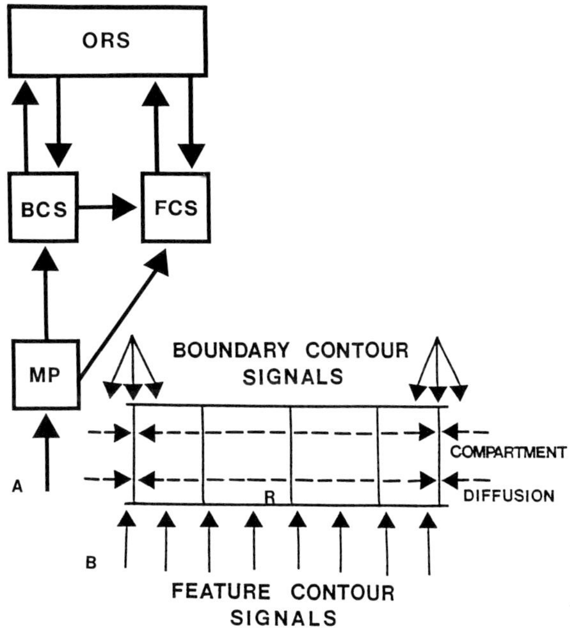

FIG. 18 (A) Macrocircuit of processing stages. Monocular preprocessed signals (MP) are sent independently to both the boundary contour system, BCS, and the feature contour system, (FCS). Interactions of BC system signals within the FC system are needed to support visible brightness and color contours. The BC system also sends bottom-up signals to and receives top-down template signals from the object recognition system (ORS). From Grossberg (1987a). (B) A monocular brightness and color stage within the FC system. Monocular FC signals activate cell compartments which permit rapid electronic diffusion of activity, or potential, across their compartment boundaries, except at those boundaries which receive BC signals from the BC system. Consequently, the FC signals are smoothed and averaged except at boundaries that are completed with the BCS.

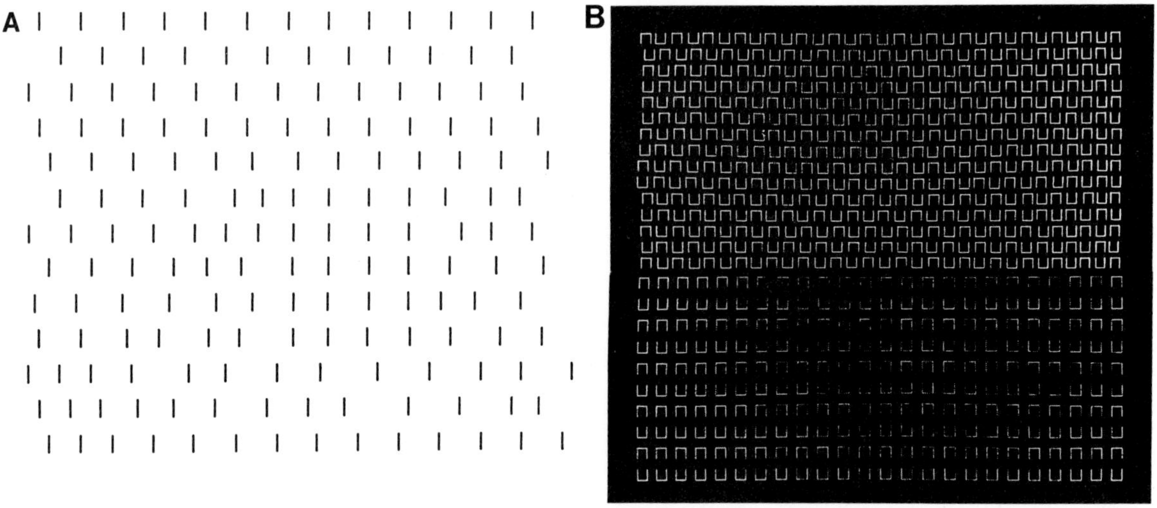

FIG. 19 (A) Emergent features. The collinear linking of short line segments into longer segments is an "emergent feature" which sustains textural grouping. (B) The diagonal grouping at the top is initiated by differential activation of diagonally oriented receptive fields, despite the absence of any diagonal edges in the picture. Horizontal cooperation of signals at the ends of vertical lines generates horizontal subjective contours at bottom. From Beck, Prazdny, and Rosenfeld (1983).

B. Emergent Features in Texture Segmentation

Beck (1983) has identified key variables affecting texture segmentation. Displays like the ones in Fig. 19 indicate that the slopes of texture elements are a critical determinant of grouping, with regions containing many features with similar slopes tending to group. If certain of these features are distributed in a regular manner, collinear groupings of these texture elements may become "emergent features" capable of segmenting one textural region from another (as in Fig. 19A). Such emergent features need not be in line with the slopes of local contrasts (Fig. 19B).

A remarkable aspect of displays such as Fig. 19 is that we see a series of short lines despite the control of perceptual grouping by the long emergent features. This may be explained as follows. Within the BCS, a boundary structure emerges corresponding to the long lines visible in Fig. 19A. This structure also includes short horizontal components near the endpoints of the lines. Within the FCS, these horizontal signals prevent featural filling-in of dark and light contrasts from crossing the boundaries corresponding to the short lines. On the other hand, the output from the BCS to the ORS reads out a long line structure without regard to which subsets of this structure will be seen as dark or light.

C. Hierarchical Resolution of the Boundary Uncertainty Induced by Orientational Sensitivity

The horizontal signals that are generated in response to the ends of vertical lines (Fig. 19B) illustrate a remarkable adaptation of the visual system, which led Grossberg and Mingolla (1985a, 1985b) to assert that *the ends of all thin lines are "illusory"*. The perceived line ends correspond to actual luminance differences and so are not illusory in that sense. However, the boundary signals indicating the position of a thin line end are weak or absent at the stage of BCS processing that corresponds to cortical complex cells (Fig. 20). The line end is detected in response to the spatial pattern of output signals from complex cells by a later stage of BCS processing that corresponds

FIG. 20 Early stages of BC system processing. At each position, cells exist with elongated receptive fields of various sizes which are sensitive to orientation, contrast, and sign of contrast. These are the simple cells at Level 3 in the BC system. Pairs of such cells sensitive to like position and orientation but opposite directions of contrast form the input to cells that are sensitive to orientation and contrast magnitude but not contrast sign. Such a complex cell neuron, at Level 4 in the model, is indicated by the empty ellipse. These cells in turn excite like-oriented hypercomplex cells corresponding to the same position and inhibit like-oriented hypercomplex cells corresponding to nearby positions at the first competitive stage (upper dashed boxes). Also, at this level, cells corresponding to the same position but different orientations inhibit each other via a push-pull competitive interaction.

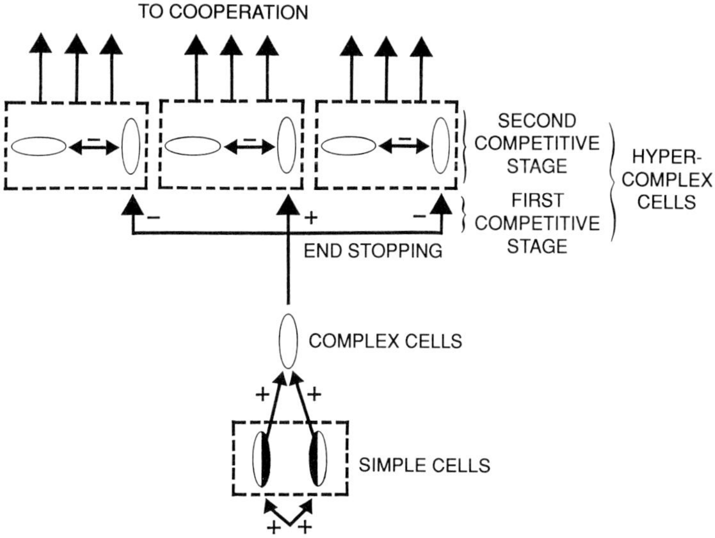

to cortical hypercomplex cells. This stage is not present in the simplified model shown in Fig. 16. Grossberg and Mingolla (1985a) called the hypercomplex responses at the line end end cuts.

Why cannot the complex cells detect the end of a thin line? The model of simple cells and complex cells developed by Cohen and Grossberg (1984) and Grossberg and Mingolla (1985a) is similar to the models proposed by Shapley and Gordon (1985) and Spitzer and Hochstein (1985). At each position, simple cells with like-oriented, but oppositely polarized, receptive fields respond to local image contrasts. Their outputs are rectified before inputting to complex cells of similar orientation. Such complex cells are not sensitive to the direction of image contrast. At the ends of thin lines and corners, these cells are insensitive to all orientations due to the very receptive field elongation that enables them to be sensitive to the orientations of scenic contrasts in edges, texture gradients, and shading that pass through the receptive field. Compensatory processing by later BCS stages is needed to generate end cuts, so that color signals cannot flow from every line end within the FCS (Fig. 18B), or for that matter from every scenic corner. Despite these precautions, colors can sometimes be seen to flow, as noted below, and the processing rules of the BCS provide an explanation of how this happens.

D. Spatial Short-Range Competitive Interactions

Within the BCS, the end cut transformation converts complex receptive fields into hypercomplex and higher-order hypercomplex receptive fields. This requires two successive stages of short-range inhibitory or competitive interactions. These interactions account for results of von der Heydt, Peterhans, and Baumgartner (1984) and have been used to explain many anomalous properties of filling-in and neon color spreading (Grossberg & Mingolla, 1985a; Grossberg, 1987a) that have been reported previously (Van Tuijl, 1975; Van Tuijl & de Weert, 1979; Redies & Spillmann 1981; Redies, Spillmann & Kunz, 1984). Hyperacuity (see Chapter 10) also depends on these inhibitory interactions in the model (Grossberg, 1987a) as does the café wall illusion shown in Fig. 16 (Grossberg & Mingolla, 1985b). Lateral inhibition is postulated between complex cells to like-oriented hypercomplex cells at nearby positions (Fig. 20). This can account for the effect of a flanking line on the perceived position of a test line, reported by Badcock and Westheimer (1985). Badcock and Westheimer's repulsion effect was independent of sign of contrast and could be generated monoptically or dichoptically, indicating that it would be due to interactions within the BCS at Level 4 or higher.

The phenomenon of end cuts illustrates that the uncertainty of retinal information is not progressively reduced by each successive stage in cortical processing. Each stage may eliminate one uncertainty while it generates yet a new uncertainty, much as in the Heisenberg uncertainty principle. For example, the elongated receptive fields of simple cells and complex cells generate "orientational certainty" in response to scenic edges and bars, but thereby generate "positional uncertainty" at line ends and corners. Subsequent short-range competitive interactions give rise to hypercomplex cell receptive fields which resolve this positional uncertainty by generating end cuts.

E. Spatially Long-Range Cooperative Interactions

Once perpendicular boundary signals are generated at line ends, they are processed by subsequent BCS stages according to the same rules as boundary signals originating in direct response to scenic luminance contrasts. Thus, in the texture displays of Fig. 19, boundary completion and grouping can occur either along the direction parallel to thin line segments or in a direction parallel to line ends. End cuts thus increase the number of potential boundary groupings for each scene. Moreover, because oriented receptive fields at Level 3 in the model are local contrast detectors, rather than edge detectors per se, certain combinations of local contrasts from disconnected scenic elements can at times trigger responses along orientations where there are no local edges. Thus, many potential groupings of parts into wholes are activated during preperceptual processes. In a final percept, a single global grouping is chosen and sharpened while all other possible groupings are actively suppressed.

The competitive interactions shown in Fig. 20 are insufficient for choosing a global grouping if only because their interactions are short-range. These competitive stages of the BCS occur between Levels 4 and 5 in the network of Fig. 16. A spatially long-range cooperative process occurs at Level 5 itself. Figure 21A schematizes the BCS model of this cooperative process. Figure 21B embeds it within the total architecture of the BCS.

A cell at Level 5 of the BCS, modeled as in Fig. 21B, can be active only if it receives sufficiently large inputs from paired populations of similarly oriented and spatially aligned cells at the competitive stage. These cooperative cells thus behave like the logical gates reported by von der Heydt et al., (1984). The cooperative cells were labeled *bipole* cells by Grossberg and Mingolla. These bipole cells (Level 5) feed back excitatory signals to competitive cells (presumed hypercomplex) at the pre-Level 5 stage. The hypercomplex cells, in turn, feed excitation backward to bipole cells. In this way, boundary completion can propagate inward rapidly in a spatially discontinuous manner.

The competitive cells whose orientations and positions receive the largest cooperative signals are favored to win out over less favored cells within the final perceptual grouping. Thus the competitive stages do double duty. They generate end cuts in response to bottom-up signals, and they help to choose the final segmentation in response to top-down signals. The cooperative–competitive feedback network which acts to choose the final segmentation is called the CC loop. Within the CC loop, boundary segments emerge at those locations and orientations that possess enough statistical inertia to survive the cooperative–competitive feedback exchange.

F. All Boundaries Are Invisible

Unless a connected boundary can be synthesized by the BCS, it cannot separate the FCS's signals into domains capable of supporting different colors or brightnesses. Thus if a later event inhibits through the CC

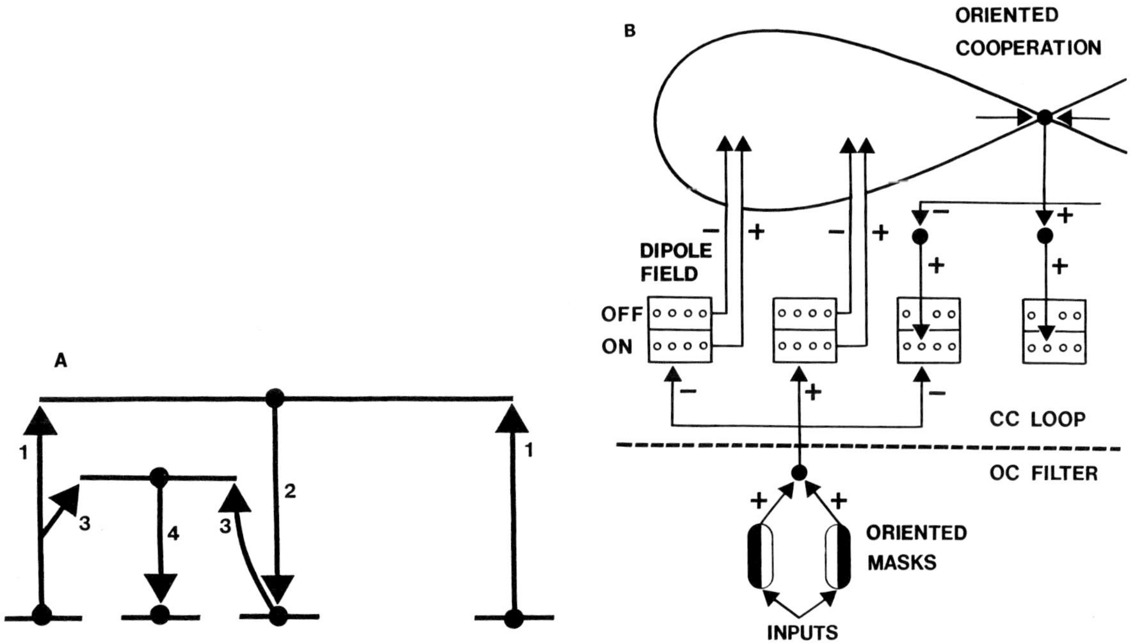

FIG. 21 (A) The pair of pathways 1 from hypercomplex cells activate a bipole cell that generates a positive boundary completion feedback along pathway 2. Then pathways such as 3 activate positive feedback along pathways such as 4. Rapid completion of a sharp boundary between pathways 1 can hereby be generated by a spatially discontinuous bisection process. (B) Circuit diagram of a monocular BCS: Inputs activate oriented simple cell receptive fields which cooperate at each position and orientation to activate complex cells before feeding into an on-center off-surround interaction. This interaction excites like-orientations at the same position and inhibits like-orientations at nearby positions, thereby giving rise to hypercomplex cells. These cells are on-cells within a dipole field: On-cells at a fixed position compete among orientations. On-cells also inhibit off-cells which represent the same position and orientation. Off-cells at each position, in turn, compete among orientations. Both on-cells and off-cells are tonically active. Net excitation of an on-cell excites a similarly oriented cooperative receptive field at a location corresponding to that of the on-cell. Net excitation of an off-cell inhibits a similarly oriented cooperative receptive field at a location corresponding to that of the off-cell. Thus, bottom-up excitation of a vertical on-cell, by inhibiting the horizontal on-cell at that position, disinhibits the horizontal off-cell at that position, which in turn inhibits (almost) horizontally oriented cooperative receptive fields that include its position. Sufficiently strong net positive activation of both receptive fields of a cooperative cell enables it to fire, as in Figure 20. Such firing generates feedback via an on-center off-surround interaction among like-oriented cells. On-cells which receive the most favorable combination of bottom-up signals and top-down signals generate the emergent boundary segmentation.

loop before a connected boundary structure is formed at Level 5, no percept may be visible. This clarifies how metacontrast might work (Breitmeyer, 1984).

Boundary signals are predicted to be invisible within the BCS. Thus, contrast sensitivity of cells within the BCS does not imply visibility of the final percept, according to Grossberg's theory. The generation within the FCS of different filled-in featural contrasts on the opposite side of a completed boundary leads to a visible percept.

G. Binocular Fusion, Rivalry, and McCollough Effect: From Ocular Dominance Columns to Multiplexed Multiple Scale Binocular Segmentation

BCS can be generalized to the binocular case (Grossberg, 1987a,b). Two steps are needed for this generalization. First, V1 cortex is organized into ocular dominance columns (Hubel & Wiesel, 1977). Binocular input is combined at the complex cell stage producing neural elements that are sensitive to position, orientation, spatial frequency, positional and orientational disparity, yet insensitive to sign of contrast (modeled by Grossberg and Marshall, 1987, 1989). Second, the model exploits the known property of multiple receptive field sizes, each feeding into its own CC loop. Within each size scale, the multiplexed data pattern represented by that scale's complex cells activates a CC loop which selects, amplifies, and coherently groups the binocularly consistent properties within that scale while suppressing the binocularly inconsistent properties. Data about binocular rivalry and the McCollough (1965) effect, respectively, are clarified by the theory's explication of how mechanisms of segmentation and stereopsis interact and of how binocular segmentation and monocular featural filling-in mechanisms interact. Of particular interest is the discovery that unoriented, monocular networks of double-opponent color cells within the FCS can, through interactions with binocular segmentations from the BCS, extract binocularly consistent brightness and color signals whose spatial organization encodes properties of oriented form, as well as of color and brightness. Such a multiplexed representation of form-and-color-and-depth, called by Grossberg a FACADE representation, has been predicted to occur in the prestriate cortical area V4.

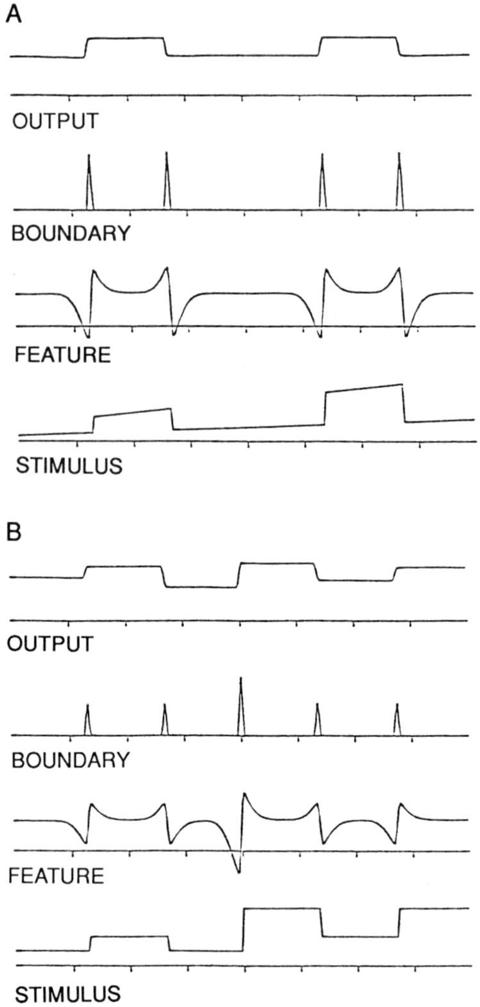

FIG. 22 Computer simulations of (A) brightness constancy and (B) brightness contrast. The rows labeled "Feature" depict the response profile of the FC system which discounts the illuminant. The rows labeled "Boundary" show the output of the BC system. Rows on top present the final filled-in pattern.

H. Explaining Monocular Brightness Data under Constant and Variable Illumination Conditions

The interactions between the BCS and FCSs can be used to account for some brightness phenomena that have not previously been explained by a single theory. Computer simulations (Fig. 21) illustrate how the model handles brightness constancy and brightness contrast. The properties of the neurons at Level 2 in the model (Fig. 16), with their center–surround organization controlled by shunting inhibition are what generates the brightness constancy of responses in the Grossberg model as illustrated in Fig. 22. This shunting network is designed to discount the illuminant. In order to accomplish this, the off–surround of the network cannot be too broad, and there must exist significant automatic gain control within the on-center to generate responses that are contrast dependent. These properties are consistent with the data summarized by Shapley and Enroth-Cugell (1984). These properties enable the model to provide a unified explanation of how different images generate brightness constancy, contrast, or assimilation when the activation patterns in which illumination is discounted activate subsequent model interactions between boundary segmentation and filling-in.

For example, Figure 22A depicts the one-dimensional cross section of the luminance distribution of an image illuminated from the right-hand side ("Stimulus" traces). The image contains two objects of equal reflectance on a less reflective background. Because of the uneven illumination, the right-hand patch has a higher luminance than the left-hand patch. The "Feature" traces represent the reaction of Level 2 neurons, center–surround retinal units with shunting excitation and inhibition that discounts the illuminant and consequently enhances high contrasts while attenuating low contrasts. The "Boundary" traces of Fig. 22A present the output of the BCS, consisting of sharp peaks corresponding to abrupt luminance steps of both polarities in the image. The "Output" traces are the model's filled-in output. The model correctly predicts brightness constancy. The filling-in process of the FCS generates the homogeneous regions with different brightness levels in the output. The importance of filling-in is also demonstrated in the model's simulation of brightness contrast in Fig. 22B.

In a simulation of a Mondrian-like image resembling Fig. 12, consisting of a number of homogeneous patches of differing luminance levels, Grossberg's model correctly predicted that local contrast would dominate over reflectance or luminance. In addition, the model has been used to simulate several classical and new variants of brightness contrast, brightness assimilation, the Craik–O'Brien–Cornsweet effect, the Koffka–Benussi ring, and the Hermann grid (see Chapter 7, this volume). The model handles a far greater variety of effects than competing computational approaches (Horn, 1974; Land, 1983; Hurlbert, 1986). These latter models are explicitly geared for reflectance recovery and must therefore fail to account for human vision on the basis of the evidence presented in Figs. 11 and 12. Also, the Retinex models alluded to have not been applied consistently to the larger selection of brightness phenomena needed to understand form from luminance adequately. In summary, neural models for cortical BCS and FCS interactions have begun to be able to account for and predict a far-reaching set of interdisciplinary data as manifestations of basic design principles, notably how the cortex achieves a resolution of uncertainties through its parallel and hierarchical interactions.

VIII. CONCLUSIONS

In order to perform the effortless act of visual perception, neural networks of substantial complexity must exist. Features, either fixed or adaptive, must be recognized by such networks. Objects are recognized and represented internally for recollection. Such tasks require spatial filters, memories, spatial organization of activity distributions in different populations of neurons, and complex competitive and cooperative interactions to regulate the network's responses. Furthermore, these interactions have a certain spatial scale intrinsic to their function that determines the stability and the characteristics of visual perception. The simplest visual tasks, such as perceiving colors and recognizing familiar faces, require elaborate computations and more neural circuitry than we have yet imagined. In the pursuit of adequate theories of vision we have learned much about the difficulty and computational requirements of the task as we have progressed toward characterizing how the task is accomplished. Theoretical progress toward the goal of understanding the visual process and how it is accomplished by nervous systems will require such a multifaceted approach for some time to come.

ACKNOWLEDGMENTS

Preparation of this chapter and the research reported by the authors were supported from many sponsors that we here acknowledge with gratitude. Robert Shapley was supported by grants from the National Eye Institute (EY1472) and National Science Foundation (BNS 8708606) and by the Sloan Foundation and MacArthur Foundation. Terry Caelli acknowledges the support of the National Research Council of Canada (Grant No. A2568). Stephen Grossberg received the support of the U.S. Air Force Office of Scientific Research (Grants F49620-86-C-0037 and F49620-87-C-0018), the U.S. Army Research Office (Grant No. DAAG-29-85-K-0095), and the National Science Foundation (IRI-84-17756). Ingo Rentschler acknowledges the Deutsche Forschungsgemeinschaft for Grant No. PO 121/13 1 Project 5.

16

BRAIN, PERCEPTION, AND MIND
A Tribute to Richard Jung, Donald M. MacKay, and Hans-Lukas Teuber

Otto D. Creutzfeldt

The aim of sensory physiology is to elucidate the brain mechanisms which underlie conscious perception. It is thus directly related to the wider problem of the relationship between the brain, conscious perception, and mind. In the context of this book, we ask the question: How much and to what extent can the phenomena of visual experience be explained by tracing the neural messages elicited by the stimuli leading to such experiences? When looking through the various chapters, one is left with "Convergences, Divergences and Lacunae," to use Hans-Lukas Teuber's words (Teuber, 1966a).

In an attempt to explain perceptual phenomena with physiological mechanisms, one must also be careful not to fall into the traps of reductionism, the "nothing butteries" of Donald MacKay, who wrote into my copy of his book, *Information, Mechanism and Meaning* (MacKay, 1969) after visiting my laboratory: "May all the information you gain on mechanism have meaning." Searching for meaning, one will quickly realize that "Physiological as well as psychological experience demonstrate two characteristics of sensory perception: (1) sensory stimuli are effective in animals and human beings mainly for their meaning to the recipient, and less because of their intensity, quality, or modality; (2) the organism learns from perception mainly during action, on the basis of emotional and instinctive motivation. Both involve an anticipation of the sensory stimulus," as Richard Jung formulated it in his last major article, entitled "Sensory Research in Historical Perspective: Some Philosophical Foundations of Perception" (Jung, 1984, p. 58).

In this concluding chapter, we wish to address these issues by referring to ideas of Richard Jung, Donald M. MacKay, and Hans-Lukas Teuber. These leaders tried to bridge the gap between the physiology of the brain and the experience of the mind, not only by leaving with us a wealth of observations and data, but also by teaching us to think deeper and further, and to avoid the traps of categorical mistakes (false linking propositions, see Chapter 3, this volume) and useless reductionism. I knew these three men since my student days in Freiburg, our ways crossed frequently, and I benefitted from their support, interest, and challenge.

The lives of Richard Jung, Hans-Lukas Teuber, and Donald MacCrimmon MacKay coincided with a marvelous period in the development of the field of vision research. Coming from different scientific, national, and cultural backgrounds, they met in the common effort to contribute to an exploration of the physiological basis of sensations. This led to a lifelong friendship and is witnessed in the joint editorship of the *Handbook of Sensory Physiology* (1973 ff). In quite different academic environments, all three founded model departments of neuroscience, at a time when this word did not even exist, and thus tried to integrate modern neurosciences into neurology, psychology, and the communication sciences (for short biographies see, respectively, Weiskrantz, 1977; Creutzfeldt, 1986; Evans, 1987).

Richard Jung (1911–1986) (shown in Fig. 1) was a neurologist and passionately dedicated to investigating the mechanism of normal and pathological perception and behavior by recording the signals accompanying such performances from the human and animal brain. The first successful recordings of the activity of single neurons in the visual cortex of cats in 1952 (Jung, von Baumgarten & Baumgartner, 1952) revealed new insights into sensory processes. Jung immediately saw the implications of this method for our understanding of visual perception. He thus initiated a whole range of studies in his laboratory in which correlations between neuronal responses and various perceptual phenomena were sought and discovered. The mechanisms underlying the Mach band phenomenon, the various types of visual afterimages, the Brücke–Bartley effect, and many others were summarized by Jung and colleagues for the first time at the Freiburg Symposium, "On the Neurophysiology and Psychophysics of the Visual System," in 1960 (Creutzfeldt, 1961; Jung & Kornhuber, 1961; Grüsser and Grüsser-Cornehls, 1973; Jung, 1973; see Chapter 7, this volume).

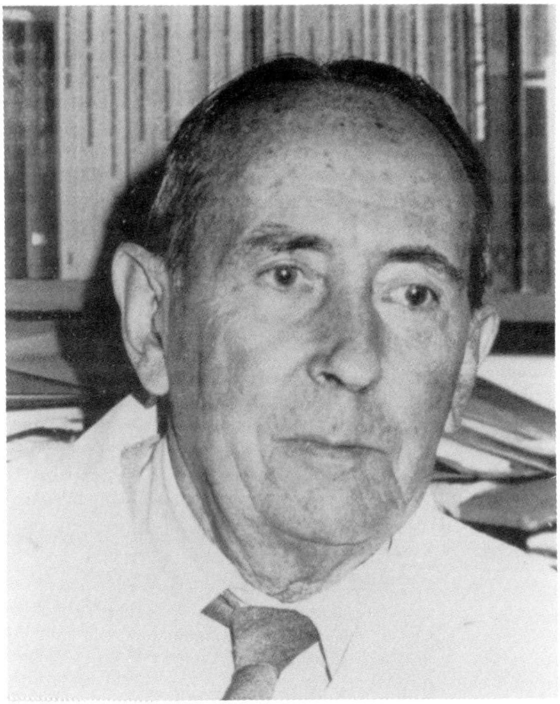

FIG. 1. **Richard Jung** (1911–1986), Professor of Neurology and Clinical Neurophysiology at the University of Freiburg, FRG.

These discoveries represented a first attempt to relate objective measures, that is, neuronal responses, with subjective experience. Of course, no questions were asked then as to whether the neuronal response patterns were sufficient for an explanation of the phenomenology of perception as this was merely a beginning. However, there was the implicit assumption and a good suspicion that, once started along this road, a final and complete picture of internal representations of sensory events might result. Jung realized that an essential step for form perception is to reduce a visual scene to its contours such as done in drawing. Such a reduction to contours could be simulated by subtracting the positive from the negative copy of a photograph. This is shown in Fig. 2. When the positive and negative copies are slightly offset relative to each other, only the lines of contrast remain (Fig. 2B). Jung writes that

A

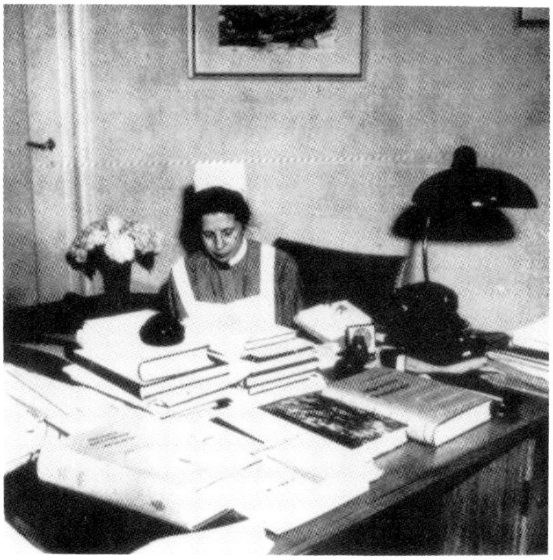

B

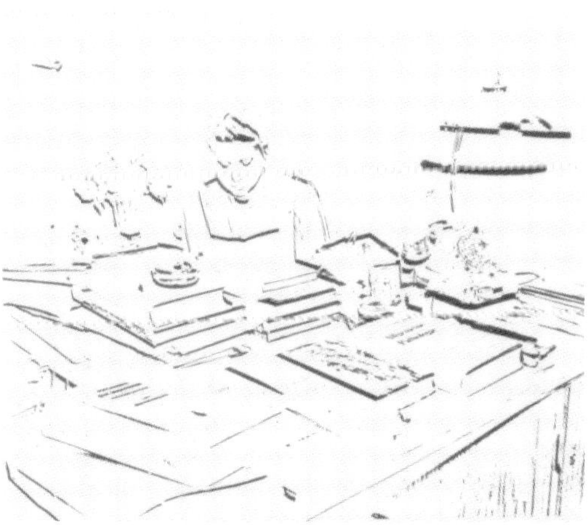

FIG. 2. Photographic simulation of the reduction of a retinal image (A) to its contours (B). This reduction is achieved by digital subtraction of the brightness values of the positive and the negative of this photograph, both slightly offset relative to each other. From Jung (1967).

> Such a reduction could be performed by a retino-geniculate neuronal system with strong lateral inhibition and after subtraction of the activities of on- and off-center neurons. . . . Although all surfaces and brightness values including the light–dark border contrast are eliminated, the . . . contour lines contain still sufficient information for recognition of the essentials of the picture. It can be assumed that the neuronal information processing in the visual cortex makes Gestalt perception possible through similar selections of the contour pattern on account of information on surfaces. [Jung, 1967, p. 537]

Such a reduction of complex images to contours is reminiscent of Marr's (1982) primal sketch and has been demonstrated experimentally in neuronal transform patterns of the lateral geniculate body and visual cortex by Creutzfeldt and Nothdurft (1978). The stimuli shown at the top of Fig. 3 were steadily moved across the receptive fields of off- and on-center geniculate cells and simple and complex cells of Area 17, as indicated on the left. Whenever a part of the figure elicited a discharge of the neuron while passing through its receptive field, a dot appeared on the appropriate place on the oscilloscope. Note that geniculate cells respond to all crossings of the line patterns with little preference for orientation. The photograph is reduced to its contours as defined by the brightness steps in the stimulus. Cortical simple cells (S) reduce these contour representations further by responding only to lines of certain orientations, while complex cells (C) respond differently to the movement of contour patterns across their receptive field. They are thus insufficient for contour representation, but mediate information on moving objects. Hypercomplex cells (S_H) respond only to short lines and line ends.

We have since learned that in the primate visual system the magnocellular geniculate cells may be largely responsible for signaling contours, while other aspects, such as color, are mediated through the parvocellular layers and represented separately in Area 17 (Tanaka, Lee & Creutzfeldt, 1983; Livingstone & Hubel, 1984; Creutzfeldt, Weber, Tanaka, & Lee, 1987; Lee, Valberg, Tigwell & Tryti, 1987).

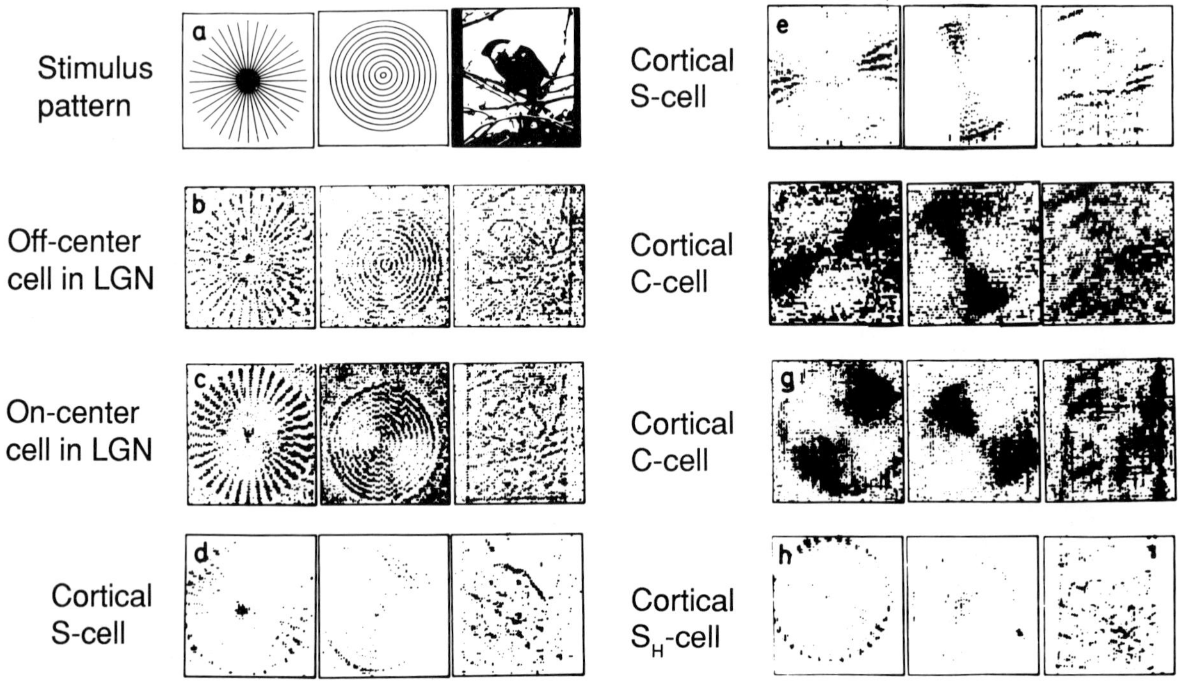

FIG. 3. Representation of complex stimuli by neurons in the lateral geniculate nucleus and in Area 17. Complex patterns (20° × 20°, top row, a) are moved across the receptive field of a single neuron along a horizontal path, line by line. Each part of the image eliciting an action potential from the cell during the scanning process is recorded as a black dot in the corresponding position. (b, c) Neurons respond to all lines of the star and to all tangent orientations of the concentric circles. They are already slightly orientation selective so that not all orientations elicit the same response. Neuron c, for example, shows almost no responses along one of the diagonals. The black-and-white photograph of the bullfinch is essentially reduced to the contrast contours in the picture, although some information is still preserved about the brightness of uniform regions. Thus, neuron b, an off-center cell, shows more activity in the region corresponding to the dark portion of the bird's body than in the region corresponding to the bright sky. Neuron c, an on-center cell, shows the reverse: more activity for the sky than for the body. (d, e) "Simple cells" of Area 17 respond selectively to lines or tangents of certain orientations. In the bird picture, the only contours represented are those with orientations conforming to the preference of the cell. Because of their small receptive fields, the spatial resolution of simple cells is sufficient to represent the details. (f, g) In comparison, complex cells of Area 17 have poor spatial resolution (large receptive fields). They respond essentially to textures moving in a certain direction. (h) Hypercomplex cells also have small receptive fields; they respond only to very short lines or to the end of a line, not to closed circles. From Creutzfeldt and Nothdurft (1978).

The optimism to fill in the gap between the perceptual phenomena and neuronal representation in the brain is still shared by many of us. It is, in fact, the necessary condition for continuing along this line, although with somewhat different expectations than those expressed by Lord E. D. Adrian (1947) and other pioneers in the 1940s and 1950s. Increasing experience, coinciding with increasing age and decreasing expectations, may make us realize that despite the immense amount of progress made in the field of visual science, a mysterious gap remains between objective physiological signals and conscious perception (Creutzfeldt, 1987). Richard Jung expressed this in the concluding sentence of his last article: "The challenge of sensory research to find the physiological correlates of the complexities of perceptual experience seems likely to remain for an indefinite future" (Jung, 1984).

In his scientific endeavors, Richard Jung avoided getting trapped in the fruitless discussion on the relation between brain and mind. He was guided by clear epistemological constraints which he had adapted from the philosophy of Nicolai Hartmann (1950), who distinguished between the various ontological levels of the anorganic, the organic–biological, and the psychological worlds. In R. Jung's words,

> Physics, biology and psychology are the basic sciences related to these three levels. Although each upper level depends on the lower, each level has its own categories. The causal laws, which are the determinants at the lower levels, apply also to the higher ones as foundations of their own causality. The task of psychiatry reaches across the three levels, as psychic disturbances may be caused by various alterations on any of the three levels. Neurophysiology, however, is restricted to the two lower levels. It works with physico-chemical methods in a narrowly defined area, the biology of the nervous system. [Jung 1967, p. 338]

Nowadays, we are aware that the distinctions between the three levels—the anorganic, the organic–biological, and the psychological—become more and more blurred as we realize that living matter is a specific form of self-organizing matter which follows general rules or natural laws that are qualitatively not different from those applicable to matter in general. Yet, they have led to a new quality, namely, life and, ultimately, mind and consciousness.

It is interesting that the phenomenon of consciousness and its implications for perception have hardly been mentioned in this book if at all. (See Chapter 11, this volume.) The reason for this is probably that, "consciousness and attention can be measured only with psychological or behavioral measures which, as such, do not give any information on neurophysiological mechanisms which could possibly underlie the regulation of consciousness and perception. Consciousness can be better illustrated by pictures and metaphors rather than defined" (Jung, 1967, p. 614). One of these metaphors is the search light hypothesis of selective attention and consciousness, proposed by Jung in 1954 (Fig. 4). The role of attention in visual perception has recently been emphasized by Julesz (1986) in his distinction between the preattentive and attentive modes of perception. (See Chapter 11, this volume.)

Nature has provided an experiment in brain pathology which sheds light on at least one aspect of conscious perception or rather of visual attention. After lesion of the right parietal lobe, attention to visual stimuli in the contralateral visual field as well as to tactile stimuli or to paralyses on the left side of the body disappears (hemineglect and hemianosognosia). Richard Jung was very interested in this syndrome and had made an important contribution to its understanding by demonstrating the failure to complete portraits in the contralateral hemifield of a painter who had suffered a stroke in his right parietal lobe

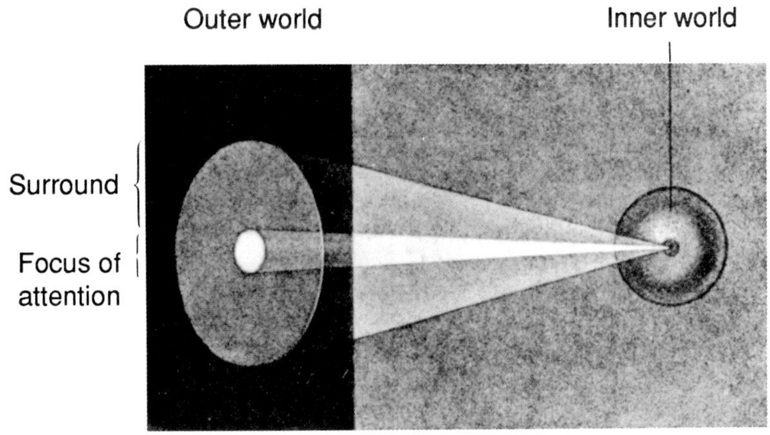

FIG. 4. The search light model of visual attention. "Pictorial scheme of the selective function of consciousness and attention as a search light. The beam of the roving search light of attention illuminates single parts of the internal and the external world and thus selects certain mental contents for consciousness. (Jung 1967, p. 614).

(Jung, 1974). It is a strange coincidence that Richard Jung himself, after lecturing on hemineglect and while visiting an art gallery, suffered from exactly this syndrome and died a few days later (without, of course, realizing that he had had this defect).

Jung shared his interest in sensory deficits in man after circumscribed cerebral lesions with Hans-Lukas Teuber. Such lesions are an experimental tool offered by nature to investigate the compartmentalization of mental functions. Hans-Lukas Teuber made this the basis for his exploration of cerebral functions and the mind. At the Black Forest conferences on neuropsychology in the 1950s, various aspects of neuropsychology were discussed, especially the agnosias and aphasias. The occasionally hair-splitting distinctions between various forms of agnosias, and the discussion whether a pure agnosia does exist at all, were sometimes bewildering to a student as they were largely based on phenomenology, with relatively little information on localization. The Black Forest discussions took place, of course, at a time before computerized tomography and electromagnetic resonance imaging were introduced, and before the peculiar and intricate representation of sensory stimuli and corresponding motor responses in the parietal cortex was discovered by Mountcastle (1976), Hyvärinen (1982), and colleagues. The situation thus was comparable to that in visual psychophysics before the structural and functional details of the visual system could be investigated and when the time-honored question of whether Hering or Helmholtz was right about the mechanisms of color and brightness perception was hotly debated, a dispute which still lingers on.

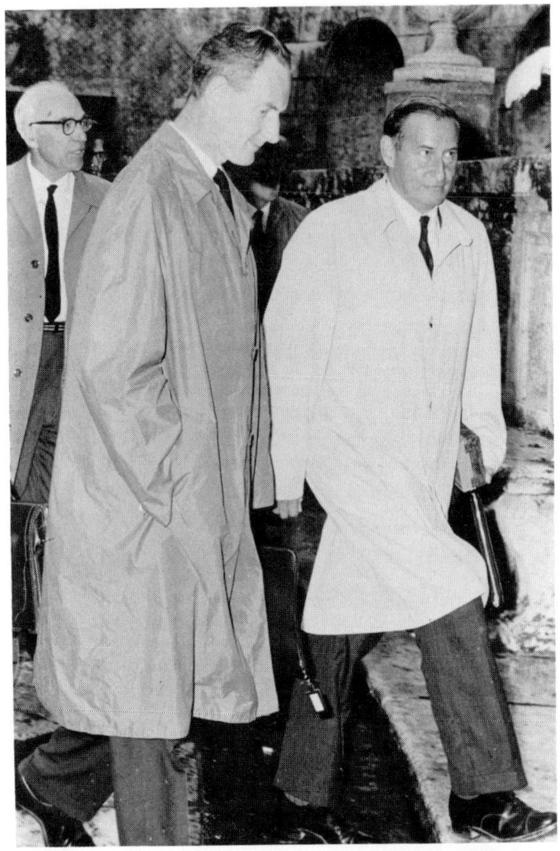

FIG. 5. **Hans-Lukas Teuber** (right) and **Donald MacKay** (left) during the conference on "Brain Mechanisms and Conscious Experience" at the Vatican Scientific Academy, 1966. In the background, Sir John C. Eccles.

Hans-Lukas Teuber (1916–1977) was a psychologist. In Fig. 5 he is seen walking with Donald MacKay through the Vatican gardens during the memorable conference on "Brain Mechanisms and Conscious Experience" (Eccles, 1966). Having been raised and educated in Berlin and Basel, imprinted by his father with the physiologically and behaviorally oriented psychology of the Wundtian tradition, he planted his scientific roots in physiological psychology in the United States under the guidance of K. S. Lashley (Lashley, 1941) and in neuropsychology under the influence of the Gestalt psychologists K. Goldstein and W. Köhler (see Teuber, 1966b, 1967) and the neurologist M. B. Bender (Bender & Teuber, 1946). In his well-known monograph (Teuber, Battersby & Bender, 1960) on the deficits of perception after localized brain injuries suffered by the unfortunate young men during the Korean war, Teuber set standards for neuropsychological research and at that same time paved the road for future work.

A major concern of his was to create a new, biologically oriented psychology, at a time when analytical or sociological biases dominated the field. For him (Teuber, 1962),

> Psychology should be that science which tries to account for the behavior of organisms (including ourselves) by methods drawn from the natural sciences, from the social sciences, and from mathematics. Such definition makes psychology more and less than some of us used to think it was. More because it makes psychology partake of methods drawn from nearly all of the other sciences, and less because psychology is not defined by some separate method that would be entirely its own. Yet, this definition . . . delineates, I believe, the crucial place of psychology, halfway between the natural and the social sciences . . . thus bridging the two cultures of . . . C. P. Snow.

In his last paper for the *Handbook of Sensory Physiology,* a lecture read at the International Psychological Congress in Paris 1976, he made it quite clear by saying,

> What we want to know is nothing less than what goes on in ourselves (and by that we mean within our central nervous system), when we perceive, when we move, when we feel or express emotions, and when we learn or remember. . . . For millennia, we have tried to comprehend the universe around us; the time has come, during this last century, and is now here, to attempt to comprehend ourselves. To this end, all the sciences have to be put into service of man's understanding of man. Psychology finds its identity, I propose, in its subject matter, not by its methods. [Teuber, 1978, pp. 880 and 913]

These are words of hope and optimism, as well as a scientific program that he carried out in setting up the Department of Psychology at MIT in Cambridge, Massachusetts, which included—in the early 1960s—sections on perception, child development, neuroanatomy, neurophysiology, and neuropsychology, attracting scientists who were leaders in their field.

This was also the spirit in which Hans-Lukas Teuber absorbed the new ideas of communication sciences, for which Norbert Wiener later coined the term cybernetics (Teuber, von Foerster & Mead, 1952). He was eager to incorporate these ideas into the study of brain and behavior, and this is when he met, at the Joshua Macy Foundation meetings, Donald MacKay. Teuber (1978) successfully implemented some of the many sensory illusion paradigms which MacKay had developed. One of them actually answers a question raised in this book as to whether illusory percepts are also seen in a scotoma, that is, whether they require Area 17 or not. Teuber reported on a patient who had a central scotoma of about 20°–30° in diameter (Fig. 6). This patient could complete the redundant pattern of radiating lines but could not see the central "eye." When a dynamic random dot pattern was superimposed onto the star, the patient even completed the field of random dots, a feature rarely observed in retinal field defects (Aulhorn & Koest, 1988). The patient failed, however, to perceive in his scotoma the induced illusory streaming motion present in his intact field of vision (Teuber, 1966a, 1978). Apparent motion, though, is still perceived across a scotoma (Teuber & Bender, 1950).

Hans-Lukas Teuber eagerly took up the neurophysiological discoveries of David Hubel and Torsten Wiesel and tried to integrate them with his observations on patients. Could the filling-in of the line patterns, just mentioned, be related to the columnar organization of orientation sensitive neurons? This question is still not answered. He realized, on the other hand, that the hierarchical principle of feature generalization had to be revised (see Teuber, 1978), and he would have been pleased to see the emphasis on parallel representations (Chapter 6) and linking propositions (Chapter 3) discussed in this book.

It would be well worth it to go back to Teuber's wonderful article "Perception" in the *Handbook of Physiology* (1960) to see how many of the problems of perception and illusions he had discussed there have actually been solved. Hans-Lukas Teuber would certainly have enjoyed the many new illusory phenomena referred to in this volume and which were made possible by "computerized television sensory physiology." Clearly, for many of the basic elements of perception, the receptor and neuronal mechanisms have now been uncovered. However, the great question as to how these elements are brought together into a Gestalt is still open. Here, Hans-Lukas Teuber

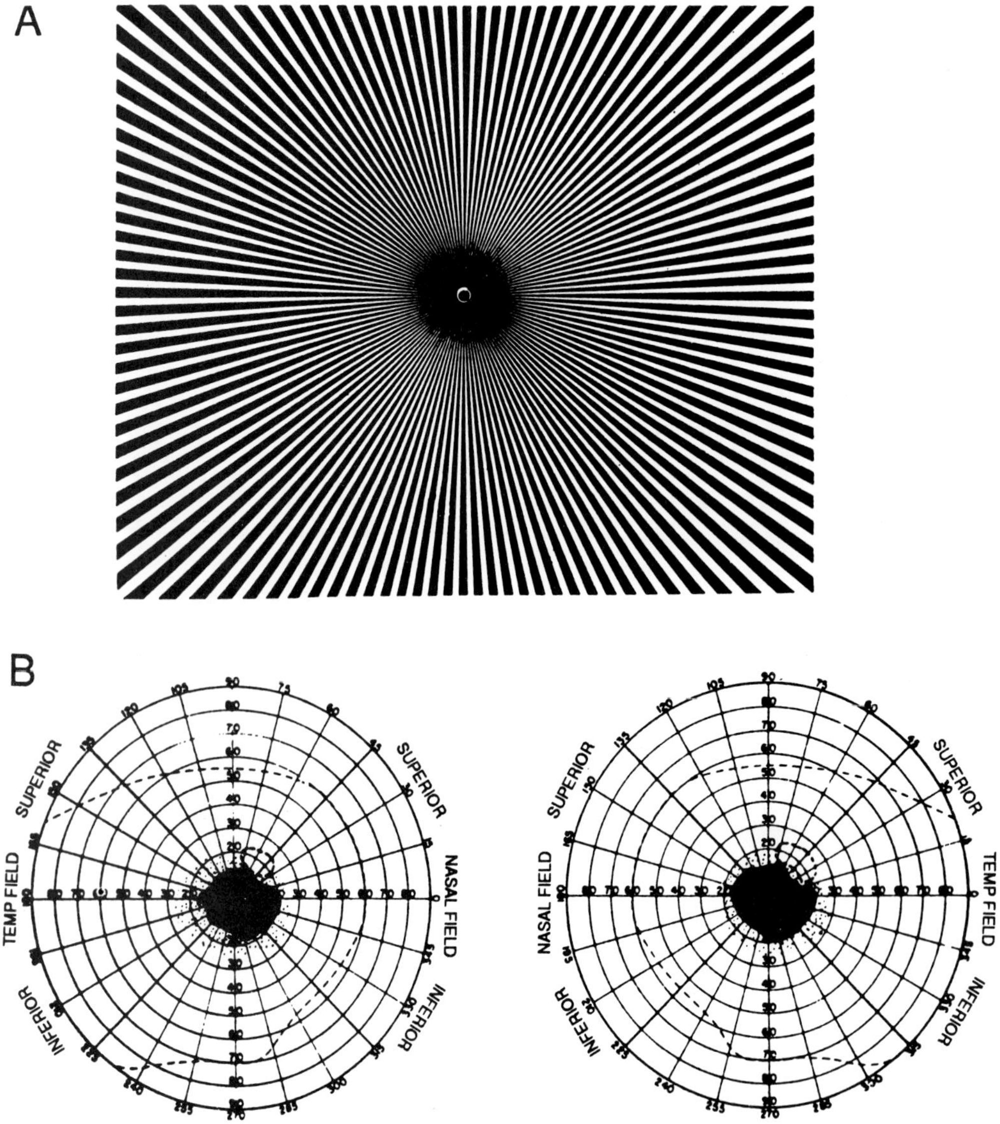

FIG. 6. Redundant patterns such as the rays in the star (A) and even a dynamic, random dot pattern will be filled in across the gap of a scotoma (B). However, the illusion of circular streaming motion resulting from the superposition of the dots onto the star pattern is not perceived in the region of the scotoma. From Teuber (1966a, 1978).

(1978) realized that "we cannot look upon perception without considering coordinated movement, with its own perceptual consequences, and both perception and movement involve memory and often mood." In view of these considerations, he advocated abandoning the classical distinction between sensory and motor fields.

The intricate link between perception and action is, of course, the theme which **Donald MacKay** (1922–1987) would have addressed in his contribution to this book. MacKay began his career in the British Admiralty as an information engineer. There he was assigned the task of developing radar-guided instrument control for targeting objects. In trying to improve the resolution of radar measurements, he soon found himself confronted with the limits of physical measurement and the problem of signal-versus-noise distinction. He realized that the information measured by an instrument is limited by the capacity of that instrument and can be calculated a priori from the specification of the instrument. A second set of information, however, could be calculated a posteriori, from a specification of what was done with the instrument, that is, how it was moved, how its lenses were adjusted for focusing, etc. (MacKay, 1969). MacKay's awareness of this truly cybernetic problem influenced his approach to understanding the visual system and the nervous system in general. He was neither blinded nor falsely attracted by formal models which describe the physical world and the perceived world in mathematical transformations, or which simply reduce it to mathematical functions or bits of information. Such formalizations of percepts do not explain why we see as we do. Rather, he considered the central nervous system as a control system that is able to steer the subject through this world. This model is illustrated in Fig. 7. He pursued this basic concept with all the rigor of deep thinking which his training as a physicist demanded, and he also made it the basis of studying perception.

Like Hans-Lukas Teuber, Donald MacKay was exposed to the ideas of biological cybernetics at the Joshua Macy Foundation meetings, and his basic ideas can be traced back to those days in the early 1950s. At the famous meeting on "Sensory Communication" organized by Walter Rosenblith in 1959, at a time when little was known about the neurophysiology of the visual system, MacKay presented some striking visual illusions producing complementary, movement afterimages. He interpreted them as indicating the presence of specific edge and movement detectors "above the retina" and of mutual inhibitory interaction between them (MacKay, 1961). Both the edge detectors and the mutual inhibition between them were later demonstrated neurophysiologically (Hubel

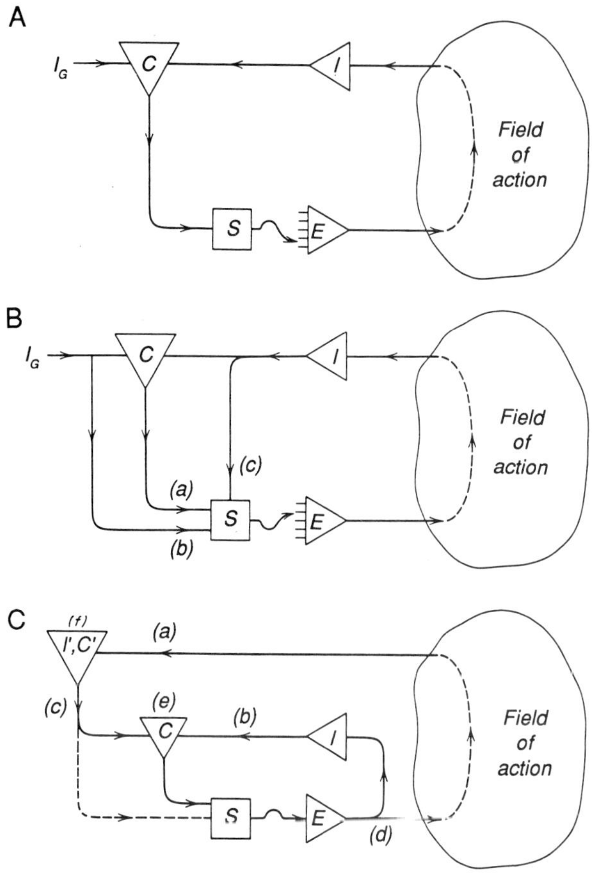

FIG. 7. Information flow model of action and perception as proposed by Donald MacKay (1966). The input–output loops of the system are closed across the "field of action." (A) In the simple feedback control loop, the intended action (goal setting) of the subject (I_G) is fed into a calculator (C), which in turn sends command signals into a selector (S), which selects the form of activity from a repertoire in the effector systems (E). The effect is a positional change of the subject in the field of action, leading to a new state which is indicated (I) and fed back into C. (B) On a further level the feedback loop (a) is controlled directly through a feed-forward loop (b) by the goal setting system (the subject) as well as by a feed-forward loop indicating the field state (c). (C) In the second-order control of steering, the simple servo-loop [e.g., the steering device (E, I, C, S) in a car with power steering] serves as the effector for a higher-order goal indicator (f), the subject, combining the functions of second-order indicator (I′), comparator (C′), and norm setter.

& Wiesel, 1963; Creutzfeldt, Kuhnt & Benevento, 1974). MacKay also demonstrated the difficulty of hand–eye coordination during discontinuous illumination by having the participants play table tennis during stroboscopic illumination, a task which turned out to be impossible.

When setting up the Department of Communication at Keele University in 1960, MacKay realized the importance of neurophysiological recordings of brain events during processes of perception. The combination of his skills in engineering, physics, and psychophysics led him, together with his colleagues, to unexpected discoveries of neuronal responses to visual noise stimuli in Area 17 that challenged the hierarchical model of an exclusive pathway from simple to complex cells (Hammond & MacKay, 1975). Already ill and under heavy cytostatic chemotherapy, he set out to examine whether evaluation processes can, in fact, be recognized as electrical signals of the brain (MacKay, 1984a,b). For this purpose, he developed a technique of evoked potential recording which employed source-density analysis and thus was able to resolve the location of evoked responses to within 1 cm on the scalp map (MacKay, 1984c). He performed many of these experiments on himself, taking advantage of his hair loss due to chemotherapy.

Donald MacKay was invited to prepare an introductory chapter for this book, but died on February 6, 1987. He had begun to prepare the chapter and left us with some notes. These notes set the stage for his intended comments as they contain the questions he wanted to ask and with which we are confronted in visual perception. He wanted to address the problem of

> The unity of the world: Two visual hemispheres, one world: "Why no gap?"—Two eyes, one world: "what if no overlap?"—*n* visual projections, one world: "How kept in register?"—Completion across retinal blind spots, cortical scotomata, etc.?—Integration of information from simple and complex cells, etc.?—Moving eyes, but a stable world?
>
> All these problems are transformed if we see the function of the visual system not as production of an image of the world nor of a description of the world, but as modulation signals, massively parallel, for the transition probability matrix governing readiness to reckon with the world. Let us begin by reminding ourselves that the perceiving self is first and foremost an agent: the possessor of a repertoire of modes of potential action in his field. Action we distinguish from mere activity by the element of evaluation, which assesses the action as less or more satisfactory, attaching a match/mismatch value to it in the light of current criteria of evaluation.

His notes end here. I shall try to indicate the way in which MacKay might have tried to answer some of the questions. Where indicated, I quote from his last paper on the subject (MacKay, 1986).

He would have first challenged the notion of a neural image being explicitly represented in the brain like on an internal map, be it a topographic representation or a feature map. He would also have questioned the hypothesis that the recognition of specific patterns depends on a kind of Fourier synthesis performed on the spatial frequencies contained in the firing pattern of so-called cortical frequency analyzers. Any neural image theory must deal with the problem of perceptual stability during exploratory eye movements and would also have to take into account the multiplicity of visual areas. Should one compare the multiple visual areas to the

> pages of a printed atlas, with repeated maps of the same area devoted, respectively, to rainfall, population, elevation and so forth? If so, people ask, how are these numerous "maps," some of them only crudely topographical, eventually recombined to form the unitary image of the visual world we perceive? How are they all kept "in register"? Is there some more central brain area in which we should expect to find once again a needle-sharp neural picture of the visual world, free of all signs of eye movement and the like? If not, then what? [p. 366] [The presupposition behind such questions is that the task of] the visual system is to generate eventually a single "explicit" internal neural image of the world. From an information-engineering standpoint, however, this presupposition is far from obvious. [Instead it could be argued] (e.g., MacKay 1956a,b, 1962, 1970) that the task of the visual system, as of other perceptual systems, should be seen first and foremost as the setting up and keeping up to date the organism's "conditional readiness for action" in its world, in

matching response to sensory input, and that on this basis the perceived world could find itself adequately represented "implicitly." [pp. 366–367] From this standpoint, perception is an adaptive exploitation of the redundancy in the pattern of demand imposed by the sensory input. . . . The main form taken by this redundancy can be termed "covariation". [p. 367]

Movement of an array of receptors relative to an object in the environment gives rise to coincident changes in signals from different channels. Such covariations between receptors within the same visual or tactile modality may betoken such things as the presence of a fixed or a moving edge, or of an object of a certain width. They could arise whether the relative motion producing the changes were caused by movement of the organism or movement of the object in question. Covariations between signals in different modalities (e.g., tactile and visual, or auditory and visual) offer the informational basis for the perception of location in space relative to the body as a whole; and so on. [p. 367]

[The functions of the multiple visual areas would be to] segregate signals in different categories such as form, motion, texture or colour so as to allow covariations between them to be "listened for" and analysed by different populations of detectors, each thus being free of the background chatter of traffic in the other populations. [p. 368] In such a model, also the function of simple and complex cells may have to be newly defined. Instead of asking what a given cell detects, we should perhaps ask "what kinds of covariation" in the signals from the retinal array it [a given cell] is equipped to sense. [p. 369]

[Thus the basic function of the CNS] is the detection and analysis of changes that occur together—asking what covaries with what? [p. 369] [If we define the visual world as] the domain within which the roving fovea has to navigate, [then the neural correlate of seeing is that] it updates our readiness for "further looking," in matching response to the demands of the current retinal input. [p. 372]

It follows that if we want to find the neural representation of the world as currently seen, the place to look, at least for its coarse-grained form, should be at the interface between the incoming visual information and the higher-level planning of ocular navigation. At this level, we should not be surprised to find objects represented only implicitly, by the conditional constraints they impose on the planning of further ocular motion. The stepping stones in a river might find themselves represented implicitly in the conditional motor programmes for jumping from one to the next, or a curved driveway might find itself represented in the matching programme of rotations of the steering wheel of a car. [p. 372]

This, of course, can be thought of as an amplification rather than a denial of the classical doctrine of local sign; but it emphasizes that what matters for perceptual experience is not where signals originate, but the kinds of conditional readiness they set up. [p. 372]

Let us now return to the questions addressed in this book, the neurophysiological basis of visual perception. It is clear that the model proposed by Donald MacKay does not explain why we actually perceive consciously, but it indicates another way of looking at what we record when we try to identify and track the signals elicited in the brain by visual stimuli. Are we recording sensory representations or potential responses of the organism to a sensory object? This question is not inappropriate, because each cortical area, whether sensory or motor, has direct access to subcortical motor control systems (Creutzfeldt, 1985).

In an attempt to bridge the gap between brain events and conscious perception we would, in fact, be well advised to realize at the start that a mystery will always remain: Why is it that certain neuronal signals in a certain area of the brain are "seen," those in another are "heard" or "felt"; why does the majority of activities in our brain not at all enter consciousness; why do only excitatory signals reach sensation while the activities of inhibitory neurons which lie next to them do not enter our sensorium as such (Creutzfeldt, 1987)? We have to accept this as a law of nature which cannot be further explained. As with other laws of nature (take gravity, for example), we can only define the causal constraints and conditions which these laws put on nature and measure their effects.

This book has demonstrated that the two approaches to measure and define the conditions and constraints of visual perception, namely, the psychophysical and the anatomical–physiological, are complementary. Psychophysics defines the limits of visual perception and can thus make certain predictions with respect to mechanisms. For example, visual resolution as determined psychophysically permits inferences about the optical quality of the refractive media of the eye and the sizes of receptive fields (see Chapter 10, this volume). Neurophysiology and neuroanatomy can show how signals are coded and where they are sent to, respectively, and thus can define the anatomical and physiological conditions of perception. Here, however, expectations are sometimes too high in that psychophysicists might assume that the neurophysiologists should be able to demonstrate that the percept is invariantly and explicitly encoded in the activity of single neurons. This approach must necessarily fail. Instead it should be realized that much of the information contained in a stimulus can be extracted only by comparing the activities of a whole population of neurons sensitive to various aspects of a complex stimulus.

Let me give an example from color vision. We can clearly distinguish the colors of two objects or fields, no matter what their relative luminances. Thus, we see a green field as green whether it is surrounded by a bright or dark achromatic, or by a bright or dark red surround, as long as the luminance ratio does not become too high. The exact quality of the color such as its hue, saturation, or brightness may change to some extent, but it still looks green. However, if we record from color-opponent cells in the parvocellular layers of the lateral geniculate nucleus, we will discover that we can always find a luminance ratio between two chromatic colors, or between an achromatic and a chromatic color, at which a given cell becomes unresponsive: A cell typically coding for green can at a given luminance difference not distinguish between grey and green or red and green. Such null positions vary between cell types, but they can be produced in each cell at a luminance ratio at which an observer would still distinguish and identify the colors (Creutzfeldt, Lee & Valberg, 1986; Chapter 8, this volume).

Thus the percept is not sufficiently defined by the activation of one type of feature-specific neuron (one type of spectrally sensitive cell in our example), but is the result of a comparison of relative excitations across neuronal populations with different feature sensitivities. These differences could enter and determine conscious perception without specific neurons signaling them as such. This view may be difficult to accept, but it does not put a greater demand on our imagination than assuming that excitatory signals, whether correlated or not, are perceived. Also, a temporary interruption of neuronal activity, such as during saccades, is not perceived as a gap, and absent signals can be interpreted as positive percepts such as in the filling-in across the optic disk or a cortical scotoma. The assumption then that the correlation of activities of certain groups of neurons may represent essential information about stimuli, as Donald MacKay has proposed, and which is also basic to other theoretical considerations (see Reichardt & Poggio, 1979; von der Malsburg, 1984), would have to include the registration of negative correlations or absence of correlations as well, each of them resulting in a different percept.

Let us now pursue the postulate that sensation can only be understood on the context of action (and vice versa), which Jung, Teuber, and MacKay have emphasized in various forms, and with which I fully agree (Creutzfeldt, 1985). We know from anatomy that every cortical area is defined not only by its specific afferent input from the thalamus and from other cortical areas, but also by its rather specific output (Creutzfeldt, 1984). The neurons which send axons out of the cortex are all located in Layer V, and all these Layers V neurons project to various subcortical motor control systems. This is obvious for the motor cortex with its corticospinal pathway, but it applies to the sensory cortices as well. Thus, in the visual cortex we find the Layer V neurons from Area 17 project into superficial layers of the superior colliculi. From extrastriate areas, they send axons into deeper collicular layers as well as into midbrain motor nuclei such as the pontine and the reticular nuclei. From these anatomical facts, we may infer that each visual cortical subfield represents not only different features of a sensory stimulus, but also the different *relations* between the subject and the objects in the visual environment (Creutzfeldt, 1984, 1985). Within such a framework one could then interpret cognitive defects due to lesions in extrastriate visual or parietotemporal association areas as a failure to represent a correct sensorimotor model of action relative to an object rather than as a failure to represent certain details which may be characteristic for that object. From there one might also argue that the perception of a Gestalt is closely related to the ability to "construct" appropriate object-related actions from these various representations of sensorimotor relationships. The analysis of agnosias supports such a view. They result from disturbances in brain regions where such representations of sensorimotor relations are most clearly seen, that is, in the parietal cortex and in some extrastriate visual association areas. Patients with an agnosia are unable to incorporate an object into their space of action; they do not know "what to do with it" or even "what to say to it" since speech is also a motor act.

Such a model may even be applied to neuronal signals recorded from Area 17. There the activation of movement-sensitive complex cells could be understood as command signals to foveate an object, such as a moving fly, a mouse, or a car appearing in the peripheral visual field, by turning the gaze toward it. These complex cells, in fact, project into the superior colliculi, the oculomotor interface between the forebrain and the mesencephalic oculomotor control system. The orientation-sensitive, contour-detecting simple cells, on the other hand, are well suited to fixate the gaze on contrasts and to align the axis of the two eyes (Creutzfeldt & Nothdurft, 1978). This alignment may be considered as a cross-correlation between the activities coming from the two eyes. The task for binocular fusion would be to reach a maximum of this cross-correlation. Extraction of contours having the same orientation would then clearly facilitate such a calculation. The organization of Area 17 with its neurons responding maximally when the contour orientations in the two eyes are identical (Li & Creutzfeldt, 1984), may be considered as a hard-wired cross-correlation matrix for binocular inputs. In such a model, we may consider complex cells as part of a command system for shifting the gaze toward a moving object and simple cells as part of a command system for holding the gaze and fixating it on the contours of objects in three-dimensional space. Experiments such as the one shown in Fig. 8 demonstrate

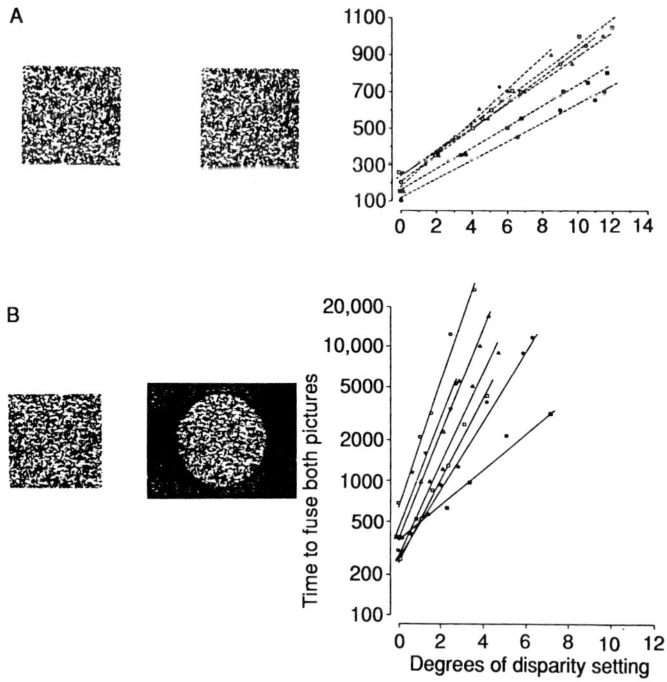

FIG. 8. Detectors for oriented contours may also be used for binocular fusion. (A) Two random dot stereograms (left) are presented dichoptically at different disparities. They are both surrounded by identical frames. When fused, a square pops out at the center. The appearance of this central square is used as the criterion for fusion. The time to reach fusion (in seconds) depends on the lateral disparity between the two stereograms (graph at right). (B) Fusion latency increases strongly when the two stereograms have different frames; at large disparities, fusion is no longer possible. This shows the importance of having identical edges and orientations (in this case the edges of the frames) seen by the two eyes. If these are missing, as in B, the two eyes will search randomly for correlated patterns; they may eventually identify the borders of the stereosquare but after a much longer search time. From R. Vaupel and O. D. Creutzfeldt (in press).

that this may, in fact, be the case. Here, binocular fusion of two random dot stereograms is shown to occur with a short latency and over a wide range of disparities if the two monocular stimuli have common edges. When frame sizes are different, the time to reach fusion greatly increases, while the disparity range decreases.

Cell classification notwithstanding, the activation of one type of neuron in the visual system may indicate different things, and its function may be defined differently depending on the context in which it is activated. For example, the simple and complex cells may not only encode contours or movement, but also texture. A characteristic feature of our environment is that it is composed of different textures varying little, if at all in color and mean luminance. Objects can be delineated and separated from each other not only because of their different luminances or colors, but also because of their different textures. Indeed, it has been demonstrated that simple and complex cells can signal texture as well as contour or movement (Nothdurft & Li, 1985). Figure 9 shows that the response of a complex cell depends on texture when line spacing is coarse, but on luminance when spacing is fine and when the gaps between elements can no longer be resolved. These results suggest that only the relative activities of various types of feature-sensitive neurons distributed over the cortex or, as Donald MacKay might have put it, the positively or negatively correlated activations of these various cell types rather than

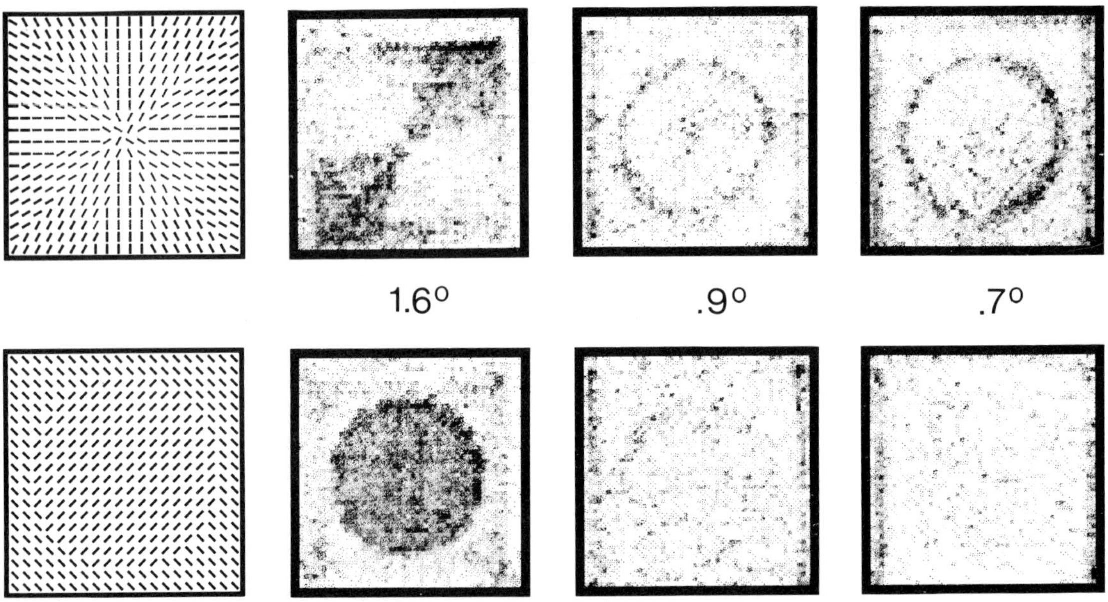

FIG. 9. Orientation-sensitive cells of Area 17 signal texture as well as contrast. Neuronal transfer diagrams (for details, see legend to Fig. 3) of a cat complex cell when textured patterns move slowly across its receptive field are shown. The pattern in the top row consists of a star of oriented line segments, but the contrast between lines and background is slightly lower within a central circle than in the periphery of the pattern. When the distances between lines are large enough (1.6°) to be discriminated by the cell, it responds to the orientation. When the gaps become smaller and cannot be resolved anymore (0.9° and 0.7°), the cell responds to the luminance contrast instead and signals the border of the circle. In the second row, the pattern consists of a central disk and a surround field with different orientations, but identical luminance contrast. The central disk is signaled as long as the cell can resolve the line pattern (1.6° line spacing) but is no longer reflected in the neuronal response pattern when the line spacing becomes too small (0.7°). With intermediate gap sizes, the border may just be marked, probably due to larger gaps between lines of different orientation (0.9°). From Nothdurft and Li (1985).

the activation of one type of feature-sensitive cells alone define a stimulus.

If one considers the cortex as a parallel set of sensorimotor or "perception–action" loops, such as alluded to above, the unification of the numerous parallel representations to a unified action would not be a serious problem (Creutzfeldt, 1984). Outputs from the various areas would be related to each other in the various subcortical and cortical motor execution systems, each of them with different weighting factors or priorities. These weighting factors may be variable to some extent, that is, adjustable to the behavioral situation or to the goal to be attained. Therefore, the corresponding weighting functions need an evaluation system by which the output signals from different parts of the visual cortex are given a certain "value" or meaning as defined by the purpose of the subject and its actions. In this way, the numerous parallel input–output lines are finally integrated to a unified action in the motor execution system.

Does this also explain a unified percept? I am afraid that it does not. Conscious perception is closely connected with our ability for symbolic representation and self-representation of the world around us and of our active relation to it. This ability is clearly coupled to the speech-dominant hemisphere. The nondominant hemisphere may be able to "respond" to stimuli, but it does not produce a conscious percept. That requires the reciprocal connections between the two hemispheres. How this is done, and through which part of the commissural pathway, is an open question, but the connections between the parietal and temporal lobes are certainly a necessary condition.

The self-representation of the symbolic abstraction of ourselves and of our environment is a necessary condition of conscious perception (for further discussion, see Creutzfeldt, 1987). This symbolic self-representation has to take into account all the various activities distributed over the brain, which represent the various subject–object relations. Such a mechanism of a symbolic loop is not only a necessary condition for conscious perception, but also the reason for the duality of our consciousness, which is evident in all descriptions of conscious perception: "I" see, "I" direct my attention toward something, as if the "I" uses the sensory organs and the brain as subordinate machinery. Such metaphors do not, of course, imply a material dualism between a conscious self and the brain, but they testify to the dual nature of conscious perception and of our mind.

This book has shown that good progress has been made in delineating and defining the conditions and constraints of perception. Many new problems have arisen which demand further efforts, and which can be solved. There are others, however, which are, by their very nature, insoluble, and therefore we may call them mysteries. These mysteries are to a large extent causal factors in conscious perception, but as with other causal factors in nature, they have to be accepted without further explanation, since they cannot be further reduced. It is the task of the experimental sciences to push their analysis as far as possible in order to confine the final causal mystery, or the mysterious cause. Yet, it is this mystery which makes the perception of our world such a wonderful experience.

REFERENCES

Numbers in parentheses indicate the pages on which the reference citations appear.

Abney, W. de W. (1913) *Researches in Colour Vision and the Trichromatic Theory,* p. 418. London: Longmans, Green. (192)

Abrahams, V. C. & Rose, P. K. (1975) Projections of extraocular neck muscle and retinal afferents to superior colliculus in cat: Their connections to cells of origin of tectospinal tract. *Journal of Neurophysiology,* **38,** 10–18. (330)

Abramov, I. (1968) Further analysis of the responses of LGN cells. *Journal of the Optical Society of America,* **58,** 574–579. (177)

Abramov, I. (1972) Retinal mechanisms of color vision. In M. G. F. Fuortes (Ed.). *Handbook of Sensory Physiology Vol. VII/2,* pp. 567–607. Berlin: Springer-Verlag. (177)

Adams, A. J. (1982a) Chromatic and luminosity processing in retinal disease. *American Journal of Optometry and Physiological Optics,* **59,** 954–960. (404–406)

Adams, A. J. (1982b) Selective loss of blue cone mechanism in central serous choroidopathy. *Investigative Ophthalmology & Visual Science, Supplement,* **22,** 62. (404)

Adams, A. J., Heron, G. & Husted, R. (1987) Clinical measures of central visual function in glaucoma and ocular hypertension. *Archives of Ophthalmology,* **105,** 782–787. (404–405, 407)

Adams, A. J., Rodic, R., Husted, R., & Stamper, R. L. (1982) Spectral sensitivity and color discrimination changes in glaucoma and glaucoma-suspect patients. *Investigative Ophthalmology & Visual Science,* **23,** 517–524. (397, 404, 407)

Adams, A. J., Schefrin, B. E., & Huie, K. (1987) A new clinical test for eye disease. *American Journal of Physiological Optics,* **64,** 29–37. (397, 404)

Adams, A. J., Zisman, F., Ai, E., & Bresnick, G. (1987) Macular edema reduces B cone sensitivity in diabetics. *Applied Optics,* **26,** 1455–1457. (397)

Adams, A. J., Zisman, F., & Cavender, J. C. (1980) Sensitivity loss in chromatic processing channels of diabetics. *Investigative Ophthalmology & Visual Science, Supplement,* **19,** 169. (405)

Adams, A. J., Zisman, F., Rodic, R. & Cavender, J. C. (1982) Chromaticity and luminosity changes in glaucoma and diabetes. *Documenta Ophthalmologica Proceedings Series,* **33,** 413–418. (397, 405)

Ade, F. (1983) Characterization of textures by "Eigenfilters." *Signal Processing,* **5,** 451–457. (425–426)

Adelson, E. A. (1982) Saturation and adaptation in the rod system. *Vision Research* **22,** 1299–1312. (71–72, 74, 76, 89)

Adelson, E. H., & Bergen, J. (1985) Spatio-temporal energy models for the perception of motion. *Journal of the Optical Society of America A,* **2,** 284–299. (212)

Adelson, E. H., & Movshon, J. A. (1982) Phenomenal coherence of moving visual patterns. *Nature (London),* **300,** 523–525. (226)

Adrian, E. D. (1928) *The Basis of Sensation; The Action of the Sense Organs.* London: Christophers. (6)

Adrian, E. D. (1947) *The Physical Background of Perception.* Oxford: Clarendon Press. (452)

Aguilar, M. & Stiles, W. S. (1954) Saturation of the rod mechanism of the retina at high levels of stimulation. *Optica Acta,* **1,** 59–65. (60, 80, 90)

Ahmed, N., & Rao, K. P. (1975) *Orthogonal Transforms for Digital Signal Processing.* Berlin: Springer-Verlag. (431)

Aho, A. C., Donner, K., Hyden, C., Larsen, L. O., & Reuter, O. (1988) Low retinal noise in animals with low body temperature allows high visual sensitivity. *Nature (London),* **334,** 348–350. (80)

Aiba, T. S., & Stevens, S. S. (1964) Relation of brightness to duration and luminance under light- and dark-adaptation. *Vision Research,* **4,** 391–401. (148)

Airaksinen, P. J., Drance, S. M., & Douglas, G. R. (1984) Diffuse and localized nerve fiber loss in glaucoma. *American Journal of Ophthalmology,* **98,** 566–571. (397)

Akita, M., Takahashi, S., & Ejima, Y. (1987) Nonlinearity of yellow–blue opponent color system: Discrepancy between deuteranope and normal trichromat. In G. Verriest (Ed.), *Colour Vision Deficiencies Vol. VIII,* pp. 485–492. New York: Academic Press. (168)

Albrecht, D. G., & De Valois, R. L. (1981) Striate cortex responses to periodic patterns with and without the fundamental harmonics. *Journal of Physiology,* **319,** 497–514. (287)

Albright, T. D. (1984) Direction and orientation selectivity of neurons in visual area MT of the macaque. *Journal of Neurophysiology,* **52,** 1106–1130. (220)

Albus, K. (1980) The detection of movement direction and effects of contrast reversal in the cat's striate cortex. *Vision Research,* **20,** 289–293. (221)

Alexander, K. R. & Fishman, G. A. (1984) Rod–cone interaction in flicker perimetry. *British Journal of Ophthalmology,* **68,** 303–309.

Allman, J., Miezin, F., & McGuinness, E. (1985) Direction- and velocity-specific responses from beyond the classical receptive field in the middle temporal visual area (MT). *Perception,* **14,** 105–126. (221, 287)

Alpern, M. (1971) Rhodopsin kinetics in the human eye. *Journal of Physiology,* **217,** 447–471. (69)

Alpern, M. (1979) Lack of uniformity in colour matching. *Journal of Physiology,* **288,** 85–105. (176)

Alpern, M., & Rushton, W. A. H. (1965) The specificity of the cone interaction in the afterflash effect. *Journal of Physiology,* **176,** 473–482. (85)

Alpern, M., Rushton, W. A. H., & Torii, S. (1970) Signals from cones. *Journal of Physiology,* **207,** 463–475. (71–72)

Amsler, M. (1947) Qualitative examination of the macular function. *Ophthalmologica,* **114,** 4–5. (398)

Amsler, M. (1949) Quantitative and qualitative vision. *Transactions of the Ophthalmological Society of the U.K.,* **69,** 397–410. (398)

Anctil, J. L., & Anderson, D. R. (1984) Early foveal involvement and generalized depression of the visual field in glaucoma. *Archives of Ophthalmology,* **102,** 363–370. (397)

Andersen, R. A. (1987) Inferior parietal lobule function in spatial perception and visuomotor integration. In V. B. Mountcastle and F. Plum (Eds.), *Handbook of Physiology: The Nervous System, V,* pp. 483–518. Bethesda, MD: American Physiological Society. (47, 365)

Andersen, R. A., & Siegel, R. M. (1987) Effects of ibotenic acid lesions in area MT on motion perception thresholds in the macaque monkey. *Investigative Ophthalmology & Visual Science Supplement,* **28,** 197. (209)

Andrews, R. W., & Pollen, D. A. (1979) Relationship between spatial frequency selectivity and receptive field profile of simple cells. *Journal of Physiology,* **287,** 163–178. (249)

Anstis, S. M. (1967) Visual adaptation to gradual change of intensity. *Science,* **155,** 710–712. (150)

Anstis, S. M. (1975) What does visual perception tell us about visual coding? In M. S. Gazzaniga & C. Blakemore (Eds.), *Handbook of Psychobiology,* pp. 267–324. New York: Academic Press. (274)

Anstis, S. M. (1979) Interaction between simultaneous contrast and adaptation to gradual change of luminance. *Perception,* **8,** 487–495. (150)

Anstis, S. M. (1986) Recovering motion information from luminance. *Vision Research,* **26,** 147–160. (150)

Anstis, S., & Harris, J. P. (1974) Movement aftereffects, contingent on binocular disparity. *Perception,* **3,** 153–168. (333)

Anstis, S., Howard, I. P., & Rogers, B. (1978) A Craik–O'Brien–Cornsweet illusion for visual depth. *Vision Research,* **18,** 213–217. (346)

Anstis, S. M. & Ramachandran, V. S. (1985) Kinetic occlusion by apparent movement. *Perception,* **14,** 145–150. (219)

Anstis, S. M., & Ramachndran, V. S. (1986a) Entrained path deflection in apparent motion. *Vision Research,* **26,** 1731–1739. (217)

Anstis, S. M., & Ramachandran, V. S. (1986b) Visual inertia in apparent motion. *Vision Research,* **26,** 755–764. (218)

Applegate, R. A. (1983) *Aperture Effects on Phototropic Orientation Properties of Human Photoreceptors.* Ph.D. Dissertation. University of California, Berkeley. (385)

Applegate, R. A., Adams, A. J., Cavender, J. C., & Zisman, F. (1987) Early color vision changes in age-related maculopathy. *Applied Optics,* **26,** 1458–1462. (400, 404)

Applegate, R. A., & Bonds, A. B. (1981) Induced movement of receptor alignment toward a new pupillary aperture. *Investigative Ophthalmology & Visual Science,* **21,** 869–873. (385)

Arden, G. B., & Jacobson, J. J. (1978) A simple grating test for contrast sensitivity: Preliminary results indicate value in screening for glaucoma. *Investigative Ophthalmology & Visual Science,* **17,** 23–32. (396)

Arden, G. B., Vaegan, B., & Hogg, H. C. (1982) Clinical and experimental evidence that the pattern electroretinogram (PERG) is generated in more proximal retinal layers than the focal electroretinogram (FERG). *Annals of the New York Academy of Science,* **388,** 580–601. (408)

Arend, L. E. (1973) Spatial differential and integral operation in human vision: Implications of stabilized retinal image fading. *Psychological Review,* **80,** 374–395. (66, 99)

Arend, L. E. (1976) Temporal determinants of the form of the spatial contrast threshold MTF. *Vision Research,* **16,** 1035–1042. (66)

Arend, L. E., & Goldstein, R. (1987) Simultaneous constancy, lightness and brightness. *Journal of the Optical Society of America A,* **4,** 2281–2285. (64, 132)

Arend, L. E., & Reeves, A. (1986) Simultaneous color constancy. *Journal of the Optical Society of America A,* **3,** 1743–1751. (68)

Arnold, R. D., & Binford, T. O. (1980) Geometric constraints in stereo vision. *Society of Photo-Optical Instrumental Engineers,* **238,** 281–292. (341)

Aslin, R. N. (1981) The development of smooth pursuit in human infants. In D. F. Fisher, R. A. Monty & J. W. Senders (Eds.), *Eye Movements: Cognition and Visual Perception,* pp. 31–52. Hillsdale, NJ: Lawrence Erlbaum. (361)

Aslin, R. N. (1987) Visual and auditory development in infancy. In J. D. Osofsky (Ed.), *Handbook of Infant Development.* New York: Wiley. (350)

Atkin, A., Bodis-Wollner, I., Wolkstein, M., Moss, A., & Podos, S. M. (1979) Abnormalities of central contrast sensitivity in glaucoma. *American Journal of Ophthalmology,* **88,** 205–211. (396–397)

Atkinson, J. (1984) Human visual development over the first 6 months of life. A review and a hypothesis. *Human Neurobiology,* **3,** 61–74. (360–361)

Atkinson, J., & Braddick, O. J. (1974) Stereoscopic discrimination in infants. *Perception,* **5,** 29–38. (361)

Atkinson, J., & Braddick, O. J. (1985) Early development of the control of visual attention. *Perception,* **14,** A25. (361, 364)

Atkinson, J., Braddick, O., & Moar, K. (1977) Development of contrast sensitivity over the first three months of life in the human infant. *Vision Research,* **17,** 1037–1044. (350–351)

Atkinson, J., Hood, B., Wattam-Bell, J., Anker, S., & Tricklebank, J. (1988) Development of orientation discrimination in infancy. *Perception,* **17,** 587–595. (363)

Atkinson, J., Wattam-Bell, J., & Braddick, O. J. (1986) Infants' development of sensitivity to pattern "textons". *Investigative Ophthalmology & Visual Science Supplement,* **27,** 265. (361)

Attneave, F. (1971) The multistability of perception. *Scientific American,* **225**(6), 62–71. (275)

Attwell, D., Werblin, F. S., & Wilson, M. (1982) The properties of single cones isolated from the tiger salamander retina. *Journal of Physiology,* **328,** 259–283. (84)

Attwell, D., Wilson, M., & Wu, S. M. (1984) A quantitative analysis of interactions between photoreceptors in the salamander (*Ambystoma*) retina. *Journal of Physiology,* **352,** 703–737. (85)

Aulhorn, E., Köst, G. (1988) Rauschfeld-Kampimetrie. *Klinische Monatsblätter für Angenheilkunde,* **192,** 284–288. (455)

Ayama, M., & Ikeda, M. (1986) Additivity of yellow chromatic valence. *Vision Research,* **26,** 763–769. (168)

Bach, M., Bouis, D., & Fischer, B. (1983) An accurate and linear infrared oculometer. *Journal of Neuroscience Methods,* **9,** 9–14. (308)

Badcock, D. R., & Schor, C. M. (1985) Depth detection function for individual spatial channels. *Journal of the Optical Society of America A,* **2,** 1211–1215. (329)

Badcock, D., & Westheimer, G. (1985) Spatial location and hyperacuity: The centre–surround localization contribution function has two substrates. *Vision Research,* **25,** 1259–1267. (444)

Bader, C. R., Bertrand, D., & Schwartz, E. A. (1982) Voltage-activated and calcium-activated currents in solitary rod inner segments from the salamander retina. *Journal of Physiology,* **331,** 253–284. (84)

Bakay Pragay, E., Mirsky, A. F., & Nakamura, R. K. (1987) Attention-related unit activity in the frontal association cortex during a go/no-go visual discrimination task. *Experimental Neurology,* **96,** 481–500. (312)

Baker, C. L. & Braddick, O. J. (1985) Eccentricity-dependent scaling of the limits for short-range apparent motion perception. *Vision Research,* **25,** 803–812. (210–211, 213–214)

Baker, H. D. (1949) The course of foveal adaptation measured by the threshold intensity increment. *Journal of the Optical Society of America,* **39,** 172–179. (75)

Baker, H. D. (1953) Instantaneous thresholds and early dark adaptation. *Journal of the Optical Society of America,* **43,** 798–803. (75)

Baker, H. D. (1966) Single-variable anomaloscope matches during recovery from artificial red blindness. *Journal of the Optical Society of America,* **56,** 686–689. (37)

Baker, H. D., & Rushton, W. A. H. (1965) The red-sensitive pigment in normal cones. *Journal of Physiology,* **176,** 56–72. (37)

Baker, H. H. (1982) *Depth from Edge and Intensity Based Stereo.* Ph.D. Thesis, University of Illinois. (341)

Baker, J. F., Petersen, S. E., Newsome, W. T., & Allman, J. M. (1981) Visual response properties of neurons in four extrastriate visual areas of the owl monkey (*Aotus trivirgatus*): A quantitative comparison of medial, dorsomedial, dorsolateral and middle temporal areas. *Journal of Neurophysiology,* **45,** 397–416. (286)

Ballard, D. H. (1986) Cortical connections and parallel processing: Structure and function. *Behavioral and Brain Sciences,* **9,** 67–120. (270)

Ballard, D. H., Hinton, G. E., & Sejnowski, T. J. (1983) Parallel visual computation. *Nature (London),* **306,** 21–26. (104)

Ballas, I., & Hoffmann, K. P. (1985) A correlation between receptive field properties and morphological structures in the pretectum of the cat. *Journal of Comparative Neurology,* **238,** 417–428. (111)

Ballas, I., Hoffmann, K.-P., & Wagner, H. J. (1981) Retinal projection to the nucleus of the optic tract in the cat as revealed by retrograde transport of horseradish peroxidase. *Neuroscience Letters,* **26,** 197–202. (111, 376)

Banks, M. S. (1980a) Infant refraction and accommodation. *International Ophthalmology Clinics,* **20,** 205–232. (351, 361)

Banks, M. S. (1980b) The development of visual accommodation during early infancy. *Child Development,* **51,** 646–666. (351, 361)

Banks, M. S., & Bennett, P. J. (1988) Optical and photoreceptor immaturities limit the spatial and chromatic vision of human neonates. *Journal of the Optical Society of America,* **5,** 2059–2079. (351–352, 354–359, 361)

Banks, M. S., & Dannemiller, J. L. (1987) Infant visual psychophysics. In P. Salapatek & L. B. Cohen (Eds.) *Handbook of Infant Perception,* pp. 115–184. New York: Academic Press. (350)

Banks, M. S., Geisler, W. S., & Bennett, P. J. (1987) The physical limits of grating visibility. *Vision Research,* **27,** 1915–1924. (351–353)

Banks, M. S., & Salapatek, P. (1978) Acuity and contrast sensitivity in 1-, 2-, and 3-month-old human infants. *Investigative Ophthalmology & Visual Science,* **17,** 361–365. (350–351)

Barbur, J. L., Ruddock, K. H., & Waterfield, V. A. (1980) Human visual responses in the absence of the geniculo-calcarine projection. *Brain,* **102,** 905–928. (414)

Barlow, H. B. (1953) Summation and inhibition in the frog's retina. *Journal of Physiology,* **119,** 69–88. (90, 110–111, 153)

Barlow, H. B. (1957) Increment threshold at low intensities considered as signal/noise discriminations. *Journal of Physiology,* **136,** 469–488. (61, 80, 84)

Barlow, H. B. (1958a) Intrinsic noise of cones. In *Visual Problems of Colour, Vol. 2,* pp. 617–630. London: Her Majesty's Stationary Office. (80)

Barlow, H. B. (1958b) Temporal and spatial summation in human vision at different background intensities. *Journal of Physiology,* **141,** 337–350. (98, 352)

Barlow, H. B. (1963) Slippage of contact lenses and other artifacts in relation to fading and regeneration of supposedly stable after images. *Quarterly Journal of Experimental Psychology,* **15(1),** 36–51. (138)

Barlow, H. B. (1964a) Dark adaptation: A new hypothesis. *Vision Research,* **4,** 47–58. (84)

Barlow, H. B. (1964b) The limits of visual discrimination. In A. C. Giese (Ed.) *Photophysiology, Vol. 2,* pp. 163–202. New York: Academic Press. (61)

Barlow, H. B. (1965) Optic nerve impulses and Weber's law. *Cold Spring Harbor Symposium on Quantitative Biology,* **30,** 539–546. (76)

Barlow, H. B. (1972a) Dark and light adaptation: Psychophysics. In D. Jameson & L. M. Hurvich (Eds.), *Handbook of Sensory Physiology, Vol. VII/4,* pp. 1–28. Berlin: Springer-Verlag. (98)

Barlow, H. B. (1972b) Single units and sensation: A neuron doctrine for perceptual psychology? *Perception,* **1,** 371–394. (46, 307)

Barlow, H. B. (1977) Retinal and central factors in human vision limited by noise. In H. B. Barlow & P. Fatt (Eds.), *Vertebrate Photoreception,* pp. 337–358. London: Academic Press. (55, 61)

Barlow, H. B. (1979) Reconstructing the visual image in space and time. *Nature (London),* **279,** 189–190. (28)

Barlow, H. B. (1981) Critical limiting factors in the design of the eye and the visual cortex. *Proceedings of the Royal Society of London, Series B,* **212,** 1–34. (422)

Barlow, H. B., & Andrews, D. P. (1973) The site at which rhodopsin bleaching raises the scotopic threshold. *Vision Research,* **13,** 903–908. (97)

Barlow, H. B., Blakemore, C., & Pettigrew, J. D. (1967) The neural mechanism of binocular depth discrimination. *Journal of Physiology,* **193,** 327–342. (23, 322, 328)

Barlow, H. B., Fitzhugh, R., & Kuffler, S. W. (1957) Change in organization in the receptive fields of the cat's retina during dark adaptation. *Journal of Physiology,* **137,** 338–354. (98, 119)

Barlow, H. B., & Levick, W. R. (1965) The mechanism of directionally selective units in rabbit's retina. *Journal of Physiology,* **178,** 477–504. (214)

Barlow, H. B., & Levick, W. R. (1969) Three factors limiting the reliable detection of light by retinal ganglion cells of the cat. *Journal of Physiology,* **200,** 1–24. (61, 88, 98)

Barlow, H. B., & Levick, W. R. (1976) Threshold settings by the surround of cat retinal ganglion cells. *Journal of Physiology,* **259,** 737–757. (98)

Barlow, H. B., & Pelli, D. S. (1987) Statistical efficiency of natural and artificial vision. Series of symposium papers edited by H. B. Barlow & D. S. Pelli, *Journal of the Optical Society of America A,* **4,** 2292–2457. (61)

Barlow, H. B., & Sakitt, B. (1973) Doubts about scotopic interactions in stabilized vision. *Vision Research,* **13,** 523–524. (100)

Barlow, H. B., & Sparrock, J. M. B. (1964) The role of afterimages in dark adaptation. *Science,* **144,** 1309–1314. (70, 138)

Barrow, H. G., & Tenenbaum, J. M. (1978) Recovering intrinsic scene characteristics from images. In A. Hanson & E. Riseman (Eds.), *Computer Vision Systems.* New York: Academic Press (344)

Bartley, S. H. (1938) Subjective brightness in relation to flash rate and the light/dark ratio. *Journal of Experimental Psychology,* **23,** 313–319. (148)

Baumgartner, G. (1960) Indirekte Grössenbestimmung der receptiven Felder der Retina beim Menschen mittels der Hermannschen Gittertäuschung. *Pflügers Archiv für die gesamte Physiologie,* **272,** 21–22. (139)

Baumgartner, G. (1961a) Der Informationswert der on-Zentrum und off-Zentrum Neurone des visuellen Systems beim Hell-Dunkel-Sehen und die informative Bedeutung von Aktivierung und Hemmung. In R. Jung & H. Kornhuber (Eds.), *Neurophysiologie und Psychophysik des visuellen Systems,* pp. 377–379. Heidelberg: Springer-Verlag. (145)

Baumgartner, G. (1961b) Neuronale Grundlagen der visuellen Kontrastverschärfung vom Auge zur Hirnrinde. In: Nachrichtentechnische Gesellschaft (Ed.), *Aufnahme und Verarbeitung von Nachrichten durch Organismen,* pp. 100–108. Stuttgart: S. Hirzel-Verlag. (135, 145)

Baumgartner, G. (1964) Neuronale Mechanismen des Kontrast- und Bewegungssehens. *Bericht der deutschen ophthalmologischen Gesellschaft,* **66,** 111–125. (134)

Baumgartner, G. (1986) Psychophysics and central processing. In A. K. Asbury, B. M. McKhann & W. J. McDonald (Eds.), *Diseases of the Nervous System. Clinical Neurobiology,* pp. 804–815. Philadelphia: W. B. Saunders. (136)

Baumgartner, G., & Hakas, P. (1962) Die Neurophysiologie des simultanen Helligkeitskontrastes. Reziproke Reaktionen antagonistischer Neuronengruppen des visuellen Systems. *Pflügers Archiv für die gesamte Physiologie,* **274,** 489–500.

Baylor, D. A. (1987) Photoreceptor signals and vision (Proctor Lecture). *Investigative Ophthalmology & Visual Science,* **28,** 34–49. (77, 80)

Baylor, D. A., Fuortes, M. G. F., & O'Bryan, P. M. (1971) Receptive field of single cones in the retina of the turtle. *Journal of Physiology,* **214,** 265–294. (85)

Baylor, D. A., & Hodgkin, A. L. (1973) Detection and resolution of visual stimuli by turtle photoreceptors. *Journal of Physiology,* **234,** 163–198. (85)

Baylor, D. A., Lamb, T. D., & Yau, K. W. (1979) Responses of retinal rods to single photons. *Journal of Physiology,* **288,** 613–634. (79)

Baylor, D. A., Matthews, G., & Yau, K. W. (1983) Two components of electrical dark noise in toad retinal rod outer segments. *Journal of Physiology,* **309,** 591–621. (80)

Baylor, D. A., Nunn, B. S., & Schnapf, S. L. (1984) The photocurrent, noise and spectral sensitivity of rods of the monkey *Macaca fascicularis. Journal of Physiology,* **357,** 575–607. (55–56, 79–80, 83, 400)

Baylor, D. A., Nunn, B. J., & Schnapf, J. L. (1987) Spectral sensitivity of cones of the monkey *Macaca fascicularis, Journal of Physiology,* **390,** 145–160. (56, 79–80, 172–174)

Bayly, E. J., Cervetto, L., Fiorentini, A., & Maffei, L. (1971) On and off retinal cells in parallel channel neural communication. *Kybernetik*, **8,** 52–58. (159)

Bear, M. F., Cooper, L. N., & Ebner, F. F. (1987) A physiological basis for a theory of synapse modification. *Science*, **237,** 42–48. (391)

Bear, M. F., & Singer, W. (1986) Modulation of visual cortex plasticity by acetylcholine and noradrenaline. *Nature (London)*, **320,** 172–176. (391)

Beaulieu, C., & Colonnier, M. (1983) The number of neurons in the different laminae of the binocular and monocular regions of area 17 in the cat. *Journal of Comparative Neurology*, **217,** 337–344. (28)

Beck, J. (1966) Effects of orientation and of shape similarity on perceptual grouping. *Perception & Psychophysics*, **1,** 300–302. (275)

Beck, J. (1967) Perceptual grouping produced by line figures. *Perception & Psychophysics*, **2,** 491–495. (275)

Beck, J. (1982) Textural segmentation. In J. Beck (Ed.), *Organization and Representation in Perception*, pp. 285–317. Hillsdale, NJ: Lawrence Erlbaum. (275)

Beck, J. (1983) Textural segmentation, second-order statistics and textural elements. *Biological Cybernetics*, **48,** 125–130. (442)

Beck, J., Prazdny, K., & Rosenfeld, A. (1983) A theory of textural segmentation. In J. Beck, B. Hope, & A. Rosenfeld (Eds.), *Human and Machine Vision*. New York: Academic Press. (442)

Becker, M F., & Knopp, J. (1978) Processing of visual illusions in the frequency and spatial domains. *Perception & Psychophysics*, **23,** 521–526. (292)

Bedell, H. E., Enoch, J. M., & Fitzgerald, C. R. (1981) A graded disturbance bordering a region of choroidal atrophy. *Archives of Ophthalmology*, **99,** 1841–1844 (400)

Bedell, H. E., & Flom, M. C. (1981) Monocular spatial distortion in strabismic amblyopia. *Investigative Ophthalmology & Visual Science*, **20,** 263–268. (265)

Békésy, von G. (1960) Neural inhibitory units of the eye and skin. Quantitative description of contrast phenomena. *Journal of the Optical Society of America*, **50,** 1060–1070. (155)

Békésy, von G. (1968) Mach- and Hering-type lateral inhibition in vision. *Vision Research*, **8,** 1483–1499. (136)

Belgum, J. H., & Copenhagen, D. R. (1988) Synaptic transfer of rod signals to horizontal and bipolar cells in the retina of the toad. (*Bufo marinus*). *Journal of Physiology*, **396,** 667–680. (85, 101)

Bender, M. B., & Bodis-Wollner, I. (1978) Visual dysfunction in optic tract lesions. *Annals of Neurology*, **3,** 187–193. (200)

Bender, M. B., & Teuber, H. L. (1946) Phenomena of fluctuation, extinction and completion in visual perception. *Archives of Neurology & Psychiatry*, **55,** 627–658. (454)

Benevento, L. A., & Fallon, J. H. (1975) The ascending projections of the superior colliculus in the rhesus monkey (*Macaca mulatta*). *Journal of Comparative Neurology*, **160,** 339–362. (411)

Bennett, P. J., & Banks, M. S. (1987) Sensitivity loss in odd-symmetric mechanisms and phase anomalies in peripheral vision. *Nature (London)*, **326,** 873–876. (270, 432)

Berardi, N., Bisti, S., & Maffei, L. (1987) The transfer of visual information across the corpus callosum: Spatial and temporal properties in the cat. *Journal of Physiology*, **384,** 619–632. (260–261)

Berardi, N., & Fiorentini, A. (1987) Interhemispheric transfer of visual information in humans: Spatial characteristics. *Journal of Physiology*, **384,** 633–647. (261)

Berardi, N., Bisti, S., Fiorentini, A., & Maffei, L. (1988) The transfer of visual information across the corpus callosum in cats, monkeys and humans: Spatial and temporal properties. In T. P. Hicks & G. Benedek (Eds.), *Progress in Brain Research*, **75,** 181–185.

Bergen, J. R., & Adelson, E. H. (1988) Early vision and texture perception. *Nature (London)*, **333,** 363–364. (425, 427)

Bergen, J. R., & Julesz, B. (1983) Parallel versus serial processing in rapid pattern discrimination. *Nature (London)*, **303,** 696–698. (276)

Berkley, M. A., Kitterle, F., & Watkins, D. W. (1975) Grating visibility as a function of orientation and retinal eccentricity. *Vision Research*, **15,** 239–244. (28–29)

Berkley, M. A., & Sprague, J. M. (1979) Striate cortex and visual acuity functions in the cat. *Journal of Comparative Neurology*, **187,** 679–702. (30)

Beverley, K. I., & Regan, D. (1973) Evidence for the existence of neural mechanisms selectively sensitive to the direction of movement in space. *Journal of Physiology*, **235,** 17–29. (333–335, 337)

Beverley, K. I., & Regan, D. (1974) Visual sensitivity to disparity pulses: Evidence for directional selectivity. *Vision Research*, **14,** 375–361. (334)

Bezold, von W. (1874) *Die Farbenlehre*, Braunschweig: Westermann. (133)

Biederman, I. (1987) Recognition-by-components: A theory of human image understanding. *Psychological Review*, **94,** 115–147. (274)

Birch, D. G., & Sandberg, M. A. (1982) Psychophysical studies of cone optical bandwidth in patients with retinitis pigmentosa. *Vision Research*, **22,** 113–117. (385–386)

Birch, D. G., Sandberg, M. A., & Berson, E. L. (1982) The Stiles–Crawford effect in retinitis pigmentosa. *Investigative Ophthalmology & Visual Science*, **22,** 157–164. (371, 400)

Birch, E. E., Gwiazda, J., & Held, R. (1982) Stereoacuity development for crossed and uncrossed disparities in human infants. *Vision Research*, **22,** 507–513. (371)

Birch, E. E., Gwiazda, J., & Held, R. (1983) The development of vergence does not account for the development of stereopsis. *Perception*, **12,** 331–336. (362)

Birch, E. E., Shimojo, S., & Held, R. (1985) Preferential looking assessment of fusion and stereopsis in infants aged 1 to 6 months. *Investigative Ophthalmology & Visual Science*, **26,** 366–370. (362, 371)

Bishop, G. H., & O'Leary, J. S. (1938) Potential records from the optic cortex of the cat. *Journal of Neurophysiology,* **3,** 308–322. (107)

Bishop, P. O., & Pettigrew, J. D. (1986) Neural mechanisms of binocular vision. *Vision Research,* **26,** 1587–1600. (24, 322)

Bishop, P. O., Coombs, J. S., & Henry, G. H. (1971) Responses to visual contours: spatio-temporal aspects of excitation in the receptive fields of simple striate neurones. *Journal of Physiology,* **219,** 625–657. (248)

Bisti, S., & Maffei, L. (1974) Behavioral contrast sensitivity of the cat in various visual meridians. *Journal of Physiology,* **241,** 201–210. (30)

Bisti, S., & Siretenau, R. (1976) Sensitivity to spatial frequency and contrast of visual cells in the cat superior colliculus. *Vision Research,* **16,** 247–251. (30)

Bjørklund, R. A., & Magnussen, S. (1979) Decrement versions of the Broca–Sulzer effect and its spatial analogue. *Vision Research,* **19,** 155–157. (146–148)

Bjorklund, R. A., & Magnussen, S. (1981) A study of the interocular transfer of spatial adaptation. *Perception,* **10,** 511–518. (152)

Blackwell, H. R. (1972) Luminance difference thresholds. In D. Jameson & L. M. Hurvich (Eds.), *Handbook of Sensory Physiology VII/4,* pp. 78–101. Berlin: Springer-Verlag. (58)

Blake, A. (1984) *Reconstructing a Visible Surface,* Proceedings of the A.A.A.I. Conference. (344)

Blake, A., & Zisserman, A. (1986a) *Weak Continuity Constraints in Computer Vision.* Internal report CSR-197-86. Department of Computer Science of University of Edinburgh, U.K. (344)

Blake, A., & Zisserman, A. (1986b) Invariant surface reconstruction using weak continuity constraints. In *Proceedings of the IEEE: Computer Vision and Pattern Recognition, Miami, FL,* pp. 62–67. (344)

Blake, A., & Zisserman, A. (1987) *Visual Reconstruction.* Cambridge, MA: M.I.T. Press. (344)

Blake, R., & Bellhorn, R. (1978) Visual acuity in cats with central retinal lesions. *Vision Research,* **18,** 15–18. (28–29)

Blake, R., & Camisa, J. (1977) Temporal aspects of spatial vision in the cat. *Experimental Brain Research,* **28,** 325–333. (31)

Blake, R., Cool, S. J., & Crawford, M. L. J. (1974) Visual resolution in the cat. *Vision Research,* **14,** 1211–1217. (26, 28, 30)

Blake, R., & DiGianfilippo, A. (1980) Spatial vision in cats with selective neural deficits. *Journal of Neurophysiology,* **43,** 1197–1205. (31)

Blake, R., & Hirsch, H. V. B. (1975) Deficits in binocular depth perception in cats after alternating monocular deprivation. *Science,* **190,** 1114–1116. (395)

Blake, R., & Holopigian, K. (1985) Orientation selectivity in cats and humans assessed by masking. *Vision Research,* **25,** 1459–1467. (31–32, 33)

Blake, R., Holopigian, K., & Wilson, H. R. (1986) Spatial frequency discrimination in cats. *Journal of the Optical Society of America A,* **3,** 1443–1449. (33)

Blake, R., & Martens, R. W. (1981) Critical bands in cat spatial vision. *Journal of Physiology,* **34,** 175–187. (31)

Blake, R., Overton, R., & Lema-Stern, S. (1981) Interocular transfer of visual aftereffects. *Journal of Experimental Psychology: Human Perception Performance,* **7,** 367–381. (152)

Blakemore, C. B. (1970) The range and scope of binocular depth discrimination in man. *Journal of Physiology,* **211,** 599–622. (324, 329)

Blakemore, C. B. (1988) The sensitive periods of the monkey's visual cortex. In G. Lennerstrand, G. K. von Noorden, & E. Campos (Eds.), *Strabismus and Amblyopia: Experimental Basis for Advances in Clinical Management,* pp. 219–234. London: MacMillan Press. (395)

Blakemore, C. B., & Campbell, F. W. (1969) On the existence of neurones in the human visual system selectively sensitive to the orientation and size of retinal images. *Journal of Physiology,* **203,** 237–260. (246, 250, 257–258, 418)

Blakemore, C. B., Garey, L. J., & Vital-Durand, F. (1978) The physiological effects of monocular deprivation and their reversal in the monkey's visual cortex. *Journal of Physiology,* **283,** 223–262. (391)

Blakemore, C. B., & Rushton, W. A. H. (1965a) Dark adaptation and increment threshold in a rod monochromat. *Journal of Physiology,* **181,** 612–628. (381)

Blakemore, C. B., & Rushton, W. A. H. (1965b) The rod increment threshold during dark adaptation in normal and rod monochromat. *Journal of Physiology,* **181,** 629–640. (70, 381)

Blakemore, C. B., & Sutton, P. (1969) Size adaptation: A new after-effect. *Science,* **166,** 245–247. (150, 296)

Blakemore, C. B., & Van Sluyters, R. C. (1974) Reversal of the physiological effects of monocular deprivation in kittens: Further evidence for a sensitive period. *Journal of Physiology,* **237,** 195–216. (391)

Blakemore, C., & Van Sluyters, R. C. (1975) Innate and environmental factors in the development of the kitten's visual cortex. *Journal of Physiology,* **248,** 663–716. (388)

Blakemore, C., & Vital-Durand, F. (1986) Organization and development of the monkey's lateral geniculate nucleus. *Journal of Physiology,* **380,** 453–491. (118)

Blakemore, C. B., Vital-Durand, F., & Garey, C. J. (1981) Recovery from monocular deprivation in the monkey. I. Recovery of physiological effects in the visual cortex. *Proceedings of the Royal Society of London, Series B,* **213,** 399–423. (391)

Blakeslee, B., Jacobs, G. H., & Neitz, J. (1988) Spectral mechanisms in the tree squirrel retina. *Journal of Comparative Physiology, A,* **162,** 773–780. (34)

Blasdel, G. G., & Lund, J. S. (1983) Termination of afferent axons in macaque striate cortex. *Journal of Neuroscience,* **3,** 1389–1413. (121)

Blasdel, G. G., & Salama, G. (1986) Voltage sensitive dyes reveal a modular organization in monkey striate cortex. *Nature (London),* **321,** 579–584. (250)

Blick, D. W., & MacLeod, D. I. A. (1978) Rod threshold: Influence of neighboring cones. *Vision Research,* **18,** 1611–1616. (100)

Bloom, M., & Berkley, M. (1977) Visual acuity and the near point of accommodation in cats. *Vision Research,* **17,** 723–730. (27–28)

Blough, D. S., & Schrier, A. M. (1963) Scotopic spectral sensitivity in the monkey. *Science,* **149,** 493–494. (43–44)

Bobak, P., Bodis-Wollner, I., Harnois, C., Maffei, L., Mylin, L., Podos, S. M., & Thornton, J. (1983) Pattern electroretinograms and visual evoked potentials in glaucoma and multiple sclerosis. *American Journal of Ophthalmology,* **96,** 72–83. (408, 410)

Boch, R. (1986) Behavioral modulation of neuronal activity in monkey striate cortex: Excitation in the absence of central fixation. *Experimental Brain Research,* **64,** 610–614. (311)

Boch, R., & Fischer, B. (1986) Further observations on the occurrence of express-saccades in the monkey. *Experimental Brain Research,* **63,** 487–494. (314)

Boch, R. A., & Goldberg, M. E. (1989) Participation of prefrontal neurons in the preparation of visually guided eye movements in the rhesus monkey. *Journal of Neurophysiology,* **61,** 1064–1084. (312)

Bodis-Wollner, I. (1981) Differences in low and high spatial frequency vulnerabilities in ocular and cerebral lesions. In L. Maffei (Ed.), *Pathophysiology of the Visual System,* pp. 195–204. The Hague: Dr. W. Junk. (408)

Bodis-Wollner, I., Bobak, P., Harnois, C., & Mylin, L. H. (1984) Methodological aspects of signal-to-noise evaluation of simultaneous pattern electroretinogram and visual evoked potential recordings. *Documenta Ophthalmologica Proceedings Series,* **40,** 39–48. (386)

Bodis-Wollner, I., & Diamond, S. P. (1976) The measurement of spatial contrast sensitivity in cases of blurred vision associated with cerebral lesions. *Brain,* **99,** 695–710. (387, 409)

Bodis-Wollner, I., Hendley, C. D., Mylin, L. H., & Thornton, J. (1979) Visual evoked potentials and the visuogram in multiple sclerosis. *Annals of Neurology,* **5,** 40–47. (409)

Bodis-Wollner, I., Marx, M., Mitra, S., Bodak, P., Mylin, L., & Yahr, M. (1987) Visual dysfunction in Parkinson's disease. *Brain,* **110,** 1675–1698. (386–388)

Bodis-Wollner, I., & Yahr, M. D. (1978) Measurements of visual evoked potentials in Parkinson's disease. *Brain,* **101,** 661–671. (386)

Bodis-Wollner, I., Yahr, M., Mylin, L., & Thornton, J. (1982) Dopamingergic deficiency and delayed visual evoked potentials in humans. *Annals of Neurology,* **11,** 478–483. (386)

Bolz, J., & Gilbert, C. D. (1986) Generation of end-inhibition in the visual cortex via interlaminar connections. *Nature (London),* **320,** 362–365. (245)

Bolz, J., Rosner, G., & Wässle, H. (1982) Response latency of brisk-sustained (X) and brisk-transient (Y) cells in the cat retina. *Journal of Physiology,* **328,** 171–190. (120)

Bonds, A. B. (1979) Development of orientation tuning in the visual cortex of kittens. In R. D. Freeman (Ed.), *Developmental Neurobiology of Vision,* pp. 31–41. New York: Plenum. (388)

Boothe, R. G., Dobson, V., & Teller, D. Y. (1985) Postnatal development of vision in humans and nonhuman primates. *Annual Review of Neuroscience,* **8,** 495–545. (350)

Boring, E. G. (1942) *Sensation and Perception in the History of Experimental Psychology.* New York: Appleton-Century-Crofts. (14–15)

Botez, M. I. (1975) Two visual systems in clinical neurology: Readaptive role of the primitive system in visual agnosis patients. *European Neurology,* **13,** 101–122. (285)

Bouman, M. A. (1950) Peripheral contrast thresholds of the human eye. *Journal of the Optical Society of America,* **40,** 825–832. (98)

Bouman, M. A. (1961) History and present status of quantum theory in vision. In W. A. Rosenblith (Ed.), *Sensory Communication,* pp. 377–402. New York: Wiley. (61)

Bouman, M. A., & Walraven, P. L. (1972) Color discrimination data. In D. Jameson & L. M. Hurvich (Eds.), *Handbook of Sensory Physiology: VII/4: Visual Psychophysics,* pp. 484–516. New York: Springer-Verlag. (255)

Bourdon, B. (1902) *La Perception Visuelle de l'Espace.* Paris: Scheicher. (239)

Bowmaker, J. K. (1984) Microspectrophotometry of vertebrate photoreceptors. *Vision Research,* **24,** 1641–1650. (170)

Bowmaker, J. K., Dartnall, H. J. A., & Mollon, J. D. (1980) Microspectrophotometric demonstration of four classes of photoreceptors in an old world primate, *Macaca fascicularis. Journal of Physiology,* **298,** 131–143. (181–182)

Bowmaker, J. K., Jacobs, G. H., & Mollon, J. D. (1987) Polymorphism of photopigments in the squirrel monkey: A sixth phenotype. *Proceedings of the Royal Society of London, Series B,* **231,** 383–390. (36)

Bowmaker, J. K., Jacobs, G. H., Spiegelhalter, D. J., & Mollon, J. D. (1985) Two types of trichromatic squirrel monkey share a pigment in the red–green spectral region. *Vision Research,* **25,** 1937–1946. (36–37, 176)

Bowmaker, J. K., Mollon, J. D., & Jacobs, G. H. (1983) Microspectrophotometric results for old and new world primates. In J. D. Mollon & L. T. Sharpe (Eds.), *Colour Vision: Physiology and Psychophysics,* pp. 57–68. New York: Academic Press.

Boycott, B. B., Dowling, J. E., Fisher, S. K., Kolb, H., & Laties, A. M. (1975) Interplexiform cells of the mammalian retina and their comparison with catecholamine-containing retinal cells. *Proceedings of the Royal Society of London, Series B,* **191,** 353–368. (88)

Boycott, B. B., Hopkins, J. M., & Sperling, H. G. (1987) Cone connections of the horizontal cells of the rhesus monkey's retina. *Proceedings of the Royal Society of London, Series B,* **229,** 345–379. (35)

Boycott, B. B., & Wässle, H. (1974) The morphological types of ganglion cells of the domestic cat's retina. *Journal of Physiology,* **240,** 397–419. (106–107, 112, 142)

Boynton, R. M. (1979) *Human Color Vision.* New York: Holt, Rinehart & Winston. (37, 66, 170)

Boynton, R. M. & Gordon, J. (1965) Bezold–Brücke hue shift measured by color-naming technique. *Journal of the Optical Society of America,* **55,** 78–86. (165)

Boynton, R. M., & Kandell, G. (1957) On responses in the human visual system as a function of adaptation level. *Journal of the Optical Society of America,* **47,** 275–286. (70)

Boynton, R. M. & Onley, J. W. (1962) A critique of the special status assigned by Brindley to the "Psychophysical linking hypothesis" of "Class A". *Vision Research,* **2,** 383–390. (15)

Boynton, R. M., & Whitten, D. N. (1970) Visual adaptation in monkey cones: Recordings of late receptor potentials. *Science,* **170,** 1423–1426. (59, 84)

Bracewell, R. N. (1965) *The Fourier Transform and Its Application.* New York: McGraw-Hill. (234)

Braddick, O. J. (1974) A short-range process in apparent motion. *Vision Research,* **14,** 519–527. (210)

Braddick, O. J., & Atkinson, J. (1983) Some recent findings on the development of human binocularity: A review. *Behavioural Brain Research,* **10,** 71–80. (361)

Braddick, O. J., & Atkinson, J. (1987) Sensory selectivity, attentional control, and cross-channel integration in early visual development. In A. Yonas (Ed.), *20th Minnesota Symposium on Child Psychology.* Hillsdale, NJ: Lawrence Erlbaum. (359, 361)

Braddick, O. J., Atkinson, J., French, J., & Howland, H. C. (1979) A photorefractive study of infant accommodation. *Vision Research,* **19,** 319–330. (351, 361)

Braddick, O. J., Atkinson, J., Julesz, B., Kropfl, W., Bodis-Wollner, I., & Raab, E. (1980) Cortical binocularity in infants. *Nature (London),* **288,** 363–365. (362)

Braddick, O. J., Atkinson, J., & Wattam-Bell, J. R. (1986) Development of the discrimination of spatial phase in infancy. *Vision Research,* **26,** 1223–1239. (361)

Braddick, O. J., Wattam-Bell, J., & Atkinson, J. (1986) Orientation-specific cortical responses develop in early infancy. *Nature (London),* **320,** 617–619. (362)

Bradley, A., Skottun, B. C., Ohzawa, I., Sclar, G., & Freeman, R. D. (1985) Neurophysiological evaluation of the differential response model for orientation and spatial-frequency discrimination. *Journal of the Optical Society of America A,* **2,** 1607–1610. (258–259)

Bradley, A., Skottun, B. C., Ohzawa, I., Sclar, G., & Freeman, R. D. (1987) Visual orientation and spatial frequency discrimination: A comparison of single neurons and behavior. *Journal of Neurophysiology,* **57,** 755–772. (25, 33, 258)

Brandt, Th. (1982) The relationship between retinal image slip, oscillopsia and postural imbalance. In G. Lennerstrand, D. S. Zee & E. L. Keller (Eds.), *Functional Basis of Ocular Motility Disorders,* pp. 379–385. Oxford: Pergamon. (228)

Brandt, Th., & Dieterich, M. (1986) Peripheral ocular motor palsy impairs motion perception. In E. L. Keller & D. S. Zee (Eds.), *Adaptive Processes in Visual and Oculomotor Systems,* pp. 457–463. Oxford: Pergamon. (228)

Brandt, Th., & Dieterich, M. (1988) Oscillopsia and motion perception. In C. Kennard & F. Clifford Rose (Eds.), *Physiological Aspects of Clinical Neuro-Ophthalmology,* pp. 321–339. London: Chapman and Hall. (227)

Braunstein, M. (1976) *Depth Perception Through Motion.* New York: Academic Press. (307)

Bravo, M., Blake, R., & Morrison, S. (1988) Cats see subjective contours. *Vision Research,* **28,** 861–865. (292)

Breitmeyer, B. G. (1975) Simple reaction time as a measure of the response properties of sustained and transient channels. *Vision Research,* **15,** 1411–1412. (120)

Breitmeyer, B. G. (1984) *Visual Masking: An Integrative Approach.* New York: Oxford University Press. (425, 445)

Breitmeyer, B., Valberg, A., Kurtenbach, W., & Neumeyer, C. (1980) The lateral effect of oscillation of peripheral luminance gratings on the foveal increment theshold. *Vision Research,* **20,** 799–805. (62)

Brewster, D. (1834) On the influence of successive impulses of light upon the retina. *Philosophical Magazine,* **4,** 241–245. (147)

Brigner, W. L., & Gallagher, M. B. (1974) Subjective contour: Apparent depth through simultaneous contrast? *Perceptual and Motor Skills,* **38,** 1047–1053. (292)

Brill, M. H., & West, G. (1986) Chromatic adaptation and color constancy: A possible dichotomy. *Color Research and Application,* **11,** 196–204. (66)

Brindley, G. (1960) *Physiology of the Retina and Visual Pathways,* 1st edition. London: Edward Arnold. (14–16, 20, 319)

Brindley, G. S. (1970) *Physiology of the Retina and Visual Pathways,* 2nd edition. Baltimore, MD: Williams & Wilkins. (138)

Brindley, G. S., DuCroz, J. J., & Rushton, W. A. H. (1966) The flicker fusion frequency of the blue-sensitive mechanism of colour vision. *Journal of Physiology,* **183,** 497–500. (184)

Brindley, G. S., Gautier-Smith, P. C., & Lewin, W. (1969) Cortical blindness and the functions of the non-geniculate fibres of the optic tracts. *Journal of Neurology, Neurosurgery and Psychiatry,* **32,** 259–264. (410)

Brindley, G. S., & Lewin, W. S. (1968) The sensations produced by electrical stimulation of the visual cortex. *Journal of Physiology,* **196,** 479–493. (238)

Broca, A., & Sulzer, D. (1902) La sensation lumineuse en fonction du temps. *Journal de Physiologie et Pathologie Générale,* **4,** 632–640. (147)

Broca, A., & Sulzer, D. (1904) La sensation lumineuse en fonction du temps. *Journal de Physiologie et Pathologie Générale,* **6,** 55–68. (147)

Bronson, G. W. (1974) The postnatal growth of visual capacity. *Child Development,* **45,** 873–890. (361)

Brown, A. M., Dobson, V., & Maier, J. (1987) Visual acuity of human infants at scotopic, mesopic, and photopic luminances. *Vision Research,* **27,** 1845–1858. (354)

Brown, P. K., & Wald, G. (1964) Visual pigments in single rods and cones of the human retina: Direct measurements reveal mechanisms of human night and color vision. *Science*, **144**, 45–52. (16)

Bruce, C. J., & Goldberg, M. E. (1985) Primate frontal eye fields. I. Single neurons discharging before saccades. *Journal of Neurophysiology*, **53**, 603–635. (312)

Bruce, V., & Green, P. (1985) *Visual Perception, Physiology, Psychology and Ecology*. London: Lawrence Erlbaum. (217, 219)

Bruesch, S. R., & Arey, L. B. (1942) The number of myelinated and unmyelinated fibers in the optic nerve of vertebrates. *Journal of Comparative Neurology*, **77**, 631–665. (110)

Brussel, E. M., Stober, S. R., & Bodinger, D. M. (1977) Sensory information and subjective contour. *American Journal of Psychology*, **90**, 145–156. (299)

Buchsbaum, G., & Gottschalk, A. (1984) Chromaticity coordinates of frequency limited functions. *Journal of the Optical Society of America A*, **1**, 885–887. (66)

Buck, S. L. (1985) Cone–rod interaction over time and space. *Vision Research*, **25**, 907–916. (383)

Buckley, D., Frisby, J. P., & Mayhew, J. E. W. (1987) *Integration of Stereo and Texture Cues in 3D Surface Interpolation: Some New Phenomena*. Paper presented to the Experimental Psychology Society, July Meeting, Oxford. (346)

Buisseret, P., & Imbert, M. (1976) Visual cortical cells: Their developmental properties in normal and dark-reared kittens. *Journal of Physiology*, **255**, 511–525. (388)

Bulens, C., Meerwaldt, J. D., van der Wildt, G. J., & Keemink, C. K. (1986) Contrast sensitivity in Parkinson's disease. *Neurology*, **36**, 1121–1125. (386)

Burbeck, C. A. (1987) Position and spatial frequency in large scale localization judgments. *Vision Research*, **27**, 417–427. (262)

Burbeck, C. A., & Regan, D. (1983) Independence of orientation and size in spatial discriminations. *Journal of the Optical Society of America*, **73**, 1691–1694. (271)

Burke, W. (1986) The function of optic nerve fibre groups in the cat, studied by means of selective block. In J. D. Pettigrew, K. J. Sanderson & W. R. Levick (Eds.), *Visual Neuroscience*, pp. 97–110. Cambridge: Cambridge University Press. (150)

Burkhalter, A., & Van Essen, D. C. (1986) Processing of color, form and disparity information in visual areas VP and V2 of ventral extrastriate cortex in the macaque monkey. *Journal of Neuroscience*, **6**, 2327–2351. (287)

Burkhardt, D. A. (1974) Sensitization to stationary flashing spots on the brisk classes of ganglion cells in the cat retina. *Journal of Physiology*, **236**, 593–610. (87)

Burns, S. A., Elsner, A. E., Lobes, L. A., & Doft, B. H. (1987) A psychophysical technique for measuring cone photopigment bleaching. *Investigative Ophthalmology & Visual Science*, **28**, 711–717. (399)

Burr, D. C. (1987) Implications of the Craik–O'Brien illusion for brightness perception. *Vision Research*, **27**, 1903–1913. (137, 160)

Burr, D. C., Fiorentini, A., & Morrone, M. C. (1987) Electrophysiological correlates of positive and negative afterimages. *Vision Research*, **27**, 201–207. (138)

Burr, D., Morrone, C., & Maffei, L. (1981) Intra-cortical inhibition prevents simple cells from responding to textured visual patterns. *Experimental Brain Research*, **43**, 455–458. (245)

Burt, P. J., & Adelson, E. H. (1983) The Laplacian pyramid as a compact image code. *IEEE Transactions on Communications*, **COM-31**, 532–540. (268)

Burt, P., & Julesz, B. (1980) A disparity gradient limit for binocular function. *Science*, **208**, 651–657. (342)

Burton, G. J. (1973) Evidence for non-linear response processes in the human visual system from measurements on the thresholds of spatial beat frequencies. *Vision Research*, **13**, 1211–1225. (97)

Burton, G. J., Nagshineh, S., & Ruddock, K. H. (1977) Processing by the human visual system of the light and dark contrast components of the retinal image. *Biological Cybernetics*, **27**, 189–197. (150, 152)

Bushnell, M. C., Goldberg, M. E., & Robinson, D. L. (1981) Behavioral enhancement of visual responses in monkey cerebral cortex. I. Modulation in posterior parietal cortex related to selective visual attention. *Journal of Neurophysiology*, **46**, 755–772. (312)

Buss, C. M., Hayhoe, M. M., & Stronmeyer, C. F. (1982) Lateral interactions in the control of visual sensitivity. *Vision Research*, **22**, 693–709. (70, 99–100)

Caelli, T. (1985) Three processing characteristics of visual texture segmentation. *Spatial Vision*, **1**, 19–30. (418, 425, 427)

Caelli, T. (1988) An adaptive computational model for texture segmentation. *IEEE Transactions on Systems, Man and Cybernetics*, **18**, 9–17. (425–427)

Caelli, T., & Hübner, M. (1983) On the efficient two-dimensional coding characteristics of spatial vision. *Vision Research*, **23**, 1053–1055. (419)

Caelli, T., Hübner, M., & Rentschler, I. (1986) On the discrimination of micropatterns and textures. *Human Neurobiology*, **5**, 129–136. (430)

Caelli, T., & Moraglia, G. (1986) On the detection of signals embedded in natural scenes. *Perception & Psychophysics*, **39**, 87–95. (424–425)

Caelli, T., Rentschler, I., & Scheidler, W. (1987) Visual pattern recognition in humans. I. Evidence for adaptive filtering. *Biological Cybernetics*, **57**, 233–240. (430)

Cajal, S. Ramón y (1892) La retina de los teleosteos y algunas observaciones sobre la de los vertebrados superiores. *Anales. Sociedad Española de Historia Natural, Madrid*, **21**, 281–305. (88)

Cajal, S. Ramón y (1893) La rétinue des vertébrés. *La Cellule*, **9**, 17–257. Translated by D. Maguire & R. W. Rodieck (1973) *The Vertebrate Retina*. San Francisco, CA: Freeman. (105)

Camisa, J., Mylin, L. H., & Bodis-Wollner, I. (1981) The effect of stimulus orientation on the visual evoked potential in multiple sclerosis. *Annals of Neurology,* **10,** 532–539. (409–410)

Campbell, F. W., & Gubisch, R. W. (1966) Optical quality of the human eye. *Journal of Physiology,* **186,** 558–578. (233)

Campbell, F. W., & Kulikowski, J. J. (1966) Orientational selectivity of the human visual system. *Journal of Physiology,* **187,** 437–445. (32, 246)

Campbell, F. W., & Maffei, L. (1971) The tilt aftereffect: A fresh look. *Vision Research,* **11,** 833–840. (296)

Campbell, F. W., Nachmias, J., & Jukes, J. (1970) Spatial frequency discrimination in human vision. *Journal of the Optical Society of America,* **60,** 555–559. (33)

Campbell, F. W., & Robson, J. G. (1968) Application of Fourier analysis to the visibility of gratings. *Journal of Physiology,* **197,** 551–566. (231, 245, 249, 351, 409, 418)

Campbell, F. W., & Rushton, W. A. H. (1955) Measurement of the scotopic pigment in the living human eye. *Journal of Physiology,* **130,** 131–147. (170)

Campbell, G., & Shatz, C. J. (1986) Synapses formed by individual retinogeniculate axons in inappropriate LGN territory during formation of eye-specific layers. *Society for Neuroscience Abstracts,* **12,** 589. (368)

Campion, J., Latto, R., & Smith, Y. M. (1983) Is blindsight an effect of scattered light, spared cortex, and near-threshold vision? *Behavioral and Brain Sciences,* **6,** 432–486. (414)

Campos, E. C., Bedell, H. E., Enoch, J. M., & Fitzgerald, C. R. (1978) Retinal receptive field-like properties and Stiles Crawford effects in a patient with traumatic choroidal rupture. *Documenta Ophthalmologica,* **45,** 381–395. (385, 399)

Canny, J. (1986) A computational approach to edge detection. *IEEE Transactions on Pattern Analysis and Machine Intelligence,* **PAMI-8,** 679–698. (268)

Carr, R. E., Ripps, H., & Siegel, I. M. (1974) Visual pigment kinetics and adaptation in fundus albipunctatus. *Eleventh ISCERG Symposium, Documenta Ophthalmologica Proceedings Series,* pp. 193–204. The Hague: Dr. W. Junk BV. (400)

Carr, R. E., Siegel, I. M., & Weale, R. A. (1966) Rhodopsin and the electrical activity of the retina in congenital night blindness. *Investigative Ophthalmology,* **5,** 497–507. (401)

Cavanagh, P. (1984) Image transforms in the visual system. In P. C. Dodwell & T. Caelli (Eds.), *Figural Synthesis,* pp. 185–218. Hillsdale, NJ: Lawrence Erlbaum. (289)

Cavanagh, P. (1985) Local log polar frequency analysis in the striate cortex as a basis for size and orientation invariance. In D. Rose & V. G. Dobson (Eds.), *Models of the Visual Cortex,* pp. 85–95. London: Wiley. (289)

Cavanagh, P. (1987) Reconstructing the third dimension: Interactions between color, texture, motion, binocular disparity and shape. *Computer Vision, Graphics and Image Processing,* **37,** 171–195. (294, 296, 298)

Cavanagh, P. (1988) Pathways in early vision. In Z. Pylyshyn (Ed.), *Computational Processes in Human Vision,* pp. 239–261. Norwood, NJ: Ablex. (285, 294–297, 299)

Cavanagh, P., & Anstis, S. M. (1986) Brightness shift in drifting ramp gratings isolates a transient mechanism. *Vision Research,* **26,** 899–908. (149)

Cavanagh, P., Arguin, M., & von Grünau, M. (1989) Interattribute apparent motion. *Vision Research,* in press. (301)

Cavanagh, P., Brussel, E. M., & Stober, S. R. (1981) Evidence against independent processing of black and white pattern features. *Perception & Psychophysics,* **29,** 423–428. (152)

Cavanagh, P., & Leclerc, Y. G. (1985) Shadow constraints. *Investigative Ophthalmology & Visual Science, Supplement,* **26,** 282. (198)

Cavanagh, P., & Leclerc, Y. G. (1989) Shape from shadows. *Journal of Experimental Psychology: Human Perception and Performance,* **15,** 3–27. (294, 298–299)

Cavanagh, P., Tyler, C. W., & Favreau, O. E. (1984) Perceived velocity of moving chromatic gratings. *Journal of the Optical Society of America A,* **1,** 893–899. (198)

Cavonius, C. R., & Hilz, R. (1973) A technique for testing visual function in the presence of opacities. *Investigative Ophthalmology,* **12,** 933–936. (397)

Chandra, S. R., Gragoudas, E. S., Freidman, E., Van Buskirk, E. M., & Klein, M. L. (1974) Natural history of disciform degeneration of the macula. *American Journal of Ophthalmology,* **78,** 579–582. (397)

Chang, J. J. (1986) Theoretical and methodological approaches to apparent movement of short-range process and pattern perception. *Behavior Research Methods, Instruments & Computers,* **18,** 542–550. (207)

Chang, J. J., & Julesz, B. (1983) Displacement limits for spatial-frequency filtered random-dot cinematograms in apparent motion. *Vision Research,* **23,** 1379–1385. (211)

Chang, J. J., & Julesz, B. (1984) Cooperative phenomena in apparent movement perception of random dot cinematograms. *Vision Research,* **24,** 1781–1788. (214)

Changeux, J. P., & Danchin, A. (1976) Selective stabilization of developing synapses as a mechanism for the specification of neuronal networks. *Nature (London),* **264,** 705–711.

Chen, B., MacLeod, D. I. A., & Stockman, A. (1987) Improvement in human vision under bright light: Grain or gain? *Journal of Physiology,* **394,** 41–66. (98)

Chevreul, M. E. (1969) *De la loi de Contraste Simultane des Couleurs.* Paris: Leon Laget. (Original work published 1839). (135)

Churchland, P. S. (1986) *Neurophilosophy.* Cambridge: MIT Press. (13, 20)

Cicerone, C. M., & Nerger, J. L. (1989) The relative numbers of long-wavelength-sensitive to middle-wavelength-sensitive cones in the fovea centralis. *Vision Research,* **29,** 115–128. (175)

Clarke, P. G. H., & Whitteridge, D. (1977) A comparison of stereoscopic mechanisms in cortical visual areas V1 and V2 of the cat. *Journal of Physiology,* **272,** 92–93P. (322)

Cleary, R. F. (1988) *Spatial Frequency Selective Processes in Short Range Motion Perception.* Ph.D. Thesis, Cambridge University. (212)

Cleary, R. F., & Braddick, O. J. (1985) Direction discrimination in narrow-band filtered kinematograms. *Perception,* **14,** A21. (211)

Cleland, B. G. (1983) Sensitivity to stationary flashing spots of the brisk classes of ganglion cells in the cat retina. *Journal of Physiology,* **345,** 15–26. (90)

Cleland, B. G., & Enroth-Cugell, C. (1968) Quantitative aspects of sensitivity and summation in the cat retina. *Journal of Physiology,* **198,** 17–38. (90)

Cleland, B. G., Dubin, M. W., & Levick, W. R. (1971) Sustained and transient neurones in the cat's retina and lateral geniculate nucleus. *Journal of Physiology,* **217,** 473–496. (112, 143)

Cleland, B. G., Harding, T. H., & Tulunay-Keesey, U. (1979) Visual resolution and receptive field size: Examination of two kinds of cat retinal ganglion cells. *Science,* **205,** 1015–1017. (30, 247)

Cleland, B. G., & Levick, W. R. (1974a) Brisk and sluggish concentrically organized ganglion cells in the cat's retina. *Journal of Physiology,* **240,** 421–456. (88)

Cleland, B. G., & Levick, W. R. (1974b) Properties of rarely encountered types of ganglion cells in the cat's retina and an overall classification. *Journal of Physiology,* **240,** 457–492. (108)

Cleland, B. G., Levick, W. R., & Sanderson, K. J. (1973) Properties of sustained and transient ganglion cells in the cat retina. *Journal of Physiology,* **228,** 649–680. (90)

Cleland, B. G., Levick, W. R., & Wässle, H. (1975) Physiological identification of a morphological class of cat retinal ganglion cells. *Journal of Physiology,* **248,** 151–171. (392)

Cohen, J. B. (1964) Dependence of the spectral reflectance curves of the Munsell color chips. *Psychonomic Science,* **1,** 369–370. (65)

Cohen, M. A., & Grossberg, S. (1984) Neural dynamics of brightness perception: Features, boundaries, diffusion, and resonance. *Perception & Psychophysics,* **36,** 428–456. (439–440–441, 443)

Coletta, N. J., & Adams, A. J. (1984) Rod–cone interaction in flicker detection. *Vision Research,* **25,** 1333–1340. (383)

Coletta, N. J., & Williams, D. R. (1987) Psychophysical estimate of extrafoveal cone spacing. *Journal of the Optical Society of America A,* **4,** 1503–1513. (234)

Collett, T. S. (1985) Extrapolating and interpolating surfaces in depth. *Proceedings of Royal Society London, Series B,* **244,** 43–56.

Collewijn, H. (1981) The oculomotor system of the rabbit and its plasticity. In V. Braitenberg, H. B. Barlow, H. Bullock, E. Florey, O.-J Grüsser, H. van der Loos (Eds.), *Studies of Brain Function, Vol. 5,* pp. 75–106. Heidelberg: Springer-Verlag. (374)

Condit, H. R., & Grum, F. (1964) Spectral energy distribution of daylight. *Journal of the Optical Society of America,* **57,** 937–944. (56)

Connolly, M., & Van Essen, D. (1984) The representation of the visual field in parvocellular and magnocellular layers of the lateral geniculate nucleus in the macaque monkey. *Journal of Comparative Neurology,* **226,** 544–564. (235–236)

Coolen, A. C. C., & Van Norren, D. (1988) Kinetics of human cone photopigment explained with a Rushton–Henry model. *Biological Cybernetics,* **58,** 123–128. (69)

Cooper, G., & Robson, J. G. (1968) Successive transformations of spatial information in the visual system. *IEE National Physiological Lab Conference Proceedings,* **42,** 134–143. (418)

Copenhagen, D. R., & Owen, W. G. (1976) Functional characteristics of lateral interactions between rods in the retina of the snapping turtle. *Journal of Physiology,* **259,** 251–282. (355–356)

Copenhagen, D. R., & Owen, W. G. (1980) Current–voltage relations in the rod photoreceptor network of the turtle retina. *Journal of Physiology,* **308,** 159–184. (85)

Copenhagen, D. R., Donner, K., & Reuter, T. (1987) Ganglion cell performance at absolute threshold in toad retina: Effects of dark events in rods. *Journal of Physiology,* **393,** 667–680. (80, 84)

Coren, S. (1972) Subjective contours and apparent depth. *Psychological Review,* **79,** 359–367. (289, 291–292)

Coren, S., & Porac, C. (1983) Subjective contours and apparent depth: A direct test. *Perception & Psychophysics,* **33,** 197–200. (292)

Cornsweet, T. N. (1970) *Visual Perception.* New York: Academic Press. (64, 99, 137, 155, 435)

Cornsweet, T. N., & Pinsker, H. M. (1965) Luminance discrimination of brief flashes under various conditions of adaptation. *Journal of Physiology,* **176,** 294–310. (61, 64)

Cornwall, M. C., MacNichol, E. F., Jr., & Fein, A. (1984) Absorptance and spectral sensitivity measurements of rod photoreceptors of the tiger salamander, *Ambystoma tigrinum. Vision Research,* **24,** 1651–1659. (172–175)

Corwin, T. R., & Giambalvo, V. (1974) Effects of simultaneous contrast on temporal brightness enhancement. *American Journal of Optometry and Physiological Optics,* **51,** 175–181. (147–148)

Coupland, S. G., & Kirkham, T. (1982) Orientation-specific visual evoked potential deficits in multiple sclerosis. *Canadian Journal of Neurological Science,* **9,** 331–337. (409)

Cowan, W. M., & O'Leary, D. D. M. (1984) Cell death and process elimination: The role of regressive phenomena in the development of vertebrate nervous system. In K. J. Isselbacher (Ed.), *Medicine, Science and Society,* pp. 643–668. New York: Wiley. (377)

Cowey, A. (1974) Atrophy of retinal ganglion cells after removal of striate cortex in a rhesus monkey. *Perception,* **3,** 257–260. (411)

Cowey, A. (1979) Cortical maps and visual perception. The Grindley Memorial Lecture. *Quarterly Journal of Experimental Psychology,* **31,** 1–17. (274)

Cowey, A., & Rolls, E. T. (1974) Human cortical magnification factor and its relation to visual acuity. *Experimental Brain Research,* **21,** 447–454. (238)

Cracco, R., & Bodis-Wollner, I. (1987) Evoked potentials. *Frontiers in Clinical Neuroscience*. New York: Alan R. Liss. (408)

Craik, K. J. W. (1939) The effect of adaptation on acuity. *British Journal of Physiology*, **29**, 252–266. (97)

Craik, K. J. W. (1940) The effect of adaptation on subjective brightness. *Proceedings of the Royal Society of London, Series B*, **128**, 232–247. (62)

Craik, K. J. W. (1966) *The Nature of Psychology. A Selection of Papers, Essays and Other Writings by the Late K. J. W. Craik*, S. L. Sherwood (Ed.). Cambridge: Cambridge University Press. (137)

Crawford, B. H. (1947) Visual adaptation in relation to brief conditioning stimuli. *Proceedings of the Royal Society of London, Series B*, **128**, 283–302. (70, 75, 89)

Crawford, B. H. (1949) The scotopic visibility function. *Proceedings of the Royal Society of London, Series B*, **62**, 321–334. (80)

Crawford, M. L. J. (1976) Behavioral control of visual fixation of the rhesus monkey. *Experimental Annals of Behavior*, **25**, 113–121. (44)

Crawford, M. L. J. (1977) Central vision of man and macaque: Cone and rod sensitivity. *Brain Research*, **119**, 345–356. (44–45)

Crawford, M. L. J., & Espinoza, S. (1978) Photic sensitivity of macaque monkey and pulvinar neurons. In S. J. Cool & E. L. Smith (Eds.), *Frontiers in Visual Science*, pp. 503–517. New York: Springer-Verlag. (46)

Crawford, M. L. J., Smith, E. L., Harwerth, R. S., & von Noorden, G. K. (1984) Stereoblind monkeys have few binocular neurons. *Investigative Ophthalmology & Visual Science*, **25**, 799–781. (24, 395)

Crawford, M. L. J., von Noorden, G. K., Meharg, L. S., Rhodes, J. W., Harwerth, R. S., Smith, E. L., & Miller, D. D. (1983) Binocular neurons and binocular function in monkeys and children. *Investigative Ophthalmology & Visual Science*, **24**, 491–495. (24)

Cremieux, J., Orban, G. A., & Duysens, J. (1984) Responses of cat visual cortical cells to continuously and stroboscopically illuminated moving light slits compared. *Vision Research*, **24**, 449–457. (223)

Creutzfeldt, O. D. (1961) General physiology of cortical neurons and neuronal information in the visual system. In M. A. B. Brazier (Ed.), *Brain and Behavior, Vol. 1*, pp. 299–358. Washington, D.C.: American Institute of Biological Sciences. (450)

Creutzfeldt, O. D. (1984) *Cortex Cerebri*. Heidelberg, Berlin: Springer-Verlag. (459–460, 463)

Creutzfeldt, O. D. (1985) Comparative aspects of representation in the visual system. In C. Chagas, R. Gattass & C. Gross (Eds.), *Pattern Recognition Mechanisms*, pp. 53–81. *Experimental Brain Research, Supplement 11*. Berlin: Springer-Verlag. (460)

Creutzfeldt, O. D. (1986) Richard Jung, 1911–1986. *Experimental Brain Research*, **64**, 1–4. (450)

Creutzfeldt, O. D. (1987) Inevitable deadlocks of the brain–mind discussion. In B. Gulyas (Ed.), *The Brain–Mind Problem. Philosophical and Neurophysiological Approaches*, pp. 3–27. Leuven: Leuven University Press. (452, 459, 463)

Creutzfeldt, O. D., & Ito, M. (1968) Functional synaptic organization of primary visual cortex neurons in the cat. *Experimental Brain Research*, **6**, 324–352. (245)

Creutzfeldt, O. D., Kuhnt, U., & Benevento, L. A. (1974) An intracellular analysis of visual cortical neurones to moving stimuli: Responses in a co-operative neuronal network. *Experimental Brain Research*, **21**, 251–274. (458)

Creutzfeldt, O. D., Lee, B. B., & Elepfandt, A. (1979) A quantitative study of chromatic organization and receptive fields of cells in the lateral geniculate body of the rhesus monkey. *Experimental Brain Research*, **35**, 527–545. (169, 180)

Creutzfeldt, O. D., Lee, B. B., & Valberg, A. (1986) Colour and brightness signals of parvocellular lateral geniculate neurons. *Experimental Brain Research*, **63**, 21–34. (460)

Creutzfeldt, O. D., & Nothdurft, H. C. (1978) Representation of complex stimuli in the brain. *Naturwissenschaften*, **65**, 307–318. (451–452, 461)

Creutzfeldt, O. D., Weber, H., Tanaka, M., & Lee, B. B. (1987) Neuronal representation of spectral and spatial stimulus aspects in foveal and parafoveal Area 17 of the awake monkey. *Experimental Brain Research*, **68**, 541–564. (451)

Crick, F. (1984) Function of the thalamic reticular complex: The searchlight hypothesis. *Proceedings of the National Academy of Sciences U.S.A.*, **81**, 4586–4590. (306)

Crick, F. H. C., Marr, D., & Poggio, T. (1980) An information processing approach to understanding the visual cortex. In F. G. Worden (Ed.), *The Cerebral Cortex*. Cambridge, MA: MIT Press. (422)

Crone, R. A., & Hardjowijoto, S. (1979) What is normal binocular vision? *Documenta Ophthalmologica*, **47**, 163–199. (331)

Crook, J. M., Lange-Malecki, B., Lee, B. B., & Valberg, A. (1988) Visual resolution of macaque retinal ganglion cells. *Journal of Physiology*, **396**, 205–224. (118, 147)

Crook, J. M., Lee, B. B., Tigwell, D. A., & Valberg, A. (1987) Thresholds to chromatic spots of cells in the macaque lateral geniculate nucleus as compared to detection sensitivity in man. *Journal of Physiology*, **392**, 193–211. (192–193)

Crumieux, J., Orban, G. A., & Duysens, J. (1984) Responses of cat visual cortical cells to continuously and stroboscopically illuminated moving light slits compared. *Vision Research*, **24**, 449–457. (223)

Cucchiaro, J. (1985) Visual abnormalities in albino mammals. In J. B. Sheffield & S. R. Hilfer (Eds.), *Heredity and Visual Development*. New York: Springer-Verlag. (265)

Curcio, C. A., Sloan, K. R., Packer, O., Hendrickson, A. E., & Kalina, R. E. (1987) Distribution of cones in human and monkey retina: Individual variability and radial asymmetry. *Science*, **236**, 579–582. (175, 232, 234, 239, 256)

Cynader, M., Berman, N., & Hein, A. (1975) Cats raised in a one-directional world: Effects on receptive fields in visual cortex and superior colliculus. *Experimental Brain Research*, **22**, 267–280. (392)

Cynader, M., Berman, N., & Hein, A. (1976) Recovery of function in cat visual cortex following prolonged deprivation. *Experimental Brain Research,* **25,** 139–156. (388, 392)

Cynader, M., & Chernenko, G. (1976) Abolition of directional selectivity in the visual cortex of the cat. *Science,* **193,** 504–505. (392)

Cynader, M., Gardner, J. C., & Mustari, M. (1984) Effects of neonatally induced strabismus on binocular responses in cat area 18. *Experimental Brain Research,* **53,** 384–399. (395)

Cynader, M., & Regan, D. (1978) Neurons in cat parastriate cortex sensitive to the direction of motion in three-dimensional space. *Journal of Physiology,* **274,** 549–569. (333, 335–337)

Cynader, M., & Regan, D. (1981) Neurons in cat visual cortex tuned to the direction of motion in depth: Effect of positional disparity. *Vision Research,* **22,** 967–982. (337)

Cynader, M., & Shaw, C. (1986) Mechanisms underlying developmental alterations of cortical ocular dominance. In E. L. Keller & D. S. Zee (Eds.), *Adaptive Processes in Visual and Oculomotor Systems,* pp. 53–61. Oxford: Pergamon. (391)

Cynader, M., Timney, B. N., & Mitchell, D. E. (1980) Period of susceptibility of kitten visual cortex to the effects of monocular deprivation extends beyond six months of age. *Brain Research,* **191,** 545–550 (390)

Dacheux, R. F., & Miller, R. F. (1981) An intracellular electrophysiological study of the ontogeny of functional synapses in the rabbit retina. I. Receptors, horizontal and bipolar cells. *Journal of Comparative Neurology,* **198,** 307–326. (87)

Dacheux, R. F., & Raviola, E. (1988) Intracellular recordings from HI horizontal cells in the monkey retina. *Investigative Ophthalmology & Visual Science Supplement,* **29,** 224. (87)

Damasio, A. R. (1985) Prosopagnosia. *Trends in Neuroscience,* **8,** 132–135. (128)

Damasio, A., Yamada, T., Damasio, H., Corbett, J., & McKee, J. (1980) Central achromatopsia: Behavioural anatomic and physiologic aspects. *Neurology,* **30,** 1064–1071. (201, 203, 285, 294)

Daniel, P. M., & Whitteridge, D. (1961) The representation of the visual field on the cerebral cortex in monkeys. *Journal of Physiology,* **159,** 203–221. (235)

Dartnall, H. J. A. (1953) The interpretation of spectral sensitivity curves. *British Medical Bulletin,* **9,** 24–30. (170)

Dartnall, H. J. A. (1957) *The Visual Pigments.* London: Methuen and Co. (172)

Darnall, H. J. A., Bowmaker, J. K., & Mollon, J. D. (1983) Microspectrophotometry of human photoreceptors. In J. D. Mollon & L. T. Sharpe (Eds.), *Colour Vision: Physiology and Psychophysics,* pp. 69–80. New York: Academic Press. (171)

Das, S. R. (1964) Foveal increment thresholds in dark adaptation. *Journal of the Optical Society of America,* **54,** 541–546. (187)

Daugman, J. G. (1980) Two-dimensional spectral analysis of cortical receptive field profiles. *Vision Research,* **20,** 847–856. (153)

Daugman, J. G. (1984) Spatial visual channels in the Fourier plane. *Vision Research,* **24,** 891–910. (248)

Daugman, J. G. (1985) Uncertainty relation for resolution in space, spatial frequency, and orientation optimized by two-dimensional visual cortical filters. *Journal of the Optical Society of America A,* **2,** 1160–1169. (249, 267–268)

Davies, S. E., Faivre, I. A., & Werner, J. S. (1983) Transient processing in chromatic induction. *Vision Research,* **23,** 707–712. (66)

Daw, N. W., & Wyatt, H. J. (1976) Kittens reared in a unidirectional environment: Evidence for a critical period. *Journal of Physiology,* **257,** 155–170. (392)

DeBruyn, B., & Orban, G. A. (1986) Human velocity discrimination measured with 2-D noise patterns. *Perception,* **15,** A8. (223)

DeMonasterio, F. M., & Gouras, P. (1975) Functional properties of ganglion cells of the rhesus monkey retina. *Journal of Physiology,* **251,** 167–195. (141, 184)

DeMonasterio, F. M., Gouras, P., & Tolhurst, D. J. (1975) Trichromatic colour opponency in ganglion cells of the rhesus monkey retina. *Journal of Physiology,* **251,** 197–216. (180)

DeMonasterio, F. M., & Schein, S. J. (1982) Spectral bandwidths of color-opponent cells of geniculocortical pathway of macaque monkey. *Journal of Neurophysiology,* **47,** 214–224. (127, 287)

Denton, E. J., & Pirenne, M. M. (1954) The absolute sensitivity and functional stability of the human eye. *Journal of Physiology,* **123,** 417–442. (55)

DeRenzi, E. (1982) *Disorders of Space Exploration and Cognition.* New York: Wiley. (306)

Derrington, A. M., & Fuchs, A. F. (1979) Spatial and temporal properties of X and Y cells in the cat lateral geniculate nucleus. *Journal of Physiology,* **293,** 347–364. (31)

Derrington, A. M., Krauskopf, J., & Lennie, P. (1984) Chromatic mechanisms in lateral geniculate nucleus of macaque. *Journal of Physiology,* **357,** 241–265. (113, 177, 185, 285)

Derrington, A. M., & Lennie, P. (1982) The influence of temporal frequency and adaptation level on receptive field organization of retinal ganglion cells in cat. *Journal of Physiology,* **333,** 343–366. (93)

Derrington, A. M., & Lennie, P. (1984) Spatial and temporal contrast sensitivities of neurones in lateral geniculate nucleus of macaque. *Journal of Physiology,* **357,** 219–240. (113, 119–120)

Desimone, R., & Schein, S. J. (1987) Visual properties of neurons in area V4 of the macaque: Sensitivity to stimulus form. *Journal of Neurophysiology,* **57,** 835–868. (284, 286–287)

Desimone, R., Schein, S. J., Moran, J., & Ungerleider, L. G. (1985) Contour, color, and shape analysis beyond the striate cortex. *Vision Research,* **25,** 441–452. (127, 202, 284)

Detwiler, P. B., & Hodgkin, A. L. (1979) Electrical coupling between cones in the turtle retina. *Journal of Physiology,* **291,** 75–100. (85)

Dev, P. (1975) Perception of depth surfaces in random dot stereograms: A neural model. *International Journal of Man–Machine Studies,* **7,** 511–528. (342)

DeValois, K. K. (1977) Independence of black and white: Phase-specific adaptation. *Vision Research,* **17,** 209–215. (150)

DeValois, K. K., DeValois, R. L., & Yund, E. W. (1979) Responses of striate cortex cells to grating and checkerboard patterns. *Journal of Physiology*, **291**, 483–505. (243–244)

DeValois, R. L. (1965) Analysis and coding of color vision in the primate visual system. *Cold Spring Harbor Symposium on Quantitative Biology*, **30**, 567–579. (13, 17, 179)

DeValois, R. L., & DeValois, K. K. (1975) Neural coding of color. In E. C. Carterette & M. P. Friedman (Eds.), *Handbook of Perception, Vol. V*, pp. 117–166. New York: Academic Press. (185)

DeValois, R. L., & DeValois, K. K. (1988) *Spatial Vision*. New York: Oxford University Press. (231, 418)

DeValois, R. L., Abramov, I., & Jacobs, G. H. (1966) Analysis of response patterns of LGN cells. *Journal of the Optical Society of America*, **56**, 966–977. (113, 179, 285)

DeValois, R. L., Albrecht, D. G., & Thorell, L. G. (1982) Spatial frequency selectivity of cells in macaque visual cortex. *Vision Research*, **22**, 545–559. (18, 240–242, 246–248, 287, 418)

DeValois, R. L., & Jacobs, G. H. (1968) Primate color vision. *Science*, **162**, 533–540. (43–44)

DeValois, R. L., Morgan, H. C., Polson, M. C., Mead, W. R., & Hull, E. M. (1974) Psychophysical studies of monkey vision. I. Macaque luminosity and color vision tests. *Vision Research*, **14**, 53–67. (31, 44, 79, 171)

DeValois, R. L., Morgan, H., & Snodderly, D. M. (1974) Psychophysical studies of monkey vision—III. Spatial luminance contrast sensitivity tests of macaque and human observers. *Vision Research*, **14**, 75–81. (118)

DeValois, R. L., Smith, C. J., Kitai, S. T., & Karoly, A. J. (1958) Responses of single cells in monkey lateral geniculate nucleus to monochromatic light. *Science*, **127**, 238–239. (163)

DeValois, R. L., Webster, M. A., DeValois, K. K., & Lingelbach, B. (1986) Temporal properties of brightness and color induction. *Vision Research*, **26**, 887–897. (148–149)

DeValois, R. L., Yund, E. W., & Hepler, N. (1982) The orientation and direction selectivity of cells in macaque visual cortex. *Vision Research*, **22**, 531–544. (287)

DeVries, H. L. (1943) The quantum character of light and its bearing upon threshold of vision, the differential sensitivity and visual acuity of the eye. *Physica*, **10**, 553–564. (61)

DeWeert, C. M. M., & Sadza, K. J. (1983) New data concerning the contribution of colour differences to stereopsis. In J. D. Mollon and L. T. Sharpe (Eds.), *Colour Vision: Physiology and Psychophysics*, pp. 553–562. London: Academic Press. (285)

DeYoe, E. A., & Van Essen, D. C. (1985) Segregation of efferent connections and receptive field properties in visual area V2 of the macaque. *Nature (London)*, **317**, 58–61. (125–127, 226, 284, 286)

DeYoe, E. A., & Van Essen, D. C. (1988) Concurrent processing streams in monkey visual cortex. *Trends in Neuroscience*, **11**, 219–226. (229)

Dieterich, M., & Brandt, T. (1987) Impaired motion perception in congenital nystagmus and acquired ocular motor palsy. *Clinical Vision Science*, **1**, 337–345. (228)

Dineen, J. T., & Hendrickson, A. E. (1981) Age-correlated differences in the amount of retinal degeneration after striate cortex lesions in monkeys. *Investigative Ophthalmology & Visual Science*, **21**, 749–752. (411)

DiStefano, J., Morrone, M. C., & Burr, D. C. (1985) Visual acuity of neurones in the cat lateral suprasylvian cortex. *Brain Research*, **331**, 282–285. (30)

Ditchburn, R. W. (1973) *Eye Movements and Visual Perception*. Oxford: Clarendon Press. (138)

Dobbins, A., Zucker, S. W., & Cynader, M. S. (1987) Endstopped neurons in the visual cortex as a substrate for calculating curvature. *Nature (London)*, **329**, 438–441. (288, 296)

Dobson, V., & Teller, D. Y. (1978) Visual acuity in human infants: A review and comparison of behavioral and electrophysiological studies. *Vision Research*, **18**, 1469–1483. (350, 360, 371)

Domenici, L., Trimarchi, C., Picolino, M., & Fiorentini, A. (1986) Dopaminergic drugs improve human visual contrast sensitivity. *Human Neurobiology*, **4**, 195–197. (387)

Dow, B. M. Snyder, A. Z., Vautin, R. G., & Bauer, R. (1981) Magnification factor and receptive field size in foveal striate cortex of the monkey. *Experimental Brain Research*, **44**, 213–228. (235, 238, 239)

Dowling, J. E. (1960) Chemistry of visual adaptation in the rat. *Science*, **188**, 114–118. (70)

Dowling, J. E. (1987) *The Retina, An Approachable Part of the Brain*. Cambridge, MA: Harvard University Press. (87)

Dowling, J. E., & Boycott, B. B. (1966) Organization of the primate retina: Electron microscopy. *Proceedings of the Royal Society of London, Series B*, **166**, 80–111. (86)

Dreher, B. (1972) Hypercomplex cells in the cat's striate cortex. *Investigative Ophthalmology*, **11**, 355–356. (244)

Dubner, R., & Zeki, S. M. (1971) Response properties and receptive fields of cells in an anatomically defined region of the superior temporal sulcus in the monkey. *Brain Research*, **35**, 528–532. (126, 284)

du Buf, J. M. H., & Roufs, J. A. J. (1986) On brightness and brightness contrast. In Stichting voor Biofysica. *Verslag Over het Jaar 1985*, pp. 228–236. Delft: De Stichting. (146)

DuCroz, J. J., & Rushton, W. A. M. (1966) The separation of cone mechanisms in dark adaptation. *Journal of Physiology*, **183**, 481–496. (85)

Duersteler, M. R., Wurtz, R. H., & Yamasaki, D. S. (1986) Pursuit and OKN deficits following ibotenic acid lesions in the medial superior temporal area (MST) of monkey. *Society for Neuroscience Abstracts*, **12**, 1182. (376)

Duke-Elder, S. S., & Wybar, K. (1973) *System of Ophthalmology, Vol. VI, Ocular Motility and Strabismus*. London: Kimpton. (390, 392)

Duwaer, A. L. (1983) Patent stereopsis with diplopia in random dot stereograms. *Perception & Psychophysics*, **33**, 443–454. (331)

Duysens, J., Maes, H. J., & Orban, G. A. (1987) The velocity dependence of direction of selectivity of visual cortical neurones, in the cat. *Journal of Physiology*, **387**, 95–113. (221)

Duysens, J., Orban, G. A., van der Glas, H. W., & deZegher, F. E. (1982) Functional properties of area 19 as compared to area 17 of the cat. *Brain Research,* **231,** 279–291. (222)

Dyer, R. S., Howell, W. E., & MacPhail, R. C. (1981) Dopamine depletion slows retinal transmission. *Experimental Neurology,* **71,** 326–340. (386)

D'Zmura, M., & Lennie, P. (1986) Mechanisms of color constancy. *Journal of the Optical Society of America A,* **3,** 1662–1672. (119, 203)

Eccles, J. C. (Ed.) (1966) *Brain and Conscious Experience.* Heidelberg, New York: Springer-Verlag. (454)

Edelman, G. M. (1987) *Neural Darwinism.* New York: Basic Books. (220)

Egeth, H., Jonides, J., & Wall, S. (1972) Parallel processing of multi-element displays. *Cognitive Psychology,* **3,** 674–698. (276)

Eggers, H. M., & Blakemore, C. (1978) Physiological basis of anisometric amblyopia. *Science,* **201,** 264–267. (30)

Ehinger, B. (1983) Functional role of dopamine in the retina. *Progress in Retinal Research,* **2,** 213–232. (386)

Ehrenstein, W. (1941) Über Abwandlungen der L. Hermannschen Helligkeitserscheinung. *Zeitschrift für Psychologie,* **150,** 83–91. (287, 293)

Ehrenstein, W. (1954) *Probleme der ganzheitspsychologischen Wahrnehmungslehre.* Leipzig: J. A. Barth. (137)

Eisner, A., Fleming, S. A., Klein, M. L., & Maudlin, W. M. (1987) Sensitivities in older eyes with good acuity: Eyes whose fellow eye has exudative AMD. *Investigative Ophthalmology & Visual Science,* **28,** 1824–1831. (404)

Ejima, Y., & Takahashi, S. (1985) Interaction between short- and longer-wavelength cones in hue cancellation codes: Nonlinearities of hue cancellation as a function of stimulus intensity. *Vision Research,* **25,** 1911–1922. (168–169, 188)

Elsner, A. (1978) Hue difference contours can be used in processing orientation information. *Perception & Psychophysics,* **24,** 451–456. (296)

Elzinga, C. H., & de Weert, C. M. M. (1984) Nonlinear codes of the yellow/blue mechanism. *Vision Research,* **24,** 911–922. (168)

Emerson, R. C., Citron, M. C., Vaughn, W. J., & Klein, S. A. (1987) Nonlinear directionally selective subunits in complex cells of cat striate cortex. *Journal of Neurophysiology,* **58,** 33–65. (214)

Enoch, J. M. (1978) Quantitative layer-by-layer perimetry. *Investigative Ophthalmology & Visual Science,* **17,** 209–257. (403)

Enoch, J. M., Baraldi, P., Lakshiminarayanan, V., Savage, G. L., & Fendick, M. (1988) The measurement of metamorphopsia in the presence of ocular media opacities. *American Journal of Optometry and Physiological Optics,* **65,** 349–353.

Enoch, J. M., & Birch, D. G. (1981) Inferred positive phototropic activity in human photoreceptors. *Philosophical Transactions of the Royal Society of London,* **291B,** 293–303. (385)

Enoch, J. M., & Campos, E. C. (1979) Analysis of patients with open angle glaucoma using perimetric techniques reflecting receptive field like properties. *Documenta Ophthalmologica Proceedings Series,* **19,** 137–149. (397, 403)

Enoch, J. M., Fitzgerald, C. R., & Campos, E. C. (1981) Quantitative layer-by-layer perimetry. An extended analysis. In J. Pokorny (Ed.), *Current Ophthalmology Monographs.* New York: Grune & Stratton. (402–403)

Enoch, J. M., Hamer, R. D., Lakshminarayanan, V., Yasuma, T., Birch, D. G., & Yamad, S. (1987) Effect of monocular light exclusion on the Stiles-Crawford function. *Vision Research,* **27,** 507–510. (385)

Enoch, J. M., & Sunga, R. N. (1969) Development of quantitative perimetric tests. *Documenta Ophthalmologica,* **26,** 215–229.

Enoch, J. M., & Tobey, Jr., F. L. (1981) *Vertebrate Photoreceptor Optics.* Berlin: Springer-Verlag. (385, 402)

Enoch, J. M., Van Loo, V. A., & Okun, E. (1973) Realignment of photoreceptors disturbed in orientation secondary to retinal detachment. *Investigative Ophthalmology,* **12,** 849–853. (399)

Enoch, J. M., & Williams, R. A. (1983) Development of clinical tests of vision: Initial data on two hyperacuity paradigms. *Perception & Psychophysics,* **33,** 314–322. (398)

Enoch, J. M., Williams, R., Essock, E., & Barricks, M. (1984) Hyperacuity perimetry: Assessment of macular function through ocular opacities. *Archives of Ophthalmology,* **102,** 1164–1168. (399)

Enoch, J. M., Williams, R., Essock, E., & Fendick, M. (1985) Hyperacuity: A promising means of evaluating vision through cataract. In N. Osborn & G. Chader (Eds.), *Progress in Retinal Research, Vol. 4,* pp. 67–88. New York: Pergamon. (398–399)

Enright, J. (1984) Changes in vergence mediated by saccades. *Journal of Physiology,* **350,** 9–31. (329)

Enroth-Cugell, C., Hertz, B. G., & Lennie, P. (1977) Cone signals in the cat's retina. *Journal of Physiology,* **269,** 273–296. (28, 100)

Enroth-Cugell, C., & Lennie, P. (1975) The control of retinal ganglion cell discharge by receptive field surrounds. *Journal of Physiology,* **247,** 551–578. (119)

Enroth-Cugell, C., Lennie, P., & Shapley, R. M. (1975) Surround contribution to light adaptation in cat retinal ganglion cells. *Journal of Physiology,* **247,** 579–588. (90)

Enroth-Cugell, C., & Robson, J. G. (1966) The contrast sensitivity of retinal ganglion cells of the cat. *Journal of Physiology,* **187,** 517–552. (25, 88, 107–108, 112, 134–135, 231, 240, 245, 435)

Enroth-Cugell, C., & Robson, J. G. (1984) Functional characteristics and diversity of cat retinal ganglion cells. *Investigative Ophthalmology,* **25,** 250–267. (91)

Enroth-Cugell, C., Robson, J. G., Schweitzer-Tong, D. E., & Watson, A. B. (1983) Spatiotemporal interactions in cat retinal ganglion cells showing linear spatial summation. *Journal of Physiology,* **341,** 279–307. (93)

Enroth-Cugell, C., & Shapley, R. M. (1973a) Adaptation and dynamics of cat retinal ganglion cells. *Journal of Physiology,* **233,** 271–309. (89, 90, 119)

Enroth-Cugell, C., & Shapley, R. M. (1973b) Flux, not retinal illumination, is what cat retinal ganglion cells really care about. *Journal of Physiology,* **233,** 311–326. (90)

Erkelens, C., & Collewijn, H. (1985a) Motion perception during dichoptic viewing of moving random-dot stereograms. *Vision Research,* **25,** 583–588. (331)

Erkelens, C., & Collewijn, H. (1985b) Eye movements and stereopsis during dichoptic viewing of moving random-dot stereograms. *Vision Research,* **25,** 1689–1700. (330–331)

Erkelens, C., & Regan, D. (1986) Ocular vergence movements induced by changing size and disparity. *Journal of Physiology,* **379,** 145–169. (330)

Essock, E. A., Lehmkuhle, S., Frascella, J., & Enoch, J. M. (1985) Temporal modulation of the background affects the sensitization response of X- and Y-cells in the dLGN of cat. *Vision Research,* **25,** 1007–1019. (100)

Essock, E., Williams, R., Enoch, J. M., & Raphael, S. (1984) The effects of retinal image degradation by cataracts on vernier acuity. *Investigative Ophthalmology & Visual Science,* **25,** 1043–1050. (398)

Estévez, O., & Spekreijse, H. (1982) The "silent substitution" method in visual research. *Vision Research,* **22,** 681–691. (17, 177)

Evans, E. F. (1987) Donald MacCrimmon MacKay, 1922–1987. *Experimental Brain Research,* **66,** 225–227. (450)

Evans, R. M. (1974) *The Perception of Color.* New York: Wiley. (193)

Evarts, E. V. (1966) Methods for recording activity of individual neurons in moving animals. *Methods in Medical Research,* **11,** 241–250. (45, 308)

Exner, S. (1868) Über die zu einer Gesichtswahrnehmung nötige Zeit. *Sitzungsberichte der mathematisch-naturwissenschaftlichen Classe der kaiserlichen Akademie der Wissenschaften,* **58II,** 601–631. (147)

Exner, S. (1888) Ueber optische Bewegungsempfindungen. *Biologisches Centralblatt,* **8,** 437–448. (2, 205)

Fach, C., & Sharpe, L. T. (1986) Assimilative hue shifts in color gratings depend on bar withs. *Perception & Psychophysics,* **40,** 412–418. (199)

Fahle, M. (1986) Curvature detection in the visual field and a possible physiological correlate. *Experimental Brain Research,* **63,** 113–124. (241)

Fain, G. L. (1976) Sensitivity of toad rods: Dependence on wavelength and background illumination. *Journal of Physiology,* **261,** 71–101. (59)

Fain, G. L., Quandt, F. N., Bastian, B. L., & Gerschenfeld, H. M. (1978) Contribution of caesium-sensitive conductance increase to the rod photoresponse. *Nature (London),* **272,** 467–469. (84)

Fairchild, M. D., & Lennie, P. (1988) Ganglion cell pathways for rod acuity. *Journal of the Optical Society of America A,* **5,** *Technical Digest,* Abstract Tu#1. (120)

Fantz, R. L., Ordy, J. M., & Udelf, M. S. (1962) Maturation of pattern vision in infants during the first six months. *Journal of Comparative Physiological Psychology,* **55,** 907–917. (351, 373)

Faugeras, O. D., Ayache, N., & Faverjon, B. (1986) Building visual maps by combining noisy stereo measurements. *IEEE Robotics Conference,* San Francisco. (346)

Favreau, O. E., & Cavanagh, P. (1981) Color and luminance: Independent frequency shifts. *Science,* **212,** 831–832. (296)

Fawcett, J. W., & O'Leary, D. D. M. (1985) The role of electrical activity in the formation of topographic maps in the nervous system. *Trends in Neuroscience,* **8,** 201–206. (376)

Fechner, G. T. (1860) *Elemente der Psychophysik.* Leipzig: Breitkopf and Härtel. (59, 64)

Feinberg, T. E., Pasik, T., & Pasik, P. (1978) Extrageniculostriate vision in the monkey. VI. Visually guided accurate reaching behavior. *Brain Research,* **152,** 422–428. (410)

Feldman, J. A. (1986) Four frames suffice: A provisional model of vision and space. *Behavioral and Brain Sciences,* **8,** 265–289. (273)

Feldman, J. A., & Ballard, D. H. (1982) Connectionist models and their properties. *Cognitive Psychology,* **6,** 205–254. (104, 215)

Felleman, D. J., & Van Essen, D. C. (1987) Receptive field properties of neurons in area V3 of macaque monkey extrastriate cortex. *Journal of Neurophysiology,* **57,** 889–920. (126, 286)

Felleman, D. J., DeYoe, E. A., Knierim, J. J., Olavarria, J., & Van Essen, D. C. (1988) Compartmental organization of projections from V2 to extrastriate areas V3, V3A, and V4t of macaque monkeys. *Investigative Ophthalmology & Visual Science, Supplement,* **29,** 115. (126)

Fender, D. H., & Julesz, B. (1967) Extension of Panum's fusional area in binocularly stabilized vision. *Journal of the Optical Society of America,* **57,** 819–830. (331, 345)

Ferree, C. E., & Rand, G. (1919) Chromatic thresholds of sensation from center to periphery of the retina and their bearing on color theory. *Psychological Review,* **26,** 16–41. (175)

Field, D., & Nachmias, J. (1984) Phase reversal discrimination. *Vision Research,* **24,** 333–340. (158, 419, 432)

Filimonoff, I. N. (1932) Über die Variabilität der Grosshirnrindenstruktur. Mitteilung II. Regio occipitalis beim erwachsenen Menschen. *Journal für Psychologie und Neurologie,* **44,** 1–96. (239)

Finkelstein, M. A., Harrison, M., & Hood, D. C. (1988) Receptoral and post-receptoral nonlinearities and foveal increment thresholds. *Investigative Ophthalmology & Visual Science, Supplement,* **29,** 300. (71)

Finkelstein, M. A., & Hood, D. C. (1981) Cone system saturation: More than one stage of sensitivity loss. *Vision Research,* **21,** 319–328. (71, 77)

Finkelstein, D., Massof, R. W., & Palmer, R. W. (1988) Retinitis pigmentosa: Design of pilot laser clinical trial in progress. *Investigative Ophthalmology & Visual Science, Supplement,* **29**(3), 142. (400)

Fiorentini, A. (1961) Sur un effet d'interaction binoculaire. *Vision Research,* **1,** 244–252. (139)

Fiorentini, A. (1972) Mach band phenomena. In D. Jameson & L. M. Hurvich (Eds.), *Handbook of Sensory Physiology Vol. VII-4, Visual Psychophysics,* pp. 188–201. Berlin: Springer-Verlag. (135, 140, 155)

Fiorentini, A., & Maffei, L. (1968) Perceptual correlates of inhibitory and facilitatory spatial interactions in the visual system. *Vision Research,* **8,** 1195–1203. (140)

Fiorentini, A., & Maffei, L. (1973) Contrast in night vision. *Vision Research,* **13,** 73–80. (134)

Fiorentini, A., & Mazzantini, L. (1966) Neural inhibition in the human fovea: A study of interactions between two line stimuli. *Atti della Fondazione G. Ronchi,* **21,** 738–747. (140, 155)

Fischer, B. (1973) Overlap of receptive field centers and representation of the visual field in the cat's optic tract. *Vision Research,* **13,** 2113–2120. (256)

Fischer, B. (1986) The role of attention in the preparation of visually guided eye movements in monkey and man. *Psychological Research,* **48,** 251–257. (308)

Fischer, B. (1987) The preparation of visually guided saccades. *Review of Physiology, Biochemistry and Pharmacology,* **106,** 1–35. (308, 315)

Fischer, B., & Boch, R. (1981a) Enhanced activation of neurons in prelunate cortex before visually guided saccades of trained rhesus monkeys. *Experimental Brain Research,* **44,** 129–137. (312)

Fischer, B., & Boch, R. (1981b) Selection of visual targets activates prelunate cortical cells in trained rhesus monkey. *Experimental Brain Research,* **41,** 431–433. (309, 312)

Fischer, B., & Boch, R. (1982) Modifications of presaccadic activation of neurons in the extrastriate cortex during prolonged training of rhesus monkeys in a visuo-oculomotor task. *Neuroscience Letters,* **30,** 127–131. (312)

Fischer, B., & Boch, R. (1983) Saccadic eye movements after extremely short reaction times in the monkey. *Brain Research,* **260,** 21–26. (312–314)

Fischer, B., & Boch, R. (1985) Peripheral attention versus central fixation: Modulation of the visual activity of prelunate cortical cells of the rhesus monkey. *Brain Research,* **345,** 111–123. (309, 311–312)

Fischer, B., & Breitmeyer, B. (1987) Mechanisms of visual attention revealed by saccadic eye movements. *Neuropsychologia,* **25,** 73–83. (308)

Fischer, B., & May, H. U. (1970) Invarianzen in der katzenretina: Gesetzmässige beziehungen zwischen empfindlichkeit, grösse und lage receptiver felder von ganglienzellen. *Experimental Brain Research,* **11,** 448–464. (90)

Fischer, B., & Ramsperger, E. (1984) Human express saccades: Extremely short reaction times of goal directed eye movements. *Experimental Brain Research,* **57,** 191–195. (314)

Fischer, B., & Ramsperger, E. (1986) Human express saccades: Effects of randomization and daily practice. *Experimental Brain Research,* **64,** 569–578. (314)

Fischer, B., Boch, R., & Ramsperger, E. (1984) Express-saccades of the monkey: Effect of daily training on probability of occurrence and reaction time. *Experimental Brain Research,* **55,** 232–242. (314)

Fitzgerald, C. R., Birch, D. G., & Enoch, J. M. (1980) Functional analysis of vision in patients following retinal detachment repair. *Archives of Ophthalmology,* **98,** 1237–1244. (400)

Fitzgerald, C. R., Enoch, J. M., Campos, E. C., & Bedell, H. E. (1979) Comparison of vision function studies in two cases of senile macular degeneration. *Albrecht von Graefes Archiv für klinische und experimentelle Ophthalmologie,* **210,** 79–91. (400)

Fitzpatrick, D., Lund, J. S., & Blasdel, G. G. (1985) Intrinsic connections of macaque striate cortex: Afferent and efferent connections of layer IVC. *Journal of Neuroscience,* **5,** 3329–3349. (123)

Flamant, F., & Stiles, W. S. (1948) The directional and spectral sensitivities of the retinal rods to adapting fields of different wavelengths. *Journal of Physiology,* **187,** 187–202. (95)

Flock, H. R., & Nusinowitz, N. (1984) Visual structures for achromatic color perceptions. *Perception & Psychophysics,* **36,** 111–130. (58)

Fodor, J. A. (1983) *The Modularity of Mind. An Essay on Faculty Psychology.* Cambridge, MA: MIT Press. (276)

Forsyth, P. M., Barbur, J. L., & Findlay, J. M. (1985) Saccadic eye movements associated with midbrain projections in human vision. *Perception,* **14,** A7. (365)

Foster, D. H. (1981) Changes in field spectral sensitivities of red-, green-, and blue-sensitive colour mechanisms obtained on small background fields. *Vision Research,* **21,** 1433–1455. (169)

Foster, K. H., Gaska, J. P., Nagler, M., & Pollen, D. A. (1985) Spatial and temporal frequency selectivity of neurons in visual cortical areas V1 and V2 of the macaque monkey. *Journal of Physiology,* **365,** 331–363. (287)

Fox, R., Aslin, R. N., Shea, S. L., & Dumais, S. T. (1980) Stereopsis in human infants. *Science,* **207,** 323–324. (362, 371)

Freeman, R. D., & Bradley, A. (1980) Monocularly deprived humans: Nondeprived eye has supernormal vernier acuity. *Journal of Neurophysiology,* **43,** 1645–1653. (395)

Freeman, R. D., & Ohzawa, I. (1988) Monocularly deprived cats: Binocular tests of cortical cells reveal functional connections from the deprived eye. *Journal of Neuroscience,* **8,** 2491–2506. (389, 395)

Freeman, R. D., & Olson, C. R. (1979) Is there a "consolidation" effect for monocular deprivation. *Nature (London),* **282,** 104–106. (389)

French, A. S., Snyder, A. W., & Stavenga, D. G. (1977) Image degradation by an irregular retinal mosaic. *Biological Cybernetics,* **27,** 229–233. (262)

Friedman, L. J., Thornton, J. E., & Pugh, E. N., Jr. (1985) Cone antagonism along visual pathways of red–green dichromats. *Vision Research,* **25,** 1647–1654. (169)

Fries, W., Keizer, K., & Kuypers, H. G. J. M. (1985) Layer VI cells in the macaque striate cortex project to both superior colliculus and prestriate visual area V. *Experimental Brain Research,* **58,** 613–616. (126)

Frisby, J. P. (1979) *Seeing: Illusion, Brain, and Mind.* Oxford: Oxford University Press. (342)

Frisby, J. P. (1984) An old illusion and a new theory of stereoscopic depth perception. *Nature (London),* **307,** 592–593. (347)

Frisby, J. P., & Clatworthy, J. L. (1975) Illusory contours: Curious cases of simultaneous brightness contrast? *Perception,* **4,** 349–357. (292)

Frisch, K. von (1913) Weitere Untersuchungen über den Farbensinn der Fische. *Zoologische Jahrbücher, Abteilung für allgemeine Zoologie und Physiologie der Tiere,* **34,** 43–68. (39)

Frisch, K. von (1914) Der Farbensinn und Formensinn der Biene. *Zoologische Jahrbücher, Abteilung für allgemeine Zoologie und Physiologie der Tiere,* **35,** 1–182. (39)

Frishman, K. J., Freeman, A. W., Troy, J. B., Schweitzer-Tong, D. E., & Enroth-Cugell, C. (1987) Spatiotemporal frequency responses of cat retinal ganglion cells. *Journal of General Physiology,* **89,** 599–628. (93)

Frost, B. J., & Nakayama, K. (1983) Single visual neurons code opposing motion independent of direction. *Science,* **220,** 744–745. (225)

Fuchs, A. F., & Robinson, D. A. (1966) A method for measuring horizontal and vertical eye movement chronically in the monkey. *Journal of Applied Physiology,* **21,** 1068–1070. (145)

Fukuda, Y., Hsiao, C. F., & Watanabe, M. (1985) Morphological correlates of Y, X and W type ganglion cells in the cat's retina. *Vision Research,* **25,** 319–327. (112)

Fuld, K., Otto, T., & Slade, C. (1986) Spectral responsivity of the white–black channel. *Journal of the Optical Society of America A,* **3,** 1182–1188. (167)

Fuld, K., Werner, J. S., & Wooten, B. R. (1983) The possible elemental nature of brown. *Vision Research,* **23,** 631–637. (166)

Fuld, K., Wooten, B. R., & Whalen, J. J. (1981) The elemental hues of short-wave and extraspectral lights. *Perception & Psychophysics,* **29,** 317–322. (165–166)

Fulton, A. B., Albert, D. M., & Craft, J. L. (1978) Human albinism. *Archives of Ophthalmology,* **96,** 305–310. (265–266)

Fuster, J. M. (1973) Unit activity in the prefrontal cortex during delayed response performance: Neuronal correlates of short-term memory. *Journal of Neurophysiology,* **36,** 61–78. (312)

Gaasterland, D., & Kupfer, C. (1974) Experimental glaucoma in the rhesus monkey. *Investigative Ophthalmology & Visual Science,* **13,** 455–457. (408)

Gallego, A. (1971) Horizontal and amacrine cells in the mammal's retina. *Vision Research, Supplement* **3,** 33–50. (88)

Galletti, C., Bataglini, P. P., & Aicardi, G. (1988) 'Real-motion' cells in visual area V2 of behaving macaque monkeys. *Experimental Brain Research,* **69,** 279–288. (227)

Gaska, J. P., Pollen, D. A., & Cavanagh, P. (1987) Diversity of complex cells responses to even- and odd-symmetric luminance profiles in the visual cortex of the cat. *Experimental Brain Research,* **68,** 249–259. (160)

Gaskill, J. D. (1978) *Linear Systems, Fourier Transforms, and Optics.* New York: Wiley. (234)

Gass, J. D. M. (1973) Drusen and disciform macular detachment and degeneration. *Archives of Ophthalmology,* **90,** 206. (397)

Geisler, W. S. (1978) Adaptation, afterimage and cone saturation. *Vision Research,* **18,** 279–289. (62, 72)

Geisler, W. S. (1979) Initial image and afterimage discrimination in the human rod and cone systems. *Journal of Physiology,* **312,** 165–179. (72, 76)

Geisler, W. S. (1981) Effects of bleaching and backgrounds on the flash response of the cone system. *Journal of Physiology,* 413–434. (65, 74–75, 77)

Geisler, W. S. (1984) Physical limits of acuity and hyperacuity. *Journal of Optical Society of America A,* **1,** 775–782. (260, 351, 358, 421–422)

Gelb, A. (1929) Die Farbenkonstanz der Sehdinge. In A. Bethe, G. V. Bergmann, G. Embden, & A. Ellinger (Eds.), *Handbuch der normalen und pathologischen Physiologie, Vol. 12,* pp. 594–678. Berlin: Springer-Verlag. (130)

Georgeson, M. A. (1973) Spatial frequency selectivity of a visual tilt illusion. *Nature (London),* **245,** 43–45. (296)

Georgeson, M. A. (1980) Spatial frequency analysis in early visual processing. *Philosophical Transactions of the Royal Society of London, Series B,* **290,** 11–22. (271)

Georgeson, M. A., & Harris, M. G. (1984) Spatial selectivity of contrast adaptation: Models and data. *Vision Research,* **24,** 729–741. (246)

Gerling, J., & Spillmann, L. (1987) Duration of visual afterimages on modulated backgrounds: Postreceptoral processes. *Vision Research,* **27,** 521–527. (138)

Gernandt, B., & Granit, R. (1947) Single fiber analysis of inhibition and the polarity of the retinal elements. *Journal of Neurophysiology,* **10,** 295–301. (145)

Gerrits, H. J. M. (1978) Differences in peripheral and foveal effects observed in stabilized vision. *Experimental Brain Research,* **32,** 225–244. (138)

Gerrits, H. J. M., Stassen, H. P. W., & van Erning, L. J. Th. O. (1984) The role of drifts and saccades for the preservation of brightness perception. In L. Spillmann and B. R. Wooten (Eds.), *Sensory Experience, Adaptation, and Perception,* pp. 439–459. Hillsdale, NJ: Lawrence Erlbaum. (138)

Gerrits, H. J. M., van Erning, L. J. Th. O., & Eijkman, E. G. J. (1988) Afterimages: A collective term for percepts of different origin. *Experimental Brain Research,* **72,** 279–286. (138)

Gerrits, H. J. M., & Vendrik, A. J. H. (1970) Simultaneous contrast, filling-in process and information processing in man's visual system. *Experimental Brain Research,* **11,** 411–430. (138, 149)

Gibson, J. J. (1966) *The Senses Considered as Perceptual Systems.* Boston: Houghton-Mifflin. (4, 307)

Gibson, J. J. (1968) What gives rise to the perception of motion? *Psychological Review,* **75,** 335–346. (4, 219)

Giffin, F., & Mitchell, D. E. (1978) The rate of recovery of vision after early monocular deprivation in kittens. *Journal of Physiology,* **274,** 511–537. (395)

Gilbert, C. D., & Wiesel, T. N. (1983) Clustered intrinsic connections in cat visual cortex. *Journal of Neuroscience,* **3,** 1116–1133. (410)

Gilchrist, A., Delman, S., & Jacobsen, A. (1983) The classification and integration of edges as critical to the perception of reflectance and illumination. *Perception & Psychophysics,* **33,** 425–436. (58, 64, 132)

Glickstein, M., & Heath, G. G. (1975) Receptors in the monochromat eye. *Vision Research,* **15,** 633–686. (383)

Gillam, B., Flagg, T., & Finlay, D. (1984) Evidence for disparity change as the primary stimulus for stereoscopic processing. *Perception & Psychophysics,* **36,** 559–564. (346)

Gillam, B., & Lawergren, B. (1983) The induced effect, vertical disparity, and stereoscopic theory. *Perception & Psychophysics,* **34,** 121–130. (346)

Ginsburg, A. P. (1975) Is the illusory triangle physical or imaginary? *Nature (London),* **257,** 219–220. (292)

Ginsburg, A. P. (1984) Visual form perception based on biological filtering. In L. Spillmann and B. R. Wooten (Eds.), *Sensory Experience, Adaptation, and Perception,* pp. 53–72. Hillsdale, NJ: Lawrence Erlbaum Associates. (423)

Glad, A., & Magnussen, S. (1972) Darkness enhancement in intermittent light: An experimental demonstration. *Vision Research,* **12,** 111–115. (148)

Glass, L., & Switkes, E. (1976) Pattern recognition in humans: Correlations which cannot be perceived. *Perception,* **5,** 67–72. (441)

Glezer, V. (1965) The receptive fields of the retina. *Vision Research,* **5,** 497–525. (154)

Glezer, V. D., Ivanoff, V. A., & Tscherbach, T. (1973) Investigation of complex and hypercomplex receptive fields of visual cortex of the cat as spatial frequency filters. *Vision Research,* **13,** 1875–1904. (418)

Goldberg, M. E. (1986) The contribution of electrophysiology to the study of attention. In K. Poeck, H.-J. Freund & H. Gänshirt (Eds.), *Neurology,* pp. 151–158. Berlin: Springer-Verlag. (311)

Goldberg, M. E., & Bruce, C. J. (1985) Cerebral cortical activity associated with the orientation of visual attention in the rhesus monkey. *Vision Research,* **25,** 471–481. (312)

Goldberg, M. E., & Bushnell, M. C. (1981) Behavioral enhancement of visual responses in monkey cerebral cortex. II. Modulation in frontal eye fields. *Journal of Neurophysiology,* **45,** 773–787. (312)

Goldberg, M. E., & Wurtz, R. H. (1972) Activity of superior colliculus in behaving monkey. II. Effect of attention on neuronal responses. *Journal of Neurophysiology,* **35,** 560–574. (309)

Goldberg, S. H., Frumkes, T. E., & Nygaared, R. W. (1983) Inhibitory influence of unstimulated rods in the human retina: Evidence provided by examining cone flicker. *Science,* **221,** 180–182. (383)

Goldmann, H., & Lotmar, W. (1970) Retinale Sehscharfenbestimmung bei Katarakt. *Ophthalmologica,* **161,** 175–179. (397)

Golomb, B., Andersen, R. A., Nakayama, K., MacLeod, D. I. A., & Wong, A. (1985) Visual thresholds for shearing motion. *Vision Research,* **25,** 813–820. (47, 49)

Gouras, P. (1968) Identification of cone mechanisms in monkey ganglion cells. *Journal of Physiology,* **199,** 533–547. (113, 184)

Gouras, P. (1972) Light and dark adaptation. In M. G. F. Fuortes (Ed.), *Handbook of Sensory Physiology Vol. VII/2,* pp. 609–634. Berlin: Springer-Verlag. (70)

Gouras, P. (1974) Opponent-colour cells in different layers of foveal striate cortex. *Journal of Physiology,* **238,** 538–602. (288)

Gouras, P., & Hoff, M. (1970) Retinal function in an isolated, perfused mammalian eye. *Investigative Ophthalmology,* **9,** 388–399. (87)

Gouras, P., & Zrenner, E. (1979) Enhancement of luminance flicker by color-opponent mechanisms. *Science,* **205,** 587–589. (184–186)

Gouras, P., & Zrenner, E. (1981) Color coding in primate retina. *Vision Research,* **21,** 1591–1598. (181)

Grafstein, B. (1971) Transneuronal transfer of radioactivity in the central nervous system. *Science,* **172,** 177–179. (366)

Graham, C. H., & Brown, J. L. (1965) Color contrast and color appearance: Brightness constancy and color constancy. In C. H. Graham (Ed.), *Vision and Visual Perception,* pp. 452–478. New York: Wiley. (66)

Graham, C. H., & Hartline, H. K. (1935) The response of single visual sense cells to lights of different wave lengths. *Journal of Physiology,* **18,** 917–931. (172–173)

Graham, C. H., & Hsia, Y. (1969) Saturation and the foveal achromatic interval. *Journal of the Optical Society of America,* **59,** 993–997. (192–193)

Graham, N. (1980) Spatial-frequency channels in human vision: Detecting edges without edge detectors. In C. S. Harris (Ed.), *Visual Coding and Adaptability.* Hillsdale, NJ: Lawrence Erlbaum. (419)

Graham, N. (1985) Detection and identification of near-threshold visual patterns. *Journal of the Optical Society of America A, 2,* 1468–1482. (156, 274)

Graham, N., & Nachmias, J. (1971) Detection of grating patterns containing two spatial frequencies: A comparison of single-channel and multiple-channel models. *Vision Research,* **11,** 251–259. (245, 250, 418)

Graham, N., & Robson, J. G. (1987) Summation of very close spatial frequencies: The importance of spatial probability summation. *Vision Research,* **27,** 1997–2007. (246)

Granrud, C. E. (1986) Binocular vision and spatial perception in

4- and 5-month-old infants. *Journal of Experimental Psychology: Human Perception and Performance,* **12,** 36–49. (371)

Green, D. G. (1970) Regional variations in the visual acuity for interference fringes on the retina. *Journal of Physiology,* **207,** 351–356. (357, 397)

Green, D. G. (1986) The search for the site of visual adaptation. *Vision Research,* **26,** 1417–1429. (84, 101)

Green, D. G., Dowling, J. E., Siegel, I. M., & Ripps, H. (1975) Retinal mechanisms of visual adaptation in the skate. *Journal of General Physiology,* **65,** 483–502. (74)

Green, D. M., & Swets, J. A. (1966) *Signal Detection Theory and Psychophysics.* New York: Wiley. (355)

Greenlee, M. W., Magnussen, S., & Nordby, K. (1988) Spatial vision of the achromat: Spatial frequency and orientation-specific adaptation. *Journal of Physiology,* **395,** 661–678. (266)

Greenstein, V., & Hood, D. C. (1986) Test of the decreased responsiveness hypothesis in retinitis pigmentosa. *American Journal of Optometry and Physiological Optics,* **63,** 22–27. (400)

Gregor, Z., Bird, A. C., & Chisholm, I. H. (1977) Senile disciform macular degeneration in the second eye. *British Journal of Ophthalmology,* **61,** 141–149. (397)

Gregory, R. L. (1972) Cognitive contours. *Nature (London),* **238,** 51–52. (289, 291–292)

Gregory, R. L. (1977) Vision with isoluminant colour contrast: 1. A projection technique and observations. *Perception,* **6,** 113–119. (198, 298–299)

Gregory, R. L., & Harris, J. P. (1974) Illusory contours and stereo depth. *Perception & Psychophysics,* **15,** 411–416. (292)

Grether, W. F. (1939) Color vision and color blindness in monkeys. *Comparative Psychology Monographs,* **15,** 1. (44)

Grimson, W. E. L. (1981) *From Images to Surfaces: A Computational Study of the Human Early Visual System.* Cambridge, MA: M.I.T. Press. (343–344)

Grimson, W. E. L. (1983) An implementation of a computational theory of visual surface interpolation. *Computer Vision, Graphics & Image Processing,* **22,** 39–69. (343)

Grinberg, D. L., & Williams, D. R. (1985) Stereopsis with chromatix signals from the blue-sensitive mechanisms. *Vision Research,* **25,** 531–537. (285)

Grind, van der, W. A., Grüsser, O.-J., & Lunkenheimer, H.-U. (1973) Temporal transfer properties of the afferent visual system. In R. Jung (Ed.), *Handbook of Sensory Physiology, Vol. VII/3A Central Processing of Visual Information,* pp. 431–573. Berlin: Springer-Verlag. (149)

Gross, C. G., Rocha-Miranda, C. E., & Bender, D. B. (1972) Visual properties of neurons in inferior temporal cortex of the macaque. *Journal of Neurophysiology,* **35,** 96–111. (288)

Grossberg, S. (1983) The quantized geometry of visual space: The coherent computation of depth, form and lightness. *Behavioral and Brain Sciences,* **6,** 625–692. (149)

Grossberg, S. (1984) Outline of a theory of brightness, color, and form perception. In E. deGreef & J. van Buggenhaut (Eds.), *Trends in Mathematical Psychology,* pp. 59–86. Amsterdam: North-Holland. (439–440)

Grossberg, S. (1987a) Cortical dynamics of three-dimensional form, color and brightness perception. I. Monocular theory. *Perception & Psychophysics,* **41,** 87–116. (440, 443, 445)

Grossberg, S. (1987b) Cortical dynamics of three-dimensional form, color and brightness perception. II. Binocular theory. *Perception & Psychophysics,* **41,** 117–158. (440, 445)

Grossberg, S. (1988) Neural networks for visual perception in variable illumination. *Optics News,* **14,** 5–10. (440)

Grossberg, S., & Marshall, J. (1987) A computational model of how cortical complex cells multiplex information about position, contrast, orientation, spatial frequency, and disparity. In M. Caudill & C. Butler (Eds.), *Proceedings of the IEEE International Conference on Neural Networks, IV,* 203–214. (446)

Grossberg, S., & Marshall, J. (1989) Stereo boundary fusion by cortical complex cells: A hybrid system of maps, filters, and feedback networks for multiplexing distributed data. *Neural Networks,* **2,** 29–51. (446)

Grossberg, S., & Mingolla, E. (1985a) Neural dynamics of form perception: Boundary completion, illusory figures, and neon color spreading. *Psychological Review,* **92,** 173–211. (292, 417, 420, 440–443)

Grossberg, S., & Mingolla, E. (1985b) Neural dynamics of perceptual grouping: Texture, boundaries, and emergent segmentations. *Perception & Psychophysics,* **38,** 141–171. (292, 417, 440–443)

Grossberg, S., & Mingolla, E. (1987) Neural dynamics of surface perception: Boundary webs, illuminants, and shape-from-shading. *Computer Vision, Graphics, and Image Processing,* **37,** 116–165. (440)

Grossberg, S., & Todorovic, D. (1988) Neural dynamics of 1-D and 2-D brightness perception: A unified model of classical and recent phenomena. *Perception & Psychophysics,* **43,** 241–277. (417, 438, 440)

Grüsser, O.-J., & Creutzfeldt, O. D. (1957) Eine neurophysiologische Grundlage des Brücke–Bartley Effektes: Maxima der Impulsfrequenz retinaler und corticaler Neurone bei Flimmerlicht mittlerer Frequenzen. *Pflügers Archiv für die gesamte Physiologie,* **263,** 668–681. (145, 148)

Grüsser, O.-J., & Grüsser-Cornehls, U. (1973) Neuronal mechanisms of visual movement perception and some psychophysical and behavioral correlations. In R. Jung, (Ed.), *Handbook of Sensory Physiology, Vol. VII/3A: Central Processing of Visual Information*, pp. 333–429. Berlin, Heidelberg, New York: Springer-Verlag. (450)

Guillery, R. W. (1972) Binocular competition in the control of geniculate cell growth. *Journal of Comparative Neurology,* **144,** 177–130. (369)

Guillery, R. W., Hickey, T. L., Kaas, J. H., Felleman, D. J., Debruyn, E. J., & Sparks, D. L. (1984) Abnormal central visual pathways in the brain of an albino green monkey (*Cercopithecus*

Aethiops). *Journal of Comparative Neurology*, **226,** 165–183. (265)

Guillery, R. W., Polley, E. H., & Torrealba, F. (1982) The arrangement of axons to fiber diameter in the optic tract of the cat. *Journal of Neuroscience*, **2,** 714–721. (200)

Guth, S. L., Massof, R. W., & Benzschawel, T. (1980) Vector model for normal and dichromatic vision. *Journal of the Optical Society of America*, **70,** d197–212. (166)

Gwiazda, J., Bauer, J., Thorn, F., & Held, R. (1986) Meridional amblyopia does result from astigmatism in early childhood. *Clinical Vision Sciences*, **1,** 145–152. (395)

Gwiazda, J., Brill, S., Mohindra, I., & Held, R. (1978) Infant visual acuity and its meridional variation. *Vision Research*, **18,** 1557–1564. (371)

Gwiazda, J., Brill, S., Mohindra, I., & Held, R. (1980) Preferential looking acuity in infants from two to fifty-eight weeks of age. *American Journal of Optometry and Physiological Optics*, **57,** 428–432. (371)

Haegerstrom-Portnoy, G., & Adams, A. J. (1983) Spatial sensitization properties of the blue-sensitive cone pathways. In J. D. Mollon & L. T. Sharpe (Eds.), *Colour Vision: Physiology and Psychophysics*, pp. 505–513. London: Academic Press. (406)

Haegerstrom-Portnoy, G., & Adams, A. J. (1988) Spatial sensitization of the B cone pathways. *Vision Research*, **28**(5), 629–638. (406)

Haegerstrom-Portnoy, G., & Brown, B. (1989) Two color increment thresholds in early age-related maculopathy. *Clinical Vision Science*, **4,** 1–8. (404)

Haegerstrom-Portnoy, G., Friedman, N., Adams, A. J., Schneck, M., & Hewlett, S. (1988) Vision of rod monochromats. *Investigative Ophthalmology & Visual Science, Supplement* **29,** 74. (383)

Haegerstrom-Portnoy, G., Verdon, W., & Adams, A. J. (1988) Cone interaction occurs in the parafovea under π_4 stimulus conditions. *Vision Research*, **28,** 397–406. (67)

Haenny, P. E., Maunsell, J. H. R., & Schiller, P. H. (1988) State dependent activity in monkey visual cortex. II. Retinal and extraretinal factors in V4. *Experimental Brain Research*, **69,** 245–259. (312–313)

Häggendal, J., & Malmfors, T. (1965) Identification and localization of the catecholamines in the retina and the choroid of the rabbit. *Acta Physiologica of Scandinavia*, **64,** 58–66. (386)

Hainline, L. (1984) Saccades in human infants. In A. G. Gale & F. Johnson (Eds.), *Theoretical and Applied Aspects of Eye Movement Research*, pp. 273–280. New York: Elsevier. (361)

Hallett, P. E. (1987) Quantum efficiency of dark-adapted human vision. *Journal of the Optical Society of America A*, **4,** 2330–2333. (55)

Halliday, A. M., McDonald, W. I., & Mushin, J. (1972) Delayed visual evoked response in optic neuritis. *Lancet*, **1,** 982–985. (409)

Halliday, A. M., McDonald, W. I., & Mushin, J. (1977) Visual evoked potential patients with demyelinating disease. In J. E. Desmedt (Ed.), *Visual Evoked Potentials in Man*, pp. 438–449. Oxford: Clarendon Press. (409)

Hamada, J. (1985) Asymmetric lightness cancellation in Craik–O'Brien patterns of negative and positive contrast. *Experimental Brain Research*, **35,** 37–46. (149)

Hamer, R. D., Lakshminarayanan, V., Enoch, J. M., & O'Donnell, J. J. (1986) Selective adaptation of the Stiles–Crawford function in a patient with gyrate atrophy. *Clinical Vision Science*, **1,** 103–106. (386)

Hammond, P. (1978) Directional tuning of complex cells in area 17 of the feline visual cortex. *Journal of Physiology*, **285,** 479–491. (285)

Hammond, P. (1985) Visual cortical processing: Textural sensitivity and its implications for classical views. In D. Rose & V. G. Dobson (Eds.), *Models of the Visual Cortex*, pp. 326–343. New York: Wiley. (285)

Hammond, P., Ahmed, B., & Smith, A. T. (1986) Relative motion sensitivity in cat cortex as a function of stimulus direction. *Brain Research*, **386,** 93–104. (224)

Hammond, P., & MacKay, D. M. (1975) Differential responses of cat visual cortical cells to textured stimuli. *Experimental Brain Research*, **22,** 427–430. (458)

Hammond, P., & MacKay, D. M. (1977) Differential responsiveness of simple and complex cells in cat striate cortex to visual texture. *Experimental Brain Research*, **30,** 275–296. (245, 269)

Hammond, P., & MacKay, D. M. (1978) Modulation of simple cell activity in cat by moving textured backgrounds. *Journal of Physiology*, **284,** 117P. (245, 269)

Hammond, P., & Mouat, G. S. V. (1985) The relationship between feline pupil size and luminance. *Experimental Brain Research*, **59,** 485–490. (27, 28)

Hammond, P., & Smith, A. T. (1982) On the sensitivity of complex cells in feline striate cortex to relative motion. *Experimental Brain Research*, **47,** 457–460. (224)

Hammond, P., & Smith, A. T. (1984) Sensitivity of complex cells in cat striate cortex to relative motion. *Brain Research*, **301,** 287–298. (224)

Hanly, M., & McKay, D. M. (1979) Polarity-sensitive perceptual adaptation to temporal sawtooth modulation of luminance. *Experimental Brain Research*, **35,** 37–46. (150, 152)

Hardin, C. L. (1988a) *Color for Philosophers: Unweaving the Rainbow*. Indianapolis, IN: Hackett Publishing Company. (20)

Hardin, C. L. (1988b) Reduction in Visual Science. *Journal of the Optical Society of America A, Technical Digest* **5,** Abstract TUD1.

Harmon, L. (1971) Some aspects of recognition of human faces. In O. J. Grüsser (Ed.), *Pattern Recognition in Biological and Technical Systems*. Berlin: Springer-Verlag. (212)

Harosi, F. (1987) Cynomolgus and rhesus monkey visual pigments. *Journal of General Physiology*, **89,** 717–743. (170, 174)

Harosi, R. I. (1976) Spectral relations of cone pigments in goldfish. *Journal of General Physiology*, **68,** 65–80. (43)

Harris, J. P., & Gregory, R. L. (1973) Fusion and rivalry of illusory contours. *Perception,* **2,** 235–247. (287)

Harris, L., Atkinson, J., & Braddick, O. J. (1976) Visual contrast sensitivity of the six-month infant measured by the evoked potential. *Nature (London),* **264,** 570–571. (360)

Hartline, H. K. (1934) Intensity and duration in the excitation of single photoreceptor units. *Journal of Cellular & Comparative Physiology,* **5,** 229–247. (6)

Hartline, H. K. (1940) The receptive fields of optic nerve fibers. *American Journal of Physiology,* **130,** 690–699. (90)

Hartline, H. K. (1949) Inhibition of activity of visual receptors by illuminating nearby retinal areas in the limulus eye. *Federation Proceedings,* **8,** 69. (179)

Hartmann, N. (1950) *Philosophie der Natur; Abrisz der speziellen Kategorienlehre.* Berlin: Verlag Walter de Gruyter. (453)

Harvey, L. O., Jr. (1986) Visual memory: What is remembered? In F. Klix and H. Hagendorf (Eds.), *Human Memory and Cognitive Capabilities,* pp. 173–187. Amsterdam: Elsevier/North Holland. (423)

Harwerth, R. S., & Levi, D. M. (1978) Reaction time as a measure of suprathreshold grating detection. *Vision Research,* **18,** 1579–1586. (120)

Harwerth, R. S., & Smith, E. L. (1985) The rhesus monkey as a model for normal vision of humans. *American Journal of Optometry and Physiological Optics,* **62,** 633–641. (44)

Hawken, M. J., & Parker, A. J. (1984) Contrast sensitivity and orientation selectivity in lamina IV of the striate cortex of Old World monkeys. *Experimental Brain Research,* **54,** 367–372. (123)

Hawken, M. J., & Parker, A. J. (1987) Spatial properties of neurons in the monkey striate cortex. *Proceedings of the Royal Society of London, Series B,* **231,** 251–288. (249, 268)

Hawken, M. J., Parker, A. J., & Lund, J. S. (1988) Laminar organization and contrast sensitivity of direction-selective cells in the striate cortex of the Old World monkey. *Journal of Neuroscience,* **8,** 3541–3548. (123)

Hayhoe, M. M. (1979a) Lateral interactions in human cone dark adaptation. *Journal of Physiology,* **296,** 125–140. (100)

Hayhoe, M. M. (1979b) After-effects of small adapting fields. *Journal of Physiology,* **296,** 125–140. (100)

Hayhoe, M. M. (1986) Spatial basis of subtractive processes in sensitivity control. *Perception,* **15,** A35. (77)

Hayhoe, M. M., & Smith, M. (1989) The role of spatial filtering in sensitivity regulation. *Vision Research,* **29,** 457–469. (100)

Hayhoe, M. M., Benimoff, N. I., & Hood, D. C. (1987) The time-course of multiplicative and subtractive adaptation process. *Vision Research,* **27,** 1981–1996. (75, 77)

Hayhoe, M. M., MacLeod, D. I. A., & Bruch, T. (1976) Rod–cone independence in dark adaptation. *Vision Research,* **26,** 591–600. (95)

Hebb, D. (1949) *The Organization of Behavior: A Neuropsychological Theory.* New York: Wiley. (307, 369, 377)

Hécaen, H., Perenin, M. T., & Jeannerod, M. (1984) The effects of cortical lesions in children: Language and visual functions. In C. R. Almli & S. Finger (Eds.), *Early Brain Damage: Research Orientations and Clinical Observations, Vol. 1.* New York: Academic Press. (414)

Hecht, S. (1928) The relation between visual acuity and illumination. *Journal of General Physiology,* **11,** 155–281. (97)

Hecht, S., Shlaer, S., & Pirenne, M. H. (1942) Energy, quanta and vision. *Journal of General Physiology,* **224,** 665–699. (79, 80)

Heggelund, P. (1974) Achromatic color vision II: Measurement of simultaneous achromatic contrast within a bidimensional system. *Vision Research,* **14,** 1081–1088. (64)

Heggelund, P. (1985) Receptive field organization of simple and complex cells. In D. Rose & V. G. Dobson (Eds.), *Models of the Visual Cortex,* pp. 358–365. New York: Wiley. (243)

Heinemann, E. G. (1955) Simultaneous brightness induction as a function of inducing- and test-field luminances. *Journal of Experimental Psychology,* **50,** 89–96. (91, 434, 436)

Held, J. R. (1968) Dissociation of visual functions by deprivation and rearrangement. *Psychologische Forschung,* **31,** 338–348. (103)

Held, R. (1985) Binocular vision—behavioral and neural development. In J. Mehler & R. Fox (Eds.), *Neonate Cognition: Beyond the Blooming Buzzing Confusion,* pp. 37–44. Hillsdale, NJ: Lawrence Erlbaum. (372)

Held, J. R., Birch, E. E., & Gwiazda, J. (1980) Stereoacuity of human infants. *Proceedings from the National Academy of Sciences U.S.A.,* **77,** 5572–5574. (362, 371)

Helmholtz, H. von (1867) *Handbuch der Physiologischen Optik,* 1st ed. Leipzig: Voss. (2, 54, 90, 129–130, 145, 163–164)

Helmholtz, H. von (1892) Versuch, das psychophysische Gesetz auf die Farbunterschiede trichromatischer Augen anzuwenden. *Zeitschrift für Psychologie und Physiologie der Sinnesorgane,* **3,** 1–20. (40)

Helson, H. (1963) Studies of anomalous contrast and assimilation. *Journal of the Optical Society of America,* **53,** 179–183. (133)

Helversen, O. von (1972) Zur spektralen Unterschiedsempfindlichkeit der Honigbiene. *Journal of Comparative Physiology,* **80,** 439–472. (38)

Hendrickson, A. E. (1985) Dots, stripes and columns in monkey visual cortex. *Trends in Neuroscience,* **8,** 406–410. (283)

Hendrickson, A. E., Wilson, J. R., & Ogren, M. P. (1978) The neuroanatomical organization of pathways between dorsal lateral geniculate nucleus and visual cortex in Old and New World primates. *Journal of Comparative Neurology,* **182,** 123–136. (121)

Hendrickson, A., & Yuodelis, C. (1984) The morphological development of the human fovea. *Ophthalmology,* **91,** 603–612. (352)

Hering, E. (1878) *Zur Lehre vom Lichtsinn.* Wien: Gerald u. Söhne. (2, 129, 130–132, 135, 137, 163–164, 166)

Hering, E. (1905) *Grundzüge der Lehre vom Lichtsinn.* Leipzig: Breitkopf & Haertel. (132)

Hering, E. (1879) Der Raumsinn und die Bewegungen der Auges.

In L. Hermann (Ed.), *Handbuch der Physiologie: Vol. 3, Part 4*, 343–602. See English translation by C. A. Radde. Baltimore: American Academy of Optometry. (332)

Hering, E. (1964, originally published 1920) *Outlines of a Theory of the Light Sense* (trans. by L. M. Hurvich & D. Jameson). Cambridge, MA: Harvard University Press. (131, 166)

Hermann, L. (1870) Eine Erscheinung des simultanen Kontrastes. *Pflügers Archiv für die gesamte Physiologie,* **3,** 13–15. (139)

Heron, G., Adams, A. J., & Husted, R. (1988) Central visual field measures of blue-sensitive pathways in glaucoma and ocular hypertension. *Investigative Ophthalmology & Visual Science,* **29**(1), 64–72. (404, 407)

Hess, R. F. (1979) Contrast sensitivity assessment of functional amblyopia in humans. *Transactions of the Ophthalmologic Society of the U.K.,* **99,** 391–397. (265)

Hess, R. F., Campbell, F. W., & Zimmern, R. (1980) Differences in the neural basis of human amblyopias: The effects of mean luminance. *Vision Research,* **20,** 295–305.(264)

Hess, R. F., & Nordby, K. (1986a) Spatial and temporal limits of vision in the achromat. *Journal of Physiology,* **371,** 365–385. (383)

Hess, R. F., & Nordby, K. (1986b) Spatial and temporal properties of human rod vision in the achromat. *Journal of Physiology,* **371,** 387–406. (383)

Hess, R. F., & Pointer, J. S. (1985) Differences in the neural basis of human amblyopia: The distribution of the anomaly across the visual field. *Vision Research,* **25,** 1577–1594. (264)

Heywood, C. A., & Cowey, A. (1987) On the role of cortical area V4 in the discrimination of hue and pattern in macaque monkeys. *Journal of Neuroscience,* **7,** 2601–2616. (127, 201–203)

Heywood, C. A., Wilson, B., & Cowey, A. (1987) A case study of cortical colour "blindness" with relatively intact achromatic discrimination. *Journal of Neurology, Neurosurgery & Psychiatry,* **50,** 22–29. (201–203)

Hickey, T. L., & Peduzzi, J. D. (1987) Structure and development of the visual system. In P. Salapatek & L. Cohen (Eds.), *Handbook of Infant Perception,* pp. 1–42. New York: Academic Press. (372)

Higgins, K. E., & Rinalducci, E. J. (1975) Suprathreshold intensity–area relationships: A spatial Broca–Sulzer effect. *Vision Research,* **15,** 129–143. (146–147)

Highman, V. N., & Weale, R. A. (1973) Rhodopsin density and visual threshold in retinitis pigmentosa. *American Journal of Ophthalmology,* **75,** 822–832. (400)

Hirsch, J., & Hylton, R. (1982) Limits of spatial frequency discrimination as evidence of neural interpolation. *Journal of the Optical Society of America,* **72,** 1367–1374. (256)

Hirsch, J., & Hylton, R. (1984) Quality of the primate photoreceptor lattice and limits of spatial vision. *Vision Research,* **24,** 347–356. (234, 262)

Hirsch, J., & Miller, W. H. (1987) Does cone positional disorder limit resolution? *Journal of the Optical Society of America A,* **4,** 1481–1492. (262)

Hitchcock, P. F., & Hickey, T. L. (1980) Ocular dominance columns: Evidence for their presence in humans. *Brain Research,* **182,** 176–179. (251–252)

Hochstein, S., & Shapley, R. M. (1976) Linear and nonlinear subunits in Y cat retinal ganglion cells. *Journal of Physiology,* **262,** 265–284. (112)

Hoff, W., & Ahuja, N. (1987) Extracting surfaces from stereo images: An integrated approach. In *Proceedings of First International Conference on Computer Vision,* pp. 284–294. New York: IEEE Computer Society Press. (345)

Hoffmann, K. P. (1981) Neuronal responses in the cat's nucleus of the optic tract related to optokinetic nystagmus. In A. Fuchs & D. P. Becker (Eds.), *Progress in Oculomotor Research,* pp. 443–454. Amsterdam: Elsevier/North Holland. (376)

Hoffmann, K. P. (1982) Cortical versus subcortical contributions to the optokinetic reflex in the cat. In G. Lennerstrand, D. Zee & E. Keller (Eds.), *Functional Basis of Ocular Motility Disorders,* pp. 303–310. Oxford: Pergamon. (374, 376)

Hoffmann, K. P. (1983) Control of the optokinetic reflex by the nucleus of the optic tract in the cat. In A. Hein & M. Jeannerod (Eds.), *Spatially Oriented Behavior,* pp. 135–153. New York: Springer. (375–376)

Hoffmann, K. P. (1986) Visual inputs relevant for optokinetic nystagmus in mammals. *Progress in Brain Research,* **64,** 75–84. (375–376)

Hoffmann, K. P. (1987) The influence of visual experience on the ontogeny of the optokinetic reflex in mammals. In J. P. Rauschecker & P. Marler (Eds.), *Imprinting and Cortical Plasticity,* pp. 267–286. New York: Wiley. (374–377)

Hoffmann, K. P., & Distler, C. (1986) The role of direction selective cells in the nucleus of the optic tract of cat and monkey during optokinetic nystagmus. In E. L. Keller & D. J. Zee (Eds.), *Adaptive Processes in Visual and Oculomotor Systems,* pp. 261–266. Oxford: Pergamon. (374)

Hoffmann, K. P., & Huber, H. P. (1983) Responses to visual stimulation in single cells in the nucleus of the optic tract (NOT) during optokinetic nystagmus (OKN) in the awake cat. *Society for Neuroscience Abstracts,* **9,** 1048. (375)

Hoffmann, K. P., & Schoppmann, A. (1975) Retinal input to direction selective cells in the nucleus tractus opticus of the cat. *Brain Research,* **99,** 359–366. (111)

Hoffmann, K. P., & Schoppmann, A. (1981) A quantitative analysis of the direction specific response of neurons in the cat's nucleus of the optic tract. *Experimental Brain Research,* **42,** 146–157. (374)

Hoffmann, K. P., & Stone, J. (1971) Conduction velocity of afferents to cat visual cortex: A correlation with cortical receptive field properties. *Brain Research,* **32,** 460–466. (245)

Hoffmann, K. P., & Stone, J. (1985) Retinal input to the nucleus of the optic tract of the cat assessed by antidromic activation of ganglion cells. *Experimental Brain Research,* **59,** 395–403. (375)

Hollins, M., & Alpern, M. (1973) Dark adaptation and visual pigment regeneration in human cones. *Journal of General Physiology,* **62,** 430–447. (69)

Holopigian, K., Blake, R., & Greenwald, M. (1986) Selective losses in binocularity in anisometropic amblyopes. *Vision Research,* **26,** 621–630. (26)

Hong, X., & Regan, D. (1989) Visual field defects for unidirectional and oscillatory motion in depth. *Vision Research,* **29,** 809–819. (334)

Hood, D. C., & Finkelstein, M. A. (1979) Comparison of changes in sensitivity and sensation: Implications for the response–intensity function of the human photopic system. *Journal of Experimental Psychology: Human Perception and Performance,* **5,** 391–405. (72)

Hood, D. C., & Finkelstein, M. A. (1983) *Colour Vision: Physiology and Psychophysics.* In J. D. Mollon & T. Sharpe (Eds.), *Color Vision.* New York: Academic Press. (13)

Hood, D. C., & Finkelstein, M. A. (1986) Visual sensitivity. In K. Boff, L. Kaufman & J. Thomas (Eds.), *Handbook of Perception and Human Performance, Vol. 1,* pp. 5-1–5-66. New York: Wiley. (56, 70, 75)

Hood, D. C., Finkelstein, M. A., & Buckingham, E. (1979) Psychophysical tests of models of the response function. *Vision Research,* **19,** 401–406. (72)

Hood, D. C., & Greenstein, V. C. (1987) Blue (S) cone vulnerability: A test of a fragile receptor hypothesis. *Applied Optics,* 1025–1029. (77)

Hood, D. C., & Greenstein, V. C. (1988) Increment threshold (t.v.i.) data and the site of disease action. *OSA Technical Digest,* **3,** 2–5. (76)

Hood, D. C., & Hock, P. A. (1974) Light adaptation of the receptors: Increment threshold functions for the frog's rods and cones. *Vision Research,* **15,** 545–553. (59)

Horn, B. K. P. (1974) Determining lightness from an image. *Computer Vision Graphics and Image Processing,* **3,** 277–299. (447)

Horn, K., & Pasternak, T. (1988) Spatial resolution of the cat: Variation with retinal eccentricity. *Investigative Ophthalmology & Visual Science, Supplement,* **29,** 141. (117)

Horton, J. C., & Hedley-White, E. T. (1984) Mapping of cytochrome oxidase patches and ocular dominance columns in human visual cortex. *Transactions of the Royal Society of London, Series B,* **304,** 255–272. (251–252)

Horton, J. C., & Hubel, D. H. (1981) A regular patchy distribution of cytochrome-oxidase staining in primary visual cortex of the macaque monkey. *Nature (London),* **292,** 762–764. (251)

Horton, J. C., & Sherk, H. (1984) Receptive field properties in the cat's lateral geniculate nucleus in the absence of ON-center retinal input. *Journal of Neuroscience,* **4,** 374–380. (143)

Howell, E. R., & Hess, R. F. (1978) The functional area for summation to threshold for sinusoidal gratings. *Vision Research,* **18,** 369–374. (351)

Howland, G. C., Atkinson, J., Braddick, O., & French, J. (1978) Infant astigmatism measured by photorefraction. *Science,* **202,** 331–333. (361)

Hoyt, N. F., Rios-Montenegro, E. N., Behrens, M. M., & Eckelhoff, R. J. (1972) Homonymous hemiooptic hypoplasia: Fundoscopic features in standard and red-free illuminations in three patients with congenital hemiplagia. *British Journal of Ophthalmology,* **56,** 537–545. (411)

Hubel, D. H., & Livingstone, M. S. (1985) Complex unoriented cells in a subregion of primate area 18. *Nature (London),* **315,** 325–327. (284)

Hubel, D. C., & Livingstone, M. S. (1987) Segregation of form, color, and stereopsis in primate area 18. *Journal of Neuroscience,* **7,** 3378–3415. (125, 131, 196, 284)

Hubel, D. H., & Wiesel, T. N. (1962) Receptive fields, binocular interaction and functional architecture in the cat's visual cortex. *Journal of Physiology,* **160,** 106–154. (25, 240–241, 244, 250, 268)

Hubel, D. H., & Wiesel, T. N. (1963) Receptive fields of cells in striate cortex of very young, visually inexperienced kittens. *Journal of Neurophysiology,* **26,** 994–1002. (388, 458)

Hubel, D. H., & Wiesel, T. N. (1965) Binocular interaction in striate cortex of kittens reared with artificial squint. *Journal of Neurophysiology,* **28,** 1041–1059. (389, 391–392)

Hubel, D. H., & Wiesel, T. N. (1968) Receptive fields and functional architecture of monkey striate cortex. *Journal of Physiology,* **195,** 215–243. (122–123, 240–241, 244, 250, 268, 288, 296)

Hubel, D. H., & Wiesel, T. N. (1969) Anatomical demonstration of columns in the monkey striate cortex. *Nature (London),* **221,** 747–750. (250)

Hubel, D. H., & Wiesel, T. N. (1970a) Cells sensitive to binocular depth in area 18 of the macaque monkey cortex. *Nature (London),* **225,** 41–42. (322, 325)

Hubel, D. H., & Wiesel, T. N. (1970b) The period of susceptibility to the physiological effects of unilateral eye closure in kittens. *Journal of Physiology,* **206,** 419–436. (390)

Hubel, D. H., & Wiesel, T. N. (1972) Laminar and columnar distribution of geniculocortical fibers in the macaque monkey. *Journal of Comparative Neurology,* **146,** 421–450. (121)

Hubel, D. H., & Wiesel, T. N. (1974) Uniformity of monkey striate cortex: A parallel relationship between field size, scatter and magnification factor. *Journal of Comparative Neurology,* **158,** 295–306. (156)

Hubel, D. H., & Wiesel, T. N. (1977) Functional architecture of macaque visual cortex. *Proceedings of the Royal Society of London, Series B,* **198,** 1–59. (250, 362, 365, 367, 445)

Hubel, D. H., Wiesel, T. N., & Stryker, M. P. (1977) Orientation columns in macaque monkey visual cortex demonstrated by the 2-deoxyglucose autoradiographic technique. *Nature (London),* **269,** 328–330. (250)

Hughes, A. (1973) Observing accommodation in the cat. *Vision Research,* **13,** 481–482. (27)

Hughes, A. (1981) Cat retina and the sampling theorem; the relation of transient and sustained brisk-unit cut-off frequency to alpha and beta mode cell density. *Experimental Brain Research,* **42,** 196–202. (28, 29)

Humphrey, A. L., & Hendrickson, A. E. (1983) Background and stimulus-induced patterns of high metabolic activity in the visual cortex (area 17) of the squirrel and macaque monkey. *Journal of Neuroscience,* **3,** 345–358. (251)

Humphrey, N. K., & Weiskrantz, L. (1967) Vision in monkeys after removal of the striate cortex. *Nature (London),* **215,** 595–597. (410)

Humphreys, G., & Riddoch, J. (1987) *To See But Not To See.* Hillsdale, NJ: Lawrence Erlbaum. (303)

Hunzelmann, N., & Spillmann, L. (1984) Movement adaptation in the peripheral retina. *Vision Research,* **24,** 1765–1769. (138)

Hurlbert, A. (1986) Formal connections between lightness algorithms. *Journal of the Optical Society of America A,* **3,** 1684–1693. (447)

Hurvich, L. M. (1981) *Color Vision.* Sunderland, MA: Sinauer Associates, Inc. (199, 434)

Hurvich, L. M., & Jameson, D. (1955) Some quantitative aspects of an opponent-colors theory. II. Brightness, saturation, and hue in normal and dichromatic observers. *Journal of the Optical Society of America,* **45,** 602–616. (168)

Hurvich, L. M. & Jameson, D. (1958) Further development of a quantified opponent-colors theory. In *Vision Problems of Colour II,* pp. 691–723. London: H.M.S.O. (74)

Hurvich, L. M., & Jameson, D. (1966) *The Perception of Brightness and Darkness.* Boston: Allyn & Bawn. (133)

Hurvich, L. M., & Jameson, D. (1974) Opponent processes as a model of neural organization. *American Psychologist,* **29,** 88–102. (133)

Ilyson, M. T., Julesz, B., & Fender, D. H. (1983) Eye movements and natural remapping during fusion of misaligned random-dot stereograms. *Journal of the Optical Society of America,* **73,** 1665–1673. (331)

Hyvärinen, J. (1982) *The Parietal Cortex of Monkey and Man.* Berlin, Heidelberg, New York: Springer-Verlag. (454)

Hyvärinen, L., & Rovamo, J. (1981) Acquired blindness for achromatic stimuli. *Documenta Ophthalmologica Proceedings Series,* **30,** 94–99. (200)

Ingle, D. (1967) Two visual mechanisms underlying the behavior of fish. *Psychologische Forschung,* **31,** 44–51. (103)

Ingling, C. R., Jr. (1977) The spectral sensitivity of the opponent-color channels. *Vision Research,* **17,** 1083–1089. (166)

Ingling, C. R., Jr., & Tsou, B. P. M. (1977) Orthogonal combination of the three visual channels. *Vision Research,* **17,** 1075–1082. (66)

Jacobs, D. S., & Blakemore, C. (1988) Factors limiting the postnatal development of visual acuity in the monkey. *Vision Research,* **28,** 947–958. (359)

Jacobs, G. H. (1981) *Comparative Color Vision.* New York: Academic Press. (34)

Jacobs, G. H. (1983a) Variations in color vision among nonhuman primates. In J. D. Mollon & L. T. Sharpe (Eds.), *Colour Vision: Physiology and Psychophysics,* pp. 39–50. London: Academic Press.

Jacobs, G. H. (1983b) Within-species variations in visual capacity among squirrel monkeys (*Saimiri sciureus*): Sensitivity differences. *Vision Research,* **23,** 239–248. (35)

Jacobs, G. H. (1984) Within species variations in visual capacity among squirrel monkeys (*Saimiri sciureus*): Color vision. *Vision Research,* **24,** 1267–1277. (35–37, 176)

Jacobs, G. H. (1987) Cone pigments and color vision polymorphism: A comparative perspective. In *Frontiers of Visual Science,* pp. 129–144. Washington, D.C.: National Academy Press. (176)

Jacobs, G. H., & Neitz, J. (1985) Color vision in squirrel monkeys: Sex-related differences suggest the mode of inheritance. *Vision Research,* **25,** 141–144. (37)

Jacobs, G. H., & Neitz, J. (1986) Spectral mechanisms and color vision in the tree shrew (*Tupaia belangeri*). *Vision Research,* **26,** 291–298. (34)

Jacobs, G. H., & Neitz, J. (1987) Inheritance of color vision in a New World monkey (*Saimiri sciureus*). *Proceedings of the National Academy of Sciences U.S.A.,* **84,** 2545–2549. (38)

Jacobs, G. H., Neitz, J., & Crognale, M. (1985) Spectral sensitivity of ground squirrel cones measured with ERG flicker photometry. *Journal of Comparative Physiology A,* **156,** 503–509. (34)

Jacobs, S. H. (1965) Effects of adaptation on lateral geniculate response to light increment and decrement. *Journal of the Optical Society of America,* **55,** 1535–1540. (89)

Jacobsen, A., & Gilchrist, A. (1988) The ratio principle holds over a million-to-one range of illumination. *Perception & Psychophysics,* **43,** 1–6. (64)

Jacobson, S. G., Franklin, K. B. J., & McDonald, W. I. M. (1976) Visual acuity of the cat. *Vision Research,* **16,** 1141–1143. (28)

Jameson, D. (1972) Theoretical issues of color vision. In D. Jameson & L. M. Hurvich (Eds.), *Handbook of Sensory Physiology, Vol. VII/4, Visual Psychophysics,* pp. 381–412. Berlin. Springer-Verlag. (167)

Jameson, D., & Hurvich, L. M. (1955) Some quantitative aspects of an opponent-colors theory: I. Chromatic responses and spectral saturation. *Journal of the Optical Society of America,* **45,** 546–552. (163, 166–167)

Jameson, D., & Hurvich, L. (1959) Perceived color and its dependence on focal, surrounding, and preceding stimulus variables. *Journal of the Optical Society of America,* **45,** 546–552. (434)

Jameson, D., & Hurvich, L. M. (1964) Theory of brightness and color contrast in human vision. *Vision Research,* **4,** 135–154. (132)

Jameson, D., & Hurvich, L. M. (1968) Opponent-response functions related to measured cone photopigments. *Journal of the Optical Society of America,* **58,** 429–430. (166, 168)

Jameson, D., & Hurvich, L. M. (1972) Color adaptation: Sensitivity control, contrast, afterimages. In D. Jameson & L. M. Hurvich (Eds.), *Handbook of Sensory Physiology, Vol. VII/4,* pp. 568–581. Berlin: Springer-Verlag. (66)

Jay, M. F., & Sparks, D. L. (1987) Sensorimotor integration in the primate superior colliculus. I. Motor convergence. *Journal of Neurophysiology,* **57,** 22–34. (311)

Jeannerod, M. (1981) Specialized channels for cognitive responses. *Cognition, 10,* 135–137. (413)

Jeannerod, M. (1988) The neural and behavioral organization of goal-directed movements. Oxford: Oxford Science Publications. (413)

Jennings, J. A. M., & Charman, W. N. (1981) Off-axis image quality in the human eye. *Vision Research,* **21,** 445–455. (233)

Johnson, C. A., Post, R. B., Chalupa, L. M., & Lee, T. J. (1982) Monocular deprivation in humans: A study of identical twins. *Investigative Ophthalmology & Visual Science,* **23,** 135–138. (395)

Johnson, E. P., Riggs, L. A., & Schick, A. M. L. (1966) Photopic retinal potentials evoked by phase alterations of a barred pattern. In H. M. Burian & J. H. Jacobson (Eds.), *Clinical Electroretinography, Proceedings of the Third International Symposium,* pp. 75–91. Oxford: Pergamon. (407)

Johnson, M. A., & Hood, D. C. (1988) A theoretical interpretation of ERG abnormalities in central retinal vein occlusion. Non-invasive assessment of the visual system. *Technical Digest of the Optical Society of America,* **3,** 84–87.

Johnson, M. A., & Massof, R. W. (1984) Evidence for temporal aliasing in the peripheral retina. *Investigative Ophthalmology & Visual Science, Supplement,* **25,** 52. (270)

Johnston, W. A., & Dark, V. J. (1982) In defense of intraperceptual theories of attention. *Journal of Experimental Psychology: Human Perception and Performance,* **8,** 407–421. (306)

Jones, K. R., Spear, P. D., & Tong, J. (1984) Critical periods for effects of monocular deprivation: Differences between striate and extrastriate cortex. *Journal of Neuroscience,* **4,** 2543–2552. (390)

Jones, R. (1977) Anomalies of disparity detection in the human visual system. *Journal of Physiology,* **264,** 621–640. (324, 330)

Julesz, B. (1960) Binocular depth perception of computer-generated patterns. *Bell Systems Technical Journal,* **39,** 1125–1162. (23, 319–320)

Julesz, B. (1964) Binocular depth perception without familiarity cues. *Science,* **145,** 356–362. (275)

Julesz, B. (1971) *Foundations of Cyclopean Perception.* Chicago: University of Chicago Press. (3, 279, 294, 299, 302, 319–322, 343, 345)

Julesz, B. (1975) Experiments in the visual perception of texture. *Scientific American,* **232**(4), 34–43. (275)

Julesz, B. (1981) Textons, the elements of texture perception, and their interactions. *Nature (London),* **290,** 91–97. (418, 425, 427)

Julesz, B. (1984) Toward an axiomatic theory of preattentive vision. In G. M. Edelman, W. E. Gall & M. Cowan (Eds.), *Dynamic Aspects of Neocortical Function,* pp. 585–611. New York: Neurosciences Research Foundation. (274–275)

Julesz, B. (1986) Stereoscopic vision. *Vision Research,* **26,** 1601–1612. (326, 343, 453)

Julesz, B., & Bergen, J. R. (1983) Textons, the fundamental elements in preattentive vision and perception of textures. *Bell System Technical Journal,* **62,** Part II: 1619–1645. (269, 425)

Julesz, B., & Chang, J. J. (1976) Interaction between pools of binocular disparity detectors tuned to different disparities. *Biological Cybernetics,* **22,** 107–119. (345)

Jung, R. (1954) Correlation of bioelectrical and anatomic phenomena with alterations of consciousness and arousal in man. In F. Delafresnaye, E. D. Adrian, F. Bremer & H. H. Jasper (Eds.), *Brain Mechanisms and Consciousness,* pp. 310–344. Oxford: Blackwell. (453)

Jung, R. (1961) Korrelationen von Neuronentätigkeit und Sehen. In R. Jung & H. H. Kornhuber (Eds.), *Neurophysiologie und Psychophysik des visuellen Systems,* pp. 410–435. Berlin, Heidelberg, New York: Springer-Verlag. (129, 132, 138, 145, 193)

Jung, R. (1967) Neurophysiologie und Psychiatrie. In H. W. Gruhle, R. Jung, W. Mayer-Gross & M. Müller (Eds.), *Psychiatrie der Gegenwart. Forschung und Praxis, Vol. 1,* pp. 325–928. Berlin: Springer-Verlag. (451, 453)

Jung, R. (1973) Visual perception and neurophysiology. In H. Autrum, R. Jung, W. Loewenstein, D. M. MacKay & H. L. Teuber (Eds.), *Handbook of Sensory Physiology, Vol. VII/3A: Central Processing of Visual Information,* pp. 1–152. Berlin, Heidelberg, New York: Springer-Verlag. (1, 132, 138, 145, 193, 410, 450)

Jung, R. (1974) Neuropsychologie und Neurophysiologie des Kontur- und Formsehens in Zeichnung und Malerei. In H. H. Wieck (Ed.), *Psychopathologie musischer Gestaltungen,* pp. 29–88. Stuttgart: Schattauer Verlag. (306)

Jung, R. (1978) Sehen. In O. H. Gauer, K. Kramer & R. Jung (Eds.), *Physiologie des Menschen, Vol. 13,* pp. 1–140. München: Urban & Schwarzenberg. (145)

Jung, R. (1984) Sensory research in historical perspective: Some philosophical foundations of perception. In J. M. Brookhart & V. B. Mountcastle (Eds.), *Handbook of Physiology, Vol. III, Sec. 1, The Nervous System,* pp. 1–74. Washington, D.C.: American Physiological Society. (449, 452)

Jung, R., Baumgarten, R. von, & Baumgartner, G. (1952) Mikroableitungen von einzelnen Nervenzellen im optischen Cortex der Katze: Die lichtaktivierten B-Neurone. *Archiv für Psychiatrie und Nervenkrankheiten. Zeitschrift für die gesamte Neurologie und Psychiatrie,* **189,** 521–539. (450)

Jung, R., & Kornhuber, H. (Eds.) (1961) *Neurophysiologie und Psychophysik des visuellen Systems.* Berlin, Göttingen, Heidelberg: Springer-Verlag. (2, 7, 11, 450)

Jung, R., & Spillmann, L. (1970) Receptive-field estimation and perceptual integration in human vision. In F. A. Young, D. B. Lindsley (Eds.), *Early Experience and Visual Information Processing in Perceptual and Reading Disorders,* pp. 181–197. Washington, D.C.: National Academy Press. (44, 139, 210)

Kahneman, D., & Chajczyk, D. (1983) Tests of the automaticity of reading: Dilution of stroop effects by color-irrelevant stimuli. *Journal of Experimental Psychology: Human Perception and Performance,* **9,** 497–508. (304)

Kahneman, D., & Treisman, A. (1984) Changing views of attention and automaticity. In R. Parasuraman & D. A. Davies (Eds.), *Varieties of Attention*, pp. 29–61. New York: Academic Press. (307)

Kaneko, A. (1970) Physiological and morphological identification of horizontal, bipolar, and amacrine cells in the goldfish retina. *Journal of Physiology,* **207,** 623–633. (87)

Kanizsa, G. (1955) Margini quasi-percettivi in campi con stimolazione omogenea. *Rivista di Psicologia,* **49,** 7–30. (137, 289)

Kanizsa, G. (1979) *Organization in Vision. Essays on Gestalt Perception.* New York: Praeger. (289)

Kaplan, E., & Shapley, R. M. (1982) X and Y cells in the lateral geniculate nucleus of macaque monkeys. *Journal of Physiology,* **330,** 125–143. (113, 119)

Kasamatsu, T. (1986) A regulatory mechanism of changes in ocular dominance. In E. L. Keller & D. S. Zee (Eds.), *Adaptive Processes in Visual and Oculomotor Systems,* pp. 71–78. Oxford: Pergamon. (391)

Kasamatsu, T., & Pettigrew, J. D. (1979) Preservation of binocularity after monocular deprivation in the striate cortex of kittens treated with 6-hydroxydopamine. *Journal of Comparative Neurology,* **185,** 139–162. (391)

Kass, M., Witkin, A., & Terzopoulos, D. (1987) Snakes: Active contour models. In *Proceedings of First International Conference on Computer Vision,* pp. 259–268. New York: IEEE Computer Society Press. (344–345–347)

Kellman, P. J., & Loukides, M. G. (1987) An object perception approach to static and kinetic subjective contours. In S. Petry & G. Meyer (Eds.), *Perception of Illusory Contours,* pp. 151–162. Berlin: Springer-Verlag. (307)

Kelly, D. H. (1969) Flickering patterns and lateral inhibition. *Journal of the Optical Society of America,* **59,** 1361–1365. (64)

Kelly, D. H. (1972a) Adaptation effects on spatio-temporal sine wave thresholds. *Vision Research,* **12,** 89–101. (232)

Kelly, D. H. (1972b) Flicker. In D. Jameson & L. M. Hurvich (Eds.), *Handbook of Sensory Physiology, Vol. VII/4, Visual Psychophysics,* pp. 273–302. Berlin: Springer-Verlag. (81)

Kelly, D. H. (1976) Pattern detection and the two-dimensional Fourier transform: Flickering checkerboards and chromatic mechanisms. *Vision Research,* **16,** 277–287. (243, 292)

Kelly, D. H. (1977) Visual contrast sensitivity. *Optica Acta,* **24,** 107–129. (359)

Kennedy, H., Martin, K. A. C., Orban, G. A., & Whitteridge, D. (1985) Receptive field properties of neurones in visual area 1 and visual area 2 in the baboon. *Neuroscience,* **14,** 405–415. (261)

Kennedy, J. M. (1978) Illusory contours and the ends of lines. *Perception,* **7,** 605–607. (292–293)

Kertesz, A. E., & Hampton, D. R. (1981) Fusional response to extrafoveal stimulation. *Investigative Ophthalmology & Visual Science,* **21,** 600–605. (330)

Kertesz, A. E., & Lee, H. J. (1988) The nature of sensory compensation during fusional response. *Vision Research,* **28,** 313–322. (331)

King-Smith, P. E. (1975) Visual detection analysed in terms of luminance and chromatic signals. *Nature (London),* **255,** 69–70. (406)

King-Smith, P. E., & Carden, D. (1976) Luminance and opponent-color contributions to visual detection and adaptation and to temporal and spatial integration. *Journal of the Optical Society of America,* **66,** 709–717. (186, 189, 192–193, 406)

King-Smith, P. E., & Kulikowski, J. J. (1975) The detection of gratings by independent activation of line detectors. *Journal of Physiology,* **247,** 237–271. (246)

King-Smith, P. E., Lubow, M., & Benes, S. C. (1984) Selective damage to chromatic mechanisms in neuro-ophthalmic diseases I. Review of published evidence. *Documenta Ophthalmologica,* 241–250. (404)

Kinnear, P. E., Jay, B., & Witkop, C. J. (1985) Albinism. *Survey of Ophthalmology,* **30,** 75–101. (265)

Kitterle, F. L., & Beard, B. L. (1983) The effects of flicker adaptation upon temporal contrast enhancement. *Perception & Psychophysics,* **33,** 75–78. (149)

Kitterle, F. L., & Corwin, T. R. (1979) Enhancement of contrast in flashed sinusoidal gratings. *Vision Research,* **19,** 33–39. (148)

Klein, S. A., & Levi, D. M. (1985) Hyperacuity thresholds of 1.0 second: Theoretical predictions and empirical validation. *Journal of the Optical Society of America A,* **2,** 1170–1190. (254, 257, 259–260, 262, 421)

Klein, S. A., & Levi, D. M. (1987) Position sense of the peripheral retina. *Journal of the Optical Society of America A,* **4,** 1543–1553.

Klein, S. A., Stromeyer, C. F., & Ganz, L. (1974) The simultaneous spatial frequency shift: A dissociation between the detection and the perception of gratings. *Vision Research,* **14,** 1421–1432. (271, 296)

Klein, S. A., & Tyler, C. W. (1981) Phase discrimination using single and compound gratings. *Investigative Ophthalmology & Visual Science, Supplement,* **20,** 124.

Kleinschmidt, J., & Dowling, J. E. (1975) Intracellular recordings from gecko photoreceptors during light and dark adaptations. *Journal of General Physiology,* **66,** 617–648. (74)

Koenderink, J. J. (1984) What does the occluding contour tell us about solid shape? *Perception,* **13,** 321–330. (288)

Koenderink, J. J. (1986) Optic flow. *Vision Research,* **26,** 161–180. (345)

Koenderink, J. J., Bouman, M. A., Bueno de Mesquita, A. E., & Slappendel, S. (1978) Perimetry of contrast detection thresholds of moving sine wave patterns. *Journal of the Optical Society of America,* **68,** 845–865.

Koenderink, J. J., Van de Grind, W. A., & Bouman, M. A. (1971) Foveal information processing at photopic luminances. *Kybernetik,* **8,** 128–144. (64)

Koenderink, J. J., & van Doorn, A. J. (1976) Geometry of binocular vision and a model for stereopsis. *Biological Cybernetics,* **21,** 29–35. (347)

Koenderink, J. J., & van Doorn, A. J. (1978) Visual detection of spatial contrast: Influence of location in the visual field, target extent and illuminance level. *Biological Cybernetics,* **30,** 157–167. (207, 225, 345)

Koffka, K. (1935) *Principles of Gestalt Psychology.* New York: Harcourt, Brace & World. (11, 133)

Kolb, H., & Nelson, R. (1984) Neural architecture of the cat retina. In N. Osborne & J. Chader (Eds.), *Progress in Retinal Research, Vol. 3,* pp. 21–60. New York: Pergamon. (87, 88)

Kolers, P. A. (1972) *Aspects of Motion Perception.* New York: Academic Press. (286)

König, A. (1894) Über den menschlichen Sehpurpur und seine Bedeutung für das Sehen. *Sitzungsberichte der Königlichen Preussischen Akademie der Wissenschaften* **30,** 577–598. (5)

Korte, A. (1915) Kinematoskopische Untersuchungen. *Zeitschrift für Psychologie,* **72,** 193–206. (209)

Kosslyn, S. M. (1987) Seeing and imagining in the cerebral hemispheres: A computational approach. *Psychological Review,* **94,** 148–175. (305)

Kratz, K. E., Sherman, S. M., & Kalil, R. (1979) A lateral geniculate nucleus in dark reared cats: Loss of Y-cells without changes in cell size. *Science,* **203,** 1353–1354. (31)

Krauskopf, J. (1963) Effect of retinal image stabilization on the appearance of heterochromatic targets. *Journal of the Optical Society of America,* **53,** 741–744. (441)

Krauskopf, J. (1980) Discrimination and detection of changes in luminance. *Vision Research,* **20,** 671–677. (150)

Kreminitzer, J. P., Vaughan, H. G., & Kurtzburg, D. (1979) Smooth pursuit eye movements in the newborn infant. *Child Development,* **50,** 442–448. (361)

Krishnan, V. V., Phillips, S., & Stark, L. (1973) Frequency analysis of accommodation, accommodative vergence and disparity vergence. *Vision Research,* **13,** 1545–1554. (330)

Krüger, J., & Fischer, B. (1973) Strong periphery effect in cat retinal ganglion cells. Excitatory responses in ON- and OFF-center neurons to single grid displacements. *Experimental Brain Research,* **18,** 316–318. (62)

Kuffler, S. W. (1952) Neurons in the retina: Organization, inhibition and excitation problems. *Cold Spring Harbor Symposium on Quantitative Biology,* **17,** 281–292. (88)

Kuffler, S. W. (1953) Discharge patterns and functional organization of mammalian retina. *Journal of Neurophysiology,* **16,** 37–68. (24, 88, 108, 142, 153, 179, 239)

Kuhn, T. S. (1970) *The Structure of Scientific Revolutions,* 2nd ed. Chicago: University of Chicago Press. (206)

Kulikowski, J. J., & King-Smith, P. E. (1973) Spatial arrangement of line, edge and grating detectors revealed by subthreshold summation. *Vision Research,* **13,** 1455–1478. (246)

Kupersmith, M. J., Seiple, W. H., Nelson, J. I., & Carr, R. E. (1984) Contrast sensitivity loss in multiple sclerosis. Selectivity by eye, orientation, and spatial frequency measured with the evoked potential. *Investigative Ophthalmology & Visual Science,* **25,** 632–639. (409–410)

Kupersmith, M. J., Shakin, E., Siegel, I. M., & Lieberman, A. (1982) Visual system abnormalities in patients with Parkinson's disease. *Archives of Neurology,* **39,** 284–286. (386–387)

Kurtenbach, W., Sternheim, C. E., & Spillmann, L. (1984) Change in hue of spectral colors by dilution with white light (Abney effect). *Journal of the Optical Society of America A,* **1,** 365–372. (193)

LaBerge, D. (1975) Acquisition of automatic processing in perceptual and associative learning. In P. M. A. Rabbit & S. Dornic (Eds.), *Attention and Performance, Vol. V* pp. 50–64. New York: Academic Press. (306)

Lamb, T. D. (1981) The involvement of rod photoreceptors in dark adaptation. *Vision Research,* **21,** 1773–1782. (70)

Land, E. H. (1983) Color vision and the natural image. III. Recent advances in the retinex theory and some implications for cortical computations. *Proceedings of the National Academy of Sciences U.S.A.,* **80,** 5163–5169. (203, 287, 438, 447)

Land, E. H. (1986) Recent advances in retinex theory. *Vision Research,* **26,** 7–21. (68)

Land, E. H., & McCann, J. J. (1971) Lightness and retinex theory. *Journal of the Optical Society of America,* **61,** 1–11. (434, 436, 438)

Lannou, J., Cazin, L., Precht, W., & LeTaillanter, M. (1984) Responses of prepositus hypoglossi neurons to optokinetic and vestibular stimulations in the rat. *Brain Research,* **301,** 39–45. (374)

Larimer, J., Krantz, D. H., & Cicerone, C. M. (1975) Opponent process additivity. II. Yellow/blue equilibria and nonlinear models. *Vision Research,* **15,** 723–731. (168)

Larsen, J. S. (1971) The sagittal growth of the eye. IV. Ultrasonic measurement of the axial length of the eye from birth to puberty. *Acta Ophthalmologica,* **48,** 873–886. (356)

Lashley, K. S. (1941) Coalescence of neurology and psychology. *Proceedings of the Philosophical Society,* **84,** 461–470. (454)

Latch, M., & Lennie, P. (1977) Rod–cone interaction in light adaptation. *Journal of Physiology,* **269,** 517–534. (100)

Laties, A. M., & Enoch, J. M. (1971) An analysis of retinal receptor orientation. I. Angular relationship of neighboring photoreceptors. *Investigative Ophthalmology,* **10,** 69–77. (385)

Laws, K. I. (1980) Rapid texture identification: Image processing for missile guidance. *SPIE, Society of Photo-optical Instrumentation for Engineers,* **238,** 376–380. (425)

Lawson, R. B., & Gulick, W. L. (1967) Stereopsis and anomalous contour. *Vision Research,* **7,** 271–297. (289)

Lee, D. N. (1979) Binocular stereopsis without spatial disparity. *Perception & Psychophysics,* **9,** 216–223. (302)

Lee, B. B., Martin, P. R., & Valberg, A. (1988) The physiological basis of heterchromatic flicker photometry demonstrated in the ganglion cells of the macaque monkey. *Journal of Physiology,* **404,** 323–347. (189)

Lee, B. B., Valberg, A., Tigwell, D. A., & Tryti, S. (1987) An account of responses of spectrally opponent neurons in macaque lateral geniculate nucleus to successive contrast. *Proceedings of the Royal Society of London, Series B,* **230,** 293–314. (451)

Legge, G. E. (1981) A power law for contrast discrimination. *Vision Research,* **21,** 457–469. (247, 254)

Legge, G. E., & Foley, J. M. (1980) Contrast masking in human vision. *Journal of the Optical Society of America,* **70,** 1458–1471. (246, 254)

LeGrand, Y. (1957) Light, color and vision. London: Chapman and Hall. (65)

Lehmkuhle, S., Kratz, K. E., Mangel, S. C., & Sherman, S. M. (1980) Spatial and temporal sensitivity of X- and Y-cells in dorsal lateral geniculate nucleus of the cat. *Journal of Neurophysiology,* **43,** 520–541. (30–31)

Lehmkuhle, S., Kratz, K. E., & Sherman, S. M. (1982) Spatial and temporal sensitivity of normal and amblyopic cats. *Journal of Neurophysiology,* **48,** 372–387. (26)

Lehmkuhle, S., Sherman, S. M., & Kratz, K. E. (1984) Spatial contrast sensitivity of dark-reared cats with striate cortex lesions. *Journal of Neuroscience,* **4,** 2419–2424. (31)

Lennie, P. (1981) The physiological basis of variations in visual latency. *Vision Research,* **21,** 815–824. (120)

Lennie, P. (1984) Recent developments in the physiology of color vision. *Trends in Neuroscience,* **7,** 243–248. (194)

Lennie, P., & D'Zmura, M. (1988) Mechanisms of color vision. *CRC Critical Reviews in Neurobiology,* **3,** 333–400. (116, 127)

Lennie, P., & MacLeod, D. I. A. (1973) Background configuration and rod threshold. *Journal of Physiology,* **233,** 143–156. (100)

Lettvin, J. Y., Maturana, H. R., McCulloch, W. S., & Pitts, W. H. (1959) What the frog's eye tells the frog's brain. *Proceedings of the Institute of Radio Engineers,* **47,** 1940–1951. (1)

Lettvin, J. Y., Maturana, H. R., Pitts, W. H., & McCulloch, W. S. (1961) Two remarks on the visual system of the frog. In W. A. Rosenblith (Ed.), *Sensory Communication,* pp. 757–776. Cambridge: MIT Press. (110)

LeVay, S., Hubel, D. H., & Wiesel, T. N. (1975) The pattern of ocular dominance columns in macaque visual cortex revealed by a reduced silver stain. *Journal of Comparative Neurology,* **159,** 559–576. (122)

LeVay, S., & Stryker, M. P. (1979) The development of ocular dominance columns in the cat. In J. A. Ferrendelli (Ed.), *Aspects of Developmental Neurobiology,* pp. 83–98. Bethesda, MD: Society for Neuroscience. (368)

LeVay, S., Stryker, M. P., & Shatz, C. J. (1978) Ocular dominance columns and their development in layer IV of the cat's visual cortex: A quantitative study. *Journal of Comparative Neurology,* **179,** 223–244. (368–369, 372)

LeVay, S., Wiesel, T. N., & Hubel, D. H. (1980) The development of ocular dominance columns in normal and visually deprived monkeys. *Journal of Comparative Neurology,* **191,** 1–51. (368–369, 390–391)

Leventhal, A. G., Rodieck, R. W., & Dreher, B. (1981) Retinal ganglion cell classes in the Old World monkey: Morphology and central projections. *Science,* **213,** 1139–1142. (113)

Levi, D. M., & Klein, S. A. (1982) Differences in vernier discrimination of gratings between strabismic and anisometropic amblyopes. *Investigative Ophthalmology & Visual Science,* **23,** 398–407. (264)

Levi, D. M., & Klein, S. A. (1985) Vernier acuity, crowding and amblyopia. *Vision Research,* **25,** 979–991. (259, 262–265)

Levi, D. M., & Klein, S. A. (1987) Sampling in spatial vision. *Nature (London),* **320,** 360–362.

Levi, D. M., Klein, S. A., & Aitsebaomo, A. P. (1985) Vernier acuity, crowding and cortical magnification. *Vision Research,* **25,** 963–977. (238, 251, 257)

Levi, D. M., Klein, S. A., & Yap, Y. L. (1987) Positional uncertainty in peripheral and amblyopic vision. *Vision Research,* **27,** 581–597. (264)

Levi, D. M., Klein, S. A., & Yap, Y. L. (1988) "Weber's law" for position: Unconfounding the role of separation and eccentricity. *Vision Research,* **28,** 597–603. (262, 264)

Levick, W. R. (1973) Maintained discharge in the visual system and its role for information processing. In R. Jung (Ed.), *Handbook of Sensory Physiology, Vol VII/3A, Central Processing of Visual Information,* pp. 575–598. Berlin, Heidelberg, New York: Springer-Verlag. (117)

Levick, W. R., & Thibos, L. N. (1980) Orientation bias of cat retinal ganglion cells. *Nature (London)* **268,** 389–390. (241)

Levine, J. S., & MacNichol, E. F., Jr. (1985) Microspectrophotometry of primate photoreceptors: Art, artifact and analysis. In A. Fein & J. S. Levine (Eds.), *The Visual System,* pp. 73–88. New York: Alan R. Liss. (170)

Lewis, T. L., Maurer, D., & Blackburn, K. (1985) The development of young infants' ability to detect stimuli in the nasal visual field. *Vision Research,* **25,** 943–950. (361)

Li, C. Y., & Creutzfeldt, O. D. (1984) The representation of contrast and other stimulus parameters by single neurons in Area 17 of the cat. *Pflügers Archiv für die gesamte Physiologie,* **401,** 304–314. (461)

Liebmann, S. (1927) Über das Verhalten farbiger Formen bei Helligkeitsgleichheit von Figur und Grund. *Psychologische Forschung,* **9,** 300–353. (298)

Linberg, K. A., & Fisher, S. K. (1986) An ultrastructural study of inter-plexiform cell synapses in the human retina. *Journal of Comparative Neurology,* **243,** 561–576. (88)

Linsenmeier, R. A., Frishman, L. J., Jakiela, H. G., & Enroth-Cugell, C. (1982) Receptive field properties of X and Y cells in the cat retina derived from contrast sensitivity measurements. *Vision Research,* **22,** 1173–1183. (90, 119)

Lisberger, S., Morris, E. J., & Tychsen, L. (1987) Visual motion processing and sensory-motor integration for smooth pursuit eye movements. *Annual Review of Neuroscience,* **10,** 97–129. (226)

Livingstone, M. S., & Hubel, D. H. (1984) Anatomy and physiology of a color system in the primate visual cortex. *Journal of Neuroscience*, **4**, 309–356. (123, 125, 194–195, 201, 251, 283, 451)

Livingstone, M. S., & Hubel, D. H. (1987a) Connections between layer 4B of area 17 and the thick cytochrome oxidase stripes of area 18 in the squirrel monkey. *Journal of Neuroscience*, **7**, 3371–3377. (125, 283)

Livingstone, M. S., & Hubel, D. H. (1987b) Psychophysical evidence for separate channels for the perception of form, color, movement and depth. *Journal of Neuroscience*, **7**, 3416–3468. (123, 283)

Livingstone, M., & Hubel, D. (1988). Segregation of form, color, movement and depth: anatomy, physiology and perception. *Science*, **240**, 740–750. (195)

Longuet-Higgins, H. C. (1982) The role of vertical dimension in vision. *Perception*, **11**, 377–386. (346)

Lotze, R. H. (1886) *Outlines of Psychology* (trans. by G. T. Ladd), Vol. IV of *Outlines of Philosophy*. Boston: Ginn. (420)

Lu, C., & Fender, D. H. (1972) The interaction of color and luminance in stereoscopic vision. *Investigative Ophthalmology*, **11**, 482–490. (198)

Ludvigh, E., & McKinnin, P. (1966) Relative effectivity of foveal and parafoveal stimuli in eliciting fusion movements of small amplitude. *Archives of Ophthalmology*, **76**, 443–449. (330)

Ludvigh, E., McKinnin, P., & Zaiteff, L. (1965) Relative effectivity of foveal and parafoveal stimuli in eliciting fusion movements. *Archives of Ophthalmology*, **73**, 115–121. (330)

Lynch, J. C., Mountcastle, V. B., Talbot, W. H., & Yin, T. C. T. (1977) Parietal lobe mechanisms for directed visual attention. *Journal of Neurophysiology*, **40**, 362–389. (312)

Mach, E. (1865) Über die Wirkung der räumlichen Verteilung des Lichtreizes auf die Netzhaut. I. *Sitzungsberichte der mathematisch-naturwissenschaftlichen Classe der kaiserlichen Akademie der Wissenschaften*, **52 II**, 303–322. (2, 134)

Mach, E. (1866a) Über den phsyiologischen Effect räumlich verteilter Lichtreize. II. *Sitzungsberichte der mathematisch-naturwissenschaftlichen Classe der kaiserlichen Akademie der Wissenschaften*, **54 II**, 131–144. (134)

Mach, E. (1866b) Über die physiologische Wirkung räumlich verteilter Lichtreize. III. *Sitzungsberichte der mathematisch-naturwissenschaftlichen Classe der kaiserlichen Akademie der Wissenschaften*, **54 II**, 393–408. (134)

Mach, E. (1897) *Die Analyse der Empfindungen*. Jena: G. Fischer. (129)

MacKay, D. M. (1956a) Towards an information-flow model of human behaviour. *British Journal of Psychology*, **47**, 30–43. (458)

MacKay, D. M. (1956b) Cerebral activity III. *Advancement of Science*, **42**, 392–395. (458)

MacKay, D. M. (1958) Perceptual stability of a stroboscopically-lit visual field. *Nature (London)* **181**, 507–508. (223)

MacKay, D. M. (1961) Interactive processes in visual perception. In W. A. Rosenblith (Ed.), *Sensory Communication*, pp. 339–355. New York, London: MIT Press, Wiley. (457)

MacKay, D. M. (1962) Theoretical models of space perception. In C. A. Muses (Ed.), *Aspects of the Theory of Artificial Intelligence*, pp. 83–104. New York: Plenum. (458)

MacKay, D. M. (1966) Cerebral organization and the conscious control of action. In J. C. Eccles (Ed.), *Brain and Conscious Experience*, pp. 422–445. Heidelberg, New York: Springer-Verlag. (457)

MacKay, D. M. (Ed.) (1969) *Information, Mechanism and Meaning*. Cambridge, London: MIT Press. (449, 457)

MacKay, D. M. (1970) Perception and brain function. In F. O. Schmitt, G. C. Quarton, T. Melnechuk & J. P. Segundo (Eds.), *The Neurosciences. Second Study Program*, pp. 303–316. New York: Rockefeller University Press. (458)

MacKay, D. M. (1984a) Source density analysis of scalp potentials during evaluated action. I. Coronal distribution. *Experimental Brain Research*, **54**, 73–85. (458)

MacKay, D. M. (1984b) Source density analysis of scalp potentials during evaluated action. II. Lateral distribution. *Experimental Brain Research*, **54**, 86–94. (458)

MacKay, D. M. (1984c) Source density mapping of human visual receptive fields using scalp electrodes. *Experimental Brain Research*, **54**, 579–581. (458)

MacKay, D. M. (1986) Vision—the capture of optical covariation. In J. D. Pettigrew, K. J. Sanderson & W. Levick (Eds.), *Visual Neuroscience*, pp. 487–500. Cambridge: Cambridge University Press. (458)

MacLeod, D. I. A. (1974) Directionally selective light adaptation: A visual consequence of receptor disarray? *Vision Research*, **14**, 369–378. (385)

MacLeod, D. I. A. (1978) Visual sensitivity. *Annual Review of Psychology*, **29**, 613–645. (62, 101)

MacLeod, D. I. A., & Boynton, R. M. (1979) A chromaticity diagram showing cone excitation by stimuli of equal luminance. *Journal of the Optical Society of America*, **69**, 1183–1185. (55)

MacLeod, D. I. A., Chen, B., & Crognale, M. (1989) Spatial organization of sensitivity regulation in rod vision. *Vision Research*, **29**, 965–978. (96)

MacLeod, D. I. A., & Hayhoe, M. M. (1974) Rod origin of prolonged afterimages. *Science*, **185**, 1171–1172. (95)

MacLeod, D. I. A., Williams, D. R., & Makous, W. (1985) Difference frequency gratings above the resolution limit. *Investigative Ophthalmology & Visual Science, Supplement*, **26**, 11. (97)

MacNichol, E. F., Jr. (1986) A unifying presentation of photopigment spectra. *Vision Research*, **26**, 1543–1556. (170–171, 174)

MacNichol, E. F., Jr., Levine, J. S., Mansfield, R. J. W., Lipetz, L. E., & Collins, B. A. (1983) Microspectrophotometry of visual pigments in primate receptors. In J. D. Mollon & L. T. Sharpe (Eds.), *Colour Vision: Physiology and Psychophysics*, pp. 13–38. New York: Academic Press. (171)

Maffei, L. (1968) Inhibitory and facilitatory spatial interactions in retinal receptive fields. *Vision Research*, **8**, 1187–1194. (142)

Maffei, L. (1985) Complex cells control simple cells. In D. Rose & V. G. Dobson (Eds.), *Models of the Visual Cortex*, pp. 334–340. New York: Wiley. (242, 245, 269)

Maffei, L., & Fiorentini, A. (1972) Retinogeniculate convergence and analysis of contrast. *Journal of Neurophysiology,* **35,** 65–72. (149)

Maffei, L., & Fiorentini, A. (1973) The visual cortex as a spatial frequency analyser. *Vision Research,* **13,** 1255–1268. (240, 247, 257, 418)

Maffei, L., & Fiorentini, A. (1976) The unresponsive regions of visual cortical receptive fields. *Vision Research,* **16,** 1131–1139. (248)

Maffei, L., & Fiorentini, A. (1977) Spatial frequency rows in the striate visual cortex. *Vision Research,* **17,** 257–264. (250)

Maffei, L., & Fiorentini, A. (1981) Electroretinographic responses to gratings before and after section of the optic nerve. *Science,* **211,** 953–955. (408)

Maffei, L., Fiorentini, A., & Bisti, S. (1973) Neural correlate of perceptual adaptation to gratings. *Science,* **182,** 1036–1038. (246, 250)

Maffei, L., Morrone, C., Pirchio, M., & Sandini, G. (1979). Responses of visual cortical cells to periodic and nonperiodic stimuli. *Journal of Physiology,* **296,** 27–47. (287)

Magnin, M., Courjon, J. H., & Flandrin, J. M. (1983) Possible visual pathways to the cat vestibular nuclei involving the nucleus prepositus hypoglossi. *Experimental Brain Research,* **51,** 298–303. (374)

Magnussen, S. (1987) Temporal aspects of vision: Psychophysical studies of B- and D-channels. In B. Lomov, Y. Zabrodin, P. Saugstad & S. Magnussen (Eds.), *Problems of Visual Perception.* Moscow: U.S.S.R. Academy of Sciences. (148)

Magnussen, S., & Glad, A. (1975a) Brightness and darkness enhancement during flicker: Perceptual correlates of neuronal B- and D-systems in human vision. *Experimental Brain Research,* **22,** 399–413. (148–149)

Magnussen, S., & Glad, A. (1975b) Temporal frequency characteristics of spatial interaction in human vision. *Experimental Brain Research,* **23,** 519–528. (148–149)

Magnussen, S., & Kurtenbach, W. (1979) A test for contrast polarity selectivity in the tilt aftereffect. *Perception,* **8,** 523–528. (152)

Makous, W. L. (1968) A transient Stiles–Crawford effect. *Vision Research,* **8,** 1271–1284. (385)

Makous, W., & Boothe, R. (1974) Cones block signals from rods. *Vision Research,* **14,** 285–294. (60, 95)

Makous, W., & Peeples, D. (1979) Rod–cone interaction: Reconciliation with Flamant and Stiles. *Vision Research,* **19,** 695–698. (60, 95)

Maloney, L. T. (1986) Evaluation of linear models of surface spectral reflectance with small numbers of parameters. *Journal of the Optical Society of America A,* **3,** 1673–1683. (65)

Malpeli, J. G., & Baker, F. H. (1975) The representation of the visual field in the lateral geniculate nucleus of *Macaca mulatta. Journal of Comparative Neurology,* **161,** 569–594. (118)

Malpeli, J. G., & Schiller, P. H. (1978) Lack of blue off-center cells in the visual system of the monkey. *Brain Research,* **141,** 385–389. (180)

Malpeli, J. G., Schiller, P., & Colby, C. L. (1981) Response properties of single cells in monkey striate cortex during reversible inactivation of individual lateral geniculate laminae. *Journal of Neurophysiology,* **46,** 1102–1119. (123)

Malsburg, C. von der (1984) Am I thinking assemblies? In G. Palm & A. Aertsen (Eds.), *Proceedings of the Trieste Meeting on Brain Theory,* pp. 161–176. Berlin, Heidelberg: Springer-Verlag. (460)

Mangel, S. C., & Dowling, J. E. (1985) Responsiveness and receptive field size of carp horizontal cells are reduced by prolonged darkness and dopamine. *Science,* **299,** 1107–1109. (386, 388)

Mansfield, R. J. W. (1976) Visual adaptation: Retinal transduction, brightness and sensitivity. *Vision Research,* **16,** 679–690. (89)

Mansfield, R. J. W. (1985) Primate photopigments and cone mechanisms. In A. Fein & J. S. Levine (Eds.), *The Visual System,* pp. 89–106. New York: Alan R. Liss. (171)

Marc, R. E., & Sperling, H. G. (1977) Chromatic organization of primate cones. *Science,* **196,** 454–456. (175–176)

Marcelja, S. (1980) Mathematical description of the responses of simple cortical cells. *Journal of the Optical Society of America,* **70,** 1297–1300. (249, 267–268)

Marks, W. B. (1965) Visual pigments of single goldfish cones. *Journal of Physiology,* **178,** 14–32. (39)

Marr, D. (1977) Analysis of occluding contour. *Proceedings of the Royal Society of London, Series B,* **197,** 441–475. (288)

Marr, D. (1982) *Vision: A Computational Investigation into the Human Representation and Processing of Visual Information.* San Francisco, CA: Freeman. (18, 68, 104, 153–154, 157, 276, 287, 307, 339, 342, 346, 419, 421, 425, 451)

Marr, D., & Hildreth, E. (1980) Theory of edge detection. *Proceedings of the Royal Society of London, Series B,* **207,** 187–217. (157, 268)

Marr, D., & Poggio, T. (1976) The cooperative computation of stereo disparity. *Science,* **194,** 283–287. (340, 342–343)

Marr, D., & Poggio, T. (1979) A computational theory of human stereovision. *Proceedings of Royal Society of London, Series B,* **204,** 301–328. (321–322, 328, 343)

Marré, M. (1973) The investigation of acquired colour vision deficiencies. In *Color 73,* pp. 99–135. London, Adam Hilger. (404–405)

Marx, M. S., May, J. G., Reed, J. L., Matteson, H. H., Van Dyk, H. J. L., & Jayarman, A. (1984) Spatio-temporal processing in multiple sclerosis. *Documenta Ophthalmologica,* **56,** 243–264. (410)

Marx, M. S., Podos, S. M., Bodis-Wollner, I., Howard-Williams, J., Siegel, M. J., Teitelbaum, C. S., Maclin, E. L., & Severin, C. (1986) Flash and pattern electroretinograms in normal and laser-induced glaucomatous primate eyes. *Investigative Ophthalmology & Visual Science,* **27,** 378–386. (408)

Mather, B., & Moulden, B. (1980) A simultaneous shift in apparent direction: Further evidence for a 'distribution-shift' model of direction coding. *Quarterly Journal of Experimental Psychology,* **32,** 325–333. (209)

Matsumoto, N., & Naka, K. I. (1972) Identification of intracellular responses in the frog retina. *Brain Research,* **42,** 59–71. (87)

Maunsell, J. H. R., & Newsome, W. T. (1987) Visual processing in monkey extrastriate cortex. *Annual Review of Neuroscience,* **10,** 363–401. (47, 124, 125, 128, 284–286, 288, 294–295)

Maunsell, J. H. R., & Van Essen, D. C. (1983a) The connections of the middle temporal visual area (MT) and their relationship to a cortical hierarchy in the macaque monkey. *Journal of Neuroscience,* **3,** 2563–2586. (222, 284, 286–287)

Maunsell, J. H., & Van Essen, D. C. (1983b) Functional properties of neurons in middle temporal visual area of the macaque monkey. I. Selectivity for stimulus direction, speed, and orientation. *Journal of Neurophysiology,* **49,** 1127–1147. (222, 284, 286–287, 337)

Maunsell, J. H., & Van Essen, D. C. (1983c) Functional properties of neurons in middle temporal visual area of the macaque monkey. II. Binocular interactions and sensitivity to binocular disparity. *Journal of Neurophysiology,* **49,** 1148–1167. (222)

Maxwell, J. C. (1856) Theory of the perception of colors. *Transactions of the Royal Scottish Society of Arts,* **4,** 394–400. (2, 163–164)

Mayer, M. J., & Kim, C. B. Y. (1986) Smooth frequency discrimination functions for foveal, high-contrast, mid spatial frequencies. *Journal of the Optical Society of America A,* **3,** 1957–1969. (256)

Mayfrank, L., Mobashery, M., Kimmig, H., & Fischer, B. (1986) The role of fixation and visual attention in the occurrence of express saccades in man. *European Archives of Psychiatry and Neurological Sciences,* **235,** 269–275. (314–315)

Mayhew, J. E. W. (1982) The interpretation of stereo-disparity information: The computation of surface orientation and depth. *Perception,* **11,** 387–403. (346)

Mayhew, J. E. W. (1983) Stereopsis. In O. J. Braddick & A. C. Sleigh (Eds.), *Physical and Biological Processing of Images.* Berlin: Springer-Verlag. (342)

Mayhew, J. E. W., & Frisby, J. P. (1978) Stereopsis masking is not orientationally tuned. *Perception,* **7,** 431–436. (321)

Mayhew, J. E. W., & Frisby, J. P. (1979a) Surfaces with steep variations in depth pose difficulties for orientationally tuned disparity filters. *Perception,* **8,** 691–698. (321)

Mayhew, J. E. W., & Frisby, J. P. (1979b) Convergent disparity discriminations in narrow-band-filtered random dot stereograms. *Vision Research,* **19,** 63–71. (343)

Mayhew, J. E. W., & Frisby, J. P. (1981) Psychophysical and computational studies toward a theory of human stereopsis. *Artificial Intelligence,* **17,** 349–386. (342)

Mayhew, J. E. W., & Longuet-Higgins, H. C. (1982) A computational model of binocular depth perception. *Nature (London)* **297,** 376–379. (347)

McCann, J. J., McKee, S. P., & Taylor, T. H. (1976) Quantitative studies in Retinex theory. A comparison between theoretical predictions and observer responses to the "Color Mondrian" experiment. *Vision Research,* **16,** 445–458. (68)

McIlwain, J. T. (1966) Some evidence concerning the periphery effect in cat's retina. *Experimental Brain Research,* **1,** 265–271. (62)

McKee, S. P., & Nakayama, K. (1984) The detection of motion in the peripheral visual field. *Vision Research,* **24,** 25–32. (239)

McLauchlan, P., Zisserman, A., & Blake, A. (1987) Knowledge source for describing stereoscopically viewed textured surfaces. *Images & Vision Computing,* **5,** 105–110. (344)

Meadows, J. C. (1974) Disturbed perception of colours associated with localized cerebral lesions. *Brain,* **97,** 615–632. (201)

Medjbeur, S., & Tulunay-Keesey, U. (1985) Spatiotemporal responses of the visual system in demyelinating disease. *Brain,* **108,** 123–138. (410)

Meeteren, A. van (1978) On the detective quantum efficiency of the human eye. *Vision Research,* **18,** 257–267. (55)

Merigan, W. H. (1989) Chromatic and achromatic vision of macaques: Role of the P pathway. *Journal of Neuroscience,* **9,** 776–783. (119)

Merigan, W. H., & Eskin, T. A. (1986) Spatio-temporal vision of macaques with severe loss of P_β retinal ganglion cells. *Vision Research,* **26,** 1751–1761. (119)

Merigan, W. H., & Pasternak, T. (1983) APB affects increment and decrement thresholds of macaques. *Investigative Ophthalmology & Visual Science, Supplement 3,* **24,** 144. (159)

Metzger, W. (1953) *Gesetze des Sehens.* Frankfurt/M: W. Kramer. (275)

Metzger, W. (1975) *Gesetze des Sehens.* Frankfurt/M: W. Kramer. (275)

Michael, C. R. (1978) Colour sensitive complex cells in monkey striate cortex. *Journal of Neurophysiology,* **41,** 1250–1266. (288)

Mikami, A., Newsome, W. T., & Wurtz, R. H. (1986) Motion selectivity in macaque visual cortex. II. Spatiotemporal range of directional interactions in MT and V1. *Journal of Neurophysiology,* **55,** 1328–1339. (213–214, 216)

Milewski, A. E. (1976) Infants' discrimination of internal and external pattern elements. *Journal of Experimental Child Psychology,* **22,** 229–246. (361)

Miller, M., Pasik, P., & Pasik, P. (1981) Extrageniculostriate vision in the monkey IV: Contrast sensitivity functions. *Journal of Neurophysiology,* **43,** 1510–1526. (410)

Miller, W. H., & Bernard, G. D. (1983) Averaging over the foveal receptor aperture curtails aliasing. *Vision Research,* **23,** 1365–1370. (116)

Minkowski, J., Palese, M., & Guyton, D. (1983) Potential acuity meter using a minute aerial pinhole aperture. *Ophthalmology,* **90,** 1360–1368. (397)

Mishkin, M. (1972) Cortical visual areas and their interactions. In A. G. Karczmar & J. C. Eccles (Eds.), *Brain and Human Behavior,* pp. 187–208. Berlin: Springer-Verlag. (284)

Mishkin, M. (1982) A memory system in the monkey. *Philosophical Transactions of the Royal Society of London, Series B*, **298,** 85–95. (127)

Mishkin, M., Ungerleider, L. G., & Macko, K. A. (1983) Object vision and spatial vision: Two critical pathways. *Trends in Neuroscience*, **6,** 414–417. (128, 196, 306)

Mitchell, D. E. (1988a) The extent of visual recovery from early monocular or binocular visual deprivation in kittens. *Journal of Physiology*, **395,** 639–660. (391)

Mitchell, D. E. (1988b) Animal models of human strabismic amblyopia: Some observations concerning the interpretation of the effects of surgically and optically induced strabismus in cats and monkeys. In. P. G. Shinkman (Ed.), *Advances in Neural and Behavioral Development, Vol. 3*, pp. 209–269. Norwood, NJ: Ablex. (392)

Mitchell, D. E., Cynader, M., & Movshon, J. A. (1977) Recovery from the effects of monocular deprivation in kittens. *Journal of Comparative Neurology*, **176,** 53–64. (391)

Mitchell, D. E., Freeman, R. D., Millodot, M., & Haegerstrom, G. (1973) Meridional amblyopia: Evidence for modification of the human visual system by early visual experience. *Vision Research*, **13,** 535–558. (395)

Mitchell, D. E., Giffin, F., & Timney, B. (1977) A behavioral technique for the rapid assessment of visual capabilities of kittens. *Perception*, **6,** 181–193. (28)

Mitchell, D. E., Murphy, K., Dzioba, H. A., & Horne, J. A. (1986) Optimization of visual recovery from early monocular deprivation: Implications for occlusion therapy in the treatment of amblyopia. *Clinical Vision Sciences*, **1,** 173–177. (393–394)

Mitchell, D. E., Murphy, K., & Kaye, M. G. (1984) The permanence of the visual recovery that follows reverse occlusion of monocularly deprived kittens. *Investigative Ophthalmology & Visual Science*, **25,** 908–917. (393)

Mitchell, D. E., & Timney, B. (1984) Postnatal development of function in the mammalian visual system. In I. Darian-Smith (Ed.), *Handbook of Physiology Section I: The Nervous System, Vol. 3, Part 1, Sensory Processes*, pp. 507–555. Bethesda, MD: American Physiological Society. (350, 389, 392, 395)

Mitchell, D. E., & Wilkinson, F. (1974) The effect of early astigmatism on the visual resolution of gratings. *Journal of Physiology*, **243,** 739–756. (395)

Mitchison, G. J., & McKee, S. P. (1985) Interpolation in stereoscopic matching. *Nature (London)* **315,** 402–404. (345)

Mitchison, G. J., & McKee, S. P. (1987a) The resolution of ambiguous stereoscopic matches by interpolation. *Vision Research*, **27,** 285–294. (345)

Mitchison, G. J., & McKee, S. P. (1987b) Interpolation and the detection of fine structure in stereoscopic matching. *Vision Research*, **27,** 295–302. (345)

Mohindra, I., Held, R., Gwiazda, J., & Brill, S. (1978) Astigmatism in infants. *Science*, **202,** 329–331. (361)

Mohler, C. W., & Wurtz, R. H. (1977) Role of striate cortex and superior colliculus in visual guidance of saccadic eye movements in monkeys. *Journal of Neurophysiology*, **40,** 74–94. (411)

Mollon, J. D., Bowmaker, J. K., & Jacobs, G. H. (1984) Variations of colour vision in a New World primate can be explained by polymorphism of retinal photopigments. *Proceedings of the Royal Society of London, Series B*, **322,** 373–399. (36, 37, 38, 176)

Mollon, J. D., & Polden, P. G. (1977) Saturation of a retinal cone mechanism. *Nature (London)* **265,** 243–246. (187–188)

Mollon, J. D., & Polden, P. S. (1979) Post-receptoral adaptation. *Vision Research*, **19,** 435–440. (67)

Mollon, J. D., Newcombe, F., Polden, P. G., & Ratcliff, G. (1980) On the presence of three cone mechanisms in a case of total achromatopsia. In G. Verriest (Ed.), *Colour Vision Deficiencies*, pp. 130–135. Bristol: A. Hilger. (201, 203)

Moran, J., & Desimone, R. (1985) Selective attention gates visual processing in the extrastriate cortex. *Science*, **229,** 782–784. (312, 316)

Morgan, M. J., & Moulden, B. (1986) The Münsterberg figure and twisted cords. *Vision Research*, **26,** 1793–1800. (420)

Morrone, M. C., & Burr, D. C. (1988) Feature detection in human vision: A phase-dependent energy model. *Proceedings of the Royal Society of London, Series B*, **235,** 221–245. (160)

Morrone, M. C., Ross, J., Burr, D. C., & Owens, R. (1986) Mach bands are phase dependent. *Nature (London)* **324,** 250–253. (135, 160)

Motter, B. C., & Mountcastle, V. B. (1981) The functional properties of the light-sensitive neurons of the posterior parietal cortex studied in waking monkeys: Foveal sparing and opponent vector organization. *Journal of Neuroscience*, **1,** 3–26. (226)

Mountcastle, V. B. (1976) The world around us. Neural command functions for selective attention. *Neuroscience Research Program Bulletin*, **14,** Supplement. (454)

Mountcastle, V. B. (1978) Brain mechanisms for directed attention. *Journal of the Royal Society of Medicine*, **71,** 14–28. (365)

Mountcastle, V. B., Andersen, R. A., & Motter, B. C. (1981) The influence of attentive fixation upon the excitability of the light-sensitive neurons of the posterior parietal cortex. *Journal of Neuroscience*, **1,** 1218–1235. (306)

Mountcastle, V. B., Motter, B. C., Steinmetz, M. A., & Sestokas, A. K. (1987) Common and differential effects of attentive fixation on the excitability of parietal and prestriate (V4) cortical visual neurons in the macaque monkey. *Journal of Neuroscience*, **7,** 2239–2255. (312)

Movshon, J. A. (1976) Reversal of the physiological effects of monocular deprivation in the kitten's visual cortex. *Journal of Physiology*, **261,** 125–174. (391)

Movshon, J. A., Adelson, E. H., Gizzi, M. S., & Newsome, W. T. (1985) The analysis of moving patterns. *Experimental Brain Research, Supplement*, **11,** 117–151. (287)

Movshon, J. A., Adelson, E. H., Gizzi, M. S., & Newsome, W. T. (1986) The analysis of moving patterns. In C. Chagas,

R. Gattass & C. Gross (Eds.), *Pattern Recognition Mechanisms,* pp. 117–151. Berlin: Springer-Verlag. (126, 208, 225–226, 288)

Movshon, J. A., Thompson, I. D., & Tolhurst, D. J. (1978a) Spatial summation in the receptive fields of simple cells in the cat's striate cortex. *Journal of Physiology,* **283,** 53–77. (26, 30, 242)

Movshon, J. A., Thompson, I. D., & Tolhurst, D. J. (1978b) Receptive field organization of complex cells in the cat's striate cortex. *Journal of Physiology,* **283,** 79–99. (30, 31, 243)

Movshon, J. A., Thompson, I. D., & Tolhurst, D. J. (1978c) Spatial and temporal contrast sensitivity of neurones in areas 17 and 18 of cat's visual cortex. *Journal of Physiology,* **283,** 101–120. (418)

Movshon, J. A., & Van Sluyters, R. C. (1981) Visual neural development. *Annual Review of Psychology,* **32,** 477–522. (26, 350, 369)

Müller, F., Wässle, H., & Voigt, T. (1988) Pharmacological manipulation of the rod pathway in the cat retina. *Journal of Neurophysiology,* **59,** 1657–1672. (145)

Müller, G. E. (1896) Zur Psychophysik der Gesichtsempfindungen. *Zeitschrift für Psychologie und Physiologie der Sinnesorgane,* **10,** 1–82. (12, 14)

Mullen, K. T. (1987) Spatial influences on colour opponent contributions to pattern detection. *Vision Research,* **27,** 829–839. (189, 193)

Murphy, K. M., & Mitchell, D. E. (1987) Reduced visual acuity in both eyes of monocularly deprived kittens following a short or long period of reverse occlusion. *Journal of Neuroscience,* **7,** 1526–1536. (393)

Nachmias, J., & Sansbury, R. V. (1974) Grating contrast: Discrimination may be better than detection. *Vision Research,* **14,** 1039–1042. (247, 254)

Naka, K. I., & Rushton, W. A. (1966) S-potentials from colour units in the retina of fish *(Cyprinidae). Journal of Physiology,* **185,** 587–599. (72, 172)

Nakayama, K. (1985) Biological image motion processing: A review. *Vision Research,* **25,** 625–660. (207, 225–226)

Nakayama, K., & Silverman, G. (1984) Temporal and spatial characteristics of the upper displacement limit for motion in random dots. *Vision Research,* **24,** 293–299. (215)

Nakayama, K., & Silverman, G. H. (1986) Serial and parallel processing of visual feature conjunctions. *Nature (London)* **320,** 264–265. (306)

Nathans, J. (1987) Molecular biology of visual pigments. *Annual Review of Neuroscience,* **10,** 163–194. (38, 176)

Nathans, J., Piantanida, T. P., Eddy, R. L., Shows, T. B., & Hogness, D. S. (1986) Molecular genetics of inherited variation in color vision. *Science,* **232,** 203–210. (163, 176, 383)

Nathans, J., Thomas, D., & Hogness, D. S. (1986) Molecular genetics of human color vision: The genes encoding blue, green, and red pigments. *Science,* **232,** 193–202. (163, 176, 383)

Neisser, U. (1963) Decision time without reaction time: Experiments in visual scanning. *American Journal of Psychology,* **76,** 376–385. (276)

Neitz, J., & Jacobs, G. H. (1986a) Polymorphism of the long-wavelength cone in normal human colour vision. *Nature (London)* **323,** 623–625. (176)

Neitz, J., & Jacobs, G. H. (1986b) Reexamination of spectral mechanisms in the rat (*Rattus norvegicus*). *Journal of Comparative Psychology,* **100,** 21–29. (34)

Neitz, J., Neitz, M., & Jacobs, G. H. (1987) Color vision polymorphism in normal males: Relation to number of X-chromosome pigment genes. *Investigative Ophthalmology & Visual Science, Supplement,* **28,** 211. (176)

Nelson, J. I. & Frost, B. J. (1978) Orientation selective inhibition from beyond the classic visual receptive field. *Brain Research,* **139,** 359–365. (62)

Nelson, R. (1977) Cat cones have rod input: A comparison of the response properties of cone-horizontal cell bodies in the retina of the cat. *Journal of Comparative Neurology,* **172,** 109–136. (85)

Nelson, R., Famiglietti, E. V., Jr., & Kolb, H. (1978) Intracellular staining reveals different levels of stratification for ON- and OFF-center ganglion cells in the cat retina. *Journal of Neurophysiology,* **41,** 472–483. (113, 143)

Neuhaus, W. (1930) Experimentelle Untersuchung der Scheinbewegung. *Archiv für die gesamte Psychologie,* **75,** 315–418. (210)

Neumeyer, C. (1980) Simultaneous color contrast in the honeybee. *Journal of Comparative Physiology,* **139,** 165–176. (38)

Neumeyer, C. (1981) Chromatic adaptation in the honeybee: Successive color contrast and color constancy. *Journal of Comparative Physiology,* **144,** 543–553. (38)

Neumeyer, C. (1984) On spectral sensitivity in the goldfish: Evidence for neural interactions between "cone mechanisms." *Vision Research,* **24,** 1123–1231. (40, 43)

Neumeyer, C. (1985) An ultra-violet receptor as a fourth receptor type in goldfish color vision. *Naturwissenschaften,* **72,** 162–163. (40, 42)

Neumeyer, C. (1986) Wavelength discrimination in the goldfish. *Journal of Comparative Physiology,* **158,** 203–213. (39, 40–41)

Neumeyer, C. (1988) *Das Farbensehen des Goldfisches. Eine verhaltensphysiologische Analyse.* Stuttgart: Thieme. (42)

Newsome, W. T., & Pare, E. B. (1988) A selective impairment of motion processing following lesions of the middle temporal visual area (MT). *Journal of Neuroscience,* **8,** 2201–2211. (126, 220, 287)

Newsome, W. T., & Wurtz, R. H. (1988) Probing visual cortical function with discrete chemical lesions. *Trends in Neuroscience,* **11,** 394–400. (230)

Newsome, W. T., Wurtz, R. H., Dursteler, M. R., & Mikami, A. (1985) Deficits in visual motion processing following ibotenic acid lesions of the middle temporal visual area of the macaque monkey. *Journal of Neuroscience,* **5,** 825–840. (126, 220)

Nielsen, K. R. K., Watson, A. B., & Ahumada, A. J. (1985) Application of a computable model of human spatial vision to phase discrimination. *Journal of the Optical Society of America A,* **2,** 1600–1606. (259–260)

Niemeyer, G., & Gouras, P. (1973) Rod and cone signals in S-potentials of the isolated perfused cat eye. *Vision Research,* **13,** 1603–1612. (87)

Nikara, T., Bishop, P. O., & Pettigrew, J. D. (1968) Analysis of retinal correspondence by studying receptive fields of binocular single units in cat striate cortex. *Experimental Brain Research,* **6,** 353–372. (322)

Nishihara, H. K. (1987) Practical real time imaging stereo matcher. In M. A. Fischler & O. Firschein (Eds.), *Readings in Computer Vision,* pp. 63–72. Los Altos, CA: Kauffman. (268)

Noorlander, C., Koonderink, J. J., Den Ouden, R. J., & Edens, B. W. (1983) Sensitivity to spatiotemporal colour contrast in the peripheral visual field. *Vision Research,* **23,** 1–11. (175)

Norcia, A. M., & Tyler, C. W. (1985) Spatial frequency sweep VEP: Visual acuity in the first year of life. *Vision Research,* **25,** 1399–1408. (350, 360)

Norcia, A. M., Tyler, C. W., & Allen, D. (1986) Electrophysiological assessment of contrast sensitivity in human infants. *American Journal of Optometry and Physiological Optics,* **63,** 12–15. (350)

Nordby, K., Stabell, B., & Stabell, U. (1984) Dark-adaptation of the human rod system. *Vision Research,* **24,** 841–849. (70)

Normann, R. A., & Anderton, P. J. (1983) The incremental sensitivity curve of turtle cone photoreceptors. *Vision Research,* **23,** 1731–1733. (59)

Normann, R. A., & Werblin, F. S. (1974) Control of retinal sensitivity. I. Light and dark adaptation of vertebrate rods and cones. *Journal of General Physiology,* **63,** 37–61. (74)

Nothdurft, H. C. (1985a) Orientation sensitivity and texture segmentation in patterns with different line orientation. *Vision Research,* **25,** 551–560. (297)

Nothdurft, H. C. (1985b) Sensitivity for structure gradient in texture discrimination tasks. *Vision Research,* **25,** 1957–1968. (297)

Nothdurft, H. C., & Li, C. Y. (1985) Texture discrimination: Representation of orientation and luminance differences in cells of the cat striate cortex. *Vision Research,* **25,** 99–113. (285, 289, 291, 462)

Nunn, B. J., Schnapf, J. L. & Baylor, D. A. (1984) Spectral sensitivity of single cones in the retina of *Macaca fascicularis. Nature (London)* **309,** 264–266. (172)

Nyman, G., Greenlee, M. W., & Laurinen, P. (1988) Sampling irregularity perturbs visual reconstruction. *Journal of the Optical Society of America A,* **5,** 628–635. (262)

O'Brien, B., & Miller, N. (1953) A study of the mechanism of visual acuity in the central retina. *Wright Air Development Center, WACD Technical Report* **5,** 53–198. Ohio: Wright-Patterson Air Force Base. (385)

O'Brien, V. (1958) Contour perception, illusion and reality. *Journal of the Optical Society of America,* **48,** 112–119. (137)

Oehler, R. (1985) Spatial interactions in the rhesus monkey retina: A behavioural study using the Westheimer paradigm. *Experimental Brain Research,* **59,** 217–225. (44, 141)

Ogden, T. E., & Miller, R. F. (1966) Studies of the optic nerve of the rhesus monkey: Nerve fiber spectrum and physiological properties. *Vision Research,* **6,** 485–506. (107, 118)

Ogle, K. N. (1950) *Reseaches in Binocular Vision.* Philadelphia: W. B. Saunders. (23, 270, 317–318, 324, 331–332, 347)

Ogle, K. N. (1964) *Researches in Binocular Vision.* New York: Hafner. (318)

Ogle, K. N., Martens, T. G., & Dyer, J. A. (1967) *Oculomotor Imbalance in Binocular Vision and Fixation Disparity.* London: Kimpton. (318)

Olson, C. R., & Freeman, R. D. (1980) Profile of the sensitive period for monocular deprivation in kittens. *Experimental Brain Research,* **39,** 17–21. (390)

Olson, R., & Attneave, F. (1970) What variables produce similarity grouping? *American Journal of Psychology,* **83,** 1–21. (275)

Olzak, L. A., & Thomas, J. (1986) Seeing spatial patterns. In K. Boff, L. Kaufman & J. Thomas (Eds.) *Handbook of Perception and Human Performance: Vol. 1, Sensory Processes and Perception,* pp. 1–7, 7–56. New York: Wiley-Interscience. (154, 156)

Onley, J. W., & Boynton, R. M. (1962) Visual responses to equally-bright stimuli of unequal luminance. *Journal of Optical Society of America,* **52,** 934–940. (62)

Oppenheim, A. V., & Lim, J. S. (1981) The importance of phase in signals. *Proceedings of the IEEE,* **69,** 529–541. (424)

Orban, G. A. (1985) Velocity tuned cortical cells and human velocity discrimination. In D. J. Ingle, M. Jeannerod & D. N. Lee (Eds.), *Brain Mechanisms and Spatial Vision,* pp. 371–388. (NATO ASI Series, Series D: Behavioural and Social Sciences, No. 21.) Dordrecht: Nijhoff. (222–223)

Orban, G. A. (1986) Processing of moving images in the geniculocortical pathway. In J. D. Pettigrew, K. J. Sanderson & W. R. Levick (Eds.), *Visual Neuroscience,* pp. 121–141. Cambridge: Cambridge University Press. (229)

Orban, G. A., DeWolf, J., & Maes, H. (1984) Factors influencing velocity coding in the human visual system. *Vision Research,* **24,** 33–39. (222)

Orban, G. A., & Gulyas, B. (1988) Image segregation by motion: Cortical mechanisms and implementation in neural networks. In R. Eckmiller & C. v.d. Malsburg (Eds.), *Neural Computers,* pp. 149–159. Heidelberg: Springer-Verlag. (223, 225)

Orban, G. A., Gulyas, B., & Spileers, W. (1988) Influence of moving textured backgrounds on responses of cat Area 18 cells to moving bars. *Progress in Brain Research,* **75,** 137–145. (221)

Orban, G. A., Gulyas, B., Spileers, W., & Maes, H. (1987) Responses of cat striate neurons to moving light and dark bars: Changes with eccentricity. *Journal of the Optical Society of America A,* **4,** 1653–1665. (221)

Orban, G. A., Gulyas, B., & Vogels, R. (1987) Influence of a moving textured background on direction selectivity of cat striate neurons. *Journal of Neurophysiology,* **57,** 1792–1812. (221, 224)

Orban, G. A., Kennedy, H., & Maes, H. (1981) Response to movement of neurons in Areas 17 and 18 of the cat: Velocity sensitivity. *Journal of Neurophysiology,* **45,** 1059–1073. (221–222)

Orban, G. A., Spileers, W., Gulyás, B., & Bishop, P. O. (1986) Motion in depth selectivity of cortical cells revisited. *Society of Neuroscience Abstracts,* **12,** 584. (338)

Orban, G. A., Van Calenbergh, F., DeBruyn, B., & Maes, H. (1985) Velocity discrimination in central and peripheral visual field. *Journal of the Optical Society of America A,* **2,** 1836–1847. (223)

Orban, G. A., Vandenbussche, E., & Vogels, R. (1984) Human orientation discrimination tested with long stimuli. *Vision Research,* **24,** 121–128. (261)

Østerberg, G. (1935) Topography of the layer of rods and cones in the human retina. *Acta Ophthalmologica, Supplement,* **6,** 1–103. (175, 232)

Ouchi, H. (1977) "Japanese and Geometrical Art." Dover, New York.

Owsley, C. (1983) The role of motion in infants' perception of solid shape. *Perception,* **12,** 707–718. (307)

Oyama, T., Furusaka, T., & Kito, T. (1979) Color vision in men and animals. *Scientific American (Japanese Edition),* December, 98–110. (171)

Oyster, C. W., & Barlow, H. B. (1967) Direction selective units in rabbit retina: Distribution of preferred directions. *Science,* **155,** 841–842. (377)

Pantle, A., & Sekuler, R. (1968) Size detecting mechanisms in human vision. *Science,* **162,** 1146–1148. (246, 250)

Parker, A., & Hawken, M. (1985) Capabilities of monkey cortical cells in spatial resolution tasks. *Journal of the Optical Society of America A,* **2,** 1101–1114. (258, 393, 421)

Parks, E., & Pendergrass, L. (1982) On the filtered-compounds approach to illusory contours. *Perception & Psychophysics,* **32,** 491–493. (292)

Parkwood, J., & Gordon, B. (1975) Stereopsis in normal domestic cats, Siamese cats, and cats raised with alternating monocular occlusion. *Journal of Neurophysiology,* **38,** 1485–1499. (395)

Partlow, G. D., Colonnier, M., & Szabo, J. (1977) Thalamic projections of the superior colliculus in the rhesus monkey *Macaca mulatta.* A light and electron microscopic study. *Journal of Comparative Neurology,* **171,** 285–318. (411)

Pasternak, T. (1986) The role of cortical directional selectivity in detection of motion and flicker. *Vision Research,* **26,** 1187–1194. (220)

Pasternak, T. (1987) Discrimination of differences in speed and flicker rate depends on directionally selective mechanisms. *Vision Research,* **27,** 1881–1890. (220, 223)

Pasternak, T., & Leinen, L. J. (1986) Pattern and motion vision in cats with selective loss of cortical directional selectivity. *Journal of Neuroscience,* **6,** 938–945. (220)

Pasternak, T., & Merigan, W. H. (1981) The luminance dependence of spatial vision in the cat. *Vision Research,* **21,** 1333–1339. (31, 94)

Pasternak, T., Schumer, R. A., Gizzi, M. S., & Movshon, J. A. (1985) Abolition of visual cortical direction selectivity affects visual behavior in cats. *Experimental Brain Research,* **61,** 214–217. (31)

Pastore, N. (1971) *Selective History of Theories of Visual Perception,* pp. 1650–1950. New York: Oxford University Press. (275)

Patel, A. (1966) Spatial resolution by the human visual system: The effect of mean retinal illuminance. *Journal of the Optical Society of America,* **56,** 689–694. (155)

Patterson, R., & Fox, R. (1984) Stereopsis during continuous head motion. *Vision Research,* **24,** 2001–2003. (331)

Peek, S. A., Mayhew, J. E. W., & Frisby, J. P. (1984) Obtaining viewing distance and angle of gaze from vertical disparity using a Hough-type accumulator. *Image & Vision Computing,* **2,** 180–190. (346)

Peichl, L., & Wässle, H. (1979) Size, scatter and coverage of ganglion cell receptive field centres in the cat retina. *Journal of Physiology,* **291,** 117–141. (92)

Peichl, L., & Wässle, H. (1981) Morphological identification of on- and off-centre brisk transient (Y) cells in the cat retina. With an appendix 'Neurofibrillar staining of cat retinae,' by B. B. Boycott & L. Peichl. *Proceedings of the Royal Society of London, Series B,* **212,** 139–156. (112, 143)

Perenin, M. T. (1978) Visual function within the hemianopic field following early cerebral hemidecortication in man. II. Pattern discrimination. *Neuropsychologia,* **16,** 697–708. (414)

Perenin, M. T., & Jeannerod, M. (1975) Residual vision in cortically blind hemifields. *Neuropsychologia,* **13,** 1–7. (411, 414)

Perenin, M. T., & Jeannerod, M. (1978) Visual function within the hemianopic field following early cerebral hemidecortication in man. I. Spatial localisation. *Neuropsychologia,* **16,** 1–13. (411–413, 415)

Perenin, M. T., & Jeannerod, M. (1983) Are extrageniculostriate pathways nonfunctional in man? *Behavioral and Brain Sciences,* **6,** 458–459. (415)

Perrett, D. I., Harries, M., Mistlin, A. J., & Chitty, A. J. (1989) Three stages in the classification of body movements by visual neurons. In H. B. Barlow, C. Blakemore & M. Weston-Smith, (Eds.), *Images and Understanding.* Cambridge: Cambridge University Press. (288)

Perrett, D. I., Rolls, E. T., & Caan, W. (1982) Visual neurons responsive to faces in the monkey temporal cortex. *Experimental Brain Research,* **47,** 329–342. (288, 307)

Perry, N. W., & Childers, D. G. (1969) *The Human Visual Evoked Response.* Springfield, Illinois: Charles C. Thomas Publishers. (408)

Perry, V. H., & Cowey, A. (1984) Retinal ganglion cells that project to the superior colliculus and pretectum in the macaque monkey. *Neuroscience,* **12,** 1125–1137. (106)

Perry, V. H., & Cowey, A. (1985) The ganglion cell and cone distributions in the monkey's retina: Implications for central magnification factors. *Vision Research,* **25,** 1795–1810. (117–118, 232, 235)

Perry, V. H., & Cowey, A. (1988) The lengths of the fibres of Henle in the retina of macaque monkeys: Implications for vision. *Neuroscience,* **25,** 225–236. (117)

Perry, V. H., Oehler, R., & Cowey, A. (1984) Retinal ganglion cells that project to the dorsal lateral geniculate nucleus in the macaque monkey. *Neuroscience,* **12,** 1101–1123. (106, 107, 113, 117–118, 141, 200)

Perry, V. H., & Silveira, L. C. L. (1988) Functional lamination in the ganglion cell layer of the macaque's retina. *Neuroscience,* **25,** 217–224. (143)

Peterhans, E., & von der Heydt, R. (1989) Mechanisms of contour perception in monkey visual cortex. II. Contours bridging gaps. *Journal of Neuroscience,* in press. (289)

Peterhans, E., von der Heydt, R., & Baumgartner, G. (1986) Neuronal responses to illusory contours stimuli reveal stages of visual cortical processing. In J. D. Pettigrew, K. J. Sanderson & W. R. Levick (Eds.), *Visual Neuroscience,* pp. 343–351. Cambridge: Cambridge University Press. (137, 292–293)

Petersik, J. T., Hicks, K. I., & Pantle, A. J. (1978) Apparent movement of successively generated subjective figures. *Perception,* **7,** 371–383. (293)

Petrig, B., Julesz, B., Kropfl, W., Baumgartner, G., & Anliker, M. (1981) Development of stereopsis and cortical binocularity in human infants: Electrophysiological evidence. *Science,* **213,** 1402–1405. (362, 371)

Petry, S., & Meyer, G. (1987) *The Perception of Illusory Contours.* New York: Springer-Verlag. (438)

Pettigrew, J. D. (1973) Binocular neurons which signal change of disparity in area 18 of cat visual cortex. *Nature (London)* **241,** 123–124. (335)

Pettigrew, J. D. (1974) The effect of visual experience on the development of stimulus specificity by kitten cortical neurones. *Journal of Physiology,* **237,** 49–74. (372)

Pettigrew, J. D., Nikara, T., & Bishop, P. O. (1968) Binocular interaction on single units in cat striate cortex: Simultaneous stimulation by single moving slits with receptive fields in correspondence. *Experimental Brain Research,* **6,** 391–410. (23)

Phillips, G. C., & Wilson, H. R. (1984) Orientation bandwidths of spatial mechanisms measured by masking. *Journal of the Optical Society of America A,* **1,** 226–232. (32, 248, 254)

Piantanida, T. P. (1986) Stereo hysteresis revisited. *Vision Research,* **26,** 431–437. (331)

Piccolino, M., Neyton, J., & Gerschenfeld, H. M. (1984) Decrease of gap junction permeability induced by dopamine and cyclic adenosine 3′5′-monophosphate in horizontal cells of turtle retina. *Journal of Neuroscience,* **10,** 2477–2488. (386)

Piotrowski, L. N., & Campbell, F. W. (1982) A demonstration of the visual importance and flexibility of spatial-frequency amplitude and phase. *Perception,* **11,** 337–346. (424)

Pirchio, M., Spinelli, D., Fiorentini, A., & Maffei, L. (1978) Infant contrast sensitivity evaluated by evoked potentials. *Brain Research,* **141,** 179–184. (350)

Pitt, F. H. G. (1935) *Characteristics of Dichromatic Vision with An Appendix on Anomalous Trichromatic Vision.* Medical Research Council Special Report, No. 200. London. (381–382)

Poggio, G. F. (1984) Processing of stereoscopic information in monkey visual cortex. In G. M. Edelman, W. E. Gall & W. M. Cowan (Eds.), *Dynamic Aspects of Neocortical Function,* pp. 613–635. New York, Wiley. (287, 322–323, 325)

Poggio, G. F. (1989) Neural responses serving stereopsis in the visual cortex of the alert macaque monkey: Position-disparity and image-correlation. In J. S. Lund. (Ed.), *Sensory Processing in the Mammalian Brain: Neural Substrates and Experimental Strategies,* pp. 226–241. Oxford: Oxford University Press. (329)

Poggio, G. F., & Fischer, B. (1977) Binocular interaction and depth sensitivity in striate and prestriate cortex of behaving rhesus monkey. *Journal of Neurophysiology,* **40,** 1392–1405. (270, 287, 321–322, 326)

Poggio, G. F., Gonzalez, F., & Krause, F. (1988) Stereoscopic mechanisms in monkey visual cortex: Binocular correlation and disparity selectivity. *Journal of Neuroscience,* **8,** 4531–4550. (328–329)

Poggio, G. F., Motter, B. C., Squatrito, S., & Trotter, Y. (1985) Responses of neurons in visual cortex (V1 and V2) of the alert macaque to dynamic random-dot stereograms. *Vision Research,* **25,** 397–406. (269, 289, 322)

Poggio, G. F., & Poggio, T. (1984) The analysis of stereopsis. *Annual Review of Neuroscience,* **7,** 379–412. (322–323, 326, 342, 347)

Poggio, T., & Reichardt, W. (1973) Considerations on models of movement detection. *Kybernetik,* **13,** 223–227. (207)

Poggio, G. F., & Talbot, W. H. (1981) Mechanism of static and dynamic stereopsis in foveal cortex of the rhesus monkey. *Journal of Physiology,* **315,** 469–492. (325–326, 335–337)

Pohl, W. (1973) Dissociation of spatial discrimination deficits following frontal and parietal lesions in monkeys. *Journal of Comparative Physiology and Psychology,* **82,** 227–239. (284)

Pokorny, J., Smith, V. C., & Ernest, J. T. (1980) Macular color vision defects: Specialized psychophysical testing in acquired and hereditary chorio-retinal diseases. *International Ophthalmology Clinics,* **20,** 53–81. (400)

Pokorny, J., Smith, V. C., Verriest, G., & Pinckers, A. J. L. G. (1979) *Congenital and Acquired Color Vision Defects.* New York: Grune & Stratton. (37, 38, 404)

Polden, P. G., & Mollon, J. D. (1980) Reversed effect of adapting stimuli on visual sensitivity. *Proceedings of the Royal Society of London, Series B,* **210,** 235–272. (187)

Pollard, S. B. (1987) The PMF stereo algorithm: Theory and implementation. *British Computer Society Parallel Architectures and Computer Vision Workshop.* Oxford: Oxford University Press. (342, 345)

Pollard, S. B., Mayhew, J. E. W., & Frisby, J. P. (1985) PMF: A stereo correspondence algorithm using a disparity gradient limit. *Perception,* **14,** 449–470. (341–342)

Pollard, S. B., Porrill, J., Mayhew, J. E. W., & Frisby, J. P. (1985) Disparity gradient, Lipschitz continuity and computing stereo correspondences. *Proceedings of the Third International Symposium of Robotics Research, Gouvieux, France,* pp. 19–26. Cambridge, MA: M.I.T. Press. (342–343, 347)

Pollard, S. B., Porrill, J., Mayhew, J. E. W., & Frisby, J. P. (1987) Matching geometrical descriptions in three-space. *Image & Vision Computing,* **5,** 73–78. (344)

Pollen, D. A., & Ronner, S. E. (1981) Phase relationships between adjacent simple cells in the visual cortex. *Science,* **212,** 1409–1411. (160, 249, 418)

Pollen, D. A., & Ronner, S. F. (1983) Visual cortical neurons as localized spatial frequency filters. *IEEE Transactions on Systems, Man, and Cybernetics,* **SMC-13,** 907–916. (249)

Polyak, S. L. (1941) *The Retina.* Chicago: University of Chicago Press. (88, 105)

Polyak, S. L. (1957) *The Vertebrate Visual System.* Chicago: University of Chicago Press. (23, 43)

Pöppel, E. (1986) Long-range colour-generating interaction across the retina. *Nature (London),* **320,** 523–525. (62)

Pöppel, E., Held, R., & Frost, D. (1973) Residual visual function after brain wounds involving the central visual pathways in man. *Nature (London)* **243,** 295–296. (411)

Pöppel, E., & Richards, W. (1974) Light sensitivity in cortical scotoma contralateral to small islands of blindness. *Experimental Brain Research,* **21,** 125–130. (414)

Porciatti, V., & von Berger, G. P. (1984) Pattern electroretinogram and visual evoked potenial in optic nerve disease: Early diagnosis and prognosis. *Documenta Ophthalmologica Proceedings Series,* **40,** 117–126. (408)

Porrill, J., Mayhew, J. E. W., & Frisby, J. P. (1987) Cyclotorsion, conformal invariance, and induced effects in stereoscopic vision. In *Frontiers of Visual Science: Proceedings of the 1985 Symposium,* pp. 90–108. Washington, D.C.: National Academy Press. (347)

Porrill, J., Pollard, S. B., Pridmore, T. P., Bowen, J. B., Mayhew, J. E. W., & Frisby, J. P. (1987) TINA: The Sheffield AIVRU vision system. *Proceedings of the Tenth International Joint Conference on Artificial Intelligence,* **2,** 1138–1144. (345)

Posner, M. I., Cohen, Y., & Rafal, R. D. (1982) Neural systems control of spatial orienting. *Philosophical Transactions of the Royal Society of London, Series B,* **298,** 187–198. (314)

Posner, M. I., Walker, J. A., Friedrich, F. J., & Rafal, R. D. (1984) Effects of parietal injury on covert orienting of attention. *Journal Neuroscience,* **4,** 1863–1874. (314)

Prablanc, C., Echallier, J. F., Komilis, E., & Jeannerod, M. (1979) Optimal response of eye and hand motor systems in pointing at a visual target. I. Spatio-temporal characteristics of eye and hand movements and their relationships when varying the amount of visual information. *Biological Cybernetics,* **35,** 113–124. (413)

Prazdny, K. (1983) Illusory contours are not caused by simultaneous brightness contrast. *Perception & Psychophysics,* **34,** 403–404. (439)

Prazdny, K. (1985a) On the nature of inducing forms generating perception of illusory contours. *Perception & Psychophysics,* **37,** 237–242. (299)

Prazdny, K. (1985b) Detection of binocular disparities. *Biological Cybernetics,* **52,** 93–99. (342)

Prazdny, K. (1986a) Psychophysical and computational studies of random-dot Moire patterns. *Spatial Vision,* **1,** 231–242. (302)

Prazdny, K. (1986b) Illusory contours from inducers defined solely by spatiotemporal correlation. *Perception & Psychophysics,* **39,** 175–178. (302)

Prazdny, K. (1987a) Three-dimensional structure from long-range apparent motion. *Perception,* **15,** 619–626. (299)

Prazdny, K. (1987b) On the coarse-to-fine strategy in stereomatching. *Bulletin of the Psychonomic Society,* **25,** 92–94. (343)

Precht, W. (1982) Anatomical and functional organisation of optokinetic pathways. In G. Lennerstrand, D. S. Zee & E. L. Keller (Eds.), *Functional Basis of Ocular Motility Disorders,* pp. 291–302. Oxford: Pergamon. (374)

Precht, W., Montarolo, P. G., & Strata, P. (1980) The role of the crossed and uncrossed retinal fibers in mediating the horizontal optokinetic nystagmus in the cat. *Neuroscience Letters,* **17,** 39–42. (374)

Probst, T., Brandt, T., & Degner, D. (1986) Object-motion detection affected by concurrent self-motion perception: Psychophysics of a new phenomenon. *Behavioral and Brain Research,* **22,** 1–11. (228)

Probst, T., Krafczyk, S., & Brandt, T. (1987) Object-motion detection affected by concurrent self-motion perception: Applied aspects for vehicle guidance. *Ophthalmology and Physiological Optics,* **7,** 309–314. (227)

Probst, T., Krafcyzk, S., Brandt, T., & Wist, E. R. (1984) Interaction between perceived self-motion and object-motion impairs vehicle guidance. *Science,* **225,** 536–538. (227)

Ptito, A., Lassonde, M., Leporé, F., & Ptito, M. (1987) Visual discrimination in hemispherectomized patients. *Neuropsychologia,* **25,** 869–879. (414)

Pugh, E. N. (1975) Rushton's paradox: Rod dark adaptation after flash photolysis. *Journal of Physiology,* **248,** 413–431. (70)

Pugh, E. N. (1976) The nature of the π_1 colour mechanism of W. S. Stiles. *Journal of Physiology,* **257,** 713–747. (66)

Pugh, E. N., Jr., & Larimer, J. (1980) Test of the identity of the site of blue/yellow hue cancellation and the site of chromatic antagonism in the π_1 pathway. *Vision Research,* **20,** 779–788. (169)

Pugh, E. N., Jr., & Mollon, J. D. (1979) A theory of the π_1 and π_3 colour mechanisms of Stiles. *Vision Research,* **19,** 293–312. (67, 96, 187, 400)

Purkinje, J. (1823) *Beobachtungen und Versuche zur Physiologie der Sinne.* Prague: J. G. Clave. (2)

Purpura, K., Kaplan, E., & Shapley, R. M. (1988a) Background light and the contrast gain of primate P and M retinal ganglion cells. *Proceedings of the National Academy of Sciences U.S.A.,* **85,** 4534–4537. (119)

Purpura, K., Kaplan, E., & Shapley, R. (1988b) Contrast gain difference between primate P and M retinal ganglion cells enhanced at low light levels. *Proceedings of the National Academy of Sciences U.S.A.,* **85,** 4534–4537. (94)

Quam, L. H. (1987) Heirarchical warp stereo. In M. A. Fischler & O. Firschien (Eds.), *Readings in Computer Vision,* pp. 80–86. Los Altos, CA: Kauffman. (268)

Quigley, H. A. (1985) Early detection of glaucomatous damage: II. Changes in the appearance of the optic disc. *Survey of Ophthalmology,* **30,** 111–126. (397)

Quigley, H. A., Sanchez, R. M., Dunkelberger, G. R., L'Hernault, N. L., & Baginski, T. A. (1987) Chronic glaucoma selectively damages large optic nerve fibers. *Investigative Ophthalmology & Visual Science,* **28,** 913–920. (408)

Rakic, P. (1977) Prenatal development of the visual system in rhesus monkey. *Philosophical Transactions of the Royal Society of London, Series B,* **278,** 245–260. (367–368)

Rakic, P. (1981) Developmental events leading to laminar and areal organization of the neocortex. In F. O. Schmidt (Ed.), *The Organization of the Cerebral Cortex,* pp. 7–28. Boston: MIT Press. (368)

Ramachandran, V. S. (1985) Apparent motion of subjective surfaces. *Perception,* **14,** 127–134. (293)

Ramachandran, V. S. (1986a) Capture of stereopsis and apparent motion by illusory contours. *Perception & Psychophysics,* **39,** 361–373. (287, 293)

Ramachandran, V. S. (1986b) The neurobiology of perception. *Perception,* **14,** 97–103. (345)

Ramachandran, V. S. (1987a) Visual perception of surfaces: A biological theory. In S. J. Petry & G. E. Meyer (Eds.), *The Perception of Illusory Contours,* pp. 93–108. New York, Berlin, Heidelberg: Springer-Verlag. (280, 284, 287, 293)

Ramachandran, V. S. (1987b) Interaction between colour and motion in human vision. *Nature (London)* **328,** 645–647. (280, 293)

Ramachandran, V. S. (1988a) Perceiving shape from shading. *Scientific American,* **256**(6), 76–83. (279)

Ramachandran, V. S. (1988b) Perception of shape from shading. *Nature (London)* **331,** 163–166. (279)

Ramachandran, V. S., & Anstis, S. M. (1985) Perceptual organization in multistable apparent motion. *Perception,* **14,** 135–144. (219)

Ramachandran, V. S., & Anstis, S. M. (1986a) The perception of apparent motion. *Scientific American,* **254**(6), 102–109. (208, 217, 286)

Ramachandran, V. S., & Anstis, S. M. (1986b) Figure ground segregation modulates apparent motion. *Vision Research,* **26,** 1969–1975. (217, 286)

Ramachandran, V. S., Ginsburg, A. P., & Anstis, S. M. (1983) Low spatial frequencies dominate apparent motion. *Perception,* **12,** 457–462. (219)

Ramachandran, V. S., & Gregory, R. L. (1978) Does color provide an input to human motion perception? *Nature (London),* **275,** 55–56. (285, 302)

Ramachandran, V. S., Rao, V. M., & Vidyasagar, T. R. (1973a) Apparent movement with subjective contours. *Vision Research,* **13,** 1399–1401. (281, 301–302)

Ramachandran, V. S., Rao, V. M., & Vidyasagar, T. R. (1973b) The role of contours in stereopsis. *Nature (London),* **242,** 412–414. (281, 301–302)

Ramachandran, V. S. & Rogers-Ramachandran, D. C. (1988) Perceptual segregation and stereopsis. *Bulletin of the Psychonomics Society,* **26,** 488. (282)

Ramoa, A. S., Freeman, R. D., & Macy, A. (1985) Comparison of response properties of cells in the cat's visual cortex at high and low luminance levels. *Journal of Neurophysiology,* **54,** 61–72. (98)

Rand, L. I., Prud'homme, G. J., Ederer, F., & Canner, P. L. (1985) Factors influencing the development of visual loss in advanced diabetic retinopathy. *Investigative Ophthalmology & Visual Science,* **26,** 983–991. (396)

Ransom-Hogg, A., & Spillmann, L. (1980) Perceptive field size in fovea and periphery of the light- and dark-adapted retina. *Vision Research,* **20,** 221–228. (141, 151) 617.7

Rashbass, C. S., & Westheimer, G. (1961) Disjunctive eye movements. *Journal of Physiology,* **159,** 339–360. (330)

Ratliff, F. (1965) *Mach Bands: Quantitative Studies of Neural Networks in the Retina.* San Francisco, CA: Holden-Day. (134–135, 155)

Ratliff, F. (1984) Why Mach bands are not seen at the edges of a step. *Vision Research,* **24,** 163–165. (135)

Ratliff, F., & Hartline, H. K. (1959) The responses of *Limulus* optic nerve fibers to patterns of illumination on the retinal mosaic. *Journal of General Physiology,* **42,** 1241–1255. (134)

Rauschecker, J. P., & Singer, W. (1981) The effects of early visual experience on the cat's visual cortex and their possible explanation by Hebb synapses. *Journal of Physiology,* **310,** 215–239. (392)

Raviola, E., & Gilula, N. B. (1973) Gap junctions between photoreceptor cells in the vertebrate retina. *Proceedings of the National Academy of Sciences U.S.A.,* **70,** 1677–1681. (101)

Redies, C., & Spillmann, L. (1981) The neon color effect in the Ehrenstein illusion. *Perception,* **10,** 667–681. (443)

Redies, C., Crook, J. M., & Creutzfeldt, O. D. (1986) Neuronal responses to borders with and without luminance gradients in cat visual cortex and dorsal lateral geniculate nucleus. *Experimental Brain Research,* **61,** 469–481. (291)

Redies, C., Spillmann, L., & Kunz, K. (1984) Colored neon flanks and line gap enhancement. *Vision Research,* **24,** 1301–1309. (292, 443)

Reese, B. E., & Cowey, A. (1988) Segregation of functionally distinct axons in the monkeys optic tract. *Nature (London)* **337,** 350–357 (200)

Reese, B. E., & Guillery, R. W. (1987) Discrimination of axons according to diameter in monkeys optic tract. *Journal of Comparative Neurology,* **260,** 453–460. (200)

Reeves, A. (1981) Transient desensitization of a red–green opponent site. *Vision Research,* **21,** 1267–1277. (188)

Regan, D. (1980) Speedy evoked potential methods for assessing vision in normal and amblyopic eyes: Pros and cons. *Vision Research,* **30,** 265–269. (361)

Regan, D. (1986) Visual processing of four kinds of relative motion. *Vision Research,* **26,** 127–145. (274, 333)

Regan, D. (1989) *Human Brain Electrophysiology: Evoked Potentials and Evoked Magnetic Fields in Science and Medicine.* New York: Elsevier. (318, 332)

Regan, D., & Beverley, K. I. (1973a) Some dynamic features of depth perception. *Vision Research,* **13,** 2369–2379. (324, 326, 329)

Regan, D., & Beverley, K. I. (1973b) Disparity detectors in human depth perception: Evidence for directional selectivity. *Science,* **181,** 877–879. (333, 335)

Regan, D., & Beverley, K. I. (1979) Binocular and monocular stimuli for motion in depth: Changing-disparity and changing-size inputs feed the same motion-in-depth stage. *Vision Research,* **19,** 1331–1342. (332, 334)

Regan, D., & Beverley, K. I. (1983a) Spatial frequency discrimination and detection: Comparison of postadaptation thresholds. *Journal of the Optical Society of America,* **73,** 1684–1690. (257–258)

Regan, D., & Beverley, K. I. (1983b) Visual fields for frontal plane motion and for changing size. *Vision Research,* **23,** 673–676. (334)

Regan, D., & Beverley, K. I. (1985) Post-adaptation orientation thresholds. *Journal of the Optical Society of America A,* **2,** 147–155. (257–258)

Regan, D., Beverley, K. I., & Cynader, M. (1978) Stereoscopic subsystems for position in depth and for motion in depth. *Proceedings of Royal Society of London, Series B,* **204,** 485–501. (334)

Regan, D., Collewijn, H., & Erkelens, C. (1986) Necessary conditions for motion in depth perception. *Investigative Ophthalmology & Visual Science,* **27,** 584–597. (331, 334)

Regan, D., & Cynader, M. (1979) Neurons in area 18 of cat visual cortex selectively sensitive to changing size: Nonlinear interactions between responses to two edges. *Vision Research,* **19,** 699–711. (307)

Regan, D., & Cynader, M. (1982) Neurons in cat visual cortex tuned to the direction of motion in depth: Effect of stimulus speed. *Investigative Ophthalmology & Visual Science,* **22,** 535–550. (336)

Regan, D., Erkelens, C. J., & Collewijn, H. (1986) Visual field defects for vergence eye movements and for stereomotion perception. *Investigative Ophthalmology & Visual Science,* **27,** 806–819. (324, 337)

Regan, D., & Heron, J. R. (1969) Clinical investigation of lesions of the visual pathway: A new objective technique. *Journal of Neurology, Neurosurgery and Psychiatry,* **32,** 479–483. (409)

Regan, D., Milner, B. A., & Heron, J. R. (1976) Delayed visual perception and delayed visual evoked potentials in the spinal form of multiple sclerosis and in retrobulbar neuritis. *Brain,* **99,** 43–66. (409)

Regan, D., & Neima, D. (1984) Visual fatigue and visual evoked potentials in multiple sclerosis, glaucoma, ocular hypertension and Parkinson's disease. *Journal of Neurology, Neurosurgery and Psychiatry,* **47,** 673–678. (386–387)

Regan, D., Silver, R., & Murray, T. J. (1977) Visual acuity and contrast sensitivity in multiple sclerosis-hidden visual loss: An auxiliary diagnostic test. *Brain,* **100,** 563–579. (409)

Regan, D., Whitlock, J. A., Murray, T. J., & Beverley, K. I. (1980) Orientation-specific losses of contrast sensitivity in multiple sclerosis. *Investigative Ophthalmology & Visual Science,* **19,** 324–327. (409)

Reichardt, W. (1961) Autocorrelation, a principle for the evaluation of sensory information by the central nervous system. In W. A. Rosenblith (Ed.), *Sensory Communication,* pp. 303–317. Cambridge: MIT Press. (206)

Reichardt, W. (1987) Evaluation of optical motion information by movement detectors. *Journal of Comparative Physiology A,* **161,** 533–547. (207)

Reichardt, W., & Poggio, T. (1979) Figure ground discrimination by relative movement in the visual system of the fly. *Biological Cybernetics,* **35,** 81–100. (460)

Reid, R. C., & Shapley, R. (1988) Brightness induction by local contrast and the spatial dependence of assimilation. *Vision Research,* **28,** 115–132. (434, 437–438)

Rentschler, I., & Fiorentini, A. (1974) Meridional anisotropy of psychophysical spatial interactions. *Vision Research,* **14,** 1467–1473. (140–141)

Rentschler, I., Hübner, M., & Caelli, T. (1988) On the discrimination of compound Gabor signals and textures. *Vision Research,* 28, 279–291. (423, 425, 428, 430, 432)

Rentschler, I., & Treutwein, B. (1985) Loss of spatial phase relationships in extrafoveal vision. *Nature (London)* **313,** 308–310. (432)

Richards, W. A. (1970) Stereopsis and stereoblindness. *Experimental Brain Research,* **10,** 380–388. (323–324)

Richards, W. A. (1971) Anomalous stereoscopic depth perception. *Journal of the Optical Society of America,* **61,** 410–414. (323, 326)

Richards, W. A. (1975) Visual space perception. In E. C. Carterette

& M. E. Freidman (Eds.), *Handbook of Perception, V: Seeing*, pp. 351–386. New York: Academic Press. (319, 324)

Richards, W. A. (1979) Quantifying sensory channels: Generalizing colorimetry to orientation and texture, touch and tones. *Sensory Processes*, **3,** 207–229. (209)

Richards, W. A., & Kaye, M. G. (1974) Local versus global stereopsis: Two mechanisms? *Vision Research,* **14,** 1345–1347. (328)

Richardson, W.A., & Regan, D. (1973) A stereofield map with implications for disparity processing. *Investigative Ophthalmology,* **12,** 904–909. (324, 334)

Richmond, B. J., Wurtz, R. H., & Sato, T. (1983) Visual responses of inferior temporal neurons in awake rhesus monkey. *Journal of Neurophysiology,* **50,** 1415–1432. (309, 312)

Riddoch, G. (1917) Dissociation of visual perceptions due to occipital injuries, with special reference to the appreciation of movement. *Brain,* **40,** 15–57. (382)

Riggs, L. A., & Niehl, E. W. (1960) Eye movements recorded during convergence and divergence. *Journal of the Optical Society of America,* **50,** 913–920. (329)

Riggs, L. A., Ratliff, F., Cornsweet, J. C., & Cornsweet, T. N. (1953) The disappearance of steadily fixated visual test objects. *Journal of the Optical Society of America,* **43,** 495–501. (138)

Riggs, L. A., & Wooten, B. R. (1972) Electrical measures and psychophysical data on human vision. In D. Jameson & L. M. Hurvich (Eds.), *Handbook of Sensory Physiology, Vol. VII/4, Visual Psychophysics,* pp. 690–731. New York: Springer-Verlag. (408)

Riklan, M. (1972) Levodopa and behavior. *Neurology,* **22,** 43–55. (386)

Ripps, H. (1982) Night blindness revisited. From man to molecules. *Investigative Ophthalmology & Visual Science,* **23,** 588–609. (400)

Ripps, H., Brin, K. P., & Weale, R. A. (1978) Rhodopsin and visual threshold in retinitis pigmentosa. *Investigative Ophthalmology & Visual Science,* **17,** 735–745. (400)

Robertson, K., & Schor, C. M. (1986) Changes in retinal correspondence induced by disparity vergence. *Investigative Ophthalmology & Visual Science, Supplement,* **27,** 79. (331)

Robinson, D. A. A. (1963) A method of measuring eye movement using a scleral search coil in a magnetic field. *IEEE Transactions on Biomedical Engineering, England,* **10,** 137–145. (308)

Robinson, D. L., Baizer, J. S., & Dow, B. M. (1980) Behavioral enhancement of visual responses of prestriate neurons of the rhesus monkey. *Investigative Ophthalmology & Visual Science,* **19,** 1120–1123. (311)

Robinson, D. L., Goldberg, M. E., & Stanton, G. B. (1978) Parietal association cortex in the primate: Sensory mechanisms and behavioral modulations. *Journal of Neurophysiology,* **41,** 910–932. (306)

Robinson, D. L., & Petersen, S. E. (1984) Posterior parietal cortex of the awake monkey: Visual responses and their modulation by behavior. In F. Reinoso-Suarez & C. Ajmone-Marsan (Eds.), *Cortical Integration,* pp. 279–290. New York: Raven Press. (306, 312)

Robson, J. G. (1966) Spatial and temporal contrast sensitivity functions of the visual system. *Journal of the Optical Society of America,* **56,** 1141–1142. (31, 116)

Robson, J. G. (1975) Receptive fields: Neural representation of the spatial and intensive attributes of the visual image. In E. C. Carterette & M. P. Freidman (Eds.), *Handbook of Perception, V: Seeing,* pp. 81–116. New York: Academic Press. (154, 267, 418–419)

Robson, J. G. (1983) Frequency domain visual processing. In O. J. Braddick & A. C. Sleigh (Eds.), *Physical and Biological Processing of Images,* pp. 73–87. New York: Springer-Verlag. (267)

Robson, J. G., & Enroth-Cugell, C. (1978) Light distribution in the cat's retinal image. *Vision Research,* **18,** 159–173. (27, 29)

Robson, J. G., & Graham, N. (1981) Probability summation and regional variation in contrast sensitivity across the visual field. *Vision Research,* **21,** 409–418. (419)

Rock, I., & Anson, R. (1979) Illusory contours as the solution to a problem. *Perception,* **8,** 665–681. (292)

Rodieck, R. W. (1965) Quantitative analysis of cat retinal ganglion cell response to visual stimuli. *Vision Research,* **5,** 583–601. (91, 92, 108, 153)

Rodieck, R. W. (1967) Receptive fields in the cat retina: A new type. *Science,* **157,** 90–92. (108)

Rodieck, R. W. (1973) *The Vertebrate Retina: Principles of Structure and Function.* San Francisco, CA: Freeman. (384)

Rodieck, R. W., & Brening, R. K. (1983) Retinal ganglion cells: Properties, types, genera, pathways and trans-species comparisons. *Brain, Behavior and Evolution,* **23,** 121–164. (105)

Rodieck, R. W., & Stone, J. (1965) Analysis of receptive fields of cat retinal ganglion cells. *Journal of Neurophysiology,* **58,** 833–849. (91)

Rodieck, R. W., Binmoeller, K. F., & Dineen, J. (1985) Parasol and midget ganglion cells of the human retina. *Journal of Comparative Neurology,* **233,** 115–132. (113)

Rogers, B. J., & Graham, M. (1979) Motion parallax as an independent cue for depth perception. *Perception,* **8,** 125–134. (346)

Rogers, B., & Graham, M. (1982) Similarities between motion parallax and stereopsis in human depth perception. *Vision Research,* **22,** 261–270. (346)

Rogers, B. J., & Koenderink, J. J. (1986) Monocular aniseikonia: A motion parallax analogue of the disparity-induced effect. *Nature (London)* **322,** 62–63. (345, 347)

Rolls, E. T., & Cowey, A. (1970) Topography of the retina and striate cortex and its relationship to visual acuity in rhesus and squirrel monkeys. *Experimental Brain Research,* **10,** 298–310. (236)

Rose, A. (1942) The relative sensitivities of television pick-up tubes, photographic film, and the human eye. *Proceeding of the Institute of Radio Engineers,* **30,** 293–300. (352)

Rose, A. (1948) The sensitivity performance of the human eye on an absolute scale. *Journal of the Optical Society of America,* **38,** 196–208. (61)

Rose, D., & Blakemore, C. (1974) An analysis of orientation selectivity in the cat's visual cortex. *Experimental Brain Research,* **20,** 1–17. (28, 32)

Ross, J., Holt, J. J., & Johnstone, J. R. (1981) High frequency limitations on Mach bands. *Vision Research,* **21,** 1165–1167. (134–136)

Roth, I., & Frisby, J. P. (1986). *Perception and Representation: A Cognitive Approach.* Milton Keynes: Open University Press. (342)

Rovamo, J., Hyvärinen, L., & Hari, R. (1982) Human vision without luminance contrast system: Selective recovery of the red–green colour-contrast system from acquired blindness. *Documenta Ophthalmologica Proceedings Series,* **33,** 457–466. (285, 294)

Rovamo, J., & Virsu, V. (1979) An estimation and application of the human cortical magnification factor. *Experimental Brain Research,* **37,** 495–510. (232, 234, 236, 238)

Rovamo, J., Virsu, V., & Näsänen, R. (1978) Cortical magnification factor predicts the photopic contrast sensitivity of peripheral vision. *Nature (London)* **271,** 54–56. (232–233)

Rovamo, J., Virsu, V., Laurinen, P., & Hyvärinen, L. (1982) Resolution of gratings oriented along and across meridians in peripheral vision. *Investigative Ophthalmology & Visual Science,* **23,** 666–670. (241)

Rubin, J. M., & Richards, W. A. (1982) Color vision and image intensities: When are changes material? *Biological Cybernetics,* **45,** 215–226. (68)

Ruddock, K. H. (1972) Light transmission through the ocular media and macular pigment and its significance for psychophysical investigation. In D. Jameson & L. M. Hurvich (Eds.), *Handbook of Sensory Physiology, Vol. VII/4,* pp. 455–469. Berlin: Springer-Verlag. (175)

Ruddock, K. H., & Naghshineh, S. (1974) Mechanisms of red–green anomalous trichromacy: Hypothesis and analysis. *Modern Problems of Ophthalmology,* **13,** 210–214. (37)

Rushton, W. A. H. (1958) Kinetics of cone pigments measured objectively in the living human fovea. *Annals of the New York Academy of Science,* **74,** 291–304. (69)

Rushton, W. A. H. (1961) Rhodopsin measurement and dark adaptation in a subject deficient in cone vision. *Journal of Physiology,* **156,** 193–205. (70)

Rushton, W. A. H. (1965) Visual adaptation. The Ferrier Lecture. *Proceedings of the Royal Society of London, Series B,* **162,** 20–46. (60, 64, 69)

Rushton, W. A. H. (1968) Rod/cone rivalry in pigment regeneration. *Journal of Physiology,* **198,** 219–236. (95)

Rushton, W. A. H. (1969) Light and dark adaptation of the retina. In W. Reichardt (Ed.), *Processing of Optical Data by Organisms and by Machines,* pp. 544–564. New York: Academic Press. (69)

Rushton, W. A. H. (1972) Visual pigments in man. In H. J. A. Dartnall (Ed.), *Handbook of Sensory Physiology, VII/1, Photochemistry of Vision,* pp. 364–394. Berlin: Springer-Verlag. (69, 382)

Rushton, W. A. H., & Henry, G. H. (1968) Bleaching and regeneration of cone pigments in man. *Vision Research,* **8,** 617–631. (69)

Rushton, W. A. H., & MacLeod, D. I. A. (1986) The equivalent background of bleaching. *Perception,* **15,** 689–703. (70)

Rushton, W. A. H., & Powell, D. S. (1972) The early phase of dark adaptation. *Vision Research,* **12,** 1083–1094. (70)

Rushton, W. A. H., Powell, D. S., & White, K. D. (1973) Exchange thresholds in dichromats. *Vision Research,* **13,** 1993–2002. (95)

Rushton, W. A. H., & Westheimer, G. (1962) The effect upon the rod threshold of bleaching neighbouring rods. *Journal of Physiology,* **164,** 318–329. (96, 97)

Sachs, M. B., Nachmias, J., & Robson, J. G. (1971) Spatial-frequency channels in human vision. *Journal of the Optical Society of America,* **61,** 1176–1186. (154, 245)

Sagi, D., & Julesz, B. (1987) Detection versus discrimination of visual orientation. *Perception,* **14,** 619–628. (277)

Saito, H.-A. (1983) Morphology of physiologically identified X-, Y- and W-type retinal ganglion cells of the cat. *Journal of Comparative Neurology,* **221,** 279–288. (112)

Saito, H., & Fukada, Y. (1986) Gain control mechanisms in X- and Y-type retinal ganglion cells of the cat. *Vision Research,* **26,** 391–408. (89, 90)

Saito, H., Yukie, M., Tanaka, K., Hikosaka, K., Fukada, Y., & Iwai, E. (1986) Integration of direction signals of image motion in the superior temporal sulcus of the macaque monkey. *Journal of Neuroscience,* **6,** 145–157. (226)

Sakitt, B. (1972) Counting every quantum. *Journal of Physiology,* **233,** 131–150. (55)

Sakitt, B., & Barlow, H. B. (1982) A model for the economical encoding of the visual image in cerebral cortex. *Biological Cybernetics,* **43,** 97–108. (33)

Sakmann, B., & Creutzfeldt, O. D. (1969) Scotopic and mesopic light adaptation in the cat's retina. *Pflügers Archiv für die gesamte Physiologie,* **313,** 168–185. (89)

Sakmann, B., & Filion, M. (1972) Light adaptation of the late receptor potential in the cat retina. In S. B. Arden (Ed.), *Advances in Experimental Medicine and Biology, Vol. 24, The Visual System—Neurophysiology, Biophysics, and Their Clinical Applications,* pp. 87–93. New York: Plenum. (87)

Salapatek, P., Banks, M. S. (1978) Infant sensory assessment: Vision. In F. D. Minifie & L. L. Lloyd (Eds.), *Communicative and Cognitive Abilities: Early Behavioral Assessment,* pp. 61–106. Baltimore: University Park Press. (350–351, 358)

Salapatek, P., Bechtold, A. G., & Bushnell, E. W. (1976) Infant visual acuity as a function of viewing distance. *Child Development,* **47,** 860–863. (351)

Sandberg, M. A., & Berson, E. L. (1977) Blue and green cone mechanisms in retinitis pigmentosa. *Investigative Ophthalmology & Visual Science,* **16,** 149. (400)

Sanders, M. D., Warrington, E. K., Marshall, J., & Weiskrantz, L. (1974) "Blindsight": Vision in a field defect. *Lancet*, 20 April, 707–708. (411)

Sarks, S. H. (1980) Drusen and their relationship to senile macular degeneration. *Australian Journal of Ophthalmology*, **8**, 117.(397)

Saslow, M. G. (1967) Effects of components of displacement-step stimuli upon latency of saccadic eye movements. *Journal of the Optical Society of America*, **57**, 1024–1029. (313)

Schefrin, B. E. (1989) *Psychophysical Vision Testing of Sites of Disease Action Secondary to Diabetes*. Ph.D. Dissertation. University of California, Berkeley. (407)

Schein, S. J. (1988) Anatomy of macaque fovea and spatial densities of neurons in foveal representation. *Journal of Comparative Neurology*, **269**, 479–505. (117)

Schein, S. J., & DeMonasterio, F. M. (1987) The mapping of retinal and geniculate neurons onto striate cortex of macaque. *Journal of Neuroscience*, **7**, 996–1009. (235)

Schein, S. J., Marrocco, R. T., & DeMonasterio, F. M. (1982) Is there a high concentration of color-selective cells in area V4 of monkey visual cortex? *Journal of Neurophysiology*, **47**, 193–213. (127, 286)

Schieting, S., & Spillmann, L. (1987) Flicker adaptation in the peripheral retina. *Vision Research*, **27**, 277–284. (138, 270)

Schiller, P. H. (1982) Central connections on the retinal ON- and OFF-pathways. *Nature (London)* **297**, 580–583. (143)

Schiller, P. H. (1984) The connections of the retinal ON- and OFF-pathways on the lateral geniculate nucleus of the monkey. *Vision Research*, **24**, 923–932. (143)

Schiller, P. H., Finlay, B. L., & Volman, S. F. (1976a) Quantitative studies of single cell properties in monkey striate cortex. II. Orientation specificity and ocular dominance. *Journal of Neurophysiology*, **39**, 1320–1333. (286–287)

Schiller, P. H., Finlay, B. L., & Volman, S. F. (1976b) Quantitative studies of single cell properties in monkey striate cortex. III. Spatial frequency. *Journal of Neurophysiology*, **39**, 1334–1351. (286–287)

Schiller, P. H., & Malpeli, J. (1977) Properties and tectal projections of monkey retinal ganglion cells. *Journal of Neurophysiology*, **40**, 428–445. (109)

Schiller, P. H., Sandell, J. H., & Maunsell, J. H. R. (1986) Functions of the ON and OFF channels of the visual system. *Nature (London)* **322**, 824–825. (143, 145, 193)

Schnapf, J. L., & Baylor, D. A. (1987) How photoreceptor cells respond to light. *Scientific American*, **256(4)**, 40–47. (78, 81, 82)

Schnapf, J. L., Kraft, T. W., & Baylor, D. A. (1987) Spectral sensitivity of human cone photoreceptors. *Nature (London)* **325**, 439–441. (79, 80, 174)

Schneider, G. E. (1967) Contrasting visuomotor functions of tectum and cortex in the golden hamster. *Psychologische Forschung*, **31**, 52–62. (103)

Schor, C. M., Robertson, K. M., & Wesson, M. (1986) Disparity vergence dynamics and fixation disparity. *American Journal of Optometry and Physiological Optics*, **63**, 611–618. (330)

Schor, C. M., & Tyler, C. W. (1981) Spatio-temporal properties of Panum's fusional area. *Vision Research*, **21**, 683–692. (327, 331)

Schor, C. M., & Wood, I. (1983) Disparity range for local stereopsis as a function of luminance spatial frequency. *Vision Research*, **23**, 1649–1654. (321, 328, 331, 343)

Schor, C. M., Wood, I., & Ogawa, J. (1984) Binocular sensory fusion is limited by spatial resolution. *Vision Research*, **24**, 661–665. (328, 331)

Schultze, M. (1866) *Ueber den gelben Fleck der Retina, seinen Einfluss auf normales Sehen und auf Farbenblindheit*. Bonn: Verlag von Max Cohen & Sohn. (2, 5)

Schumann, F. (1900) Beiträge zur Analyse der Gesichtswahrnehmungen. Erste Abhandlung. Einige Beobachtungen über die Zusammenfassung von Gesichtseindrücken zu Einheiten. *Zeitschrift für Psychologie*, **23**, 1–32. (289)

Schwartz, E. A. (1974) Responses of bipolar cells in the retina of the turtle. *Journal of Physiology*, **236**, 211–224. (87)

Schwartz, E. A. (1975) Cones excite rods in the retina of the turtle. *Journal of Physiology*, **246**, 639–651. (85)

Schwartz, E. L. (1980) Computational anatomy and functional architecture of striate cortex: A spatial mapping approach to perceptual coding. *Vision Research*, **20**, 645–669. (236)

Schwartz, E. L. (1984) Spatial mapping and spatial vision in primate striate and inferotemporal cortex. In L. Spillmann and B. R. Wooten (Eds.), *Sensory Experience, Adaptation, and Perception*, pp. 73–104. Hillsdale, NJ: Lawrence Erlbaum. (236, 288)

Sclar, G., Maunsell, J. H. R., & Lennie, P. (1989) Coding of image contrast in central visual pathways of the macaque monkey. *Vision Research* in press. (120)

Sejknowski, T. J., Koch, C., & Churchland, P. S. (1988) Computational neuroscience. *Science*, **241**, 1299–1306. (339)

Sekuler, R., & Blake, R. (1985) *Visual Perception*. New York: A. Knopf. (150)

Sekuler, R., Pantle, A., & Levinson, E. (1978) Physiological basis of motion perception. In R. Held, H. W. Leibowitz & H.-L. Teuber (Eds.), *Handbook of Sensory Physiology, Vol. VIII, Perception*, pp. 67–96. Berlin: Springer-Verlag. (207)

Shapere, D. (1974) Scientific theories and their domains. In F. Suppe (Ed.), *The Structure of Scientific Theories*, pp. 518–565. Urbana: University of Illinois Press.

Shapley, R. (1986) The importance of contrast for the activity of single neurons, the VEP and perception. *Vision Research*, **26**, 45–61. (89, 436–437)

Shapley, R., & Enroth-Cugell, C. (1984) Visual adaptation and retinal gain controls. In N. Osborne & G. Chader (Eds.), *Progress in Retinal Research, Vol. 3*, pp. 263–346. Oxford: Pergamon. (58, 76, 90, 132, 434–436, 446)

Shapley, R., & Gordon, J. (1985) Nonlinearity in the perception of form. *Perception & Psychophysics*, **37**, 84–88. (417, 438–439, 441, 443)

Shapley, R., & Gordon, J. (1987) Nonlinearity in the perception of form. In S. J. Petry & G. E. Meyer (Eds.), *The Percep-*

tion of Illusory Contours, pp. 109–115. New York: Springer. (438, 441)

Shapley, R., & Perry, V. H. (1986) Cat and monkey retinal ganglion cells and their visual functional roles. *Trends in Neuroscience,* **9,** 229–235. (120, 160, 200–201)

Shapley, R., & Reid, R. C. (1985) Contrast and assimilation in the perception of brightness *Proceedings of the National Academy of Science U.S.A.,* **82,** 5983–5986. (436–437)

Shapley, R., & So, Y. T. (1980) Is there an effect of monocular deprivation on the proportion of X- and Y-cells in the cat lateral geniculate nucleus? *Experimental Brain Research,* **39,** 41–48. (31)

Shapley, R., & Victor, J. D. (1986) Hyperacuity in cat retinal ganglion cells. *Science,* **231,** 999–1002. (421–422)

Sharpe, L. T. (1989) The light-adaptation of the rods. In R. F. Hess, L. T. Sharpe and K. Nordby (Eds.), *Night Vision: Basic, Clinical and Applied Aspects.* Cambridge: Cambridge University Press, in press. (60)

Sharpe, L. T., & Nordby, K. (1989a) Total colour-blindness: an introduction. In R. F. Hess, L. T. Sharpe, & K. Nordby (Eds.), *Night Vision: Basic, Clinical and Applied Aspects,* Chapter I. Cambridge: Cambridge University Press. (383)

Sharpe, L. T., & Nordby, K. (1989b) The photoreceptors in the achromat. In R. F. Hess, L. T. Sharpe, & K. Nordby (Eds.), *Night Vision: Basic, Clinical and Applied Aspects,* Chapter III. Cambridge: Cambridge University Press. (383)

Sharpe, L. T., Fach, C., Nordby, K., & Stockman, A. (1989) The incremental threshold of the rod visual system and Weber's Law. *Science,* **244,** 354–356. (60, 90)

Shatz, C. J. (1983) The prenatal development of the cat's retinogeniculate pathway. *Journal of Neuroscience,* **3,** 482–499. (367)

Shatz, C. J., & Kirkwood, P. A. (1984) Prenatal development of functional connections in the cat's retinogeniculate pathway. *Journal of Neuroscience,* **5,** 1378–1397. (370)

Shatz, C. J., Lindstrom, S. H., & Wiesel, T. N. (1977) The distribution of afferents representing the right and left eyes in the cat's visual cortex. *Brain Research,* **131,** 103–116. (366)

Shatz, C. J., & Sretavan, D. W. (1986) Interactions between retinal ganglion cells during the development of the mammalian visual system. *Annual Review of Neuroscience,* **9,** 171–207. (367, 370, 377)

Shatz, C. J., & Stryker, M. P. (1978) Ocular dominance in layer IV of the cat's visual cortex and the effects of monocular deprivation. *Journal of Physiology,* **281,** 267–283. (369)

Shatz, C. J., & Stryker, M. P. (1988) Formation fo the eye-specific layers in the lateral geniculate nucleus is blocked by tetrodotoxin. *Science,* **242,** 87–89. (370)

Sherk, H., & Horton, J. C. (1984) Receptive field properties in the cat's area 17 in the absence of ON-center geniculate input. *Journal of Neuroscience,* **4,** 381–393. (143)

Sherman, S. M., & Spear, P. D. (1982) Organization of visual pathways in normal and visually deprived cats. *Annual Review of Physiology,* **62,** 738–855. (350, 369)

Shevell, S. K. (1977) Saturation in human cones. *Vision Research,* **17,** 427–434. (71)

Shevell, S. K. (1978) The dual role of chromatic backgrounds in color perception. *Vision Research,* **18,** 1649–1661. (66, 74)

Shiffrin, R., & Schneider, W. (1977) Controlled and automatic human information processing. II. Perceptual learning, automatic attending and a general theory. *Psychological Review,* **84,** 127–190. (306)

Shimojo, S., Bauer, J. A., O'Connell, K. M., & Held, R. (1986) Pre-stereoptic binocular vision in infants. *Vision Research,* **26,** 501–510. (373)

Shimojo, S., Birch, E. E., Gwiazda, J., & Held, R. (1984) Development of vernier acuity in infants. *Vision Research,* **24,** 721–728. (371, 373)

Shimojo, S., & Held, R. (1987) Vernier acuity is less than grating acuity in 2- and 3-month-olds. *Vision Research,* **27,** 77–86. (373)

Shipp, S. D., & Zeki, S. (1984) Specificity of connections is related to cytochrome oxidase architecture in area V2 of macaque monkey. *Journal of Physiology,* **353,** 23. (196, 201)

Shipp, S., & Zeki, S. (1985) Segregation of pathways leading from area V2 to areas V4 and V5 of macaque monkey visual cortex. *Nature (London)* **315,** 322–325. (125–127, 196, 201, 284)

Sidley, N. A., & Sperling, H. G. (1967) Photopic spectral sensitivity in the rhesus monkey. *Journal of the Optical Society of America,* **57,** 816–818. (43, 44)

Sidley, N. A., Sperling, H. G., Bedarf, E. W., & Hiss, R. H. (1965) Photopic spectral sensitivity in the monkey: Methods for determining and initial results. *Science,* **150,** 1837–1839. (44)

Siegel, R. M., & Andersen, R. A. (1986) Motion perceptual deficits following ibotenic acid lesions of the middle temporal area (MT) in the behaving rhesus monkey. *Society of Neuroscience Abstracts,* **12,** 1183. (49)

Siegel, R. M., & Andersen, R. A. (1988) Perception of three-dimensional structure from motion in monkey and man. *Nature (London)* **331,** 259–261 (47–48, 209, 287)

Sillito, A. M. (1975) The contribution of inhibitory mechanisms to the receptive field properties of neurones in the striate cortex of the cat. *Journal of Physiology,* **250,** 305–329. (245)

Sillito, A. M. (1979) Inhibitory mechanisms influencing complex cell orientation selectivity and their modification at high resting discharge levels. *Journal of Physiology,* **289,** 33–53. (245)

Sillito, A. M. (1985) Inhibitory circuits and orientation selectivity in the visual cortex. In D. Rose & V. G. Dobson (Eds.), *Models of the Visual Cortex,* pp. 396–407. New York: Wiley. (245)

Singer, W., & Rauschecker, J. P. (1982) Central core control of developmental plasticity in the kitten visual cortex. II. Electrical activation of mesencephalic and diencephalic projections. *Experimental Brain Research,* **47,** 223–233. (391)

Sirovich, L., & Abramov, I. (1977) Photopigments and pseudopigments. *Vision Research,* **17,** 5–16. (172–173, 178)

Slaughter, M. M., & Miller, R. F. (1981) 2-Amino-4-phosphonobutyric acid: A new pharmacological tool for retina research. *Science,* **211,** 182–184. (143)

Smiddy, W. E., & Fine, S. L. (1984) Prognosis of patients with bilateral macular drusen. *Ophthalmology,* **91,** 271. (397)

Smith, D. C. (1985) Behavioral and electrophysiological effects of visual deprivation and their reversal. In R. N. Aslin (Ed.), *Advances in Neural and Behavioral Development, Vol. 1,* pp. 131–156. Norwood, NJ: Ablex. (394)

Smith, D. C., Holdefer, R. N., & Reeves, T. M. (1982) Visual acuity following unequal alternating monocular deprivation in the cat. *Investigative Ophthalmology & Visual Science, Supplement,* **22,** 90. (394)

Smith, K. U. (1936) Visual discrimination in the cat: IV. The visual acuity of the cat in relation to stimulus distance. *Journal of Genetic Psychology,* **49,** 297–313. (28)

Smith, R. A., & Cass, P. F. (1987) Aliasing in the parafovea with incoherent light. *Journal of the Optical Society of America A,* **4,** 1530–1534. (234)

Smith, V. C., & Pokorny, J. (1975) Spectral sensitivity of the foveal cone photopigments between 400 and 500 nm. *Vision Research,* **15,** 161–171. (174)

Smith, V. C., & Pokorny, J. (1977) Large-field trichromacy on protanopes and deuteranopes. *Journal of the Optical Society of America,* **67,** 213–220. (170)

Smith, V. C., Pokorny, J., & Van Norren, D. (1983) Densitometric measurement of human cone photopigment kinetics. *Vision Research,* **13,** 517–524. (69)

Snowden, R. J., & Braddick, O. J. (1987) Extension of displacement limits in multiple exposure sequences of apparent motion. *Perception,* **16,** 263. (215–216)

Snowden, R. J., & Braddick, O. J. (1989). Extension of displacement limits in multiple-exposure sequences of apparent motion. *Vision Research,* **29.** (216)

Snyder, A. W., & Miller, W. H. (1977) Photoreceptor diameter and spacing for highest resolving power. *Journal of the Optical Society of America,* **67,** 696–698. (354)

So, Y. T., & Shapley, R. M. (1979) Spatial properties of X and Y cells in the lateral geniculate nucleus of the cat and conduction velocities of their inputs. *Experimental Brain Research,* **36,** 533–550. (31)

Sparrock, J. M. B. (1969) Stabilized images: Increment thresholds and subjective brightness. *Journal of the Optical Society of America,* **59,** 872–874. (100)

Spekreijse, H., Estévez, O., & van der Tweel, L. H. (1973) Luminance response to pattern reversal. In J. T. Pearlman (Ed.), *Documenta Ophthalmologica Proceedings Series, 2,* pp. 205–211. The Hague: Dr. W. Junk BV. (407)

Sperling, H. G., Crawford, M. L. J., & Espinoza, S. (1978) Threshold spectral sensitivity of single neurons in the lateral geniculate nucleus and of performing monkeys. *Modern Problems in Ophthalmology,* **19,** 2–18. (45–46)

Sperling, H. G., & Harwerth, R. S. (1971) Red–green cone interactions in the increment-threshold spectral sensitivity of primates. *Science,* **172,** 180–184. (43, 186, 189)

Sperling, H. G., Sidley, N. A., Dockens, W. S., & Jolliffe, C. L. (1968) Increment threshold spectral sensitivity of the rhesus monkey as a function of the spectral composition of the background field. *Journal of the Optical Society of America,* **58,** 263–268. (44)

Spillmann, L. (1971) Foveal receptive fields in the human visual system measured with simultaneous contrast in grids and bars. *Pflügers Archiv für die gesamte Physiologie,* **326,** 281–299. (139, 155, 193)

Spillmann, L., & Conlon, J. (1972) Photochromatic interval during dark adaptation and as a function of background illumination. *Journal of the Optical Society of America,* **62,** 182–185. (193)

Spillmann, L., Ransom-Hogg, A., & Oehler, R. (1987) A comparison of perceptive and receptive fields in man and monkey. *Human Neurobiology,* **6,** 51–62. (44, 100, 140–141, 147)

Spillmann, L., & Roberge, W. (1972) Evaluation of visual function in a case of traumatic leukoma and cataract. *Graefes Archiv für Klinische und Experimentelle Ophthalmologie,* **184,** 267–277. (398)

Spillmann, L., & Seneff, S. (1971) Photochromatic intervals as a function of retinal eccentricity for stimuli of different size. *Journal of the Optical Society of America,* **61,** 267–270. (193)

Spillmann, L., Wolf, E., & Nowlan, A. T. (1971) Dark and light adaptation with opposite time courses. *Journal of the Optical Society of America,* **61,** 1122–1123. (70)

Spitzer, H., & Hochstein, S. (1985) A complex-cell receptive field model. *Journal of Neurophysiology,* **53,** 1266–1286. (418, 443)

Sprague, J. M., Berkley, M. A., & Hughes, H. C. (1979) Visual acuity functions and pattern discrimination in the destriate cat. *Acta Neurobiologiae Experimentalis,* **39,** 643–682. (30)

Sretavan, D. W., & Shatz, C. J. (1986) Prenatal development of retinal ganglion cell axons: Segregation into eye-specific layers. *Journal of Neuroscience,* **6,** 234–251. (368)

Sretavan, D. W., Shatz, C. J., & Stryker, M. P. (1989) Modification of retinal ganglion cell axon morphology by prenatal infusion of tetrodotoxin. *Nature,* **336,** 468–471. (370)

St. Cyr, G. J., & Fender, D. H. (1969) The interplay of flicks and drifts in binocular fixation. *Vision Research,* **9,** 245–265. (329)

Stabell, U,. & Stabell, B. (1982) Color vision in the peripheral retina under photopic conditions. *Vision Research,* **22,** 839–844. (170, 175)

Steinberg, R. H. (1969) Rod and cone contributions to S-potentials from the cat retina. *Vision Research,* **9,** 1319–1329. (183)

Steinberg, R. H. (1971) Incremental responses to light recorded from pigment epithelial cells and horizontal cells of the cat retina. *Journal of Physiology,* **217,** 93–110. (87, 90)

Steinberg, R. H, Reid, M., & Lacy, P. L. (1973) The distribution of rods and cones in the retina of the cat (*Felis domesticus*). *Journal of Comparative Neurology,* **148,** 229–248. (27, 28)

Steinman, R. M., & Collewijn, H. (1980) Binocular retinal image motion during active head rotation. *Vision Research,* **20,** 415–429. (331)

Steinman, R. M., Cushman, W. B., & Martins, A. J. (1982) The precision of gaze. *Human Neurobiology,* **1,** 97–109. (329–330)

Steinman, R. M., Levinson, J. Z., Collewijn, H., & Van der Steen, J. (1985) Vision in the presence of known natural retinal image motion. *Journal of the Optical Society of America A*, **2**, 226–233. (331)

Stensaas, S. S., Eddington, D. K., & Dobelle, W. H. (1974) The topography and variability of the primary visual cortex in man. *Journal of Neurosurgery*, **40**, 747–755. (239)

Sterling, P., Freed, M. A., & Smith, R. G. (1988) Architecture of the rod and cone circuits to the on-beta ganglion cell. *Journal of Neuroscience*, **8**, 623–642. (105)

Sternheim, C. E., & Boynton, R. M. (1966) Uniqueness of perceived hues investigated with a continuous judgemental technique. *Journal of Experimental Psychology*, **72**, 770–776. (165)

Sternheim, C. E., Stromeyer, C. F. III, & Khoo, M. C. K. (1979) Visibility of chromatic flicker upon spectrally mixed adapting fields. *Vision Research*, **19**, 175–183. (67)

Stevens, K. A., & Brookes, A. (1987) Depth reconstruction in stereopsis. In *Proceedings of the First International Conference on Computer Vision*, pp. 682–686. New York: IEEE Computer Society Press. (339, 346)

Stigmar, G. (1971) Blurred visual stimuli. II. The effect of blurred visual stimuli on vernier and stereo acuity. *Acta Ophthalmology*, **49**, 364–379. (397)

Stiles, W. S. (1939) The derectional sensitivity of the retina and the spectral sensitivities of the rods and cones. *Proceedings of the Royal Society of London, Series B*, **127**, 64–105. (60)

Stiles, W. S. (1949) Increment thresholds and the mechanisms of colour vision. *Documenta Opthalmologica*, **3**, 138–165. (403)

Stiles, W. S. (1959) Color vision: The approach through increment thresholds. *Proceedings of the National Academy of Sciences U.S.A.*, **45**, 100–114. (177, 187)

Stiles, W. S. (1961) Adaptation, chromatic adaptation, colour transformation. *Anales. Real Sociedad Española de Fisica y Quimica*, **57**, 149–175. (66–67)

Stiles, W. S. (1978) In J. D. Mollon (Ed.), *Mechanisms of Colour Vision*. London: Academic Press. (59, 66)

Stiles, W. S., & Crawford, B. H. (1932) Equivalent adaptation levels in localised retinal areas. *Report of Discussions of the Vision Physiology Society of London*, **194**. (70)

Stiles, W. S., & Crawford, B. H. (1933) The luminous efficiency of rays entering the eye pupil at different points. *Proceedings of the Royal Society*, **112**, 428–450. (383, 399)

Stockham, T. (1972) Image processing in the context of a visual model. *Proceedings of the IEEE*, **60**, 828–842. (435)

Stoerig, P., Hübner, M., & Pöppel, E. (1985) Signal detection analysis of residual vision in a field defect due to a post-geniculate lesion. *Neuropsychology*, **23**, 589–599. (415)

Stone, J. (1983) *Parallel Processing in the Visual System*. New York: Plenum. (109)

Stone, J., & Freeman, R. B. (1971) Conduction velocity as a parameter in the organization of the afferent relay in the cat's lateral geniculate nucleus. *Experimental Brain Research*, **13**, 489–497. (107)

Stork, D., & Wilson, H. R. (1988) Analysis of Gabor function descriptions of visual receptive fields. *Investigative Ophthalmology & Visual Science, Supplement*, **29**, 398. (249)

Stromeyer, C. F., & Julesz, B. (1972) Spatial frequency masking in vision: Critical bands and the spread of masking. *Journal of the Optical Society of America*, **62**, 1221–1232. (32, 247)

Stromeyer, C. F., & Klein, S. (1975) Evidence against narrow-band spatial frequency channels in human vision: The detectability of frequency modulated gratings. *Vision Research*, **15**, 899–910. (246)

Stromeyer, C. F. III, Kranda, K., & Sternheim, C. E. (1978) Selective chromatic adaptation at different spatial frequencies. *Vision Research*, **18**, 427–437. (66)

Stromeyer, C. F. III, Kronauer, R. E., & Madsen, J. C. (1979) Response saturation of short-wavelength cone pathways controlled by color-opponent mechanisms. *Vision Research*, **19**, 1025–1040. (71, 77)

Stroop, J. R. (1935) Studies of interference in serial verbal reactions. *Journal of Experimental Psychology*, **18**, 643–662. (304)

Stryker, M. P., & Harris, W. A. (1986) Binocular impulse blockade prevents the formation of ocular dominance columns in cat visual cortex. *Journal of Neuroscience*, **6**, 2117–2133. (370)

Stryker, M. P., & Strickland, S. L. (1984) Physiological segregation of ocular dominance columns depends on the pattern of afferent electrical activity. *Investigative Ophthalmology & Visual Science, Supplement*, **25**, 278. (370)

Suppe, F. (Ed.) (1977) *The Structure of Scientific Theories*. Urbana, IL: University of Illinois Press. (11, 13–14)

Svaetichin, G., & MacNichol, E. F., Jr. (1958) Retinal mechanisms for chromatic and achromatic vision. *Annals of the New York Academy of Sciences*, **74**, 385–404. (163)

Swanson, W. H., & Wilson, H. R. (1985) Eccentricity dependence of contrast matching and oblique masking. *Vision Research*, **25**, 1285–1295. (232, 238, 261–262)

Szamier, R. B., & Berson, E. L. (1977) Retinal ultrastructure in advanced retinitis pigmentosa. *Investigative Ophthalmology & Visual Science*, **16**, 947–962. (400)

Takahashi, S., & Ejima, Y. (1984) Spatial properties of red–green and yellow–blue perceptual opponent-color response. *Vision Research*, **24**, 987–994. (169)

Takahashi, S., & Ejima, Y. (1987) Effect of surround configuration on increment thresholds of a tiny violet flash. *Vision Research*, **27**, 537–546. (169)

Tanaka, K., Hikosaka, H., Saito, H., Yukie, Y., Fukuda, Y., & Iwai, E. (1986) Analysis of local and wide-field movements in the superior temporal visual areas of the macaque monkey. *Journal of Neuroscience*, **6**, 134–144. (287)

Tanaka, M., Lee, B. B., & Creutzfeldt, O. D. (1983) Spectral tuning and contour representation in area 17 of the awake monkey. In J. D. Mollon & L. T. Sharpe (Eds.), *Colour Vision: Physiology and Psychophysics*, pp. 269–276. New York: Academic Press. (451)

Tansley, B. W., & Boynton, R. M. (1978) Chromatic border perception: The role of red- and green-sensitive cones. *Vision Research*, **18**, 683–697. (169)

Teich, M. C., Prucnal, P. R., Vanucci, G., Breton, M. E., & McGill, W. J. L. (1982) Multiplication noise in the human visual system at threshold: 3, The role of non-Poisson quantum fluctuations. *Biological Cybernetics*, **44,** 157–165. (61)

Teller, D. Y. (1980) Locus questions in visual science. In C. S. Harris (Ed.), *Visual Coding and Adaptability* Hillsdale, NJ: Lawrence Erlbaum. (14)

Teller, D. Y. (1984) Linking propositions. *Vision Research*, **24,** 1233–1246. (13, 14, 15, 229, 319)

Teller, D. Y., & Bornstein, M. H. (1986) Infant color vision and color perception. In P. Salapatek & L. B. Cohen (Eds.), *Handbook of Infant Perception*, pp. 185–236. New York: Academic Press. (350)

Teller, D. Y., & Gestrin, P. J. (1969) Sensitization by annular surrounds: Sensitization and dark adaptation. *Vision Research*, **9,** 1481–1490. (70, 100)

Teller, D. Y., & Movshon, J. A. (1986) Visual development. *Vision Research*, **26,** 1483–1506. (350)

Teller, D. Y., & Pugh, E. N., Jr. (1983) Linking propositions in color vision. In J. D. Mollon & T. Sharpe (Eds.), *Colour Vision: Physiology and Psychophysics*, New York: Academic Press. (12, 14)

Teranishi, T., Negishi, K., & Kato, S. (1984) Regulatory effect of dopamine on spatial properties of horizontal cells in carp retina. *Journal of Neuroscience*, **4,** 1271–1280. (386)

Terzopoulos, D. (1984) *Multiresolution Computations of Visible Surface Representation.* Ph.D. Thesis, M.I.T., Cambridge, MA. (344)

Teuber, H. L. (1960) Perception. In J. Field, H. W. Magoun & V. E. Hall (Eds.), *Handbook of Physiology, Section 1: Neurophysiology*, Chapter 65, pp. 1595–1668. Washington, D.C.. American Physiological Society (455)

Teuber, H. L. (1962) *Talk on Psychology to the M.I.T. Corporation*, Oct. 1, 1962 (unpublished). (455)

Teuber, H. L. (1966a) Alterations of perception after brain injury. In C. J. Eccles (Ed.), *Brain and Conscious Experience*, pp. 182–216. New York: Springer-Verlag. (449, 455–456)

Teuber, H. L. (1966b) Kurt Goldstein's role in the development of neuropsychology. *Neuropsychologia*, **4,** 299–310. (454)

Teuber, H. L. (1967) Wolfgang Köhler zum Gedenken. *Psychologische Forschung*, **31,** 11–14. (454)

Teuber, H. L. (1978) The brain and human behavior. In R. Held, H. W. Leibowitz, & H. L. Teuber (Eds.) *Handbook of Sensory Physiology, Vol. VIII: Perception*, pp. 879–920. Berlin: Springer-Verlag. (455–456)

Teuber, H. L., Battersby, N. S., & Bender, M. F. (1960) *Visual Field Defects After Penetrating Missile Wounds of the Brain.* Cambridge, MA: Harvard University Press. (382, 411, 414, 454)

Teuber, H. L., & Bender, M. B. (1950) Perception of apparent movement across acquired scotomata in the visual field. *American Psychologist*, **5,** 271. (455)

Teuber, H. L., von Foerster, H., & Mead, M. (1952) *Introduction to Cybernetics.* New York: Macy. (455)

Thibos, L. N., Cheney, F. E., & Walsh, D. J. (1987) Retinal limits to the detection and resolution of gratings. *Journal of the Optical Society of America A*, **4,** 1524–1529. (234)

Thibos, L. N., & Werblin, F. S. (1978a) The response properties of the steady antagonistic surround in the mudpuppy retina. *Journal of Physiology*, **278,** 79–99. (87)

Thibos, L. N., & Werblin, F. S. (1978b) The properties of surround antagonism elicited by spinning windmill patterns in the mudpuppy retina. *Journal of Physiology*, **278,** 101–116. (87)

Thijssen, J. M., & Vendrik, A. J. H. (1971) Differential luminance sensitivity of the human visual system. *Perception & Psychophysics*, **10,** 58–64. (61)

Thomas, J. (1966). Brightness variations in stimuli with ramp-like contours. *Journal of the Optical Society of America*, **56,** 238–242. (155)

Thomas, J. (1968) Linearity of spatial integrations involving inhibitory interactions. *Vision Research*, **8,** 49–60. (155)

Thomas, J. (1970) Model of the function of receptive fields in human vision. *Psychological Review*, **77,** 121–134. (154, 268)

Thomas, J., & Kovar, C. (1965) The effect of contour sharpness on perceived brightness. *Vision Research*, **5,** 381–384. (155)

Thomas, J., Rourke, D., & Wilder, D. (1968) Inhibitory effect of less intense stimuli upon the increment threshold for a narrow test line. *Vision Research*, **8,** 537–542. (155)

Thompson, P. (1980) Margaret Thatcher; A new illusion. *Perception*, **9,** 483–484. (303)

Thorell, L. G., De Valois, R. L., & Albrecht, G. (1984) Spatial mapping of monkey V1 cells with pure color and luminance stimuli. *Vision Research*, **24,** 751–769. (288)

Tieman, D. B., McCall, M. A., & Hirsch, H. V. B. (1983) Physiological effects of unequal alternating monocular exposure. *Journal of Neurophysiology*, **49,** 804–817. (394)

Timney, B. N. (1981) Development of binocular depth perception in kittens. *Investigative Ophthalmology & Visual Science*, **21,** 493–496. (372)

Tolhurst, D. J. (1972) On the possible existence of edge detector neurons in the human visual system. *Vision Research*, **12,** 797–804. (135)

Tolhurst, D. J. (1973) Separate channels for the analysis of the shape and the movement of a moving visual stimulus. *Journal of Physiology*, **231,** 385–402. (120)

Tolhurst, D. J., & Thompson, I. D. (1981) On the variety of spatial frequency selectivities shown by neurons in area 17 of the cat. *Proceedings of the Royal Society of London, Series B*, **213,** 183–199. (247)

Tomita, T. (1965) Electrophysiological study of the mechanisms subserving color coding in fish retina. *Cold Spring Harbor Symposium on Quantitative Biology*, **30,** 559–566. (39)

Tootell, R. B. H., Hamilton, S. L., & Switkes, E. (1988) Functional anatomy of macaque striate cortex. IV. Contrast and magno–parvo streams. *Journal of Neuroscience*, **8,** 1594–1609. (123)

Tootell, R. B. H., Silverman, M. S., & DeValois, R. L. (1981)

Spatial frequency columns in primary visual cortex. *Science,* **214,** 813–815. (250)

Tootell, R. B. H., Silverman, M. S., DeValois, R. L., & Jacobs, G. H. (1983) Functional organization of the second cortical visual area in primates. *Science,* **220,** 737–739. (125)

Tootell, R. B. H., Silverman, M. S., Hamilton, S. L., DeValois, R. L., & Switkes, E. (1988) Functional anatomy of macaque striate cortex. III. Color. *Journal of Neuroscience,* **8,** 1569–1593. (123)

Tootell, R. B. H., Silverman, M. S., Hamilton, S. L., Switkes, E., & DeValois, R. L. (1988) Functional anatomy of macaque striate cortex. V. Spatial frequency. *Journal of Neuroscience,* **8,** 1610–1624. (123)

Tootell, R. B. H., Silverman, M. S., Switkes, E., & DeValois, R. L. (1982) Deoxyglucose analysis of retinotopic organization in primate striate cortex. *Science,* **218,** 902–904. (236–237)

Torjussen, T. (1978) Residual function in cortically blind hemifields. *Neuropsychology,* **16,** 15–21. (414)

Torre, V., & Owen, W. G. (1981) Ionic basis of high-pass filtering of small signals by network of retinal rods in the toad. *Proceedings of the Royal Society of London, Series B,* **212,** 253–261. (84)

Torrealba, F., Guillery, R. W., Eysel, U., Polley, E. H., & Mason, C. A. (1983) Studies of retinal representations within the cat's optic tract. *Journal of Comparative Neurology,* **211,** 377–396. (200)

Toyama, K. Komatsu, Y., Kasai, H., Fujii, K., & Umetani, K. (1985) Responsiveness of Clare–Bishop neurons to visual cues associated with motion of a visual stimulus in three-dimensional space. *Vision Research,* **25,** 407–417. (337)

Treisman, A. (1982) Perceptual grouping and attention in visual search for features and for objects. *Journal of Experimental Psychology: Human Perception and Performance,* **8,** 194–214. (304–305, 418, 425–426)

Treisman, A. (1985) Preattentive processing in vision. *Computer Vision and Image Processing.* **31,** 156–177. (275, 304)

Treisman, A. (1986a) Features and objects in visual processing. *Scientific American,* **255**(5), 114–126. (274, 282, 305)

Treisman, A. (1986b) Properties, parts and objects. In K. R. Boff, L. Kaufman & J. P. Thomas (Eds.), *Handbook of Perception and Human Performance*, pp. 1–70. New York: Wiley. (274, 305)

Treisman, A. (1988) Features and objects: The fourteenth Bartlett Memorial lecture. *Quarterly Journal of Experimental Psychology,* **40A,** 201–237. (104, 276–277, 305–306)

Treisman, A., & Gelade, G. (1980) A feature integration theory of attention. *Cognitive Psychology,* **12,** 97–136. (275–276, 304)

Treisman, A., & Gormican, S. (1988) Feature analysis in early vision: Evidence from search asymmetries. *Psychological Review,* **95,** 15–48. (274, 276–278)

Treisman, A., Kahneman, D., & Burkell, J. (1983) Perceptual objects and the cost of filtering. *Perception & Psychophysics*, **33,** 527–532. (304)

Treisman, A., & Paterson, R. (1984) Emergent features, attention and object perception. *Journal of Experimental Psychology: Human Perception and Performance,* **10,** 12–31. (275)

Treisman, A., & Schmidt, H. (1982) Illusory conjunctions in the perception of objects. *Cognitive Psychology,* **14,** 107–141. (307)

Treisman, A., & Souther, J. (1985) Search asymmetry: A diagnostic for preattentive processing of separable features. *Journal of Experimental Psychology: General,* **114,** 285–310. (277–278)

Treisman, M. (1964) Noise and Weber's law: The discrimination of brightness and other dimensions. *Psychological Review,* **71,** 314–330. (76)

Trevarthen, C. B. (1968) Two mechanisms of vision in primates. *Psychologische Forschung,* **31,** 229–337. (103)

Trezona, P. W. (1976) Aspects of peripheral colour vision. *Modern Problems in Ophthalmology,* **17,** 52–70. (170)

Trick, G. L. (1985) Retinal potentials in patients with primary open angle glaucoma: Physiological evidence for temporal frequency tuning defects. *Investigative Ophthalmology & Visual Science,* **26,** 1750–1758. (408)

Trick, G. L. (1986) PRRP abnormalities in glaucoma and ocular hypertension. *Investigative Ophthalmology & Visual Science,* **27,** 1730–1736. (408)

Trivedi, H. P., & Lloyd, S. A. (1985) The role of disparity gradient in stereo vision. *Perception,* **14,** 685–690. (343)

Troxler, D. (1804) Ueber das Verschwinden gegebener Gegenstände innerhalb unseres Gesichtskreises. In K. Himly and J. A. Schmidt (Eds.), *Ophthalmische Bibliothek Vol. 2,* pp. 51–53. Jena: Fromann. (138)

Troy, J. B. (1987) Do Y Geniculate neurons have greater contrast sensitivity than X geniculate neurons at all locations in the visual field? *Vision Research,* **17,** 1733–1735. (119)

Troy, J. B., Enroth-Cugell, C., & Robson, J. G. (1987) Do X and Y retinal ganglion cells signal contrast? *Proceedings of the IEEE International Conference on Systems, Man and Cybernetics,* 1070–1074. (83–94)

Troy, J. B., & Lennie, P. (1987) Detection latencies of X and Y type cells of the cat's dorsal lateral geniculate nucleus. *Experimental Brain Research,* **65,** 703–705. (120)

Troy, J. B., Robson, J. G., & Enroth-Cugell, C. (1986) Retinal ganglion cell processing of spatial information in cats. *Proceedings of the IEEE International Conference on Systems, Man and Cybernetics,* 498–503. (119)

Tsai, R. Y. (1986) An efficient and accurate camera calibration technique for 3D machine vision. In *Proceedings of the IEEE: Computer Vision Pattern Recognition, Miami, FL,* pp. 364–374. (341)

Ts'o, D. Y., & Gilbert, C. D. (1988) The organization of chromatic and spatial interactions in the primate striate cortex. *Journal of Neuroscience,* **8,** 1712–1727. (104, 123)

Tulunay-Keesey, U., & Jones, R. M. (1977) Spatial sensitization as a function of delay. *Vision Research,* **17,** 1191–1199. (100)

Tyler, C. W. (1973) Periodic vernier acuity. *Journal of Physiology,* **227,** 637–647. (257)

Tyler, C. W. (1974) Depth perception in disparity gratings. *Nature (London),* **251,** 140–142. (326, 342)

Tyler, C. W. (1975a) Characteristics of stereomovement suppression. *Perception & Psychophysics,* **17,** 225–230. (321)

Tyler, C. W. (1975b) Spatial organization of binocular disparity sensitivity. *Vision Research,* **15,** 583–590. (327)

Tyler, C. W. (1975c) Stereoscopic tilt and size aftereffects. *Perception,* **4,** 187–192. (296, 298)

Tyler, C. W. (1977) Stereomovement from interocular delay in dynamic visual noise: A random spatial disparity hypothesis. *American Journal of Optometry,* **54,** 374–386. (321)

Tyler, C. W. (1981) Specific defects of flicker sensitivity in glaucoma and ocular hypertension. *Investigative Ophthalmology & Visual Science,* **20,** 204–212. (397)

Tyler, C. W. (1983) Sensory processing of binocular disparity. In C. M. Schor & K. J. Cuiffreda (Eds.), *Vergence Eye Movements,* pp. 199–295. Boston: Butterworths. (319–320–321, 326–327, 345)

Tyler, C. W. (1985) Analysis of visual modulation sensitivity. II. Peripheral retina and the role of photoreceptor dimensions. *Journal of the Optical Society of America A,* **2,** 393–398. (270)

Tyler, C. W., & Raibert, M. (1975) Generation of random-dot stereogratings. *Behavior Research Methods and Instrumentation,* **7,** 37–41. (326)

Uchikawa, H., Kaiser, P. K., & Uchikawa, K. (1982) Color-discrimination perimetry. *Color Research and Application,* **7,** 264–272. (175)

Ullman, S. (1979a) The interpretation of structure from motion. *Proceedings of the Royal Society of London, Series B,* **203,** 405–426. (286)

Ullman, S. (1979b) *The Interpretation of Visual Motion.* Cambridge, MA: MIT Press. (286)

Ullman, S. (1984) Visual routines. *Cognition,* **18,** 97–159. (282)

Ullman, S., & Schechtman, G. (1982) Adaptation and gain normalization. *Proceedings of the Royal Society of London, Series B,* **216,** 299–313. (64)

Ungerleider, L. G., & Desimone, R. (1986) Cortical connections of visual area MT in macaque. *Journal of Comparative Neurology,* **248,** 190–222. (126)

Ungerleider, L. G., & Mishkin, M. (1982) Two cortical visual systems. In D. J. Ingle, M. A. Goodale & R. J. W. Mansfield (Eds.), *Analysis of Visual Behavior,* pp. 549–586. Cambridge, MA: MIT Press. (128, 284)

Vaegan, & Taylor, D. (1980) Critical period for deprivation amblyopia in children. *Transactions of the Ophthalmological Society of the United Kingdom,* **99,** 432–439. (390)

Vakkur, G. J., & Bishop, P. O. (1963) The schematic eye in the cat. *Vision Research,* **3,** 357–381. (27)

Vakkur, G. J., Bishop, P. O., & Kozak, W. (1963) Visual optics in the cat including posterior nodal distance and retinal landmarks. *Vision Research,* **3,** 289–314. (27)

Valberg, A., & Lee, B. B. (1989) Detection and discrimination of colour, a comparison of physiological and psychophysiological data. *Physica Scripta* **39,** 178–186. (190–192)

Valberg, A., Lee, B. B., & Tigwell, D. A. (1986) Neurones with strong inhibitory S-cone inputs in the macaque lateral geniculate nucleus. *Vision Research,* **26,** 1061–1064. (180)

Valberg, A., Lee, B. B., Tigwell, D. A., & Creutzfeldt, O. D. (1985) A simultaneous contrast effect of steady remote surrounds on responses of cells in macaque lateral geniculate nucleus. *Experimental Brain Research,* **58,** 604–608. (62)

Valberg, A., Lee, B. B., & Tryti, J. (1987) Simulation of responses of spectrally-opponent neurones in the macaque lateral geniculate nucleus to chromatic and achromatic light stimuli. *Vision Research,* **27,** 867–882. (190)

Valberg, A., Seim, T., Lee, B. B., & Tryti, J. (1986) Reconstruction of equidistant color space from responses of visual neurones of macaques. *Journal of the Optical Society of America A,* **3,** 1726–1734. (193)

Valeton, J. M. (1983) Photoreceptor light adaptation models: An evaluation. *Vision Research,* **23,** 1549–1554. (59)

Valeton, J. M., & Van Norren, D. (1983) Light adaptation of primate cones: An analysis based on extracellular data. *Vision Research,* **23,** 1539–1547. (84, 101)

Van Buren, J. M. (1963) Trans-synaptic retrograde degeneration in the visual system of primates. *Journal of Neurology, Neurosurgery and Psychiatry,* **26,** 402–409. (410)

Van den Brink, G., & Bouman, M. A. (1957) Visual contrast thresholds of moving point sources. *Journal of the Optical Society of America,* **47,** 612–618. (61)

Van der Horst, G. J. C., & Bouman, M. A. (1969) Spatiotemporal chromaticity discrimination. *Journal of the Optical Society of America,* **59,** 1482–1488. (116)

Van Essen, D. C. (1985) Functional organization of primate visual cortex. In A. A. Peters & E. G. Jones (Eds.), *Cerebral Cortex, Vol. 3,* pp. 259–329. New York: Plenum. (47, 201, 283–284, 293–294)

Van Essen, D. C., & Maunsell, J. H. R. (1980) Two-dimensional maps of the cerebral cortex. *Journal of Comparative Neurology,* **191,** 255–281. (110)

Van Essen, D. C., & Maunsell, J. H. R. (1983) Hierarchical organization and functional streams in the visual cortex. *Trends in Neuroscience,* **6,** 370–375. (229)

Van Essen, D. C., Newsome, W. T., & Maunsell, J. H. R. (1984) The visual representation in striate cortex of macaque monkey: Asymmetries, anisotropies and individual variability. *Vision Research,* **24,** 429–448. (121, 235, 239)

Van Essen, D. C., Newsome, W. T., Maunsell, J. H. R., & Bixby, J. L. (1986) The projections form striate cortex (V1) to areas V2 and V3 in the macaque monkey: Asymmetries, areal boundaries, and patchy connections. *Journal of Comparative Neurology,* **244,** 451–480. (124)

Van Hof-van Duin, J., & Mohn, G. (1986) Visual field measurements, optokinetic nystagmus, and the visual threatening response: Normal and abnormal development. *Documenta Ophthalmologica Proceedings Series,* **45,** 305–315. (364)

Van Loo, J. A., & Enoch, J. M. (1975) The scotopic Stiles Crawford effect. *Vision Research,* **15,** 1005–1009. (385)

Van Santen, J. P. H., & Sperling, G. (1985) Elaborated Reichardt detectors. *Journal of the Optical Society of America A,* **2,** 300–321. (212)

Van Tuijl, H. F. G. M. (1975) A new visual illusion: Neonlike color spreading and complementary color induction between subjective contours. *Acta Psychologia,* **39,** 441–445. (287, 441, 443)

Van Tuijl, H. F. G. M., & de Weert, C. M. M. (1979) Sensory conditions for the occurrence of the neon spreading illusion. *Perception,* **8,** 211–215. (443)

Vandenbussche, E., & Orban, G. A. (1983) Meridional variations in the line orientation discrimination of the cat. *Behavioral Brain Research,* **9,** 237–255. (28, 32)

Vandenbussche, E., & Orban, G. A. (1984) Line length and meridional variations in orientation discrimination of the cat: Behavioural and physiological data. *Investigative Ophthalmology & Visual Science, Supplement,* **25,** 143.

Vandenbussche, E., Orban, G. A., & Maes, H. (1986a) Velocity discrimination in the cat. *Vision Research,* **26,** 1835–1849. (222)

Vandenbussche, E., Orban, G. A., & Maes, H. (1986b) Velocity discrimination in the monkey. *Society for Neuroscience Abstracts,* **12,** 1183. (222)

Verdon, W., Adams, A. J., & Haegerstrom-Portnoy, G. (1986) Assessment of post-receptoral integrity in diabetics. *Investigative Ophthalmology & Visual Science, Supplement,* **27,** 308. (406)

Virsu, V. (1978) Retinal mechanisms of visual adaptation and afterimages. *Medical Biology,* **56,** 84–96. (60)

Virsu, V., & Lee, B. B. (1983) Light adaptation in cells of macaque lateral geniculate nucleus and its relation to human light adaptation. *Journal of Neurophysiology,* **50,** 864–877. (89)

Virsu, V., & Rovamo, J. (1979) Visual resolution, contrast sensitivity, and the cortical magnification factor. *Experimental Brain Research,* **37,** 475–494. (232)

Volbrecht, V. J., Werner, J. S., & Wooten, B. R. (1989) Temporal induction of blackness: 1. Color appearance. *Vision Research,* **29,** in press. (167)

von der Heydt, R. (1987) Approaches to visual cortical function. *Review of Physiology, Biochemistry and Pharmacology,* **108,** 69–150. (287)

von der Heydt, R., Adorjani, C., Hänny, P., & Baumgartner, G. (1978) Disparity sensitivity and receptive field incongruity of units in the cat striate cortex. *Experimental Brain Research,* **31,** 523–545. (322)

von der Heydt, R., & Peterhans, E. (1989a) Mechanisms of contour perception in monkey visual cortex. I. Lines of pattern discontinuity. *Journal of Neuroscience,* **9,** 1731–1748. (289–290)

von der Heydt, R., & Peterhans, E. (1989b) Ehrenstein and Zöllner illusions in a neuronal theory of contour processing. In C. M. Dickinson & J. J. Kulikowski (Eds.), *Seeing Contour and Color. Proceedings of the Third Symposium of the Northern Eye Institute, Manchester, Aug 9–13, 1987.* London: Pergamon, in press. (293)

von der Heydt, R., Peterhans, E., & Baumgartner, G. (1984) Illusory contours and cortical neuron responses. *Science,* **224,** 1260–1262. (137, 289–291, 443–444)

Von Grünau, M., & Frost, B. J. (1983) Double-opponent-process mechanism underlying RF-structure of directionally specific cells of cat lateral suprasylvian visual area. *Experimental Brain Research,* **49,** 84–92. (221)

Von Kries, J., (1905) Die Gesichtsempfindungen. In W. Nagel (Ed.), *Handbuch der Physiologie des Menschen, Vol. 3,* pp. 109–282. Vieweg; Braunschweig. (2, 66)

Von Noorden, G. K. (1967) Classification of amblyopia. *American Journal of Ophthalmology,* **63,** 238–244. (390)

Vos, J. J. (1978) Colorimetric and photometric properties of a 2° fundamental observer. *Color Research and Application,* **3,** 125–128. (55, 80)

Vos, J. J., & Walraven, P. L. (1971) On the derivation of the foveal cone primaries. *Vision Research,* **11,** 799–818. (175)

Vos, J. J., & Walraven, P. L. (1972) An analytical description of the line element in the zone-fluctuation model of colour vision. II. The derivation of the line element. *Vision Research,* **12,** 1345–1365. (166)

Wagner, H. G., MacNichol, E. F., Jr., & Wolbarsht, M. L. (1963) Functional basis for "on"-center and "off"-center receptive fields in the retina. *Journal of the Optical Society of America,* **53,** 66–70. (91)

Wald, G. (1964) The receptors of human color vision. *Science,* **145,** 1007–1016. (177, 404)

Wallach, H. (1948) Brightness constancy and the nature of achromatic colors. *Journal of Experimental Psychology,* **38,** 310–324. (91)

Wallach, H. (1976) *On Perception.* New York: Quandrangle. (434)

Wallach, H., & O'Connell, D. N. (1953) The kinetic depth effect. *Journal of Experimental Psychology,* **45,** 205–217. (287)

Walraven, J. (1973) Spatial characteristics of chromatic induction: The segregation of lateral effects from straylight artefacts. *Vision Research,* **13,** 1739–1753. (66)

Walvaren, J. (1976) Discounting the background—the missing link in the explanation of chromatic induction. *Vision Research,* **16,** 289–295. (66, 74, 98)

Walraven, J. (1977) Color signals form incremental and decremental light stimuli. *Vision Research,* **17,** 71–76. (66)

Walraven, J. (1980) The derivation of nerve signals from contrast flash data: A re-analysis. *Biological Cybernetics,* **38,** 23–29. (72)

Walraven, J. (1981) Perceived color under conditions of chromatic adaptation: Evidence for gain control by π-mechanisms. *Vision Research,* **21,** 611–620. (66)

Walraven, J., Benzschawel, T. L., & Rogowitz, B. E. (1989) Color constancy interpretation of chromatic induction. *Die Farbe*. (67–68)

Walraven, P. L., & Bouman, M. A. (1966) Fluctuation theory of color discrimination of normal trichromat. *Vision Research*, **6**, 567–586. (61)

Walraven, J., & Valeton, J. M. (1984) Visual adaptation and response saturation. In A. J. Van Doorn, W. A. Van de Grind & J. J. Koenderink (Eds.), *Limits in Perception*. Utrecht: VNU Science Press. (60, 63–64, 74, 76)

Wanger, P., & Persson, H. E. (1983) Pattern-reversal electroretinograms in unilateral glaucoma. *Investigative Ophthalmology & Visual Science*, **24**, 749–753. (408)

Wanger, P., & Persson, H. E. (1985) Pattern-reversal electroretinograms in ocular hypertension. *Documenta Ophthalmologica*, **61**, 27–31. (408)

Warrington, E. K. (1962) The completion of visual forms across hemianopic field defects. *Journal of Neurology, Neurosurgery and Psychiatry*, **25**, 208–217. (414)

Wässle, H. (1982) Morphological types and central projections of ganglion cells in the cat retina. In N. Osborne & G. Chader (Eds.), *Progress in Retinal Research, Vol. 1*, pp. 125–152. (112)

Wässle, H. (1988) Sampling of visual space by retinal ganglion cells. *Investigative Ophthalmology & Visual Science, Supplement*, **29**, 117. (143)

Wässle, H., Boycott, B. B., & Illing, R.-B. (1981) Morphology and mosaic of on- and off-beta cells in the cat retina and some functional considerations. *Proceedings of the Royal Society of London, Series B*, **212**, 177–195. (113)

Wässle, H., Levick, W. R., & Cleland, B. G. (1975) The distribution of the alpha-type of ganglion cells in the cat's retina. *Journal of Comparative Neurology*, **159**, 419–437. (112)

Wässle, H., Peichl, L., & Boycott, B. B. (1983) A spatial analysis of on- and off-ganglion cells in the cat retina. *Vision Research*, **23**, 1151–1160. (117, 143–144)

Wässle, H., & Riemann, H. J. (1978) The mosaic of nerve cells in the mammalian retina. *Proceedings of the Royal Society of London, Series B*, 441–461. (27)

Watamaniuk, S. N. J., Sekuler, R., & Williams, D. W. (1989). Direction perception in complex dynamic displays: The integration of direction information. *Vision Research*, **29**, 47–60. (209)

Watanabe, S. (1981) Pattern recognition as a quest for minimum entropy. *Pattern Recognition*, **13**, 381–387. (430)

Watanabe, S. (1985) *Pattern Recognition, Human and Mechanical*. New York: Wiley. (429, 432)

Watson, A. B. (1983) Detection and recognition of simple spatial forms. In O. J. Braddick & A. C. Sleigh (Eds.), *Physical and Biological Processing of Images*, pp. 100–114. New York: Springer-Verlag. (153, 260)

Watson, A. B. (1987) Estimation of local spatial scale. *Journal of the Optical Society of America A*, **4**, 1579–1582. (239)

Watson, A., Barlow, H. B., & Robson, J. G. (1893) What does the eye see best? *Nature (London)* **302**, 419–422. (419)

Watt, R. J., & Morgan, M. J. (1983) Mechanisms responsible for the assessment of visual location: Theory and evidence. *Vision Research*, **23**, 97–109. (420–421)

Watt, R. J., & Morgan, M. J. (1984) Spatial filters and the localization of luminance changes in human vision. *Vision Research*, **24**, 1387–1397. (417, 420–421)

Watt, R. J., & Morgan, M. J. (1985) A theory of the primitive spatial code in human vision. *Vision Research*, **25**, 1661–1674. (156–157, 159, 254, 260, 420–421)

Wattam-Bell, J. (1987) Motion-specific VEPs in adults and infants. *Perception*, **16**, 231. (361, 364)

Wattam-Bell, J., Braddick, O., Atkinson, J., & Day, J. (1987) Measures of infant binocularity in a group at risk for strabismus. *Clinical Vision Sciences*, **1**, 327–336. (362)

Weale, R. A. (1959) Photo-sensitive reactions in foveae of normal and cone-monochromatic observers. *Optica Acta*, **6**, 158–174. (37, 170)

Weale, R. A. (1965) Vision and fundus reflectometry: A review. *Photochemistry and Photobiology*, **4**, 67–87. (170, 382)

Webster, M., & DeValois, R. (1985) Relationship between spatial-frequency and orientation tuning of striate-cortex cells. *Journal of the Optical Society of America A*, **2**, 1124–1132. (153, 158)

Weiskrantz, L. (1977) Hans-Lukas Teuber. *Nature (London)*, **266**, 485. (450)

Weiskrantz, L. (1986) *Blindsight. A Case Study and Implications*. Oxford: Oxford University Press. (361, 411, 414–415)

Weiskrantz, L., Warrington, E. K., Sanders, M. D., & Marshall, J. (1974) Visual capacity in the hemianopic field following a restricted occipital ablation. *Brain*, **97**, 709–728. (411–414)

Weisstein, N. (1980) The joy of Fourier analysis. In C. S. Harris (Ed.), *Visual Coding and Adaptability*, pp. 365–380. Hillsdale, NJ: Lawrence Erlbaum. (92)

Werblin, F. S. (1972) Lateral interactions at the inner plexiform layer of the retina: Antagonistic response to change. *Science*, **175**, 1008–1009. (402)

Werblin, F. S. (1974) Control of retinal sensitivity: II. Lateral interaction at the outer plexiform layer. *Journal of General Physiology*, **63**, 62–87. (74)

Werblin, F. S., & Dowling, J. E. (1969) Organization of the retina of the mudpuppy, *Necturus maculosus*. II. Intracellular recording. *Journal of Neurophysiology*, **32**, 339–355. (87, 142)

Werner, J. S. (1982) Development of scotopic sensitivity and the absorption spectrum of the human ocular media. *Journal of the Optical Society of America*, **72**, 247–258. (175, 352)

Werner, J. S., Cicerone, C. M., Kliegl, R., & DellaRosa, D. (1984) Spectral efficiency of blackness induction. *Journal of the Optical Society of America A*, **1**, 981–986. (130, 167)

Werner, J. S., Donnelly, S. K., & Kliegl, R. (1987) Aging and human macular pigment density; Appended with translations from the work of Max Schultze and Ewald Hering. *Vision Research*, **27**, 257–268. (175)

Werner, J. S., & Lipsitt, L. P. (1981) The infancy of human sensory systems. In E. S. Gollin (Ed.), *Developmental Plasticity: Behavioral and Biological Aspects of*

Variation in Development (pp. 35–68). New York: Academic Press. (350)

Werner, J. S., & Walraven, J. (1982) Effect of chromatic adaptation on the achromatic locus: The role of contrast, luminance and background color. *Vision Research,* **22,** 929–943. (66)

Werner, J. S., & Wooten, B. R. (1979) Opponent chromatic mechanisms: Relation to photopigments and hue naming. *Journal of the Optical Society of America,* **69,** 422–434. (165, 168)

Wertheim, T. (1894) Über die indirekte Sehschärfe. *Zeitschrift für Psychologie und Physiologie der Sinnesorgane,* **7,** 172–189. (118)

Wertheimer, M. (1912) Experimentelle Studien über das Sehen von Bewegung. *Zeitschrift für Psychologie,* **61,** 161–265. (3, 205, 209–210, 213, 218)

Wertheimer, M. (1923) Untersuchungen zur Lehre von der Gestalt II. *Psychologische Forschung,* **4,** 301–350. (275, 287)

Wertheimer, M. (1938) Laws of organization in perceptual forms. In W. D. Ellis (Ed. and Trans.), *A Source-book of Gestalt Psychology,* pp. 71–88. New York: Harcourt, Brace and Co. (275, 287)

Westheimer, G. (1965) Spatial interaction in the human retina during scotopic vision. *Journal of Physiology,* **181,** 812–894. (17, 99, 100, 402)

Westheimer, G. (1967) Spatial interaction in human cone vision. *Journal of Physiology,* **190,** 139–154. (140, 402)

Westheimer, G. (1968) Bleached rhodopsin and retinal interaction. *Journal of Physiology,* **195,** 97–105. (70, 100)

Westheimer, G. (1979a) The spatial sense of the eye. *Investigative Ophthalmology & Visual Science,* **18,** 893–912. (254, 256, 421)

Westheimer, G. (1979b) Cooperative neural processes involved in stereoscopic acuity. *Experimental Brain Research,* **26,** 585–597. (329–330, 397)

Westheimer, G. (1982) The spatial grain of the perifoveal visual field. *Vision Research,* **22,** 157–162. (239)

Westheimer, G., & Hauske, G. (1975) Temporal and spatial interference with vernier acuity. *Vision Research,* **15,** 1137–1141. (251)

Westheimer, G., & McKee, S. P. (1977) Spatial configurations for visual hyperacuity. *Vision Research,* **17,** 941–947. (238, 256–257)

Westheimer, G., & Mitchell, D. E. (1969) The sensory stimulus for disjunctive eye movements. *Vision Research,* **9,** 749–755. (330)

Weymouth, F. W. (1958) Visual sensory units and the minimal angle of resolution. *American Journal of Ophthalmology,* **46,** 102–113. (238)

Wheatstone, C. (1838) Some remarkable phenomena of vision. I. *Philosophical Transactions of Royal Society,* **13,** 371–395. (23, 318)

Wheatstone, C. (1852) Contributions to the physiology of vision. II. *Philosophical Transactions of Royal Society,* **142,** 1–18. (318, 332)

Wheeler, T. G. (1982) Color vision and retinal chromatic information processing in teleost: A review. *Brain Research Reviews,* **4,** 177–235. (39)

White, T. W., Irwin, G. E., & Williams, M. (1980) Asymmetry in the brightness and darkness Broca–Sulzer effects. *Vision Research,* **20,** 723–726. (148)

Whittle, P. (1986) Increments and decrements: Luminance discrimination. *Vision Research,* **26,** 1677–1691. (57)

Whittle, P., & Challands, P. D. C. (1969) The effect of background luminance on the brightness of flashes. *Vision Research,* **9,** 1095–1110. (62, 66, 98, 435)

Whittle, P., & Swanston, M. T. (1974) Luminance discrimination of separated flashes: The effect of background luminance and the slope of the t.v.i. curves. *Vision Research,* **14,** 713–719. (61)

Wienrich, M., & Zrenner, E. (1984) Cone mechanisms and the colour-opponent interaction in monkey and cat. *Ophthalmic Research,* **16,** 40–47. (181)

Wiesel, T. N., & Hubel, D. H. (1963a) Single cell responses in striate cortex of kittens deprived of vision in one eye. *Journal of Neurophysiology,* **26,** 1003–1017. (388–389)

Wiesel, T. N., & Hubel, D. H. (1963b) Effects of visual deprivation on morphology and physiology of cells in the cat's lateral geniculate body. *Journal of Neurophysiology,* **26,** 978–993. 388–389)

Wiesel, T. N., & Hubel, D. H. (1964) Comparison of the effects of unilateral and bilateral eye closure on cortical unit responses in kittens. *Journal of Neurophysiology,* **28,** 1029–1040. (369, 389, 391)

Wiesel, T. N., & Hubel, D. H. (1966) Spatial and chromatic interactions in the lateral geniculate body of the rhesus monkey. *Journal of Neurophysiology,* **29,** 1115–1156. (113, 179, 184)

Wild, H. M., Butler, S. R., Garden, D. & Kulikowski, J. J. (1985) Primate cortical area V4 important for colour constancy but not wavelength discrimination. *Nature (London)* **313,** 133–135. (203)

Williams, D., & Gassel, M. M. (1962) Visual function in patients with homonymous hemianopia. I. The visual fields. *Brain,* **85,** 175–250. (411, 414)

Williams, D. R. (1985a) Aliasing in human foveal vision. *Vision Research,* **25,** 195–205. (234, 256)

Williams, D. R. (1985b) Visibility of interference fringes near the resolution limit. *Journal of the Optical Society of America A,* **2,** 1087–1093. (234, 357)

Williams, D. R. (1986) Seeing through the photoreceptor mosaic. *Trends in Neuroscience,* **9,** 193–198. (116–117, 234)

Williams, D. R., & MacLeod, D. I. A. (1979) Interchangeable backgrounds for cone afterimages. *Vision Research,* **19,** 867–878. (95)

Williams, D. R., MacLeod, D. I. A., & Hayhoe, M. M. (1981) Punctate sensitivity of the blue-sensitive mechanism. *Vision Research,* **21,** 1357–1375. (175)

Williams, D. W., & Sekuler, R. (1984) Coherent global motion percepts from stochastic local motions. *Vision Research,* **24,** 55–62. (209, 214–215)

Williams, D. W., Phillips, G., & Sekuler, R. (1986) Hysteresis in perception of motion direction as evidence for neural cooperativity. *Nature (London)* **324,** 253–254. (206, 214–215)

Williams, R. A., Enoch, J. M., & Essock, E. (1984) The resistance of selected hyperacuity configurations to retinal image degradation. *Investigative Ophthalmology & Visual Science,* **25,** 389–399. (398)

Willmer, E. N. & Wright, W. D. (1945) Colour sensitivity of the fovea centralis. *Nature (London),* **156,** 119–121. (170)

Wilson, H. R. (1985) Discrimination of contour curvature: Data and theory. *Journal of the Optical Society of America A,* **2,** 1191–1199. (257)

Wilson, H. R. (1986) Responses of spatial mechanisms can explain hyperacuity. *Vision Research,* **26,** 453–469. (254, 256, 262, 419, 421–422)

Wilson, H. R. (1988) Development of spatiotemporal mechanisms in infant vision. *Vision Research,* **28,** 611–628. (266, 361)

Wilson, H. R. (1989a) Model of peripheral and amblyopic hyperacuity. *Vision Research,* in press. (262, 265)

Wilson, H. R. (1989b) Psychophysical models of spatial vision and hyperacuity. In D. Regan (Ed.), *Spatial Form Vision,* in press. London: MacMillan Press. (249, 256, 262)

Wilson, H. R., & Bergen, J. R. (1979) A four mechanism model for threshold spatial vision. *Vision Research,* **19,** 19–32. (153, 246)

Wilson, H. R., & Gelb, D. J. (1984) Modified line element theory for spatial frequency and width discrimination. *Journal of the Optical Society of America A,* **1,** 124–131. (18, 153, 247, 254–257, 271, 419, 425)

Wilson, H. R., McFarlane, D. K., & Phillips, G. C. (1983) Spatial frequency tuning of orientation selective units estimated by oblique masking. *Vision Research,* **23,** 873–882. (247, 254, 258, 425)

Wilson, H. R., Mets, M. B., Nagy, S. E., & Kressel, A. (1988) Albino spatial vision as an instance of arrested visual development. *Vision Research,* **28,** 979–990. (265–266)

Wilson, H. R., & Regan, D. (1984) Spatial frequency adaptation and grating discrimination: Predictions of a line element model. *Journal of the Optical Society of America A,* **1,** 1091–1096. (256–258)

Wilson, H. R., & Richards, W. A. (1988) Curvature and separation discrimination at texture boundaries. *Investigative Ophthalmology & Visual Science Supplement,* **29,** 408. (269)

Wilson, H. R., & Richards, W. A. (1989) Mechanisms of contour curvature discrimination. *Journal of the Optical Society of America A,* **6,** 106–115.

Wisowaty, J. J. (1981) Estimates for the temporal response characteristics of chromatic pathways. *Journal of the Optical Society of America,* **71,** 970–977. (116)

Witkin, A. (1983) Scale-space filtering. *Proceedings of the Eighth International Joint Conference on Artificial Intelligence,* **2,** 1019–1022. (157)

Witkin, A. (1984) Space-scale filtering: A new approach to multiscale description. In S. Ullman (Ed.), *Image Understanding 1983: Advances in Computational Vision.* Norwood, NJ: Ablex. (157)

Witkin, S. R., Bresnick, G. H., Freidberg, M., Palta, M., Adams, A. J., & Huie, K. E. (1986) Blue cone sensitivity and hue discrimination in diabetic retinopathy. *Investigative Ophthalmology & Visual Science Supplement,* **26**(3), 74. (404)

Witkop, C., Jay, B., Creel, D., & Guillery, R. W. (1982) Optic and optic neurologic abnormalities in oculocutaneous and ocular albinism. *Birth Defects: Original Article Series,* **18,** 299–318. (265)

Wolfe, J. M., Cave, K. R., & Franzel, S. L. (1989) A modified feature integration model for visual search. *Journal of Experimental Psychology: Human Perception and Performance,* in press.

Wolfe, J. M., Cave, K. R., & Franzel, S. L., (1989) Parallel visual search for conjunctions of color and form. **15.** (306)

Wolff, H. (1925) Das Farbunterscheidungsvermögen der Ellritze. *Zeitschrift für Vergleichende Physiologie,* **3,** 279–329. (39)

Wong-Riley, M. T. T. (1979) Changes in the visual system of monocularly sutured or enucleated cats demonstratable with cytochrome oxidase histochemistry. *Brain Research,* **171,** 11–28. (195–196)

Wooten, B. R. (1984) The effects of successive chromatic contrast on spectral hue. In L. Spillmann & B. R. Wooten (Eds.), *Sensory experience, adaptation, and perception.* Hillsdale, London: Lawrence Erlbaum. (166)

Worthey, J. A., & Brill, N. H. (1986) Heuristic analysis of von Kries color constancy. *Journal of the Optical Society of America A,* **3,** 1708–1712. (66)

Wright, M. J. (1987) Spatiotemporal properties of grating motion detection in the center and the periphery of the visual field. *Journal of the Optical Society of America A,* **4,** 1627–1633. (239)

Wright, W. D. (1967) *The Rays Are not Coloured, Vol. 3.* London: Hilger. (53)

Wurtz, R. H. (1969) Comparison of effects of eye movements and stimulus movements on striate cortex neurons of the monkey. *Journal of Neurophysiology,* **32,** 987–994. (308–309)

Wurtz, R. H., & Goldberg, M. E. (1972) The primate superior colliculus and the shift of visual attention. *Investigative Ophthalmology,* **11,** 441–449. (310)

Wurtz, R. H., Goldberg, M. E., & Robinson, D. L. (1982) Brain mechanisms of visual attention. *Scientific American,* **246**(6), 124–135. (306, 310)

Wurtz, R. H., & Mohler, C. W. (1976a) Organization of monkey superior colliculus: Enhanced visual response of superfinal layer cells. *Journal of Neurophysiology,* **39,** 745–765. (309–310)

Wurtz, R. H., & Mohler, C. W. (1976b) Enhancement of visual responses in monkey striate cortex and frontal eye fields. *Journal of Neurophysiology,* **39,** 766–772. (311)

Wyszecki, G., & Stiles, W. S. (1982) *Color Science: Concepts and*

Methods, Quantitative Data and Formulae, Second Edition. New York: Wiley. (40, 54, 55, 59, 130, 255)

Yamane, S., Maske, R., & Bishop, P. O. (1985) Direction selectivity of simple cells in cat striate cortex to moving light bars. II. Relation to moving dark bar responses. *Experimental Brain Research,* **57,** 523–536. (221)

Yap, Y. L., Levi, D. M., & Klein, S. A. (1987) Peripheral hyperacuity: Three-dot bisection scales to a single factor from 0 to 10 degrees. *Journal of the Optical Society of America A,* **4,** 1557–1561. (253)

Yarbus, A. L. (1967) *Eye Movements and Vision* (Translation editor, L. A. Riggs). New York: Plenum. (138, 441)

Yarczower, M., & Bitterman, M. (1965) Stimulus generalization in the goldfish. In D. J. Mostofsky (Ed.), *Stimulus Generalization,* pp. 179–192. Stanford, California: Stanford University Press. (39)

Yellott, J. I. (1982) Spectral analysis of spatial sampling by photoreceptors: Topological disorder prevents aliasing. *Vision Research,* **22,** 1205–1210. (117, 234, 262, 270)

Yellott, J. I. (1984) Image sampling properties of photoreceptors: A reply to Miller and Bernard. *Vision Research,* **24,** 281–282. (234, 262, 270)

Yerkes, R. M. (1903) The instincts, habits and reactions of the frog. Part I. The associative processes of the green frog. *Psychological Review Monographs Supplement,* **4,** 579–597. (110)

Yo, C. & Wilson, H. R. (1987) Temporal frequency matching and discrimination in peripheral vision. *Investigative Ophthalmology & Visual Science, Supplement,* **28,** 355. (270)

Yo, C., Wilson, H. R., Mets, M. B., & Ritacco, D. G. (1989) Human albinos can discriminate spatial frequency and phase as accurately as normal subjects. *Vision Research,* in press. (266)

Young, R. S. L., & Fishman, G. A. (1980) Color matches of patients with retinitis pigmentosa. *Investigative Ophthalmology & Visual Science,* **19,** 967. (400)

Young, R. S. L., & Fishman, G. A. (1982) Sensitivity losses in a long wavelength sensitive mechanism of patients with retinitis pigmentosa. *Vision Research,* **22,** 163. (400)

Yuille, A. L., & Grzywacz, N. M. (1988) A computational theory for the perception of coherent motion. *Nature (London),* **333,** 71–74. (214)

Yuodelis, C., & Hendrickson, A. (1986) A qualitative and quantitative analysis of the human fovea during development. *Vision Research,* **26,** 847–855. (266, 352–356, 361)

Zeki, S. M. (1973) Color coding in rhesus monkey prestriate cortex. *Brain Research,* **53,** 422–427. (127, 202, 284)

Zeki, S. M. (1974) Cells responding to changing image size and disparity in the cortex of rhesus monkey. *Journal of Physiology,* **243,** 827–841. (284, 335)

Zeki, S. M. (1977) Color coding in the superior temporal sulcus of the rhesus monkey visual cortex. *Proceedings of the Royal Society of London, Series B,* **197,** 195–223. (127)

Zeki, S. M. (1978a) Uniformity and diversity of structure and function in rhesus monkey prestriate visual cortex. *Journal of Physiology,* **277,** 273–290. (194, 202, 285–286, 288, 294)

Zeki, S. M. (1978b) Functional specialization in the visual cortex of the rhesus monkey. *Nature (London),* **274,** 423–428. (194, 202, 285–286, 288, 294)

Zeki, S. M. (1979) Functional specialization and binocular interaction in the visual areas of rhesus monkey prestriate cortex. *Proceedings of the Royal Society of London, Series B,* **204,** 379–397. (294)

Zeki, S. M. (1980) The representation of colours in the cerebral cortex. *Nature (London),* **284,** 412—418. (287)

Zeki, S. M. (1983a) Colour coding in the cerebral cortex: The reaction of cells in monkey visual cortex to wavelengths and colours. *Neuroscience,* **9,** 741–765. (127, 202–203, 287)

Zeki, S. M. (1983b) Colour coding in the cerebral cortex: The response of wavelength-selective and colour-coded cells in monkey visual cortex to changes in wavelength composition. *Neuroscience,* **9,** 767–781. (202–203, 287)

Zeki, S. M. (1983c) The distribution of wavelength and orientation selective cells in different areas of monkey visual cortex. *Proceedings of the Royal Society of London, Series B,* **217,** 449–470. (284, 286)

Zemon, V., Gordon, J., & Welch, J. (1988) Asymmetries in ON- and OFF-visual pathways of humans revealed using contrast-evoked cortical potentials. *Visual Neuroscience,* **1,** 145–150. (147)

Zihl, J. (1980) Blindsight: Improvement of visually guided eye movements by systematic practice in patients with cerebral blindness. *Neuropsychologia,* **18,** 71–77. (412)

Zihl, J., von Cramon, D., & Mai, N. (1983) Selective disturbance of movement vision after bilateral brain damage. *Brain,* **106,** 313–340. (104, 196, 230, 285, 294)

Zihl, J., & Werth, R. (1984a) Contributions to the study of "blindsight." I. Can stray light account for saccadic localization in patients with postgeniculate field defects? *Neuropsychologia,* **22,** 1–11. (413)

Zihl, J., & Werth, R. (1984b) Contributions to the study of "blindsight." II. The role of specific practice for saccadic localizations in patients with postgeniculate visual field defects. *Neuropsychologia,* **22,** 13–22. (413)

Zisman, F., & Adams, A. J. (1982) Spectral sensitivity of cone mechanisms in juvenile diabetics. *Documenta Ophthalmologica Proceedings Series,* **33,** 127–132. (404–405)

Zisman, F., King-Smith, P. E., & Bhargava, S. K. (1978) Spectral sensitivities of acquired color defects analysed in terms of color opponent theory. *Modern Problems in Ophthalmology,* **19,** 254–257. (404)

Zrenner, E. (1977) Influence of stimulus duration and area on the spectral luminosity function as determined by sensory and VECP measurements. *Documenta Ophthalmologica Proceedings Series,* **13,** 21–30. (186)

Zrenner, E. (1983a) Neurophysiological aspects of color mechanisms in the primate retina. In J. Mollon & L. T. Sharpe (Eds.), *Colour Vision: Physiology and Psychophysics*, pp. 195–210. New York: Academic Press. (169, 180, 182, 184, 189, 201)

Zrenner, E. (1983b) *Neurophysiological Aspects of Color Vision in Primates*. Berlin: Springer-Verlag. (179, 182, 184–185, 187–188, 201)

Zrenner, E. & Gouras, P. (1978) Luminous and chromatic flicker functions are based on the phase relations between center and surround responses of color opponent ganglion cells. *Pflügers Archiv für die gesamte Physiologie, Supplement,* **337,** R 48. (184–186)

Zrenner, E. & Gouras, P. (1980) The blue sensitive mechanism in ganglion cells of macaque retina. *Investigative Ophthalmology & Visual Science, Supplement*, **19,** 7. (180)

Zrenner, E. & Gouras, P. (1981) Characteristics of the blue sensitive cone mechanism in primate retinal ganglion cells. *Vision Research,* **21,** 1605–1609. (169, 180, 183–184, 188)

Zrenner, E. & Gouras, P. (1983) Cone opponency in tonic ganglion cells and its variation with eccentricity in rhesus monkey retina. In J. Mollon & T. Sharpe (Eds.), *Colour Vision: Physiology and Psychophysics*, pp. 211–223. New York: Academic Press. (185)

Zrenner, E. & Krüger, C. J. (1981) Ethambutol mainly affects the function of red/green opponent neurons. *Documenta Ophthalmologica Proceedings Series,* **27,** 25. (186–187)

Zrenner, E., Magnussen, S., & Lorenz, B. (1988). Blauzapfen Monochromasie: Diagnose, genetische beratung und optische *Hilfsmittel. Klinische Monatsbläter für Augenheilkunde* **193,** 510–517. (183)

Zumbroich, T. J., & Blackmore, C. (1987) Spatial and temporal selectivity in the suprasylvian visual cortex of the cat. *Journal of Neuroscience*, **7,** 482–500. (30–31)

INDEX